ANESTHESIA
REVIEW

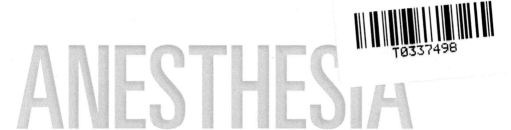

1000
QUESTIONS AND ANSWERS
TO BLAST THE BASICS
AND ACE THE ADVANCED

ANESTHESIA
REVIEW

1000
QUESTIONS AND ANSWERS
TO BLAST THE BASICS
AND ACE THE ADVANCED

Sheri M. Berg, MD
Instructor of Anesthesia
Harvard Medical School
Medical Director, PACUs
Department of Anesthesia, Critical Care, and
Pain Medicine
Massachusetts General Hospital
Boston, MA

Maricela Schnur, MD, MBA
Resident Physician
Department of Anesthesia, Critical Care, and
Pain Medicine
Massachusetts General Hospital
Boston, MA

Rebecca I. Kalman, MD
Clinical Instructor of Anesthesia
Department of Anesthesia, Critical Care, and
Pain Medicine
Massachusetts General Hospital
Boston, MA

Edward A. Bittner, MD, PhD
Associate Professor of Anesthesia
Harvard Medical School
Program Director, Critical Care-Anesthesiology Fellowship
Associate Director, Surgical Intensive Care Unit
Department of Anesthesia, Critical Care, and
Pain Medicine
Massachusetts General Hospital
Boston, MA

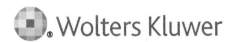

Philadelphia • Baltimore • New York • London
Buenos Aires • Hong Kong • Sydney • Tokyo

Acquisitions Editor: Keith Donnellan
Editorial Coordinator: Tim Rinehart
Editorial Assistant: Levi Bentley
Marketing Manager: Stacy Malyil
Production Project Manager: Kim Cox
Design Coordinator: Elaine Kasmer
Manufacturing Coordinator: Beth Welsh
Prepress Vendor: TNQ Books and Journals

9   8   7   6   5   4

Printed in the United States of America

Library of Congress Cataloging-in-Publication Data

Names: Berg, Sheri M., editor. | Schnur, Maricela, editor. | Kalman, Rebecca I., editor. | Bittner, Edward A., 1967- editor.
Title: Anesthesia review : 1000 questions and answers to blast the basics and ace the advanced / [edited by] Sheri M. Berg, Maricela Schnur, Rebecca I. Kalman, Edward A. Bittner.
Description: Philadelphia : Wolters Kluwer, [2019] | Includes bibliographical references.
Identifiers: LCCN 2018017425 | ISBN 9781496383501 (pbk.)
Subjects: | MESH: Anesthesia | Examination Questions
Classification: LCC RD82.3 | NLM WO 218.2 | DDC 617.9/6076—dc23 LC record available at
    https://lccn.loc.gov/2018017425

LWW.com

DEDICATION

To the fellows and residents who go to work every day and still find time to prepare themselves for the next chapter in their lives.

To my husband and son who always motivate me to be my best each and every day.

—Maricela Schnur

This book is dedicated to two of the most amazingly incredible people I know, my parents, Anne and Gary. Thank you for everything, but above all, thank you for writing a book of eternal love, infinite generosity, and exceptional kindness—I never read this book—because of you, this story is my life. Your endless support in everything I have done, and continue to do, puts me at a loss for words. I am forever grateful.

—Sheri M. Berg

CONTRIBUTORS

Alexandra Raisa Adler, MD, MPhil
Resident (PGY-3)
Anesthesiology
Massachusetts General Hospital
Harvard University
Boston, MA

Aditi Balakrishnan, MD
Resident Physician
Anesthesia, Critical Care and Pain Medicine
Massachusetts General Hospital
Boston, MA

Christine Choi, MD
Critical Care Fellow
Department of Anesthesia
Critical Care and Pain Medicine, Massachusetts
General Hospital
Boston, MA

Jennifer Cottral, MD
Resident Physician
Anesthesia, Critical Care and Pain Medicine
Massachusetts General Hospital
Boston, MA

Jerome Crowley, MD, MPH
Clinical Instructor
Anesthesiology
Harvard Medical School
Boston, MA

Michael Fitzsimons, MD
Chief Cardiac Anesthesia
Department of Anesthesia, Critical Care and
Pain Medicine
Massachusetts General Hospital
Boston, MA

Ryan Joseph Horvath, MD, PhD
Instructor of Anesthesia
Anesthesia, Critical Care and Pain Medicine
Harvard University
Boston, MA

Rebecca I. Kalman, MD
Clinical Instructor of Anesthesia
Department of Anesthesia, Critical Care, and
Pain Medicine
Massachusetts General Hospital
Boston, MA

Mara Kenger, MD
Resident Physician
Anesthesia, Critical Care and Pain Medicine
Massachusetts General Hospital
Boston, MA

Jean Kwo, MD
Clinical Instructor
Anesthesia, Critical Care and Pain Medicine
Massachussetts General Hospital
Boston, MA

Nathan Lee, MD
Critical Care Fellow
Department of Anesthesia, Critical Care and
Pain Medicine
Massachusetts General Hospital
Boston, MA

Lydia Miller, MD
Critical Care Fellow
Anesthesia, Critical Care and Pain Medicine
Massachusetts General Hospital
Boston, MA

Christoph Nabzdyk, MD
Critical Care Fellow
Department of Anesthesia, Critical Care and
Pain Medicine
Massachusetts General Hospital
Boston, MA

Alexander Nagrebetsky, MD
Critical Care Fellow
Department of Anesthesia, Critical Care and
Pain Medicine
Massachusetts General Hospital
Boston, MA

Emily Naoum, MD
Resident Physician
Department of Anesthesia, Critical Care and
Pain Medicine
Massachusetts General Hospital
Boston, MA

Matthieu A. Newton, MD, DPT
Resident Physician
Anesthesia, Critical Care and Pain Medicine
Massachusetts General Hospital
Boston, MA

Alexandra Plichta, MD
Resident Physcian
Anesthesia, Critical Care and Pain Medicine
Massachussetts General Hospital
Boston, MA

Katarina Ruscic, MD
Resident Physician
Anesthesia, Critical Care and Pain Medicine
Massachusetts General Hospital
Boston, MA

Kyan Safavi, MD, MBA
Crical Care Fellow
Department of Anesthesia, Critical Care and
Pain Medicine
Massachusetts General Hospital
Boston, MA

Maricela Schnur, MD, MBA
Resident Physician
Department of Anesthesia, Critical Care and
Pain Medicine
Massachusetts General Hospital
Boston, MA

Lauren Smith, MD
Resident Physician
Anesthesia, Critical Care and Pain Medicine
Massachusetts General Hospital
Boston, MA

Abraham Sonny, MD
Clinical Instructor
Department of Anesthesia, Critical Care and
Pain Medicine
Harvard Medical School
Boston, MA

Jamie L. Sparling, MD
Resident Physician
Department of Anesthesia, Critical Care and
Pain Medicine
Massachusetts General Hospital
Boston, MA

Nicole Zaneta Spence, MD
Fellow
Department of Anesthesia, Critical Care and
Pain Medicine
Massachusetts General Hospital
Boston, MA

Amanda Xi, MD, MSE
Resident Physician
Anesthesia, Critical Care and Pain Medicine
Massachusetts General Hospital
Boston, MA

Qing Yang, MD
Resident Physician
Anesthesia, Critical Care and Pain Medicine
Massachusetts General Hospital
Boston, MA

TABLE OF CONTENTS

BASIC SECTION

1

MONITORS AND ANESTHESIA DELIVERY DEVICES

Matthieu A. Newton

1. **The concentration of a specific gas in solution depends on which of the following?**

   A. Temperature of the solution
   B. Volume of the system
   C. Solubility of the specific gas in that solution
   D. Molecular weight of the gas

2. **Which of the following statements is true about the partial pressure of a gas at equilibrium?**

   A. Directly proportional to its concentration of gas in solution
   B. Inversely proportional to its concentration of gas in solution
   C. Less than its concentration of gas in solution
   D. Greater than its concentration of gas in solution

3. **A vaporizer is mishandled and accidentally tipped on its side. Which of the following is the best course of action to take?**

   A. Run high fresh gas flows with the dial set to a high concentration for 30 minutes.
   B. Run high fresh gas flows with the dial set to a low concentration for 30 minutes.
   C. Run low fresh gas flows with the dial set to a low concentration for 30 minutes.
   D. Run low fresh gas flows with the dial set to a high concentration for 30 minutes.

4. **Which of the following would *increase* the output concentration of a volatile anesthetic from a vaporizer?**

   A. Fresh gas flow rate of 100 mL/min
   B. Fresh gas flow rate of 20 L/min
   C. Decreased operating room temperature
   D. Significantly increasing the ratio of oxygen to nitrous oxide

5. **To *decrease* temperature fluctuations while delivering an anesthetic agent, manufacturers seek to use vaporizer materials that have which of the following properties?**

   A. Low specific heat, high thermal conductivity
   B. Low specific heat, low thermal conductivity
   C. High specific heat, high thermal conductivity
   D. High specific heat, low thermal conductivity

6. **A portable E-cylinder of oxygen has 1760 psig. In approximately what time frame will the cylinder be depleted if used at 8 L/min?**

   A. 30 minutes
   B. 45 minutes
   C. 60 minutes
   D. 85 minutes

7. **Which of the following statements defines the critical temperature?**

   A. The temperature at which a liquid will boil
   B. The highest temperature at which a gas can exist in liquid form
   C. The temperature at which a substance can exist as a gas or liquid
   D. The temperature at which a solid becomes a liquid

8. **Which of the following describes the partial pressure of inhaled anesthetics in the central nervous system (CNS), blood, and alveoli at equilibrium?**

   A. CNS partial pressure (PCNS) = blood partial pressure (Pblood) = alveolar partial pressure (Palveolar)
   B. PCNS > Pblood = Palveolar
   C. PCNS < Pblood = Palveolar
   D. PCNS = Pblood < Palveolar

9. **Which of the following would *increase* the rate of rise of Fa/Fi?**

   A. A high blood:gas solubility
   B. A high cardiac output
   C. A low minute ventilation
   D. A high anesthetic concentration

10. **After an 8-hour general anesthetic case with volatile agents, which tissue group plays the greatest role in determining emergence time?**

    A. Vessel-rich tissue
    B. Muscle
    C. Fat
    D. Each is equal

11. **Which of the following is the purpose of the check valve on the anesthesia machine?**

    A. To prevent hypoxic gas mixtures
    B. To prevent gas flow from the common gas outlet to the vaporizers
    C. To prevent overly high flows of oxygen
    D. To ensure adequate ratios of oxygen to nitrogen

12. **Which of the following flowmeter arrangements would be the *most likely* to lead to a *hypoxic* gas mixture?**

    A. N_2O, Air, O_2
    B. Air, N_2O, O_2
    C. N_2O, O_2, Air
    D. O_2, Air, N_2O

13. **Standards for basic anesthetic monitoring during general anesthesia include which of the following?**

    A. Continuous display of MAC
    B. Continuous display of electrocardiogram
    C. Continuous display of tidal volume
    D. Continuous display of temperature

14. Which of the following would cause an abrupt *decrease* in the end-tidal CO_2 ($ETCO_2$) during general anesthesia?

   A. Hyperthermia
   B. Sepsis
   C. Shivering
   D. Pulmonary embolism

15. To mitigate the effects of attenuation during ultrasonography, an anesthesiologist would perform which of the following maneuvers?

   A. Use a low-frequency signal.
   B. Use a high-frequency signal.
   C. Increase the amplitude.
   D. Decrease the amplitude.

16. To maximize the axial resolution of an ultrasound image, an anesthesiologist would use which of the following?

   A. Long pulses of low frequency
   B. Long pulses of high frequency
   C. Short pulses of low frequency
   D. Short pulses of high frequency

17. Flow proportioning systems of anesthesia machines were designed to prevent which of the following?

   A. Inconsistent proportions of volatile anesthetic gases
   B. Hypoxic mixtures of nitrogen and oxygen
   C. Inaccurate proportions of gas flow to the common gas outlet
   D. Direct communication between the high-pressure and low-pressure circuits

18. Which of the following devices prevents the delivery of a hypoxic mixture by ensuring appropriate connections from the hospitals' pipeline gas supply to the anesthesia machine?

   A. Second-stage oxygen pressure regulator
   B. Pin Index Safety System
   C. Diameter Index Safety System
   D. Check valve

19. An isolated power system (IPS) acts to prevent which of the following situations?

   A. Prevention of operating room power loss
   B. Prevention of an ungrounded operating room
   C. Prevention of macroshock
   D. Prevention of microshock

20. All of the following are functions of the equipment ground wire EXCEPT which one?

   A. Provides a low-resistance path for fault currents to decrease the risk of macroshock.
   B. Minimizes leakage currents that may cause microshock in certain patients.
   C. Provides information to the line isolation monitor on the status of an ungrounded system.
   D. Acts to eliminate the need for ground fault circuit interrupters (GFCIs).

Chapter 1 ▪ Answers

1. Correct answer: C

Inhaled anesthetics accumulate to specific concentrations in the CNS by creating a certain partial pressure of the gas in the lung. Solubility is the tendency of a gas to equilibrate with a solution. Partial pressure of a gas in solution is the pressure of the gas in the gas phase when in equilibrium with the liquid. The concentration of gas in a mixture of gases depends on the partial pressures in the gas phase in equilibrium with the solution and its solubility within that solution. As anesthetic gases move from the alveoli to the blood, the partial pressures of the blood and alveoli equilibrate. The final concentration of anesthetic depends on the partial pressure it exerts at equilibrium and at its blood solubility. This same process occurs from blood to the target tissue, brain. Given that this system (from alveoli to blood to target tissue) is closed, the concentration of a gas in the alveoli is theoretically the same as the concentration of the said gas in the brain. Thus, minimum alveolar concentration is a proxy for the concentration of the gas in the brain. This is expressed via the Henry law; the concentration of gas in solution is proportional to its partial pressure in the gas phase: $C_g = kP_g$. C_g is the concentration of the gas in solution, k is a solubility constant, and P_g is the partial pressure of the gas.

Reference:

1. Ebert TJ, Lindebaum L. Inhaled anesthetics. In: Barash PG, Cullen BF, Stoelting RK, et al, eds. *Clinical Anesthesia*. 7th ed. Philadelphia: Wolters Kluwer Health; 2013:447-477.

2. Correct answer: A

See answer explanation given for question 1.

Inhaled anesthetics accumulate to specific concentrations in the CNS by creating a certain partial pressure of the gas in the lung. Solubility is the tendency of a gas to equilibrate with a solution. Partial pressure of a gas in solution is the pressure of the gas in the gas phase when in equilibrium with the liquid. The concentration of gas in a mixture of gases depends on the partial pressures in the gas phase in equilibrium with the solution and its solubility within that solution. As anesthetic gases move from the alveoli to the blood, the partial pressures of the blood and alveoli equilibrate. The final concentration of anesthetic depends on the partial pressure it exerts at equilibrium and at its blood solubility. This same process occurs from blood to the target tissue, brain. Given that this system (from alveoli to blood to target tissue) is closed, the concentration of a gas in the alveoli is theoretically the same as the concentration of the said gas in the brain. Thus, minimum alveolar concentration is a proxy for the concentration of the gas in the brain. This is expressed via the Henry law; the concentration of gas in solution is proportional to its partial pressure in the gas phase: $C_g = kP_g$. C_g is the concentration of the gas in solution, k is a solubility constant, and P_g is the partial pressure of the gas.

Reference:

1. Ebert TJ, Lindebaum L. Inhaled anesthetics. In: Barash PG, Cullen BF, Stoelting RK, et al, eds. *Clinical Anesthesia*. 7th ed. Philadelphia: Wolters Kluwer Health; 2013:447-477.

3. Correct answer: A

Excessive tipping of a vaporizer allows liquid anesthetic to leak into the bypass chamber, causing increased vapor concentrations when delivering an anesthetic. Tipping rarely occurs when the vaporizer is connected to the machine and most often occurs during transportation or connection of a vaporizer to the machine. After being tipped, the vaporizer should be taken out of service and run at a high fresh gas flow with the vaporizer concentration set to a high concentration and should continue until all liquid anesthetic has evaporated. This allows the majority of the flow to pass through the bypass chamber. Several types of vaporizers now have a transport mode, which isolates the liquid anesthetic from the bypass chamber to eliminate the risk of tipping.

Reference:

1. Riutort KT, Eisenkraft JB. The anesthesia workstation and delivery systems for inhaled anesthetics. In: Barash PG, Cullen BF, Stoelting RK, et al, eds. *Clinical Anesthesia*. 7th ed. Philadelphia: Wolters Kluwer Health; 2013:641-696.

4. **Correct answer: D**

Several factors affect the output concentration of vaporizers. These include fresh gas flow rate, temperature, and the composition of fresh gas. At low fresh gas flow rates, there is not enough turbulence to pick up the anesthetic vapors, whereas at high flow rates >15 L/min, the output is less than the actual dial setting, as there is not enough time to saturate the carrier gas. Modern vaporizers accommodate varying temperatures by using a bimetallic strip or expansion element to direct a greater portion of gas flow through the bypass chamber when temperature increases and less when temperature decreases. When the fresh gas is changed from 100% oxygen to 100% nitrous oxide, a rapid decrease in the vaporizer output occurs, as the nitrous is more soluble in anesthetic liquid than is the oxygen. When the ratio of oxygen to nitrous oxide is increased, the reverse occurs such that output increases as the amount of oxygen increases.

Reference:
1. Riutort KT, Eisenkraft JB. The anesthesia workstation and delivery systems for inhaled anesthetics. In: Barash PG, Cullen BF, Stoelting RK, et al, eds. *Clinical Anesthesia*. 7th ed. Philadelphia: Wolters Kluwer Health; 2013:641-696.

5. **Correct answer: C**

Temperature fluctuations of the anesthetic agent while in the vaporizer can lead to varying amounts of agent being delivered at a given amount of concentration per the dial. Thus it is imperative that the vaporizer maintain a constant temperature. Specific heat is the number of calories needed to increase 1 g of a substance by 1°C. High specific heat minimizes the temperature changes with vaporization. Thermal conductivity is the measure of speed with which heat flows through a substance. A high thermal conductivity allows for the uniformity of temperature throughout the vaporizer.

Reference:
1. Riutort KT, Eisenkraft JB. The anesthesia workstation and delivery systems for inhaled anesthetics. In: Barash PG, Cullen BF, Stoelting RK, et al, eds. *Clinical Anesthesia*. 7th ed. Philadelphia: Wolters Kluwer Health; 2013:641-696.

6. **Correct answer: C**

Oxygen E-cylinders are small and portable and are on the back of every anesthesia machine. It is imperative to know the amount of time left in the tank in case the wall supply fails or perhaps when providing offsite anesthetic services. The E-cylinders contain 625 L and have a pressure of 2000 psig. A quick way to determine the amount of time left in an oxygen tank can be derived via the following equation:

$$T \text{ (hours)} = \text{Oxygen cylinder pressure (psig)} / 200 \times \text{Oxygen flow rate (L/min)}$$

Therefore, using our example:

$$T = 1760/200 \times 8$$
$$= 1760/1600$$
$$= 1.1 \text{ hours}$$

Reference:
1. Riutort KT, Eisenkraft JB. The anesthesia workstation and delivery systems for inhaled anesthetics. In: Barash PG, Cullen BF, Stoelting RK, et al, eds. *Clinical Anesthesia*. 7th ed. Philadelphia: Wolters Kluwer Health; 2013:641-696.

7. **Correct answer: B**

The critical temperature is the highest temperature at which a gas can exist in liquid form. The critical temperature of nitrous oxide (36.5°C) is just above room temperature (20°C), which means that it can remain a liquid at room temperature. Nitrous tanks are filled with liquid with a small amount of gas near the top of the tank. As the tank is opened and gas leaves, more liquid is vaporized to maintain its equilibrium within the tank. The ratio of liquid to gas remains the same, maintaining the same pressure within the tank until the tank is almost empty. The only way to determine the volume of nitrous remaining in the tank is to weigh the tank and subtract the weight of an empty tank. Once the tank is near empty and contains only gas, the volume of gas remaining can adequately be calculated from the pressure. Full E-cylinders of nitrous contain approximately 1600 L of gas and exert a pressure of approximately 750 psig.

Reference:

1. Riutort KT, Eisenkraft JB. The anesthesia workstation and delivery systems for inhaled anesthetics. In: Barash PG, Cullen BF, Stoelting RK, et al, eds. *Clinical Anesthesia*. 7th ed. Philadelphia: Wolters Kluwer Health; 2013:641-696.

8. Correct answer: A

See answer explanation given for question 1.

Inhaled anesthetics accumulate to specific concentrations in the CNS by creating a certain partial pressure of the gas in the lung. Solubility is the tendency of a gas to equilibrate with a solution. Partial pressure of a gas in solution is the pressure of the gas in the gas phase when in equilibrium with the liquid. The concentration of gas in a mixture of gases depends on the partial pressures in the gas phase in equilibrium with the solution and its solubility within that solution. As anesthetic gases move from the alveoli to the blood, the partial pressures of the blood and alveoli equilibrate. The final concentration of anesthetic depends on the partial pressure it exerts at equilibrium and at its blood solubility. This same process occurs from blood to the target tissue, brain. Given that this system (from alveoli to blood to target tissue) is closed, the concentration of a gas in the alveoli is theoretically the same as the concentration of the said gas in the brain. Thus, minimum alveolar concentration is a proxy for the concentration of the gas in the brain. This is expressed via the Henry law; the concentration of gas in solution is proportional to its partial pressure in the gas phase: $C_g = kP_g$. C_g is the concentration of the gas in solution, k is a solubility constant, and P_g is the partial pressure of the gas.

Reference:

1. Ebert TJ, Lindebaum L. Inhaled anesthetics. In: Barash PG, Cullen BF, Stoelting RK, et al, eds. *Clinical Anesthesia*. 7th ed. Philadelphia: Wolters Kluwer Health; 2013:447-477.

9. Correct answer: D

Uptake is the mechanism by which volatile agents entering the alveoli are mixed with blood in the lungs. Uptake can be assessed by the ratio of fractional concentration of alveolar anesthetic to inspired anesthetic (Fa/Fi). The faster the Fa rises, the faster the speed of induction. Distribution is the mechanism by which the volatile agents from the blood are taken up by 3 physiologic tissue groups: the vessel-rich group (VRG) (which includes brain, heart, kidney, liver, gastrointestinal tract, and glandular tissue), muscle groups, and fat groups. Uptake of the anesthetic depends on the partial pressure the gas exerts at equilibrium, its blood solubility, and pulmonary blood flow. Partial pressure differences determine the rate of flow to and from alveoli, blood, and physiologic tissue. Higher pulmonary blood flow allows for increased uptake, and decreased flow allows for lower and slower uptake. The partition coefficient is the ease with which anesthetic agent moves from the alveoli to blood, and a high coefficient means there is a higher concentration in the blood and vice versa. While blood concentrations of the gas are equilibrating with the alveoli, the same is happening in the 3 physiologic tissues. The tissues equilibrate at different speeds, however, owing primarily to their differences in perfusion. The VRG perfuses at about 75 mL/min per 100 g of tissue, whereas muscle and fat perfuse at 3 mL/min per 100 g. Fat is further limited by its lower percentage of cardiac output. Thus, fat plays little to no role in the speed of induction but may be a factor in delayed emergence in cases longer than 4 hours.

Reference:

1. Ebert TJ, Lindebaum L. Inhaled anesthetics. In: Barash PG, Cullen BF, Stoelting RK, et al, eds. *Clinical Anesthesia*. 7th ed. Philadelphia: Wolters Kluwer Health; 2013:447-477.

10. Correct answer: C

See answer explanation given for question 9.

Uptake is the mechanism by which volatile agents entering the alveoli are mixed with blood in the lungs. Uptake can be assessed by the ratio of fractional concentration of alveolar anesthetic to inspired anesthetic (Fa/Fi). The faster the Fa rises, the faster the speed of induction. Distribution is the mechanism by which the volatile agents from the blood are taken up by 3 physiologic tissue groups: the VRG (which includes brain, heart, kidney, liver, gastrointestinal tract, and glandular tissue), muscle groups, and fat groups. Uptake of the anesthetic depends on the partial pressure the gas exerts at equilibrium, its blood solubility, and pulmonary blood flow. Partial pressure differences determine the rate of flow to and from alveoli, blood, and physiologic tissue. Higher pulmonary blood flow allows for increased uptake, and decreased flow allows for lower and slower uptake. The partition coefficient is the ease with which anesthetic agent moves from the alveoli to blood, and a high coefficient means there is a higher concentration in the blood and vice versa. While blood concentrations of the gas are equilibrating with the alveoli, the same is happening in the 3 physiologic tissues. The tissues equilibrate at different speeds, however, owing primarily to their differences in perfusion. The VRG perfuses at about 75 mL/min per 100 g of tissue, whereas muscle and fat perfuse at 3 mL/min per 100 g. Fat is further limited by its lower percentage of cardiac output. Thus, fat plays little to no role in the speed of induction but may be a factor in delayed emergence in cases longer than 4 hours.

Reference:
1. Ebert TJ, Lindebaum L. Inhaled anesthetics. In: Barash PG, Cullen BF, Stoelting RK, et al, eds. *Clinical Anesthesia*. 7th ed. Philadelphia: Wolters Kluwer Health; 2013:447-477.

11. Correct answer: B

The check valve is located downstream from the vaporizers and upstream from the oxygen flush valve and common gas outlet. It serves to prevent back pressure into the vaporizers from either the common gas outlet or the oxygen flush valve. Back pressure can occur with oxygen flushing, with positive pressure ventilation, and during leak tests.

Reference:
1. Riutort KT, Eisenkraft JB. The anesthesia workstation and delivery systems for inhaled anesthetics. In: Barash PG, Cullen BF, Stoelting RK, et al, eds. *Clinical Anesthesia*. 7th ed. Philadelphia: Wolters Kluwer Health; 2013:641-696.

12. Correct answer: D

The arrangement of flowmeters must be such that a hypoxic mixture does not result in the event of a leak. Hypoxic mixtures are most likely to occur when nitrous is the most downstream flowmeter and least likely to occur when the oxygen flowmeter is located downstream from both the air and nitrous oxide flowmeters. A hypoxic mixture is less likely when oxygen is furthest downstream because nitrous would also advance the oxygen toward the common gas outlet.

Reference:
1. Riutort KT, Eisenkraft JB. The anesthesia workstation and delivery systems for inhaled anesthetics. In: Barash PG, Cullen BF, Stoelting RK, et al, eds. *Clinical Anesthesia*. 7th ed. Philadelphia: Wolters Kluwer Health; 2013:641-696.

13. Correct answer: B

During all anesthetics, the patient's oxygenation, ventilation, circulation, and temperature should be continually evaluated. This includes the use of an inspired oxygen analyzer with a low oxygen concentration limit alarm and a quantitative method of assessing oxygenation, such as pulse oximetry. Continuous monitoring for the presence of expired carbon dioxide, unless limited by the patient, procedure, or equipment, should be available and visible throughout the case. A breathing system disconnection alarm with an audible signal must be in use when using a mechanical ventilator. During regional or local anesthesia, adequacy of ventilation should be monitored by continual observation of qualitative clinical signs. Continuous electrocardiogram is displayed from the beginning of anesthesia until preparing to leave the anesthetizing location. Arterial blood pressure and heart rate are evaluated at least every 5 minutes. Furthermore, every patient should be evaluated by at least one of the following: palpation of pulse, auscultation of heart sounds, intra-arterial pressure tracing, ultrasound peripheral pulse monitoring, or pulse plethysmography or oximetry. Every patient should have temperature monitored when clinically significant changes in body temperature are intended, anticipated, or suspected.

Reference:
1. Connor CW. Commonly used monitoring techniques. In: Barash PG, Cullen BF, Stoelting RK, et al, eds. *Clinical Anesthesia*. 7th ed. Philadelphia: Wolters Kluwer Health; 2013:699-722.

14. Correct answer: D

An abrupt decrease in the $ETco_2$ is often linked with a life-threatening predicament and is almost always associated with either a ventilation or perfusion issue. Examples include sudden severe hypotension, endotracheal tube migration, massive pulmonary embolism, and cardiac arrest. When an abrupt decrease in $ETco_2$ is noted, it should be quickly verified and addressed. During cardiopulmonary resuscitation, adequacy of circulation can be monitored via return of the $ETco_2$.

Factors that decrease ETco$_2$ during anesthesia include hypothermia, hypothyroidism, hyperventilation, hypoperfusion, and pulmonary embolism. Factors that increase ETco$_2$ include hyperthermia, sepsis, malignant hyperthermia, shivering, hyperthyroidism, hypoventilation, and rebreathing.

Reference:

1. Connor CW. Commonly used monitoring techniques. In: Barash PG, Cullen BF, Stoelting RK, et al, eds. *Clinical Anesthesia*. 7th ed. Philadelphia: Wolters Kluwer Health; 2013:699-722.

15. Correct answer: A

Ultrasound technology uses sound waves to produce a real-time image of body structures. Sound waves are characterized by their amplitude, frequency, wavelength, and velocity. Amplitude is perceived, as loudness of a sound wave represents its peak pressure. Frequency is the number of cycles per second used by the sound wave. Wavelength is the distance between the peaks of each wave. Lastly, velocity is the product of wavelength and frequency and is determined by the medium through which the sound wave passes.

As sound travels through tissues, the sound waves diminish in intensity because of dispersion and absorption; this is known as attenuation and decreases the energy returned to the ultrasound probe. To diminish attenuation, low frequencies, which better penetrate tissues, are used.

Reference:

1. Perrino AC, Popescu WM, Skubas NJ. Echocardiography. In: Barash PG, Cullen BF, Stoelting RK, et al, eds. *Clinical Anesthesia*. 7th ed. Philadelphia: Wolters Kluwer Health; 2013:723-761.

16. Correct answer: D

Resolution of ultrasound images is evaluated using their axial resolution, lateral resolution, and elevational resolution. Axial resolution evaluates objects lying along the axis of the ultrasound beam, lateral resolution evaluates objects horizontal to the beam, and elevational resolution evaluates objects vertical to the beam's orientation. Short, high-frequency pulses have the greatest axial resolution but decreased tissue penetration. As a result, the best ultrasound images are taken parallel to the beam's axis.

Reference:

1. Perrino AC, Popescu WM, Skubas NJ. Echocardiography. In: Barash PG, Cullen BF, Stoelting RK, et al, eds. *Clinical Anesthesia*. 7th ed. Philadelphia: Wolters Kluwer Health; 2013:723-761.

17. Correct answer: B

Modern anesthesia machines have multiple mechanisms to prevent the administration of a hypoxic gas mixture; one of these is the flow proportioning system. The flow proportioning system links the administration of nitrous oxide and oxygen such that the minimum oxygen concentration delivered is between 23% and 25%. Traditionally this was done via a mechanical link between the 2 flowmeters such that a nitrous oxide to oxygen ratio of 3:1 would be maintained. Because there are limitations to this system, all anesthesia machines are equipped with an oxygen or multigas analyzer with an alarm for hypoxic mixture delivery.

Reference:

1. Riutort KT, Eisenkraft JB. The anesthesia workstation and delivery systems for inhaled anesthetics. In: Barash PG, Cullen BF, Stoelting RK, et al, eds. *Clinical Anesthesia*. 7th ed. Philadelphia: Wolters Kluwer Health; 2013:641-696.

18. Correct answer: C

Multiple mechanisms exist to prevent the administration of a hypoxic mixture of gases to a patient; one of these is the Diameter Index Safety System. This system provides uniformly threaded, noninterchangeable hose connections for nitrous oxide and oxygen from the wall pipeline system to the anesthesia machine. Via this mechanism, the only way a hypoxic mixture could result is if the hospital pipelines were somehow crossed. The Pin Index Safety System prevents nitrous oxide cylinders from connecting to the oxygen yoke on the anesthesia machine and vice versa.

Reference:

1. Riutort KT, Eisenkraft JB. The anesthesia workstation and delivery systems for inhaled anesthetics. In: Barash PG, Cullen BF, Stoelting RK, et al, eds. *Clinical Anesthesia*. 7th ed. Philadelphia: Wolters Kluwer Health; 2013:641-696.

19. Correct answer: C

Macroshock is the application of a strong electric shock to the body, which is often large enough to cause ventricular fibrillation. As a safety mechanism to prevent macroshock, the power supply to most operating rooms is ungrounded with the current isolated from the ground potential. This is termed the IPS and ensures that there is no circuit between the ground and either of the isolated power lines.

Reference:
1. Ehrenwerth J, Seifert HA. Electrical and fire safety. In: Barash PG, Cullen BF, Stoelting RK, et al, eds. *Clinical Anesthesia*. 7th ed. Philadelphia: Wolters Kluwer Health; 2013:189-218.

20. Correct answer: D

All equipment parts of the IPS have an equipment ground wire. The equipment ground wire is attached to the piece of equipment and gives electric current a low-resistance pathway, allowing dangerous current to flow to the ground instead of to patients or personnel. The role of the equipment ground wire is to provide a low-resistance path for fault currents to decrease the risk of macroshock, minimize leakage currents that may cause microshock in certain patients, and lastly to provide information to the line isolation monitor on the status of an ungrounded system. Notably, the line isolation monitor (which monitors the IPS) is unable to detect faulty ground wires, which could make a compromised system appear safe. GFCIs can be combined with an IPS. GFCI systems monitor both sides of a circuit for equal current flow. If there is a difference detected, the GFCI trips and cuts off power to that outlet, removing the flow of current. Often this is caused by a surge; however, if after being reset, the GFCI trips again, the offending piece of equipment should be removed and taken in for servicing.

Reference:
1. Ehrenwerth J, Seifert HA. Electrical and fire safety. In: Barash PG, Cullen BF, Stoelting RK, et al, eds. *Clinical Anesthesia*. 7th ed. Philadelphia: Wolters Kluwer Health; 2013:189-218.

2

BASIC ANATOMY

Lauren Smith

1. When preparing to place a thoracic epidural, you palpate the inferior border of the scapula. This landmark corresponds to which level of the vertebral column?

   A. C7-T1
   B. T4-T6
   C. T10-T11
   D. T7-T8

2. Assuming normal anatomy, which of the following landmarks is appropriate for gaining subclavian venous access?

   A. Needle insertion medial to the sternocleidomastoid muscle, just medial to the carotid artery
   B. Needle insertion above the inguinal ligament, lateral to the femoral artery
   C. Needle insertion at the midpoint of the clavicle with the needle directed toward the suprasternal notch
   D. Needle insertion at the lateral border of the clavicular head of the sternocleidomastoid muscle in the interscalene groove

3. While providing anesthesia for a 15-month-old, 5-kg girl undergoing strabismus surgery, you notice that the patient suddenly becomes hypotensive and bradycardic while the surgeons are applying direct pressure to the globe. Despite release of pressure, the patient continues to be hypotensive and bradycardic. After treatment with atropine, the patient becomes normotensive with a normal rhythm. The afferent limb of this reflex is mediated by which of the following?

   A. CN VII
   B. CN VI
   C. CN V
   D. CN III

4. Which of the following treatments for glaucoma has been shown to increase the duration of action of succinylcholine?

   A. Echothiophate
   B. Dipivefrin
   C. Betaxolol
   D. Cyclopentolate

5. The muscles of the larynx are innervated by the recurrent laryngeal nerve EXCEPT which of the following?

    A. Thyroarytenoid
    B. Thyroepiglotticus
    C. Cricothyroid
    D. Transverse arytenoids

6. The glossopharyngeal nerve (CN IX) provides sensory innervation to all of the following structures EXCEPT which one?

    A. Posterior 1/3 of tongue
    B. Rostral epiglottis
    C. Pharynx
    D. Vocal cords

7. Which of the following structures would be effectively anesthetized by injection of lidocaine into the anterior tonsillar pillars bilaterally?

    A. Soft palate and oropharynx
    B. Anterior 2/3 of tongue
    C. Hypopharynx
    D. Vocal cords

8. Which of the following structures would be effectively anesthetized by injection of lidocaine inferior to the greater cornu of the hyoid bone?

    A. Recurrent laryngeal nerve
    B. Glossopharyngeal nerve
    C. Superior laryngeal nerve, internal branch
    D. Superior laryngeal nerve, external branch

9. While performing a preoperative assessment of your patient, you note that on recent transthoracic echocardiogram (TTE) there was abnormal movement of the inferior wall with increased heart rates, whereas all other portions were noted to move normally. Which of the following arteries most likely has a stenotic lesion?

    A. Posterior descending artery
    B. Left circumflex artery
    C. Left anterior descending artery
    D. Right coronary artery

10. The leaflets of the aortic valve are named which of the following?

    A. Anterior and posterior
    B. Anterior, posterior, and septal
    C. Right coronary, left coronary, and noncoronary
    D. Right, left, and anterior

11. The nipple line is at what dermatomal level?

    A. T2
    B. T4
    C. T6
    D. T8

12. **In regard to the trachea, all of the following are true EXCEPT which one?**

    A. Normally half of the trachea is intrathoracic and half is extrathoracic.
    B. Normal tracheal movement in an adult can result in endotracheal movement of 4 cm with neck flexion and extension.
    C. The tracheal rings are located anteriorly.
    D. The trachea is the only part of the bronchial tree that does not participate in gas exchange.

13. **During bronchoscopy, where does the right upper lobe bronchus usually take off?**

    A. 5 cm past the carina
    B. Located farther away from the carina than the lingular bronchus on the left
    C. 2.5 cm past the carina
    D. It has little anatomic variation

14. **You are taking care of a 10-month-old boy presenting for bilateral orchiopexy. You plan to perform a caudal block for postoperative pain. All of the following sacral anatomic landmarks are used to identify the proper location for the block EXCEPT which one?**

    A. Posterior superior iliac spines (PSISs)
    B. Sacral ala
    C. Sacral cornu
    D. Sacral hiatus

15. **When performing a single-shot caudal block, you must first pierce through which ligament?**

    A. Sacrococcygeal
    B. Sacrotuberous
    C. Sacrospinous
    D. Sacroiliac

16. **All of the following are true of the femoral triangle EXCEPT which one?**

    A. Superior border: formed by the inguinal ligament
    B. Lateral border: formed by the medial border of the sartorius muscle
    C. Medial border: formed by the medial border of the adductor longus muscle
    D. Medial to lateral structures: femoral nerve, artery, vein, lymphatics

17. **A fracture of the proximal humerus can result in all of the following EXCEPT which one?**

    A. Inability to abduct the arm at the shoulder
    B. Decreased sensation over the shoulder
    C. Wrist drop
    D. Atrophy of shoulder muscles

18. **What is the anatomic location of the cords of the brachial plexus?**

    A. Above the clavicle, at the lateral border of the clavicular head of the sternocleidomastoid muscle
    B. At the clavicle, lateral to the subclavian artery
    C. Below the clavicle, closely related to the axillary artery
    D. Below the clavicle, closely related to the axillary vein

19. You are taking care of a 27-year-old G3P2 woman for whom you placed an epidural in early labor. Her labor has progressed slowly and she has been pushing for many hours. She ultimately has an unremarkable vaginal delivery of a health baby boy. The epidural is removed post delivery and she is eventually sent to the floor. During postdelivery rounds the next day, the patient complains of continued numbness on the anterolateral aspect of her thighs bilaterally. Injury to which nerve is responsible for her discomfort?

    A. Obturator nerve
    B. Lateral femoral cutaneous nerve
    C. Femoral nerve
    D. Sciatic nerve

20. While in preparation for placement of a central line, you perform ultrasonography on the patient's neck and notice the internal jugular vein (IJV) overlying the common carotid artery. Which of the following maneuvers will aid in decreasing the overlap between the IJV and the common carotid artery?

    A. Neck flexion
    B. Trendelenburg position
    C. Rotation of head 0°-45° to contralateral side
    D. Ultrasound probe placement toward clavicle

Chapter 2 ▪ Answers

1. Correct answer: D

Utilization of topographic anatomic landmarks to assist anesthesiologists during procedural care relies on a thorough understanding of anatomic relationships to effectively deliver anesthesia and to avoid potential morbidity and mortality. Common topographic landmarks are as follows:

LEVEL	LANDMARK
C7	Vertebra prominens
T4	Nipple line
T7	Xiphoid process
T8	Inferior border of scapula
T10	Umbilicus
L2	Termination of spinal cord adults
L4	Iliac crest

Reference:
1. Freeman BS, Berger JS. Topographical anatomy as landmarks. In: *Anesthesiology Core Review: Part One, Basic Exam*. New York: McGraw-Hill; 2014:1-2.

2. Correct answer: C

Needle insertion at the midpoint of the clavicle with the needle directed toward the suprasternal notch describes the correct approach for obtaining subclavian venous access. For IJV access, needle insertion is between the sternal and clavicular heads of the sternocleidomastoid muscle, lateral to the carotid artery. For femoral venous access, needle insertion is medial to the femoral artery below the inguinal ligament. Needle insertion at the lateral border of the clavicular head of the sternocleidomastoid muscle in the interscalene groove describes the landmarks for interscalene nerve block.

Reference:
1. Freeman BS, Berger JS. Topographical anatomy as landmarks. In: *Anesthesiology Core Review: Part One, Basic Exam*. New York: McGraw-Hill Education; 2014:1-2.

3. Correct answer: C

The oculocardiac reflex (OCR) is defined, clinically, as a 10% decrease in heart rate associated with traction applied to the extraocular muscles (especially the medial rectus), direct pressure on the globe, ocular manipulation, and ocular pain. The reflex most commonly leads to hypotension and sinus bradycardia but may also lead to junctional rhythm, ectopic beats, atrioventricular block, or asystole. The incidence of OCR decreases with age and tends to be more prominent in young, healthy patients, especially in the pediatric population, with the highest incidence in neonates and infants undergoing strabismus surgery.

The afferent limb of the OCR is mediated by the trigeminal nerve (ciliary ganglion → ophthalmic division of the trigeminal nerve → Gasserian ganglion → main trigeminal sensory nucleus). The afferents synapse with visceral motor nucleus of the vagus nerve. The efferent limb of the OCR is then vagally mediated. Efferent signals travel to the heart and decrease output from the sinoatrial node.

Reference:
1. Gonzalez RM, Louca K, Maldonado-Villalba S. Anesthesia for otolaryngologic and ophthalmic surgery. In: Barash PG, Cullen BF, Stoelting RK, et al, eds. *Clinical Anesthesia Fundamentals*. Philadelphia: Lippincott; 2015:539-556.

4. **Correct answer: A**

Echothiophate is an anticholinesterase agent used to treat refractory glaucoma that results in a reduction of pseudocholinesterase activity. This known side effect can last up to several weeks, increasing the duration of action of succinylcholine and ester-type local anesthetics. Dipivefrin is a prodrug of epinephrine that reduces production of aqueous humor and increases outflow. It has fewer side effects than epinephrine, which include hypertension, headaches, and dysrhythmias. Betaxolol is a newer antiglaucoma agent that is more oculoselective than Timolol and thus has minimal systemic effects. It may potentiate effects of systemic β-blockers and is contraindicated in patients with sinus bradycardia, first-degree AV block, CHF, and cardiogenic shock. Cyclopentolate is a mydriatic agent. It is associated with concentration-dependent CNS toxicity, eg, dysarthria, disorientation, seizures (in children), and psychotic episodes.

Reference:
1. Gonzalez RM, Louca K, Maldonado-Villalba S. Anesthesia for otolaryngologic and ophthalmic surgery. In: Barash PG, Cullen BF, Stoelting RK, et al, eds. *Clinical Anesthesia Fundamentals*. Philadelphia: Lippincott; 2015:539-556.

5. **Correct answer: C**

All of the intrinsic muscles of the larynx are innervated by the recurrent laryngeal nerve with the exception of the cricothyroid muscle, which is innervated by the external branch of the superior laryngeal nerve.

Reference:
1. Gonzalez RM, Louca K, Maldonado-Villalba S. Anesthesia for otolaryngologic and ophthalmic surgery. In: Barash PG, Cullen BF, Stoelting RK, et al, eds. *Clinical Anesthesia Fundamentals*. Philadelphia: Lippincott; 2015:539-556.

6. **Correct answer: D**

The glossopharyngeal nerve (CN IX) is responsible for the sensory innervation to the posterior 1/3 of the tongue, rostral epiglottis, and pharynx. The vagus nerve supplies sensory innervation to the mucosal surface of the larynx and trachea via the recurrent laryngeal nerve, and dorsal epiglottis and vocal cords via the superior laryngeal nerve.

Reference:
1. Gonzalez RM, Louca K, Maldonado-Villalba S. Anesthesia for otolaryngologic and ophthalmic surgery. In: Barash PG, Cullen BF, Stoelting RK, et al, eds. *Clinical Anesthesia Fundamentals*. Philadelphia: Lippincott; 2015:539-556.

7. **Correct answer: A**

Innervation:
Anterior 2/3 of tongue: trigeminal, mandibular branch (V3)
Posterior 1/3 of tongue: glossopharyngeal (IX)
Soft palate: glossopharyngeal (IX)
Oropharynx: glossopharyngeal (IX)
Hypopharynx (below the level of the epiglottis): internal branch of the superior laryngeal nerve (vagus (X))
Vocal cords: internal branch of superior laryngeal nerve and recurrent laryngeal nerve
Larynx (below the vocal cords, above the trachea): recurrent laryngeal nerve
Trachea: recurrent laryngeal nerve

Regional Anesthesia for Intubation:
1. Glossopharyngeal block: Intraoral approach instills local anesthetic submucosally at the caudal portion of the posterior tonsillar pillar.
2. Superior laryngeal nerve block: Local anesthetic is instilled at the level of the thyrohyoid membrane at the inferior aspect of greater cornu of hyoid bone. (This blocks the internal branch of superior laryngeal nerve.)
3. Transtracheal block: The recurrent laryngeal nerve is blocked by instilling local anesthetic into the trachea at the level of the cricothyroid membrane.

References:
1. Abrons RO, Rosenblatt WH. Airway management. In: Barash PG, Cullen BF, Stoelting RK, et al, eds. *Clinical Anesthesia Fundamentals*. Philadelphia: Lippincott; 2015:373-394.
2. Miller RD, Cohen NH, Eriksson LI, et al. Airway management. In: *Miller's Anesthesia: Airway Management*. New York: Elsevier; 2005:222-223.
3. Morgan GE, Mikhail MS, Murray MJ. Airway management. In: *Clinical Anesthesiology*. New York: McGraw Hill Medical; 2006:309-342.

8. Correct answer: C

The superior laryngeal nerve branches into internal and external components. The internal branch provides sensory input to the larynx above the level of the vocal cords and is the target for the superior laryngeal nerve block. The external branch provides motor innervation to the cricothyroid muscle. The superior laryngeal nerve block is performed by instilling local anesthetic at the level of the thyrohyoid membrane at the inferior aspect of greater cornu of hyoid bone. The recurrent laryngeal nerve provides sensory innervation to the larynx below the vocal cords and motor innervation to all intrinsic muscles of the larynx except for the cricothyroid. The glossopharyngeal nerve supplies taste and innervation to the posterior 1/3 of the tongue, motor innervation to the pharynx, and sensory innervation to the pharynx with contribution also from the vagus nerve.

References:
1. Abrons RO, Rosenblatt WH. Airway management. In: Barash PG, Cullen BF, Stoelting RK, et al, eds. *Clinical Anesthesia Fundamentals*. Philadelphia: Lippincott; 2015:373-394.
2. Miller RD, Cohen NH, Eriksson LI, et al. Airway management. In: *Miller's Anesthesia: Airway Management*. New York: Elsevier; 2005:222-223.
3. Morgan GE, Mikhail MS, Murray MJ. Airway management. In: *Clinical Anesthesiology*. New York: McGraw Hill Medical; 2006:309-342.

9. Correct answer: D

Echocardiographic and anatomic segmental analysis divides the left ventricle into various sections. In simplest terms, the left ventricle can be divided into 6 walls: anteroseptal, inferoseptal, inferior, inferolateral, anterolateral, and anterior walls. In general, the anteroseptal wall is supplied by the left anterior descending artery (LAD), the inferoseptal wall is supplied by the right coronary artery (RCA) and the LAD, the inferior wall is supplied by the RCA, the inferolateral wall is supplied by the RCA and the left circumflex artery (LCX), the anterolateral wall is supplied by the LCX, and the anterior wall is supplied by the LAD.

References:
1. Sharar SR, von Homeyer P. Cardiovascular anatomy and physiology. In: Barash PG, Cullen BF, Stoelting RK, et al, eds. *Clinical Anesthesia Fundamentals*. Philadelphia: Lippincott; 2015:41-67.
2. Freeman BS, Berger JS. Cardiac anatomy. In: *Anesthesiology Core Review: Part One, Basic Exam*. New York: McGraw-Hill; 2014:443-446.
3. Butterworth JF, Mackey DC, Wasnick JD. Cardiovascular physiology and anesthesia. In: *Morgan and Mikhail's Clinical Anesthesiology*. New York: McGraw-Hill; 2013: 343-374.

10. Correct answer: C

The aortic valve is a trileaflet valve with each leaflet named for its corresponding coronary artery. The right coronary leaflet lies near the ostium of the right coronary artery. The left coronary leaflet lies near the ostium of the left main coronary artery. The noncoronary cuff is not associated with a coronary artery.

The mitral valve has posterior and anterior leaflets.

The tricuspid valve is composed of anterior, posterior, and septal leaflets.

The leaflets of the pulmonic valve are named for their anatomic location: right, left, and anterior.

Reference:
1. Bernards CM, Hostetter LS. Spinal and epidural anesthesia. In: Barash PG, Cullen BF, Stoelting RK, et al, eds. *Clinical Anesthesia*. Philadelphia: Lippincott; 2013:905-935.

11. Correct answer: B

Utilization of topographic anatomic landmarks to assist anesthesiologists during procedural care relies on a thorough understanding of anatomic relationships to effectively deliver anesthesia and to avoid potential morbidity and mortality. Common topographic landmarks are as follows:

LEVEL	LANDMARK
C7	Vertebra prominens, level of stellate ganglion
T1-T4	Cardioaccelerator fibers
T3	Axilla
T4	Nipple line
T7	Xiphoid process
T8	Inferior border of scapula
T9-L2	Origin of artery of Adamkiewicz in 85% of patients
T10	Umbilicus
T12-L4	Lumbar plexus
L1	Level of celiac plexus
L2	Termination of spinal cord (adults)
L3	Termination of spinal cord (pediatrics)
L4	Iliac crest
L4-S3	Sacral plexus
S2	PSIS, termination of subarachnoid space (adults)

Reference:
1. Freeman BS, Berger JS. Topographical anatomy as landmarks. In: *Anesthesiology Core Review: Part One, Basic Exam*. New York: McGraw-Hill; 2014:1-2.

12. Correct answer: D

The trachea, mainstem bronchi, and terminal bronchioles do NOT participate in gas exchange. The first site of gas exchange occurs at the respiratory bronchiole.

Reference:
1. Bernards CM, Hostetter LS. Spinal and epidural anesthesia. In: Barash PG, Cullen BF, Stoelting RK, et al, eds. *Clinical Anesthesia*. Philadelphia: Lippincott; 2013:905-935.

13. Correct answer: C

The adult right upper lobe bronchus is usually 2.5 cm from the carina, much closer than the left upper lobe takeoff, which is approximately 5 cm from the carina. In 10% of adults, the right upper lobe takeoff is less than 2.5 cm from carina, and in 2%-3% of people, the right upper lobe takeoff is directly from the trachea.

Reference:
1. Bernards CM, Hostetter LS. Spinal and epidural anesthesia. In: Barash PG, Cullen BF, Stoelting RK, et al, eds. *Clinical Anesthesia*. Philadelphia: Lippincott; 2013:905-935.

14. **Correct answer: B**

Caudal anesthesia involves the injection of local anesthetics into the caudal epidural space, the lowest portion of the epidural system accessed through the sacral hiatus. The sacral hiatus is a defect in the lower part of the posterior wall of the sacrum formed by the failure of the laminae of S5 and/or S4 to meet and fuse in the midline and is bound by the sacral cornu (palpable on either side of the midline about 1 cm apart). The sacral hiatus can be located by drawing/visualizing an equilateral triangle between the bilateral PSIS and sacral hiatus. Once the sacral hiatus is identified, a short beveled needle is directed at about 45° to skin and inserted till a pop is felt, as the sacrococcygeal ligament is pierced. The needle is then carefully directed in a cephalad direction at an angle approaching the long axis of the spinal canal.

Reference:
1. Rodes ME, Ahmad S. Ambulatory anesthesia, monitored anesthesia care, and office-based anesthesia. In: Barash PG, Cullen BF, Stoelting RK, et al, eds. *Clinical Anesthesia Fundamentals*. Philadelphia: Lippincott; 2015:469-488.

15. **Correct answer: A**

See answer explanation given for question 14.

Caudal anesthesia involves the injection of local anesthetics into the caudal epidural space, the lowest portion of the epidural system accessed through the sacral hiatus. The sacral hiatus is a defect in the lower part of the posterior wall of the sacrum formed by the failure of the laminae of S5 and/or S4 to meet and fuse in the midline and is bound by the sacral cornu (palpable on either side of the midline about 1 cm apart). The sacral hiatus can be located by drawing/visualizing an equilateral triangle between the bilateral PSIS and sacral hiatus. Once the sacral hiatus is identified, a short beveled needle is directed at about 45° to skin and inserted till a pop is felt, as the sacrococcygeal ligament is pierced. The needle is then carefully directed in a cephalad direction at an angle approaching the long axis of the spinal canal.

Reference:
1. Rodes ME, Ahmad S. Ambulatory anesthesia, monitored anesthesia care, and office-based anesthesia. In: Barash PG, Cullen BF, Stoelting RK, et al, eds. *Clinical Anesthesia Fundamentals*. Philadelphia: Lippincott; 2015:469-488.

16. **Correct answer: D**

All are true except D. The **lateral to medial** structures are femoral nerve, artery, vein, and lymphatics.

Reference:
1. Drake RL, Vogl AW, Mithcell AW. Regional anatomy. In: *Gray's Basic Anatomy E-Book*. 2nd ed. Philadelphia: Elsevier; 2016.

17. **Correct answer: C**

The axillary nerve (C5-6) originates from the brachial plexus (upper trunk, posterior division, posterior cord) at the level of the axilla and travels with the posterior circumflex humeral artery and vein. The nerve can be injured with anterior-inferior dislocations of the shoulder often because of stretch and during fracture of the surgical neck of the humerus. Injury results in both motor and sensory deficits. Motor deficits include the loss of abduction of arm, weak flexion, extension, and rotation of shoulder. Sensory deficits include loss of sensation in the skin over the deltoid muscle. Wrist drop is due to radial nerve injury more commonly associated with mid to distal humerus fractures.

Reference:
1. Warner ME. Patient positioning and potential injuries. In: Barash PG, Cullen BF, Stoelting RK, et al, eds. *Clinical Anesthesia Fundamentals*. Philadelphia: Lippincott; 2015:413-426.

18. **Correct answer: C**

The cords of the brachial plexus are closely related to the axillary artery, at or below the level of the clavicle. An infraclavicular brachial plexus block is performed at the level of the cords, as the plexus emerges from beneath the clavicle and enters the axilla. An infraclavicular block provides reliable anesthesia to the hand, forearm, elbow, and upper arm. The lateral border of the clavicular head of the sternocleidomastoid muscle is a landmark used to identify the interscalene groove for interscalene block. During this block, the roots of the brachial plexus are anesthetized. The supraclavicular block is performed just above the clavicle, lateral to the subclavian artery, and targets the trunks/divisions of the brachial plexus.

Reference:

1. DeLeon AM, Asher YG. Regional anesthesia. In: Barash PG, Cullen BF, Stoelting RK, et al, eds. *Clinical Anesthesia Fundamentals*. Philadelphia: Lippincott; 2015:395-412.

19. Correct answer: B

The lateral femoral cutaneous nerve, a pure sensory nerve, is susceptible to compression, as it courses from the lumbosacral plexus under the inguinal ligament into the thigh. This clinical syndrome of pain is known as meralgia paresthetica, which describes the pain and/or dysesthesia in the anterolateral thigh associated with compression of the nerve. A myriad of factors have been identified as associated with the development of meralgia paresthetica, including but not limited to obesity, diabetes mellitus, and older age. Additional associations include large abdomens with overlying panniculus, tight belts or garments around the waist, scar tissue near the lateral aspect of the inguinal ligament, surgical position (eg, prolonged lithotomy position > 2 hours), and pregnancy.

References:

1. Warner ME. Patient positioning and potential injuries. In: Barash PG, Cullen BF, Stoelting RK, et al, eds. *Clinical Anesthesia Fundamentals*. Philadelphia: Lippincott; 2015:413-426.
2. Parisi TJ, Mandrekar J, Dyck PJ, Klein CJ. Meralgia paresthetica: relation to obesity, advanced age, and diabetes mellitus. *Neurology*. 2011;77:1538.
3. Sax TW, Rosenbaum RB. Neuromuscular disorders in pregnancy. *Muscle Nerve*. 2006; 34:559.
4. Van Diver T, Camann W. Meralgia paresthetica in the parturient. *Int J Obstet Anesth*. 1995;4:109.

20. Correct answer: C

Greater overlap of the IJV and the common carotid artery during ultrasonography for IJV cannulation is generally a result of excessive rotation of the patient's head toward the contralateral side. When positioning a patient for IJV cannulation, greater overlap of the IJV and the common carotid artery can be minimized when the head is rotated less than 45° from the neutral position; conversely, greater overlap is exhibited with rotation greater than 45° from the neutral position. Mild neck flexion, over extension of the neck, placement of the patient in the Trendelenburg position and placement of the probe close to the clavicle all serve to increase the IJV diameter. None of these maneuvers however affect the degree of IJV and carotid artery overlap.

Reference:

1. Troianos CA, Hartman GS, Glas KE, et al. Guidelines for performing ultrasound guided vascular cannulation: Recommendations of the American Society of Echocardiography and the Society of Cardiovascular Anesthesiologists. *J Am Soc Echocardiogr*. 2011;24(12):1291-1318.

3

CENTRAL AND PERIPHERAL NERVOUS SYSTEMS

Lauren Smith

1. After performing an interscalene block, your patient complains of pain in his fourth and fifth digits. Which dermatomes are not adequately covered with an interscalene block?

   A. C5-C6
   B. C6-C7
   C. C7-C8
   D. C8-T1

2. During neuraxial blockade, the level of sympathetic blockade is generally how far away from the sensory level?

   A. 1-2 dermatomes above
   B. 4-6 dermatomes above
   C. 1-2 dermatomes below
   D. 4-6 dermatomes below
   E. 0 dermatome change

3. During neuraxial blockade, the level of sensory blockade, in general, is how many dermatomes away from the level of motor blockade?

   A. 0
   B. 2
   C. 4
   D. 6
   E. 8

4. Cutaneous infiltration of a local anesthetic to block the intercostobrachial nerve provides anesthesia to which dermatome(s)?

   A. C7
   B. C8
   C. T1
   D. T2

5. **Each respiratory center is correctly paired with its function EXCEPT which one of the following?**

    A. Dorsal respiratory center: provides ventilatory rate
    B. Ventral respiratory center: coordinates exhalation
    C. Apneustic center: prolongs exhalation via signals to ventral respiratory center
    D. Pneumotaxic center: limits inspiration

6. **All of the following are examples of reflex or higher cortical structures that exert an influence on the respiratory centers/control of respiration EXCEPT which one?**

    A. Cough reflex
    B. Hering-Breuer reflex
    C. Reticular activating system
    D. Bezold-Jarisch reflex

7. **Carotid body chemoreceptors communicate with the respiratory centers via which nerve?**

    A. Trigeminal
    B. Glossopharyngeal
    C. Vagus
    D. Hypoglossal

8. **An infarct involving the hypothalamus would most likely result from occlusion of which artery?**

    A. Anterior spinal artery
    B. Vertebral artery
    C. Anterior cerebral artery
    D. Middle cerebral artery
    E. Posterior cerebral artery

9. **Regarding the gray matter in the spinal cord, all of the following are correct EXCEPT which one?**

    A. Consists of neurons, neuronal processes, and neuroglia
    B. Butterfly or H-shaped
    C. Categorized into columns and laminae
    D. Ratio of gray to white matter is least at the cervical and lumbar regions
    E. Each of the 10 Rexed laminae involved in sensory or motor pathways

10. **Which of the following pathways carries fibers that control fine touch, vibration, proprioception, and pressure?**

    A. Dorsal column
    B. Spinothalamic
    C. Corticospinal
    D. Reticulospinal

11. **All of the following are true regarding the descending motor tracts EXCEPT which one?**

    A. They originate in either the cerebral cortex or brainstem.
    B. The pathways are generally made of a two-neuron system.
    C. The upper motor neuron fibers target lower motor neurons of the spinal cord or cranial nerves.
    D. They are involved in assisting with voluntary movement.

12. **Which of the following pathways carries fibers that are involved in pain and temperature sensation?**

    A. Dorsal column
    B. Spinothalamic
    C. Corticospinal
    D. Reticulospinal

13. **The main functions of the meninges include all of the following EXCEPT which one?**

    A. Protecting the brain and spinal cord from mechanical injury
    B. Providing blood supply to the skull and to the hemispheres
    C. Providing a space for the flow of cerebrospinal fluid (CSF)
    D. Producing cerebral spinal fluid

14. **Which layer of the meninges is pain sensitive?**

    A. Dura
    B. Pia
    C. Arachnoid
    D. Subarachnoid

15. **What is the potential space between the arachnoid and pia mater?**

    A. Epidural
    B. Subarachnoid
    C. Subdural
    D. Arachnoid

16. **What is the potential space between the dura and arachnoid mater?**

    A. Epidural
    B. Subarachnoid
    C. Subdural
    D. Arachnoid

17. **Cerebral perfusion pressure (CPP), in the absence of intracranial pathology, is MOST closely correlated with which parameter?**

    A. Intracranial pressure (ICP)
    B. Central venous pressure (CVP)
    C. Cerebral blood volume (CBV)
    D. Mean arterial blood pressure (MAP)

18. **Which of the following situations has the *least* significant effect on cerebral blood flow (CBF)?**

    A. $Paco_2$ of 80
    B. Temperature of 34°C
    C. Increased blood viscosity
    D. Acute metabolic acidosis

19. **The diagram below shows the autoregulation curve for CBF. Which of the following changes occurs in patients with long-standing hypertension?**

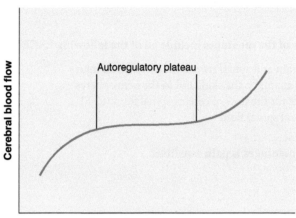

(From Dagal A, Lam AL. Anesthesia for neurosurgery. In: Barash PG, Cullen BF, Stoelting RK, et al. *Clinical Anesthesia*. Philadelphia: Lippincott Williams and Wilkins; 2013:999, with permission.)

    A. Leftward shift
    B. Rightward shift
    C. Downward shift
    D. No change

20. **In regard to cerebral blood flow (CBF), cerebral metabolic rate (CMR), and volatile anesthetics, which of the following is a potential detrimental adverse effect?**

    A. Increase in blood flow and a decrease in metabolic demand
    B. Increase in ICP
    C. Redistribution of blood flow away from ischemic areas of brain
    D. Decreased formation of cerebral spinal fluid

21. **All of the following medications can be used to decrease elevated ICP EXCEPT which one?**

    A. Hypertonic saline
    B. Furosemide
    C. Propofol
    D. Ketamine
    E. Acetazolamide

22. **Which of the following agents can cause an increase in CBF and $CMRo_2$?**

    A. Nitrous oxide
    B. Desflurane
    C. Halothane
    D. Sevoflurane

23. **Which of the following inhalational agents facilitates CSF absorption?**

    A. Halothane
    B. Isoflurane
    C. Sevoflurane
    D. Desflurane

24. **Clinical goals for preventing or limiting neuronal tissue damage include all of the following EXCEPT which one?**

    A. Optimizing CPP
    B. Decreasing metabolic requirements (basal and electrical)
    C. Limiting effects of mediators of cellular injury
    D. Tight glucose control

25. **What is the approximate total CSF volume?**

    A. 350-500 mL
    B. 100-150 mL
    C. 200-250 mL
    D. 50-100 mL

26. **Which of the following pairings is correct with respect to the production or absorption of CSF?**

    A. Choroid plexus; cerebral venous sinuses
    B. Arachnoid villi; third ventricle
    C. Choroid plexus; subarachnoid space
    D. Choroid plexus; lateral ventricles
    E. Arachnoid villi; lateral ventricles

27. **All of these medications decrease CSF production EXCEPT which one?**

    A. Acetazolamide
    B. Furosemide
    C. Thiopental
    D. Ketamine

28. **Which of the following inhalational agents impedes CSF absorption?**

    A. Halothane
    B. Isoflurane
    C. Sevoflurane
    D. Desflurane

29. **Which intravenous (IV) anesthetic has been shown to provide some protection against focal ischemia?**

    A. Phenobarbital
    B. Propofol
    C. Etomidate
    D. Fentanyl
    E. Midazolam

30. **In patients undergoing neurosurgery, all of the following are acceptable ventilator strategies EXCEPT which one?**

    A. Tidal volumes 6-8 cc/kg
    B. Peak pressure <30 cm H_2O
    C. High positive end expiratory pressure
    D. Avoidance of hypoventilation

31. **All of the following are acceptable ways to decrease elevated ICP EXCEPT which one?**

    A. Total IV anesthesia
    B. Mannitol administration
    C. Opioid administration
    D. Elevation of the head of the bed

32. **In regard to skeletal muscle contraction, all of the following are true EXCEPT which one?**

    A. Calcium triggers contraction by reaction with regulatory proteins that, in the absence of calcium, prevent interaction of actin and myosin.
    B. Calcium entry into nerve terminals triggers the release of acetylcholine into the synaptic cleft.
    C. The binding of calcium to actin controls the movement of tropomyosin.
    D. Myosin head releases ADP and Pi and triggers the power stroke of muscle contraction.

33. **All of the following are potential substrates for immediately replenishing ATP within the muscle fiber EXCEPT which one?**

    A. Creatine phosphate
    B. Glycogen
    C. Free fatty acids (FFA)
    D. Lactate

34. **Binding of which molecule(s) is required for the myosin head to release its binding to actin?**

    A. ATP
    B. GTP
    C. ADP
    D. cAMP

35. **Activation of which opioid receptor types can provide relief from opioid-induced itching?**

    A. Mu
    B. Delta
    C. Sigma
    D. Kappa

36. **Which of the following drugs does not exhibit *N*-methyl-D-aspartate (NMDA) receptor antagonism?**

    A. Methadone
    B. Meperidine
    C. Ketamine
    D. Memantine

37. **Which of the following conditions describes the process of activation of Aβ fibers via tactile, nonnoxious stimuli causing inhibition of interneurons in the dorsal horn of the spinal cord, leading to inhibition of pain signals transmitted via C fibers?**

    A. Stimulation produces analgesia
    B. Stress-induced analgesia
    C. Gate control theory
    D. Hyperanalgesia

38. **Which of the following statements is false with regard to the pain experience of elderly patients as compared with younger patients?**

    A. Elderly patients may be undertreated because of stoicism or perceived different pain threshold.
    B. Elderly patients may be more likely to experience confusion and delirium from treatment with opioids.
    C. Elderly patients metabolize drugs more effectively than younger patients.
    D. Neuraxial techniques can help circumvent the use of systemic opioids.

39. **Which of the following statements most accurately describes the Monro-Kellie doctrine?**

    A. Given the nondistensible cranial vault, the volume of blood, CSF, and brain tissue must be in equilibrium to maintain ICP and CPP.
    B. The cranial vault is distensible; therefore, there is adequate room for a space-occupying lesion without altering ICP.
    C. Given the nondistensible cranial vault, brain tissue and CSF must remain in equilibrium to maintain ICP. CSF volume has no impact.
    D. There is no relationship between brain tissue, CSF, and CBV and ICP.

40. **Which of the following is the most ubiquitous material in the epidural space?**

    A. Veins
    B. Arteries
    C. Fat
    D. Lymphatics

Chapter 3 ▪ Answers

1. Correct answer: D

An interscalene block targets the roots of the brachial plexus and is an ideal technique for surgery of the shoulder and the proximal arm. Roots C5-C7 are most densely blocked with this approach. The ulnar nerve originates from C8 and T1 roots and may be spared; thus, this block is not ideal for hand surgery and can spare the caudad border of the forearm.

It is common for the local anesthetic to spread to contiguous nerves during interscalene nerve block. Spread to the sympathetic chain on the anterior vertebral body often leads to Horner syndrome. Spread to the cervical plexus often leads to blockade of the motor fibers to the diaphragm. This should be taken into account when considering the upper extremity block in patients with significant underlying pulmonary disease.

References:
1. DeLeon AM, Asher YG. Regional anesthesia. In: Barash PG, Cullen BF, Stoelting RK, et al, eds. *Clinical Anesthesia Fundamentals*. Philadelphia: Lippincott; 2015:395-412.
2. Madison SJ, Ilfeld BM. Peripheral nerve blocks. In: Butterworth J, Mackey DC, Wasnick JD. *Morgan and Mikhail's Clinical Anesthesiology*. 5th ed. New York: McGraw-Hill; 2013:975-1022.

2. Correct answer: A

The sympathetic level is generally 1-2 dermatome levels higher than the sensory level. This phenomenon is referred to as differential blockade and is seen in both neuraxial and peripheral nerve blocks. In general, sympathetic nerve fibers are blocked by the lowest concentration of the local anesthetic, followed by sensory fibers, and then by motor fibers. It is thought that this observation is due in part to nerve fiber diameter and degree of myelination, with smaller diameter and unmyelinated fibers being more sensitive to the effects of the local anesthetic. However, this is unlikely to be the sole explanation for the observation of differential blockade, which is likely a multifactorial phenomenon. Sympathetic blockade is usually 1-2 dermatomes above the sensory blockade, which is generally 1-3 levels beyond the motor blockade.

Reference:
1. Butterworth J, Mackey DC, Wasnick JD. Spinal, epidural and caudal blocks. In: *Morgan and Mikhail's Clinical Anesthesiology*. 5th ed. New York: McGraw-Hill; 2013:937-974.

3. Correct answer: B

The sensory level is generally between 1 and 3 dermatome levels higher than the motor level.
See full explanation in the previous question.

Reference:
1. Butterworth J, Mackey DC, Wasnick JD. Spinal, epidural and caudal blocks. In: *Morgan and Mikhail's Clinical Anesthesiology*. 5th ed. New York: McGraw-Hill; 2013:937-974.

4. Correct answer: D

The intercostobrachial nerve is a lateral cutaneous branch of the second intercostal nerve that supplies sensation to the skin of the proximal arm, T2 dermatome. It is unreliably blocked (often spared) during an axillary brachial plexus approach; to ensure complete blockade, additional infiltration of local anesthesia can be added superficially. This superficial block is often performed when tourniquet use is planned.

Reference:
1. Madison SJ, Ilfeld BM. Butterworth J, Mackey DC, Wasnick JD. *Morgan and Mikhail's Clinical Anesthesiology*. 5th ed. New York: McGraw-Hill; 2013:975-1022.

5. Correct answer: C

Ventilation is primarily controlled by respiratory centers in the brainstem, specifically the medulla and pons, which process information and set a respiratory rate. The medulla contains basic respiratory centers: the dorsal and ventral respiratory centers. The dorsal respiratory center provides the ventilator rate by stimulating inspiration. Conversely, the ventral respiratory center terminates the dorsal respiratory center stimulus and ends inspiration, allowing for passive exhalation. The pontine respiratory centers are the apneustic and pneumotaxic centers, which communicate with the medulla centers and alter ventilatory patterns and rate. The apneustic center sends signals to the dorsal respiratory group to sustain inspiration. The pneumotaxic center functions to limit the depth of inspiration.

Reference:

1. DeLeon AM, Asher YG. Regional anesthesia. In: Barash PG, Cullen BF, Stoelting RK, et al, eds. *Clinical Anesthesia Fundamentals*. Philadelphia: Lippincott; 2015:395-412.

6. Correct answer: D

The midbrain and cerebral cortex are secondary centers of respiratory control and also affect ventilatory patterns. The reticular activating center in the midbrain increases the ventilatory rate and volume of inspiration. Additionally, various reflexes exert influence on respiration. For example, cough reflex stimulates both a deep inspiration and forceful exhalation. The Hering-Breuer reflex is an inhibition of inspiration with lung stretch (though thought to be weak in humans). Vomiting and swallowing reflexes also alter ventilator patterns.

Take-home point: Although the medulla and pons are the primary sites that control respiration, there are reflexes and higher cortical structures that exert an influence on the control of ventilation through a myriad of mechanisms. The Bezold-Jarisch reflex is an inhibitory parasympathetic characterized by bradycardia, vasodilation, and hypotension triggered by intense stimulation of cardiac myocytes.

Reference:

1. Al-Qamari A, Nava RD. The respiratory system. In: Barash PG, Cullen BF, Stoelting RK, et al, eds. *Clinical Anesthesia Fundamentals*. Philadelphia: Lippincott; 2015:15-40.

7. Correct answer: B

Carotid body chemoreceptors communicate with the respiratory centers via the glossopharyngeal nerve. Carotid body chemoreceptors signal to the respiratory centers in response to oxygen, carbon dioxide, and acidosis. Aortic arch chemoreceptors deliver signals to the respiratory centers via the vagus nerve.

Reference:

1. Al-Qamari A, Nava RD. The respiratory system. In: Barash PG, Cullen BF, Stoelting RK, et al, eds. *Clinical Anesthesia Fundamentals*. Philadelphia: Lippincott; 2015:15-40.

8. Correct answer: C

The anterior portion of the hypothalamus, which consists largely of the preoptic region, obtains its blood supply from branches of the anterior cerebral arteries, where they lie above the optic nerves. There may be an element of blood supply from the anterior communicating artery as well.

The anterior cerebral artery supplies a part of the frontal lobe, specifically its medial surface and the upper border. It also supplies the front four-fifths of the corpus callosum and provides blood to deep structures such as the anterior limb of the internal capsule, part of the caudate nucleus, and the anterior part of the globus pallidus.

The middle cerebral artery supplies the bulk of the lateral surface of the hemisphere, except for the superior inch of the frontal and parietal lobes (anterior cerebral artery) and the inferior part of the temporal lobe. The superior division supplies the lateroinferior frontal lobe (location of Broca area, ie, language expression). The inferior division supplies the lateral temporal lobe (location of Wernicke area, ie, language comprehension). Deep branches supply the basal ganglia as well as the internal capsule. The posterior cerebral artery supplies the occipital lobe and inferior temporal gyrus.

Reference:

1. Pare JR, Kahn JH. Basic neuroanatomy and stroke syndromes. *Emerg Med Clin North Am*. 2012;30(3):601-615.

9. **Correct answer: D**

The proportion of gray to white matter varies at different levels of the spinal cord. The ratio of gray to white matter is greatest at the cervical and lumbar regions.

Reference:
1. Uddeen S, Moy G. Spinal cord: organization and tracts. In: Freeman BS, Berger JS. *Anesthesiology Core Review: Part One, Basic Exam*. New York: McGraw-Hill; 2014:343-346.

10. **Correct answer: A**

The dorsal column tract represents an ascending spinal pathway that contains nerve bundles that communicate through a three-neuron system. First-order neurons have sensory receptor endings and cell bodies in the dorsal root ganglion of the spinal nerve. They synapse with second-order neurons in the dorsal horn, which cross the spinal cord to the opposite side as they ascend to higher levels. Third-order neurons are located in the thalamus, which then project to sensory areas in the sensory cortex. The dorsal column pathway carries fibers that control fine touch, vibration, proprioception, and pressure.

The spinothalamic tract, an anterolateral system, carries fibers involved in pain and temperature sensation. It is also an ascending spinal tract that contains nerve bundles that communicate through a three-neuron system. The corticospinal tract is a descending pathway that innervates skeletal muscles and muscle stretch receptors. The reticulospinal tract is a descending pathway that influences voluntary movement and reflexes and is involved in the hypothalamic control of autonomic activity.

Reference:
1. Uddeen S, Moy G. Spinal cord: organization and tracts. In: Freeman BS, Berger JS. *Anesthesiology Core Review: Part One, Basic Exam*. New York: McGraw-Hill; 2014:343-346.

11. **Correct answer: B**

Similar to the ascending pathways, the descending pathways are generally composed of a three-neuron system. For tracts originating in the cortex that travel to the spinal cord, the first-order neuron is in the cerebral cortex, which then synapses with a second-order neuron (usually an interneuron) located in the anterior gray column of the spinal cord. Finally, the third-order neuron, or the lower motor neuron, is the final destination.

Reference:
1. Uddeen S, Moy G. Spinal cord: organization and tracts. In: Freeman BS, Berger JS. *Anesthesiology Core Review: Part One, Basic Exam*. New York: McGraw-Hill; 2014:343-346.

12. **Correct answer: B**

The spinothalamic tract in an ascending spinal pathway carries fibers involved in pain and temperature sensation. Axons from the periphery travel to the spinal cord and ascend or descend one to two segments before synapsing at the dorsal root ganglion. Second-order fibers then cross over to the anterolateral portion of the contralateral spinal cord and travel to synapse with third-order neurons in the thalamus. From there, third-order neurons carry signals to the cortex.

The dorsal columnar tract represents an ascending spinal tract that carries fibers that control fine touch, vibration, proprioception, and pressure. The corticospinal tract is a descending pathway, which innervates skeletal muscles and muscle stretch receptors. The reticulospinal tract is a descending pathway that influences voluntary movement and reflexes and is involved in the hypothalamic control of autonomic activity.

Reference:
1. Uddeen S, Moy G. Spinal cord: organization and tracts. In: Freeman BS, Berger JS. *Anesthesiology Core Review: Part One, Basic Exam*. New York: McGraw-Hill; 2014:343-346.

13. **Correct answer: D**

The brain and spinal cord are surrounded by three layers of membranes called meninges: the outer dura mater, middle arachnoid mater, and inner pia matter. They serve to protect the brain and spinal cord from mechanical injury, provide blood supply to the skull and to the hemispheres, and provide a space for the flow of CSF. The production of CSF occurs in the lateral cerebral ventricles by the choroid plexus.

Reference:
1. Taheripour M. Anatomy of the meninges. In: Freeman BS, Berger JS. *Anesthesiology Core Review: Part One, Basic Exam*. New York: McGraw-Hill; 2014: 371-372.

14. Correct answer: A

The innervation of the dura mater is via small meningeal branches of all three divisions of the trigeminal nerve (V1, V2, and V3), the vagus nerve, and cranial nerves I-III. The pia and arachnoid matter are not innervated. The subarachnoid describes the space between the arachnoid and pia mater and contains the subarachnoid fluid.

Reference:
1. Taheripour M. Anatomy of the meninges. In: Freeman BS, Berger JS. *Anesthesiology Core Review: Part One, Basic Exam*. New York: McGraw-Hill; 2014: 371-372.

15. Correct answer: B

The subarachnoid cavity is the interval between the arachnoid and pia mater and contains the subarachnoid fluid. The arachnoid space refers to the middle meninges. The spinal dura mater is separated from the arachnoid by a potential cavity, the *subdural cavity*. The two membranes are, in fact, in contact with each other, except where they are separated by a minute quantity of fluid, which serves to moisten the surfaces. The epidural space describes the space between the wall of the vertebral canal and the dura and contains a venous plexus and loose areolar tissue.

Reference:
1. Taheripour M. Anatomy of the meninges. In: Freeman BS, Berger JS. *Anesthesiology Core Review: Part One, Basic Exam*. New York: McGraw-Hill; 2014: 371-372.

16. Correct answer: C

The spinal dura mater is separated from the arachnoid by a potential cavity, the *subdural cavity*. The two membranes are, in fact, in contact with each other, except where they are separated by a minute quantity of fluid, which serves to moisten the surfaces.

Reference:
1. Taheripour M. Anatomy of the meninges. In: Freeman BS, Berger JS. *Anesthesiology Core Review: Part One, Basic Exam*. New York: McGraw-Hill; 2014: 371-372.

17. Correct answer: D

CPP is MAP—ICP or CVP, whichever is greatest. Because the ICP (and CVP) is usually less than 10 mm Hg, CPP is primarily determined by MAP. Normal CPP is approximately 80-100 mm Hg. CPP progressively decreases as ICP or CVP increases. Likewise, CPP decreases as MAP decreases. CPP less than 50 mm Hg shows slowing on EEG, CPP of 25-40 mm Hg shows flat EEG, and CPP sustained at less than 25 mm Hg results in irreversible brain damage. CBV refers to cerebral blood volume.

References:
1. Butterworth J, Mackey DC, Wasnick JD. Neurophysiology and anesthesia. In: *Morgan and Mikhail's Clinical Anesthesiology*. 5th ed. New York: McGraw-Hill; 2013:575-592.
2. Lewis CRA. Cerebral blood flow determinants. In: Freeman BS, Berger JS. *Anesthesiology Core Review: Part One, Basic Exam*. New York: McGraw-Hill; 2014:333-334.

18. Correct answer: D

Acute metabolic acidosis has little effect on CBF because hydrogen ions cannot readily cross the blood-brain barrier. $Paco_2$ affects CBF. CBF increases approximately 1-2 mL/100 g/min per mm Hg increase in $Paco_2$. This effect is thought to be due to CO_2 diffusing across the blood-brain barrier and inducing changes in the pH of the CSF and the cerebral tissue. CBF changes 5%-7% per 1°C change in temperature. Hypothermia decreases both CMR and CBF, whereas hyperthermia has the reverse effect. The most important determinant of blood viscosity is hematocrit. A decrease in hematocrit decreases viscosity and can improve CBF though probably not to an appreciable extent. Conversely, elevated hematocrit increases blood viscosity and can reduce CBF to an appreciable extent.

References:
1. Butterworth J, Mackey DC, Wasnick JD. Neurophysiology and anesthesia. In: *Morgan and Mikhail's Clinical Anesthesiology.* 5th ed. New York: McGraw-Hill; 2013:575-592.
2. Lewis CRA. Cerebral blood flow determinants. In: Freeman BS, Berger JS. *Anesthesiology Core Review: Part One, Basic Exam.* New York: McGraw-Hill; 2014:333-334.

19. Correct answer: B

CPP equals MAP—ICP (or CVP), and in the absence of intracranial pathology, CPP is primarily determined by MAP. In patients with chronic systemic hypertension, both the upper and lower limits of the cerebral autoregulation curve are shifted to the right. The brain normally tolerates a wide range of blood pressures, with little change in blood flow. In normal individuals, CBF remains nearly constant between MAPs of about 60 and 160 mm Hg. Beyond these limits, blood flow becomes pressure dependent.

References:
1. Butterworth J, Mackey DC, Wasnick JD. Neurophysiology and anesthesia. In: *Morgan and Mikhail's Clinical Anesthesiology.* 5th ed. New York: McGraw-Hill; 2013:575-592.
2. Lewis CRA. Cerebral blood flow determinants. In: Freeman BS, Berger JS. *Anesthesiology Core Review: Part One, Basic Exam.* New York: McGraw-Hill; 2014:333-334.
3. Bebway JF, Koht A. Anesthesia in neurosurgery. In: Barash PG, Cullen BF, Stoelting RK, et al. *Clinical Anesthesia Fundamentals.* Philadelphia: Lippincott; 2015:557-576.

20. Correct answer: C

This is known as the circulatory steal phenomenon. As previously discussed, in the absence of pathologic conditions or anesthetics, CBF and metabolic rate are coupled. At normocarbia, volatile anesthetics alter, but do not uncouple, the normal relationship of CBF and CMR. They dilate cerebral vessels and impair autoregulation in a dose-dependent and time-dependent manner. While increasing CBF, volatile anesthetics also cause a decrease in the neuronal metabolic demand; the combination of decreased metabolic demand with an increased blood flow has been termed luxury perfusion. In contrast to luxury perfusion, the circulatory steal phenomenon leads to an increase in blood flow to normal areas of the brain rather than ischemic areas, where vessels are already maximally dilated, which results in the redistribution of blood flow away from ischemic areas of brain.

References:
1. Butterworth J, Mackey DC, Wasnick JD. Neurophysiology and anesthesia. In: *Morgan and Mikhail's Clinical Anesthesiology.* 5th ed. New York: McGraw-Hill; 2013:575-592.
2. Lewis CRA. Cerebral blood flow determinants. In: Freeman BS, Berger JS. *Anesthesiology Core Review: Part One, Basic Exam.* New York: McGraw-Hill; 2014:333-334.

21. Correct answer: D

In general,
1. IV agents—IV induction agents generally decrease CBF. Ketamine *is the only exception in that it increases CBF.*
2. Opioids generally either have no effect or decrease CBF. Remifentanil increases CBF at low sedative doses.
3. Benzodiazepines reduce CBF.
4. Volatile-inhaled anesthetics increase CBF at greater than or equal to 1 minimum alveolar concentration (MAC) (halothane > enflurane > desflurane = isoflurane > sevoflurane).
5. Nitrous oxide increases CBF. The effect is exaggerated when used in conjunction with volatile agents and less when used with IV induction agents other than ketamine.

References:
1. Butterworth J, Mackey DC, Wasnick JD. Neurophysiology and anesthesia. In: *Morgan and Mikhail's Clinical Anesthesiology.* 5th ed. New York: McGraw-Hill; 2013:575-592.
2. Lewis CRA. Cerebral blood flow determinants. In: Freeman BS, Berger JS. *Anesthesiology Core Review: Part One, Basic Exam.* New York: McGraw-Hill; 2014:333-334.

22. Correct answer: A

In the absence of pathologic conditions or anesthetics, CBF and metabolic rate are coupled. At normocarbia, volatile anesthetics alter, but do not uncouple, the normal relationship of CBF and CMR. They dilate cerebral vessels and impair autoregulation in a dose-dependent and time-dependent manner. With continued administration over 2-5 h, effects may normalize. Volatile anesthetics increase CBF at greater than or equal to 1 MAC. Halothane produces the greatest increase in blood flow, whereas sevoflurane produces the least (halothane > desflurane > isoflurane > sevoflurane). While increasing CBF, volatile anesthetics also cause a decrease in the $CMRo_2$. Nitrous oxide, however, is an exception. When combined with IV agents, nitrous oxide has minimal effects on CBF, CMR, and ICP. Adding this agent to a volatile anesthetic, however, can further increase CBF. When given alone, nitrous oxide causes mild cerebral vasodilation and an increase in both CBF and $CMRo_2$.

References:
1. Butterworth J, Mackey DC, Wasnick JD. Neurophysiology and anesthesia. In: *Morgan and Mikhail's Clinical Anesthesiology.* 5th ed. New York: McGraw-Hill; 2013:575-592.
2. Lewis CRA. Cerebral blood flow determinants. In: Freeman BS, Berger JS. *Anesthesiology Core Review: Part One, Basic Exam.* New York: McGraw-Hill; 2014:333-334.

23. Correct answer: B

Volatile anesthetics affect both formation and absorption of CSF. Halothane impedes absorption of CSF but only causes a minimal decrease in CSF formation. Isoflurane facilitates CSF absorption.

Reference:
1. Butterworth J, Mackey DC, Wasnick JD. Neurophysiology and anesthesia. In: *Morgan and Mikhail's Clinical Anesthesiology.* 5th ed. New York: McGraw-Hill; 2013:575-592.

24. Correct answer: D

Cerebral protection limits brain tissue injury by attempting to maximize oxygen delivery and decrease cerebral metabolism. Strategies for cerebral protection aimed at preventing or limiting neuronal tissue damage are usually similar despite focal or global ischemia; they include both physiologic and medical interventions. Overall clinical goals are usually to optimize CPP, decrease metabolic requirements (basal and electrical), and possibly block mediators of cellular injury.

Elevated blood glucose concentrations have been linked to increased mortality and worse neurologic outcomes: however, clinical studies of tight glucose control revealed that it is associated with an increased risk of hypoglycemic episodes and cellular injury when compared with conventional glucose control protocols. Increased rates of hypoglycemic episodes have also been associated with detrimental effects on the injured brain. At this current point, there is little conclusive evidence to support the use of tight glucose control.

References:
1. Butterworth J, Mackey DC, Wasnick JD. Neurophysiology and anesthesia. In: *Morgan and Mikhail's Clinical Anesthesiology.* 5th ed. New York: McGraw-Hill; 2013:575-592.
2. Alshaeri T, David MD. Cerebral protection. In: Freeman BS, Berger JS. *Anesthesiology Core Review: Part One, Basic Exam.* New York: McGraw-Hill; 2014:341-342.
3. Bebway JF, Koht A. Anesthesia in neurosurgery. In: Barash PG, Cullen BF, Stoelting RK, et al, eds. *Clinical Anesthesia Fundamentals.* Philadelphia: Lippincott; 2015:557-576.
4. Fukuda S, Warner DS. Cerebral protection. *Br J Anaesth.* 2007;99:10-17.
5. Marion DW. Optimum serum glucose levels for patients with severe traumatic brain injury. *F1000 Med Rep.* 2009;1:42.
6. Jauch-Chara K, et al. Glycemic control after brain injury: boon and bane for the brain. *Neuroscience.* 2014;283:202-209.

25. Correct answer: B

Production of CSF occurs in the lateral cerebral ventricles by the choroid plexus. About 20 mL/h (500 mL/d) is produced, but absorption at arachnoid villi in cerebral venous sinuses maintains total CSF volume at 100-150 mL.

References:
1. Butterworth J, Mackey DC, Wasnick JD. Neurophysiology and anesthesia. In: *Morgan and Mikhail's Clinical Anesthesiology.* 5th ed. New York: McGraw-Hill; 2013:575-592.
2. Alshaeri T, David MD. Cerebrospinal fluid. In: Freeman BS, Berger JS. *Anesthesiology Core Review: Part One, Basic Exam.* New York: McGraw-Hill; 2014:339-340.

26. **Correct answer: A**

See answer explanation given for question 25.

Production of CSF occurs in the lateral cerebral ventricles by the choroid plexus. About 20 mL/h (500 mL/d) is produced, but absorption at arachnoid villi in cerebral venous sinuses maintains total CSF volume at 100-150 mL.

References:

1. Butterworth J, Mackey DC, Wasnick JD. Neurophysiology and anesthesia. In: *Morgan and Mikhail's Clinical Anesthesiology.* 5th ed. New York: McGraw-Hill; 2013:575-592.
2. Freeman BS, Berger JS. Cerebrospinal fluid. In: *Anesthesiology Core Review: Part One, Basic Exam.* New York: McGraw-Hill; 2014:339-340.

27. **Correct answer: D**

Changes in CSF formation in response to medications largely depend on the net effect of factors that increase CSF production (such as increased CPP, dilation of choroidal blood vessels, and decreased sympathetic tone) versus factors that inhibit production (such as decreased CPP and increased sympathetic tone). Ketamine is thought to increase CSF production through increased systemic blood pressure and dilation of choroidal blood vessels. Ketamine has also been shown to increase CBV concomitant with increases in CSF pressure.

References:

1. Butterworth J, Mackey DC, Wasnick JD. Neurophysiology and anesthesia. In: *Morgan and Mikhail's Clinical Anesthesiology.* 5th ed. New York: McGraw-Hill; 2013:575-592.
2. Alshaeri T, David MD. Cerebrospinal fluid. In: Freeman BS, Berger JS. *Anesthesiology Core Review: Part One, Basic Exam.* New York: McGraw-Hill; 2014:339-340.

28. **Correct answer: A**

Volatile anesthetics affect both formation and absorption of CSF. Halothane impedes absorption of CSF but only causes a minimal decrease in CSF formation.

Reference:

1. Butterworth J, Mackey DC, Wasnick JD. Neurophysiology and anesthesia. In: *Morgan and Mikhail's Clinical Anesthesiology.* 5th ed. New York: McGraw-Hill; 2013:575-592.

29. **Correct answer: A**

Barbiturates have been shown to provide some protection against focal (NOT global) ischemia. With the exception of ketamine and etomidate, nearly all IV anesthetics can lower $CMRo_2$ and protect the brain; however, none have been shown to provide protection against global ischemia.

Reference:

1. Bebway JF, Koht A. Anesthesia in neurosurgery. In: Barash PG, Cullen BF, Stoelting RK, et al, eds. *Clinical Anesthesia Fundamentals.* Philadelphia: Lippincott; 2015:557-576.

30. **Correct answer: C**

High positive end expiratory pressure should be avoided, if possible, because it increases intrathoracic pressure and may impede cerebral venous drainage, worsening ICP. Low tidal volume ventilation and peak pressures <30 cm H_2O are used to decrease the risk of acute respiratory distress syndrome. Avoidance of hypoventilation is aimed at preventing cerebral vasodilation and increase in ICP.

Reference:

1. Bebway JF, Koht A. Anesthesia in neurosurgery. In: Barash PG, Cullen BF, Stoelting RK, et al, eds. *Clinical Anesthesia Fundamentals.* Philadelphia: Lippincott; 2015:557-576.

31. **Correct answer: C**

The administration of opioids in a ventilated patient will have minimal effect on CBF and ICP. All other techniques listed are acceptable. In general, IV induction agents generally decrease CBF. Ketamine is an exception in that it increases CBF. Benzodiazepines reduce CBF. Volatile-inhaled anesthetics are generally protective; however, they increase CBF at greater than or equal to 1 MAC (halothane > enflurane > desflurane = isoflurane > sevoflurane). Nitrous oxide increases CBF. The effect is exaggerated when used in conjunction with volatile agents and less when used with IV induction agents other than ketamine.

Mannitol decreases ICP by decreasing cerebral parenchymal cell water via osmotic diuresis.

Elevation of the head of the bed can decrease ICP by promoting venous drainage and decreasing CBV.

References:

1. Butterworth J, Mackey DC, Wasnick JD. Neurophysiology and anesthesia. In: *Morgan and Mikhail's Clinical Anesthesiology*. 5th ed. New York: McGraw-Hill; 2013:575-592.
2. Lewis CRA. Cerebral blood flow determinants. In: Freeman BS, Berger JS. *Anesthesiology Core Review: Part One, Basic Exam*. New York: McGraw-Hill; 2014:333-334.
3. Bebway JF, Koht A. Anesthesia in neurosurgery. In: Barash PG, Cullen BF, Stoelting RK, et al, eds. *Clinical Anesthesia Fundamentals*. Philadelphia: Lippincott; 2015:557-576.

32. Correct answer: C

In actin-linked regulation, troponin and tropomyosin regulate actin by blocking sites on actin required for complex formation with myosin. Depolarization in muscle cell plasma membrane spreads to T tubules and opens voltage-gated calcium channels (dihydropyridine receptors). Dihydropyridine receptor in T tubule membrane is coupled to the ryanodine receptor in sarcoplasmic reticulum membrane. Opening of dihydropyridine receptors causes a conformational change that transiently opens ryanodine receptors and releases sarcoplasmic reticulum calcium stores into the cytosol. Cytosolic Ca^{2+} binds troponin C and displaces tropomyosin, exposing myosin-binding sites on actin filaments. Myosin head releases ADP and inorganic phosphate and triggers a power stroke of muscle contraction.

References:

1. de Jesus M. Skeletal muscle contraction. In: Freeman BS, Berger JS. *Anesthesiology Core Review: Part One, Basic Exam*. New York: McGraw-Hill; 2014:353-354.
2. Clark M. Milestone 3 (1954): sliding filament model for muscle contraction. Muscle sliding filaments. *Nat Rev Mol Cell Biol*. 2008;9:s6-s7.
3. Goody RS. The missing link in the muscle cross-bridge cycle. *Nat Struct Mol Biol*. 2003;10:773-775.
4. Hoyle G. Comparative aspects of muscle. *Annu Rev Physiol*. 1969;31:43-82.

33. Correct answer: D

Lactic acid must be reconverted to pyruvic acid and metabolized aerobically, either in the muscle cell itself or in the liver. Muscle cells, like all others, use ATP as their energy; however, muscle cells can only store a very limited amount of ATP. Additionally, some muscle activity limits or exhausts the cell's ability to generate ATP as fast as consumed; hence, muscle cells have developed several mechanisms to provide for their energy requirements. In resting muscle fibers, the demand for ATP is relatively low. Resting muscle fibers absorb glucose and fatty acids from the bloodstream. These fatty acids are broken down in the mitochondria, and ATPs are generated; these ATPs are used to convert glucose to glycogen and creatine to creatine phosphate. Creatine phosphate can be stored and is broken down quickly during periods of high activity, and its energy is converted to ATP. During strenuous activity, skeletal muscles generate ATP through glycolysis under anaerobic conditions. Glycolysis slows down as its product, pyruvic acid, builds up. To extend glycolysis, lactate dehydrogenase converts pyruvic acid to lactic acid. Lactic acid eventually builds up, slowing metabolism and contributing to muscle fatigue. During recovery from strenuous activity, when oxygen is plentiful, lactic acid is converted back to pyruvic acid. Some of the pyruvic acid is broken down aerobically, by the tricarboxylic acid cycle to produce ATP. The rest is converted back to glucose. Lactic acid recycling is divided between the liver and the muscles in the Cori cycle. The liver absorbs the circulating lactic acid and produces glucose for discharge into the bloodstream. Muscle fibers then use the glucose to rebuild their glycogen reserves.

References:

1. de Jesus M. Skeletal muscle contraction. In: Freeman BS, Berger JS. *Anesthesiology Core Review: Part One, Basic Exam*. New York: McGraw-Hill; 2014:353-354.
2. Clark M. Milestone 3 (1954): sliding filament model for muscle contraction. Muscle sliding filaments. *Nat Rev Mol Cell Biol*. 2008; 9:s6-s7.

3. Goody RS. The missing link in the muscle cross-bridge cycle. *Nat Struct Mol Biol*. 2003;10:773-775.
4. Hoyle G. Comparative aspects of muscle. *Annu Rev Physiol*. 1969;31:43-82.

34. Correct answer: A

Binding of ATP to contracted myosin head allows for detachment to occur, whereas hydrolysis of ATP cocks the myosin head for another contraction.

References:

1. de Jesus M. Skeletal muscle contraction. In: Freeman BS, Berger JS. *Anesthesiology Core Review: Part One, Basic Exam*. New York: McGraw-Hill; 2014:353-354.
2. Clark M. Milestone 3 (1954): sliding filament model for muscle contraction. Muscle sliding filaments. *Nat Rev Mol Cell Biol*. 2008;9:s6-s7.

35. Correct answer: D

Four major opioid receptor types have been identified: mu (μ), kappa (κ), delta (δ), and sigma (σ). All opioid receptors couple to G proteins; binding of an agonist to an opioid receptor causes primarily inhibitory effects that decrease neuronal excitability. In the spinal cord, opioids inhibit the release of nociceptive and inflammatory mediators P from dorsal horn sensory neurons attenuating transmission of painful stimuli (periphery to cortex). In the brainstem, opioids act on descending inhibitory pathways to attenuate the transmission of painful stimuli. Activation of opioid receptor types has various effects. Activation of spinal kappa receptors is responsible for the antipruritic effect.

References:

1. Butterworth J, Mackey DC, Wasnick JD. Analgesic agents. In: *Morgan and Mikhail's Clinical Anesthesiology*. 5th ed. New York: McGraw-Hill; 2013:189-198.
2. Badri S, Desai M. Opioids. In: Freeman BS, Berger JS. *Anesthesiology Core Review: Part One, Basic Exam*. New York: McGraw-Hill; 2014:145-148.
3. Thackeray EM, Egan TD. Analgesics. In: Barash PG, Cullen BF, Stoelting RK, et al, eds. *Clinical Anesthesia Fundamentals*. Philadelphia: Lippincott; 2015:165-184.

36. Correct answer: B

Cells in the dorsal horn possess specific receptors for a plethora of neuromediators. NMDA is a receptor for the excitatory neurotransmitter glutamate that is widely distributed in the dorsal horn. The activation of NMDA receptors has been associated with hyperalgesia, neuropathic pain, and reduced functionality of opioid receptors. The NMDA receptor antagonists reduce central sensitization, hyperalgesia, and opioid tolerance. Common NMDA receptor antagonists include ketamine, methadone, memantine, amantadine, and dextromethorphan. The use of NMDA receptor antagonists to treat acute pain can theoretically reduce the postoperative and postsurgical chronic pain by reducing central sensitization. Meperidine does not act on the NMDA receptor.

Reference:

1. Ballantyne J, Ryder E. Postoperative pain in adults. In: Ballantye J. *The Massachusetts General Hospital handbook of Pain Management*. 3rd ed. Philadelphia: Lippincott; 2005:279-301.

37. Correct answer: C

The gate control theory describes how nonpainful input closes the gates to painful input, which results in attenuation of the pain sensation from traveling to the CNS (ie, nonnoxious input [stimulation] suppresses pain). The theory suggests that collaterals of the large sensory fibers carrying cutaneous sensory input activate inhibitory interneurons, which modulate pain transmission information carried by the pain fibers. Nonnoxious input suppresses pain, or sensory input "closes the gate" to noxious input. The gate theory predicts that, at the spinal cord level, nonnoxious stimulation will produce presynaptic inhibition on dorsal root nociceptor fibers that synapse on nociceptor spinal neurons and that this presynaptic inhibition will block incoming noxious information from reaching the CNS. Other possible mechanisms may be in play in the neuromodulation of pain, eg, increased dorsal horn inhibitory action via GABA, or activation of descending analgesia pathways via serotonin or norepinephrine.

Reference:

1. Stojanovic MP. Neuromodulation techniques for the treatment of pain. In: Ballantyne J. *The Massachusetts General Hospital Handbook of Pain Management*. 3rd ed. Philadelphia: Lippincott; 2005:193-203.

38. **Correct answer: C**

Elderly patients are more likely to have decreased liver and kidney function, as well as disease. Given this knowledge, elderly patients are perceived to metabolize drugs less effectively than younger patients and may be more susceptible to systemic adverse effects from parent compounds and their metabolites.

Reference:
1. Stojanovic MP. Neuromodulation techniques for the treatment of pain. In: Ballantyne J. *The Massachusetts General Hospital Handbook of Pain Management*. 3rd ed. Philadelphia: Lippincott; 2005:193-203.

39. **Correct Answer: A**

The Monro-Kellie doctrine refers to the fact that the cranial vault is nondistensible; thus, CBV, CSF, and brain tissue must be in equilibrium to maintain ICP and CPP. Efforts to decrease ICP can focus on decreasing CBV (elevating the head of the bed to allow drainage), decreasing brain tissue (through diuresis), and decreasing CSF volume (through drainage).

Reference:
1. Bebway JF, Koht A. Anesthesia in neurosurgery. In: Barash PG, Cullen BF, Stoelting RK, et al, eds. *Clinical Anesthesia Fundamentals*. Philadelphia: Lippincott; 2015:557-576.

40. **Correct answer: C**

The most ubiquitous material in the epidural space is fat. This has clinically important effects on the pharmacology of epidurally and intrathecally administered drugs. A rich network of veins course through the epidural space along with lymphatics and segmental arteries running between the aorta and the spinal cord.

Reference:
1. Bernards CM, Hostetter LS. Spinal and Epidural Anesthesia. In: Barash PG, Cullen BF, Stoelting RK, et al, eds. *Clinical Anesthesia*. Philadelphia: Lippincott; 2013:905-936.

4

THE RESPIRATORY SYSTEM

Amanda Xi

1. **Which of the following is a typical tidal volume (TV) range during quiet breathing?**

   A. 4-6 mL/kg
   B. 6-8 mL/kg
   C. 8-10 mL/kg
   D. 10-12 mL/kg

2. **Forced expiratory volume within the first second divided by forced vital capacity (FEV1/FVC) is typically greater than or equal to which one of the following?**

   A. 75%
   B. 65%
   C. 55%
   D. 45%

3. **FVC is normally equal to which one of the following?**

   A. Inspiratory capacity (IC)
   B. Vital capacity (VC)
   C. Functional residual capacity (FRC)
   D. Total lung capacity (TLC)

4. **Which lung volume is the primary determinant of oxygen reserve when apnea occurs?**

   A. Inspiratory capacity
   B. Vital capacity
   C. Functional residual capacity
   D. Total lung capacity

5. **What is the name of the lung volume at passive end expiration?**

   A. Residual volume (RV)
   B. Expiratory reserve volume (ERV)
   C. Vital capacity (VC)
   D. Functional residual capacity (FRC)

6. **What volumes comprise TLC?**

    A. Inspiratory reserve volume (IRV) + TV + ERV
    B. IRV + TV
    C. ERV + RV
    D. VC + RV

7. **What volumes comprise IC?**

    A. IRV + TV + ERV
    B. IRV + TV
    C. ERV + RV
    D. VC + RV

8. **What volumes comprise FRC?**

    A. IRV + TV + ERV
    B. IRV + TV
    C. ERV + RV
    D. VC + RV

9. **Which of the following statements is false regarding maximum voluntary ventilation (MVV)?**

    A. MVV is the largest volume that can be breathed in 1 minute voluntarily.
    B. MVV measures the endurance of ventilatory muscles.
    C. MVV is increased in patients with restrictive disease.
    D. MVV is decreased in patients with obstructive disease.

10. **Which of the following statements is false regarding FRC?**

    A. FRC increases 10% when a healthy subject lies down.
    B. When FRC decreases, increased venous admixture results in arterial hypoxemia.
    C. The midportion of the pulmonary volume-pressure curve at FRC defines lung compliance.
    D. FRC may be used to quantify the degree of pulmonary restriction.

11. **The amount of net pressure required for inflation of an alveolus is dependent on which of the following?**

    A. Surface tension
    B. Density of gas
    C. Radius of the alveolus
    D. A and C

12. **Which of the following "laws" describes the pressure required within the alveolus to remain inflated?**

    A. Laplace's law
    B. Boyle's law
    C. The ideal gas law
    D. Henry's law

13. **Which type of alveolar cells produces surfactant?**

    A. Type I
    B. Type II
    C. Type III
    D. Type IV

For questions 14-17, select the correct flow-volume loop.

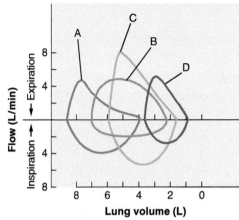

(From Eisenkraft JB, Cohen E, Neustein SM. Anesthesia for thoracic surgery. In: Barash PG, Cullen BF, Stoelting RK, et al, eds. *Clinical Anesthesia*. 7th ed. Philadelphia: Wolters Kluwer; 2013:1030-1075, with permission.)

14. **Chronic obstructive pulmonary disease**

15. **Tracheal stenosis**

16. **Normal lung**

17. **Pulmonary fibrosis**

18. **Type II alveolar cells:**

    A. Produce surfactant in the lungs
    B. Modulate local electrolyte balance
    C. Provide for immunologic lung defense
    D. A and B
    E. All of the above

19. **Which of the following is/are depicted in a flow-volume loop?**

    A. Total lung capacity
    B. Functional residual capacity
    C. Tidal volume
    D. All of the above

20. **Which of the following statements about flow-volume loops is false?**

    A. Shape and peak airflow rates during expiration at high lung volumes are effort dependent.
    B. Flow-volume loops provide more precise and useful information in the diagnosis of upper airway and extrathoracic obstruction compared with MRI.
    C. A flow-volume loop graphically demonstrates the flow generated during a forced expiratory maneuver followed by a forced inspiratory maneuver, plotted against the volume of gas expired.
    D. Flow-volume loops provide information about total lung volume, TV, FRC, and RV.

21. **Which of the following pulmonary structures participates in gas exchange?**

    A. Terminal bronchioles
    B. Alveoli
    C. Alveolar ducts
    D. A and B
    E. B and C

22. **Which of the following statements regarding the distribution of ventilation in the lung is true?**

    A. There is an alveolar pressure gradient in the lung.
    B. The negative intrapleural pressure results in more distended alveoli at the base of the lung.
    C. More ventilation is delivered to dependent pulmonary areas.
    D. The largest portion of TV reaches the apex of the lung.

23. **Which of the following statements regarding the distribution of blood flow in the lung is false?**

    A. Blood flow into the lung is mainly gravity dependent.
    B. West Zone 1 is the most gravity-dependent portion of the lung.
    C. Blood flow depends on the relationship between pulmonary artery pressure, alveolar pressure, and pulmonary venous pressure.
    D. West Zone 1 receives ventilation in the absence of perfusion.

24. **Select the correct relationship between the pulmonary artery pressure (Ppa), alveolar pressure (PA), and pulmonary venous pressure (Ppv) in West Zone 3:**

    A. Ppa > Ppv > PA
    B. Ppa = Ppv = PA
    C. Ppa > PA > Ppv
    D. PA > Ppa > Ppv

25. **The ideal V/Q ratio of 1 is believed to occur at approximately the level of which one of the following?**

    A. First rib
    B. Third rib
    C. Fifth rib
    D. Seventh rib

26. **A V/Q ratio of 1:0 is known as which one of the following?**

    A. Normal
    B. Dead space
    C. Shunt
    D. Silent unit

27. **A V/Q ratio of 0:0 is known as which one of the following?**

    A. Normal
    B. Dead space
    C. Shunt
    D. Silent unit

28. **A V/Q ratio of 0:1 is known as which one of the following?**

    A. Normal
    B. Dead space
    C. Shunt
    D. Silent unit

29. **Which of the following statements regarding hypoxic pulmonary vasoconstriction (HPV) is false?**

    A. HPV leads to bronchiolar constriction.
    B. HPV is stimulated by alveolar hypoxia.
    C. HPV decreases blood flow.
    D. HPV causes areas that were previously shunted to effectively become silent units.

30. **Which of the following is/are direct inhibitor(s) of HPV?**

    A. Infection
    B. Vasodilator drugs
    C. Hypocarbia
    D. A and C
    E. All of the above

31. **Which of the following medical conditions shift(s) the oxyhemoglobin dissociation curve to the right?**

    A. Hypocapnia
    B. Acidosis
    C. Hyperthermia
    D. B and C
    E. A and B

32. **In a normal patient, the Po_2 drops from 100 to 40 mm Hg. What do you expect the pulse oximeter to read?**

    A. 99%
    B. 95%
    C. 85%
    D. <75%

33. **Which of the following medical conditions cause(s) a leftward shift to the oxyhemoglobin dissociation curve?**

    A. Hypothermia
    B. Alkalosis
    C. Fetal hemoglobin
    D. All of the above

34. **Which of the following statements regarding respiratory acidosis is false?**

    A. It is improved with laparoscopic procedures.
    B. It is always characterized by hypercarbia ($Paco_2$ > 45 mm Hg).
    C. It occurs because of a decrease in minute alveolar ventilation.
    D. It is usually characterized by a low pH (<7.35).

35. **Which of the following statements is/are true regarding systemic effects of hypercapnia?**

    A. Arteriolar dilation
    B. Increased sympathetic output
    C. Pulmonary vasoconstriction
    D. All of the above

36. **Which of the following statements is false regarding hyperoxia?**

    A. It contributes to atelectasis.
    B. Prolonged exposure may increase the risk of secondary infections.
    C. It increases intracranial pressure.
    D. It increases systemic vascular resistance.

37. **Which of the following is/are the systemic effect(s) of hypoxia?**

    A. Peripheral vessels dilate
    B. Increased ventilation
    C. Increased cardiac output
    D. All of the above

38. **Interpret this arterial blood gas (ABG): pH = 7.27, CO_2 = 53, HCO_2 = 24.**

    A. Metabolic acidosis
    B. Metabolic alkalosis
    C. Respiratory acidosis
    D. Respiratory alkalosis

39. **Interpret this ABG: pH = 7.18, CO_2 = 38, HCO_3 = 16**

    A. Metabolic acidosis
    B. Metabolic alkalosis
    C. Respiratory acidosis
    D. Respiratory alkalosis

40. **Interpret this ABG: pH = 7.60, CO_2 = 37, HCO_3 = 35**

    A. Metabolic acidosis
    B. Metabolic alkalosis
    C. Respiratory acidosis
    D. Respiratory alkalosis

41. **The respiratory centers in the brain are located in which one of the following?**

    A. Cerebrum
    B. Cerebellum
    C. Brainstem
    D. Spinal cord

42. **Which of the following structures comprise(s) the peripheral chemoreceptors?**

    A. Carotid bodies
    B. Carotid sinus
    C. Aortic bodies
    D. A and C
    E. All of the above

43. **Central chemoreceptors are primarily sensitive to changes in which one of the following?**

    A. Carbon dioxide
    B. Hydrogen ion concentration
    C. Oxygen
    D. Bicarbonate

44. **The sources of ventilatory rhythmicity are located in which one of the following?**

    A. Dorsal respiratory group
    B. Ventral respiratory group
    C. Apneustic center
    D. Pneumotaxic respiratory center

45. **Which of the following is/are known as cause(s) of true hyperventilation?**

    A. Arterial hypoxemia
    B. Metabolic acidemia
    C. A and B
    D. None of the above
    E. All of the above

46. **According to the diagram of the carbon dioxide response curve, the slope of curve B represents which one of the following?**

    A. The apneic threshold
    B. The set point
    C. Carbon dioxide sensitivity
    D. None of the above

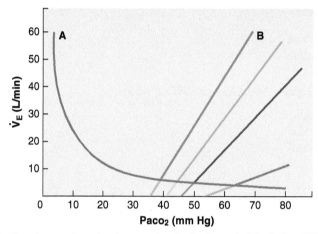

(From Tamul PC, Ault ML. Respiratory function in anesthesia. In: Barash PG, Cullen BF, Stoelting RK, et al, eds. *Clinical Anesthesia*. 7th ed. Philadelphia: Wolters Kluwer; 2013:263-286, with permission.)

47. **At what level does Pao_2 lack any influence on the carbon dioxide response curve?**

    A. <65 mm Hg
    B. 65 mm Hg
    C. 85 mm Hg
    D. 100 mm Hg

48. **Changes in physiology that can displace the carbon dioxide response curve to the right include which of the following?**

    A. Normal sleep
    B. Opioids
    C. Inhaled anesthetics
    D. All of the above

49. **Which of the following statements is true regarding the oxyhemoglobin dissociation curve?**

    A. Left shift leads to lower O_2 affinity.
    B. Left shift leads to higher O_2 affinity.
    C. Right shift leads to higher O_2 affinity.
    D. None of the above.

50. **How does fetal hemoglobin impact the hemoglobin dissociation curve?**

    A. Shifts it to the left.
    B. Shifts it to the right.
    C. Shifts it up.
    D. Shifts it down.

51. **With regards to smoking, which of the following statements is/are true?**

    A. Smoking leads to V/Q mismatch, bronchitis, and airway hyperreactivity.
    B. Smoking leads to increased carboxyhemoglobin concentration.
    C. Smoking is one of the main risk factors associated with postoperative morbidity.
    D. All of the above.

52. **Which of the following statements about smoking cessation is true?**

    A. Patients who quit smoking less than 8 weeks preoperatively have a significantly higher complication rate compared with those who quit more than 8 weeks preoperatively.
    B. Smokers who decrease cigarette consumption in an attempt to quit without nicotine replacement therapy decrease their nicotine intake.
    C. Smokers should be advised to stop smoking 3 months before elective operations to maximize the effect of smoking cessation.
    D. If smokers stop for at least 2 weeks preoperatively, they benefit from improved mucociliary function.

53. **Bronchodilators, such as albuterol, act on which type of receptor?**

    A. α1-Adrenergic
    B. α2-Adrenergic
    C. β1-Adrenergic
    D. β2-Adrenergic

54. **With regard to the action of anticholinergic bronchodilators, which of the following statements is/are true?**

    A. They act to block nicotinic receptors.
    B. They block the formation of cyclic guanosine monophosphate.
    C. They are muscarinic agonists.
    D. B and C.

55. **Which of the following statements describes the correct mechanism of action of β2-agonist bronchodilators?**

    A. Receptor activation leads to increased production of cyclic guanosine monophosphate.
    B. Receptor activation leads to decreased production of cyclic guanosine monophosphate.
    C. Receptor activation leads to increased production of cyclic adenosine monophosphate (cAMP).
    D. Receptor activation leads to decreased production of cAMP.

56. **Which of the following is the mechanism of action of leukotriene modifiers?**

    A. Decreasing the production of leukotrienes
    B. Increasing the production of leukotrienes
    C. Agonizing the leukotriene receptor agonist
    D. Antagonizing the leukotriene receptor antagonist

57. **Which of the following statements is/are true regarding immunoglobulin E (IgE) blockers?**

    A. They inhibit binding of IgE to the receptor on the surface of mast cells and basophils.
    B. One agent is a monoclonal antibody.
    C. They can be used for the treatment of asthma.
    D. All of the above.

58. **Which of the following is the mechanism of action of first-generation medications that target mast cells?**

    A. Enhancement of mast cell chemical mediator release
    B. Stabilization of mast cells to inhibit release of chemical mediators
    C. Antagonizing the H1 receptor
    D. Agonizing the H1 receptor

59. **Which of the following statements is/are true about the mechanism of action of exogenous glucocorticoids?**

    A. They directly bind to glucocorticoid receptors to exert their action.
    B. They inhibit molecules such as cytokines, chemokines, and arachidonic acid metabolites.
    C. They upregulate anti-inflammatory mediators.
    D. All of the above.

60. **Select the correct order of greatest to least anti-inflammatory properties of the following glucocorticoids:**

    A. Hydrocortisone > prednisone > methylprednisolone > dexamethasone
    B. Dexamethasone > methylprednisolone > prednisone > hydrocortisone
    C. Dexamethasone > hydrocortisone > methylprednisolone > prednisone
    D. Hydrocortisone > dexamethasone > prednisone > methylprednisolone

Chapter 4 ▪ Answers

1. **Correct answer: B**

TV is the volume of gas that moves in and out of the lungs during quiet breathing and typically is 6-8 mL/kg.

Reference:
1. Tamul PC, Ault ML. Respiratory function in anesthesia. In: Barash PG, Cullen BF, Stoelting RK, et al, eds. *Clinical Anesthesia.* 7th ed. Philadelphia: Wolters Kluwer; 2013:263-286.

2. **Correct answer: A**

Forced expiratory volume over a given time interval is a measurement of flow over a designated interval (typically 1 second). Measurement of expiratory flow over a given time interval can provide indication of degree of airway obstruction. Normal subjects can expire 75%-85% of FVC in 1 second.

Reference:
1. Tamul PC, Ault ML. Respiratory function in anesthesia. In: Barash PG, Cullen BF, Stoelting RK, et al, eds. *Clinical Anesthesia.* 7th ed. Philadelphia: Wolters Kluwer; 2013:263-286.

3. **Correct answer: B**

FVC is normally equal to VC. FVC is defined as the volume of gas expired forcefully and quickly after maximal inspiration. In chronic obstructive diseases, FVC may be decreased, whereas in restrictive diseases, FVC is nearly always decreased. Patient effort and cooperation are vital to obtaining an accurate FVC measurement.

Reference:
1. Tamul PC, Ault ML. Respiratory function in anesthesia. In: Barash PG, Cullen BF, Stoelting RK, et al, eds. *Clinical Anesthesia.* 7th ed. Philadelphia: Wolters Kluwer; 2013:263-286.

For answers to questions 4 through 8, refer to the following figure:

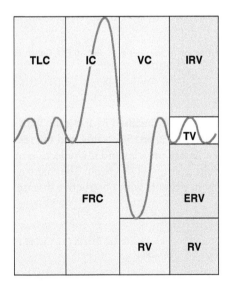

(From Tamul PC, Ault ML. Respiratory function in anesthesia. In: Barash PG, Cullen BF, Stoelting RK, et al, eds. *Clinical Anesthesia.* 7th ed. Philadelphia: Wolters Kluwer; 2013:263-286, with permission.)

4. **Correct answer: C**

FRC is the volume of gas remaining within the lungs at passive end expiration. It is the resting expiratory volume of the lung, and thus during apnea, it is the primary determinant of oxygen reserve in humans. FRC determines elastic pressure-volume relationships within the lung and greatly influences ventilation-perfusion relationships. Diseases that decrease FRC include acute lung injury, pulmonary edema, pulmonary fibrosis, and atelectasis. Pregnancy, obesity, pleural effusion, and posture are mechanical factors that also reduce FRC.

Reference:
1. Tamul PC, Ault ML. Respiratory function in anesthesia. In: Barash PG, Cullen BF, Stoelting RK, et al, eds. *Clinical Anesthesia.* 7th ed. Philadelphia: Wolters Kluwer; 2013:263-286.

5. Correct answer: D

FRC is defined as the volume of gas remaining in the lungs at the end of a quiet or TV breath. FRC is also the sum of ERV and RV. RV is the gas remaining within the lungs at the end of forced expiration. VC correlates with the capacity of deep breathing and is made up of IRV, TV, and ERV.

Reference:
1. Tamul PC, Ault ML. Respiratory function in anesthesia. In: Barash PG, Cullen BF, Stoelting RK, et al, eds. *Clinical Anesthesia.* 7th ed. Philadelphia: Wolters Kluwer; 2013:263-286.

6. Correct answer: D

TLC is the sum of VC and reserve volume. VC comprises IRV, TV, and ERV.

Reference:
1. Tamul PC, Ault ML. Respiratory function in anesthesia. In: Barash PG, Cullen BF, Stoelting RK, et al, eds. *Clinical Anesthesia.* 7th ed. Philadelphia: Wolters Kluwer; 2013:263-286.

7. Correct answer: B

IC is the sum of IRV and TV.

Reference:
1. Tamul PC, Ault ML. Respiratory function in anesthesia. In: Barash PG, Cullen BF, Stoelting RK, et al, eds. *Clinical Anesthesia.* 7th ed. Philadelphia: Wolters Kluwer; 2013:263-286.

8. Correct answer: C

FRC is the sum of ERV and TV.

Reference:
1. Tamul PC, Ault ML. Respiratory function in anesthesia. In: Barash PG, Cullen BF, Stoelting RK, et al, eds. *Clinical Anesthesia.* 7th ed. Philadelphia: Wolters Kluwer; 2013:263-286.

9. Correct answer: C

MVV is the largest volume that can be breathed in 1 minute with voluntary effort. Subjects breathe as deeply and rapidly as possible for 10, 12, or 15 seconds, and the result is extrapolated to 1 minute. MVV measures the endurance of ventilatory muscles and is a reflection of lung-thorax compliance and airway resistance. Healthy, young adults average ~170 L/min. The maneuver exaggerates air trapping, which is why MVV is decreased greatly in patients with obstructive disease. MVV is usually normal in patients with restrictive disease.

Reference:
1. Tamul PC, Ault ML. Respiratory function in anesthesia. In: Barash PG, Cullen BF, Stoelting RK, et al, eds. *Clinical Anesthesia.* 7th ed. Philadelphia: Wolters Kluwer; 2013:263-286.

10. Correct answer: A

FRC decreases 10% when a healthy subject lies down. When FRC is reduced, it leads to increased venous admixture (low V/Q), which results in arterial hypoxemia.

The zero line on the lung volume-pressure curve defines FRC. Severe restrictive lung disease (red curve) profoundly decreases FRC (and thus, the lungs are less compliant). FRC can thus be used to quantify lung restriction. Obstructive disease is depicted by the orange line and leads to an increase in FRC and compliance.

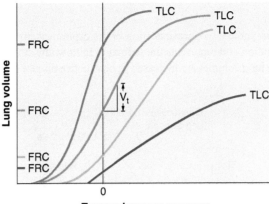

Transpulmonary pressure

(From Tamul PC, Ault ML. Respiratory function in anesthesia. In: Barash PG, Cullen BF, Stoelting RK, et al, eds. *Clinical Anesthesia*. 7th ed. Philadelphia: Wolters Kluwer; 2013:263-286, with permission.)

Reference:
1. Tamul PC, Ault ML. Respiratory function in anesthesia. In: Barash PG, Cullen BF, Stoelting RK, et al, eds. *Clinical Anesthesia*. 7th ed. Philadelphia: Wolters Kluwer; 2013:263-286.

11. Correct answer: D

The amount of net pressure required for inflation of an alveolus is dependent on the Laplace equation—$P = 2T/R$, where P = the pressure within the alveolus, T = the surface tension of the liquid, and R = the radius of the alveolus. Density of gas is not a variable in the Laplace equation.

Reference:
1. Tamul PC, Ault ML. Respiratory function in anesthesia. In: Barash PG, Cullen BF, Stoelting RK, et al, eds. *Clinical Anesthesia*. 7th ed. Philadelphia: Wolters Kluwer; 2013:263-286.

12. Correct answer: A

Laplace's law or equation describes the pressure the alveolus requires to remain inflated. It is $P = 2T/R$, where P = the pressure within the alveolus, T = the surface tension of the liquid, and R = the radius of the alveolus. Boyle's law states that for a fixed mass of gas at constant temperature, the product of pressure and volume is constant. The equation is $P_1V_1 = P_2V_2$, where P = pressure and V = volume. The ideal gas law is written as $PV = nRT$, where P = pressure, V = volume, n = amount of substance, R = constant, and T = temperature. Henry's law expresses the relationship of concentration of gas in solution to the partial pressure of gas. It is written as $C = kP$, where C = concentration of gas, k = solubility constant, and P = partial pressure of the gas.

References:
1. Tamul PC, Ault ML. Respiratory function in anesthesia. In: Barash PG, Cullen BF, Stoelting RK, et al, eds. *Clinical Anesthesia*. 7th ed. Philadelphia: Wolters Kluwer; 2013:263-286.
2. Riutort KT, Eisenkraft JB. The anesthesia workstation and delivery systems for inhaled anesthetics. In: Barash PG, Cullen BF, Stoelting RK, et al, eds. *Clinical Anesthesia*. 7th ed. Philadelphia: Wolters Kluwer; 2013:641-696.
3. Ebert TJ, Lindenbaum L. Inhaled anesthetics. In: Barash PG, Cullen BF, Stoelting RK, et al, eds. *Clinical Anesthesia*. 7th ed. Philadelphia: Wolters Kluwer; 2013:447-477.

13. Correct answer: B

Type I cells are flattened, squamous cells that cover ~80% of the alveolar surface. They contain flattened nuclei and are extremely thin to promote gas exchange. They are highly susceptible to injury, and when they are damaged, type II cells replicate and form new type I cells. Type II alveolar cells are polygonal cells that manufacture surfactant. Type III alveolar cells are macrophages and are an important part of immunologic lung defense. Type IV alveolar cells do not exist.

Reference:
1. Tamul PC, Ault ML. Respiratory function in anesthesia. In: Barash PG, Cullen BF, Stoelting RK, et al, eds. *Clinical Anesthesia*. 7th ed. Philadelphia: Wolters Kluwer; 2013:263-286.

14. **Correct answer: A**

In obstructive lung disease, note the concave portion of the expiratory curve. This illustrates the effort-independent portion of expiration and represents the reduction in flow rate at 25%-75% FVC seen in obstructive disease. Additionally, the lung volumes are increased in obstructive disease secondary to increases in RV.

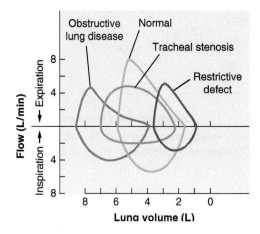

Reference:
1. Eisenkraft JB, Cohen E, Neustein SM. Anesthesia for thoracic surgery. In: Barash PG, Cullen BF, Stoelting RK, et al, eds. *Clinical Anesthesia*. 7th ed. Philadelphia: Wolters Kluwer; 2013:1030-1075.

15. **Correct answer: C**

In a fixed or static obstruction such as tracheal stenosis, both the inspiratory and expiratory curves are decreased compared with baseline.

Reference:
1. Eisenkraft JB, Cohen E, Neustein SM. Anesthesia for thoracic surgery. In: Barash PG, Cullen BF, Stoelting RK, et al, eds. *Clinical Anesthesia*. 7th ed. Philadelphia: Wolters Kluwer; 2013:1030-1075.

16. **Correct answer: B**

It is important to be able to recognize a normal flow-volume loop, as it can provide a significant amount of information such as the VC, RV, and TLC.

Reference:
1. Eisenkraft JB, Cohen E, Neustein SM. Anesthesia for thoracic surgery. In: Barash PG, Cullen BF, Stoelting RK, et al, eds. *Clinical Anesthesia*. 7th ed. Philadelphia: Wolters Kluwer; 2013:1030-1075.

17. **Correct answer: D**

In patients with restrictive lung disease such as pulmonary fibrosis and scoliosis, the flow-volume curves are normal in shape, but the lung volumes and peak flow rates are decreased.

Reference:
1. Eisenkraft JB, Cohen E, Neustein SM. Anesthesia for thoracic surgery. In: Barash PG, Cullen BF, Stoelting RK, et al, eds. *Clinical Anesthesia*. 7th ed. Philadelphia: Wolters Kluwer; 2013:1030-1075.

18. **Correct answer: D**

Type II alveolar cells are primarily located at alveolar-septal junctions and are polygonal in shape. They have metabolic and enzymatic activities that contribute to their role in producing surfactant as well as modulation of local electrolyte balance. They also contribute to endothelial and lymphatic cell functions.

Reference:
1. Tamul PC, Ault ML. Respiratory function in anesthesia. In: Barash PG, Cullen BF, Stoelting RK, et al, eds. *Clinical Anesthesia*. 7th ed. Philadelphia: Wolters Kluwer; 2013:263-286.

19. Correct answer: D

Flow-volume loops can provide an estimate of TLC, FRC, TV, and RV. These loops are effort dependent, but valuable information about pathologies such as a fixed obstruction or restrictive lung disease can be elucidated from them.

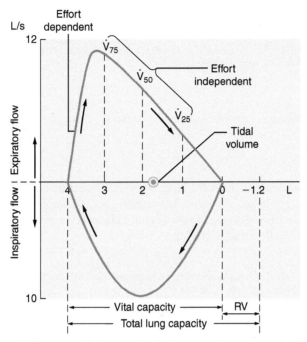

(From Eisenkraft JB, Cohen E, Neustein SM. Anesthesia for thoracic surgery. In: Barash PG, Cullen BF, Stoelting RK, et al, eds. *Clinical Anesthesia*. 7th ed. Philadelphia: Wolters Kluwer; 2013:1030-1075, with permission.)

Reference:
1. Eisenkraft JB, Cohen E, Neustein SM. Anesthesia for thoracic surgery. In: Barash PG, Cullen BF, Stoelting RK, et al, eds. *Clinical Anesthesia*. 7th ed. Philadelphia: Wolters Kluwer; 2013:1030-1075.

20. Correct answer: B

Flow-volume loops were formerly useful in the diagnosis of large airway and extrathoracic airway obstruction before the availability of precise imaging techniques such as MRI.

Reference:
1. Tamul PC, Ault ML. Respiratory function in anesthesia. In: Barash PG, Cullen BF, Stoelting RK, et al, eds. *Clinical Anesthesia*. 7th ed. Philadelphia: Wolters Kluwer; 2013:263-286.

21. Correct answer: E

The lung parenchyma can be subdivided into functional airway divisions. Only respiratory bronchioles, alveolar ducts, alveoli, and alveolar sacs participate in gas exchange. The trachea, mainstem bronchi, lobar bronchi, and terminal bronchioles are responsible for basic gas transport without exchange. Respiratory bronchioles and alveolar ducts participate in gas movement and exchange.

Functional Airway Divisions

TYPE	FUNCTION	STRUCTURE
Conductive	Bulk gas movement	Trachea to terminal bronchioles
Transitional	Bulk gas movement	Respiratory bronchioles
Respiratory	Limited gas exchange Gas exchange	Alveolar ducts Alveoli Alveolar sacs

From Tamul PC, Ault ML. Respiratory function in anesthesia. In: Barash PG, Cullen BF, Stoelting RK, et al, eds. Clinical Anesthesia. *7th ed. Philadelphia: Wolters Kluwer; 2013:263-286, with permission.*

Reference:
1. Tamul PC, Ault ML. Respiratory function in anesthesia. In: Barash PG, Cullen BF, Stoelting RK, et al, eds. *Clinical Anesthesia.* 7th ed. Philadelphia: Wolters Kluwer; 2013:263-286.

22. Correct answer: C

Alveolar pressure is same throughout the lung; however, there is more negative intrapleural pressure at the apex, which results in larger, more distended apical alveoli. Despite the smaller alveoli at the base of the lung, more ventilation is delivered to dependent pulmonary areas. Thus, the largest portion of TV reaches the gravity-dependent part of the lung.

Reference:
1. Tamul PC, Ault ML. Respiratory function in anesthesia. In: Barash PG, Cullen BF, Stoelting RK, et al, eds. *Clinical Anesthesia.* 7th ed. Philadelphia: Wolters Kluwer; 2013:263-286.

23. Correct answer: B

West Zone 1 conditions occur in the most gravity-independent part of the lung (the apex). In this portion of the lung, alveolar pressure exceeds pulmonary artery pressure, and no flow occurs because of vessel collapse.

Reference:
1. Tamul PC, Ault ML. Respiratory function in anesthesia. In: Barash PG, Cullen BF, Stoelting RK, et al, eds. *Clinical Anesthesia.* 7th ed. Philadelphia: Wolters Kluwer; 2013:263-286.

24. Correct answer: A

West Zone 3 occurs in the most gravity-dependent areas of the lung. Gravity increases both the arterial and venous pressures, therefore exceeding alveolar pressure (Ppa > Ppv > PA). There is no zone where all three pressures are equivalent. West Zone 2 is defined as the portion of the lung where the pressure difference between the pulmonary artery and alveolar pressure determines the amount of blood flow; pulmonary venous pressure has little influence here. In West Zone 1, the alveolar pressure is approximately equal to atmospheric pressure, and both the pulmonary artery pressure and pulmonary venous pressure are subatmospheric. Alveolar pressure transmitted to the pulmonary capillaries promotes collapse, theoretically leading to zero flow in this region, hence ventilation without perfusion.

Reference:
1. Tamul PC, Ault ML. Respiratory function in anesthesia. In: Barash PG, Cullen BF, Stoelting RK, et al, eds. *Clinical Anesthesia.* 7th ed. Philadelphia: Wolters Kluwer; 2013:263-286.

25. Correct answer: B

The ideal V/Q ratio of 1:1 (where ventilation and perfusion match) occurs approximately at the level of the third rib. Above this level, ventilation occurs slightly in excess of perfusion, whereas below this level, the V/Q ratio becomes less than 1.

Reference:
1. Tamul PC, Ault ML. Respiratory function in anesthesia. In: Barash PG, Cullen BF, Stoelting RK, et al, eds. *Clinical Anesthesia.* 7th ed. Philadelphia: Wolters Kluwer; 2013:263-286.

26. Correct answer: B

When ventilation exceeds perfusion to a significant amount, it is called dead space. Although this model of gas exchange units is helpful in understanding V/Q relationships and their influences on gas exchange, most dead space units are not absolute (truly zero blood flow).

Reference:
1. Tamul PC, Ault ML. Respiratory function in anesthesia. In: Barash PG, Cullen BF, Stoelting RK, et al, eds. *Clinical Anesthesia.* 7th ed. Philadelphia: Wolters Kluwer; 2013:263-286.

27. Correct answer: D

When there is no ventilation or perfusion, it is defined as a silent unit. This could theoretically be the result of a combination of a pulmonary vaso-hypoxic response in addition to a pulmonary bronchiolar-constrictive response.

Reference:
1. Tamul PC, Ault ML. Respiratory function in anesthesia. In: Barash PG, Cullen BF, Stoelting RK, et al, eds. *Clinical Anesthesia.* 7th ed. Philadelphia: Wolters Kluwer; 2013:263-286.

28. Correct answer: C

When a unit has no ventilation but there is blood flow, it is called a shunt. Although this model of gas exchange units is helpful in understanding V/Q relationships and their influences on gas exchange, most shunted units are not absolute (truly zero ventilation).

Reference:
1. Tamul PC, Ault ML. Respiratory function in anesthesia. In: Barash PG, Cullen BF, Stoelting RK, et al, eds. *Clinical Anesthesia.* 7th ed. Philadelphia: Wolters Kluwer; 2013:263-286.

29. Correct answer: A

Bronchiolar constriction occurs in areas of reduced regional pulmonary flow to decrease the degree of dead space ventilation. HPV is stimulated by alveolar hypoxia and decreases blood flow to areas of poorly ventilated alveoli. When there is little oxygenation to an alveolar unit, HPV effectively causes these units to be silent.

Reference:
1. Tamul PC, Ault ML. Respiratory function in anesthesia. In: Barash PG, Cullen BF, Stoelting RK, et al, eds. *Clinical Anesthesia.* 7th ed. Philadelphia: Wolters Kluwer; 2013:263-286.

30. Correct answer: E

In addition to potent inhaled agents, factors such as mitral stenosis, volume overload, thromboembolism, hypothermia, vasoconstrictor drugs, and a large hypoxic lung segment may be indirect inhibitors of HPV. Direct inhibitors of HPV include infection, vasodilator drugs such as nitroglycerin and nitroprusside, hypocarbia, and metabolic alkalemia.

Reference:
1. Eisenkraft JB, Cohen E, Neustein SM. Anesthesia for thoracic surgery. In: Barash PG, Cullen BF, Stoelting RK, et al, eds. *Clinical Anesthesia.* 7th ed. Philadelphia: Wolters Kluwer; 2013:1030-1075.

31. **Correct answer: D**

Conditions that shift the oxyhemoglobin dissociation curve to the right decrease the affinity of hemoglobin for oxygen. They include hypercapnia, acidosis, hyperthermia, and high 2-3 diphosphoglycerate (DPG). Conditions that shift the oxyhemoglobin dissociation curve to the left increase the affinity of hemoglobin for oxygen and include low 2-3 DPG, hypothermia, alkalosis, and fetal hemoglobin.

Reference:
1. Tamul PC, Ault ML. Respiratory function in anesthesia. In: Barash PG, Cullen BF, Stoelting RK, et al, eds. *Clinical Anesthesia.* 7th ed. Philadelphia: Wolters Kluwer; 2013:263-286.

32. **Correct answer: D**

Oxygen saturation is a function of the partial pressure of oxygen and the affinity that hemoglobin has for oxygen. The oxyhemoglobin dissociation curve (shown below) is sigmoidal in shape and demonstrates that in a normal state, decreasing Po_2 to 80 mm Hg, the saturation remains in the 90s. However, decreasing oxygen saturation to a level between 20 and 40 mm Hg, there is a steep decline from 75% down to 25% saturation.

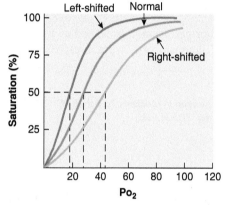

(From Connor CW. Commonly used monitoring techniques. In: Barash PG, Cullen BF, Stoelting RK, et al, eds. *Clinical Anesthesia.* 7th ed. Philadelphia: Wolters Kluwer; 2013:699-722, with permission.)

Reference:
1. Eisenkraft JB, Cohen E, Neustein SM. Anesthesia for thoracic surgery. In: Barash PG, Cullen BF, Stoelting RK, et al, eds. *Clinical Anesthesia.* 7th ed. Philadelphia: Wolters Kluwer; 2013:1030-1075.

33. **Correct answer: D**

Conditions that shift the oxyhemoglobin dissociation curve to the left increase the affinity of hemoglobin for oxygen and include low 2-3 DPG, hypothermia, alkalosis, and fetal hemoglobin. Conditions that shift the oxyhemoglobin dissociation curve to the right decrease the affinity of hemoglobin for oxygen and include hypercapnia, acidosis, hyperthermia, and high 2-3 DPG.

Reference:
1. Rosenblatt WH, Sukhupragarn W. Airway management. In: Barash PG, Cullen BF, Stoelting RK, et al, eds. *Clinical Anesthesia.* 7th ed. Philadelphia: Wolters Kluwer; 2013:762-802.

34. **Correct answer: A**

Respiratory acidosis is always associated with hypercarbia ($Paco_2$ > 45 mm Hg). It occurs due to decreased minute alveolar ventilation or an increase in production of carbon dioxide (eg, laparoscopic procedures) or both. Respiratory acidosis is typically worsened in laparoscopic procedures due to insufflation with carbon dioxide.

Reference:
1. Prough DS, Funston JS, Svensén CH, Wolf SW. Fluids, electrolytes, and acid-base physiology. In: Barash PG, Cullen BF, Stoelting RK, et al, eds. *Clinical Anesthesia.* 7th ed. Philadelphia: Wolters Kluwer; 2013:327-361.

35. **Correct answer: D**

The impact of hypercapnia includes stimulation of ventilation via central and peripheral chemoreceptors, arteriolar dilation (of note, including cerebral vasodilation), stimulation of the sympathetic nervous system, and pulmonary vasoconstriction (making it important to watch in patients with pulmonary hypertension).

Reference:
1. Joshi GP, Cunningham A. Anesthesia for laparoscopic and robotic surgeries. In: Barash PG, Cullen BF, Stoelting RK, et al, eds. *Clinical Anesthesia*. 7th ed. Philadelphia: Wolters Kluwer; 2013:1257-1273.

36. **Correct answer: C**

Excessive oxygenation causes absorptive atelectasis because of nitrogen displacement. Prolonged hyperoxic exposure alters upper airway flora and may increase the risk of secondary infections. Arterial hyperoxia induces vasoconstriction and increases systemic vascular resistance. Cerebral vasoconstriction leads to a decrease in intracranial pressure, not an increase.

Reference:
1. Helmerhorst HJF, Schultz MJ, Van Der Voort PH, de Jonge E, van Westerloo DJ. Bench-to-bedside review: the effects of hyperoxia during critical illness. *Crit Care*. 2015;19(1).

37. **Correct answer: D**

Peripheral vessels respond to low oxygenation by vasodilating. The pulmonary vasculature responds in an opposite manner by vasoconstricting to decrease V/Q mismatch. Cells also respond to hypoxia by increasing ventilation and cardiac output to enhance oxygenation to tissues.

Reference:
1. Michiels C. Physiological and pathological responses to hypoxia. *Am J Pathol*. 2004;164(6):1875-1882.

38. **Correct answer: C**

Respiratory acidosis is characterized by hypercarbia ($Paco_2$ > 45 mm Hg) and typically a low pH (pH < 7.35). It occurs either from a decrease in ventilation or an increase in production of carbon dioxide or both.

Reference:
1. Prough DS, Funston JS, Svensén CH, Wolf SW. Fluids, electrolytes, and acid-base physiology. In: Barash PG, Cullen BF, Stoelting RK, et al, eds. *Clinical Anesthesia*. 7th ed. Philadelphia: Wolters Kluwer; 2013:327-361.

39. **Correct answer: A**

Metabolic acidosis is characterized by low bicarbonate (<21 mEq/L) and a low pH (<7.35). It occurs either as a result of buffering by bicarbonate or abnormal external loss of bicarbonate.

Reference:
1. Prough DS, Funston JS, Svensén CH, Wolf SW. Fluids, electrolytes, and acid-base physiology. In: Barash PG, Cullen BF, Stoelting RK, et al, eds. *Clinical Anesthesia*. 7th ed. Philadelphia: Wolters Kluwer; 2013:327-361.

40. **Correct answer: B**

Metabolic alkalosis is characterized by high bicarbonate level and increased pH (>7.45). Causes of metabolic alkalosis include loss of acid from extracellular space, excessive bicarbonate loads, and posthypercapnic states.

Reference:
1. Prough DS, Funston JS, Svensén CH, Wolf SW. Fluids, electrolytes, and acid-base physiology. In: Barash PG, Cullen BF, Stoelting RK, et al, eds. *Clinical Anesthesia*. 7th ed. Philadelphia: Wolters Kluwer; 2013:327-361.

41. Correct answer: C

The respiratory center is located in the brainstem (both the pons and medulla). Breathing depends on a small area of the medulla near the origin of the vagus nerves.

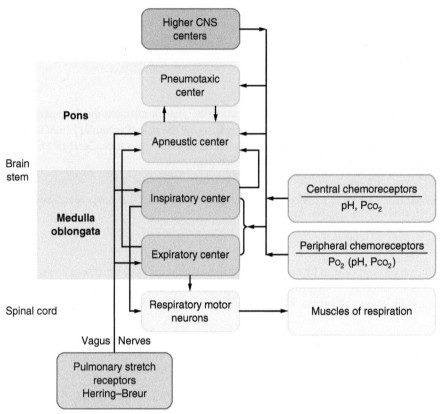

(From Tamul PC, Ault ML. Respiratory function in anesthesia. In: Barash PG, Cullen BF, Stoelting RK, et al, eds. *Clinical Anesthesia.* 7th ed. Philadelphia: Wolters Kluwer; 2013:263-286.)

Reference:
1. Tamul PC, Ault ML. Respiratory function in anesthesia. In: Barash PG, Cullen BF, Stoelting RK, et al, eds. *Clinical Anesthesia.* 7th ed. Philadelphia: Wolters Kluwer; 2013:263-286.

42. Correct answer: D

Both carotid and aortic bodies comprise the peripheral chemoreceptors. Carotid bodies are located at the bifurcation of the common carotid artery, whereas aortic bodies are located throughout the aortic arch and its branches. Both carotid and aortic bodies are stimulated by decreases in Pao_2. Pao_2 values less than 100 mm Hg lead to increased neural activity from these receptors, but augmentation of minute ventilation (via increased ventilatory rate and TV) does not occur until Pao_2 falls to 60-65 mm Hg.

Reference:
1. Tamul PC, Ault ML. Respiratory function in anesthesia. In: Barash PG, Cullen BF, Stoelting RK, et al, eds. *Clinical Anesthesia.* 7th ed. Philadelphia: Wolters Kluwer; 2013:263-286.

43. Correct answer: B

Although the central response is a contributing factor in regulation of breathing by carbon dioxide, central chemoreceptors are actually primarily sensitive to changes in hydrogen ion concentration. Carbon dioxide's effect is indirect—it reacts with water to form carbonic acid and thus hydrogen and bicarbonate ions when dissociated.

Reference:
1. Tamul PC, Ault ML. Respiratory function in anesthesia. In: Barash PG, Cullen BF, Stoelting RK, et al, eds. *Clinical Anesthesia.*
7th ed. Philadelphia: Wolters Kluwer; 2013:263-286.

44. **Correct answer: A**

The dorsal medullary reticular formation contains the dorsal respiratory group (DRG), which contains the inspiratory centers. Ventilatory rhythmicity is generated by the DRG. The ventral respiratory group is located in the ventral medullary reticular formation and coordinates expiratory efforts. The apneustic center is located in the middle or lower pons and sends impulses to the DRG to sustain inspiration. The pneumotaxic respiratory center is located in the rostral pons, and its function is to limit the depth of inspiration.

Reference:
1. Tamul PC, Ault ML. Respiratory function in anesthesia. In: Barash PG, Cullen BF, Stoelting RK, et al, eds. *Clinical Anesthesia.*
7th ed. Philadelphia: Wolters Kluwer; 2013:263-286.

45. **Correct answer: E**

The three situations that are causes of true hyperventilation include arterial hypoxemia, metabolic acidemia, and alterations in CNS activity, including drug administration, increased intracranial pressure, hepatic cirrhosis, and anxiety/fear. These situations also cause a left shift and/or steepen the slope of the carbon dioxide response curve.

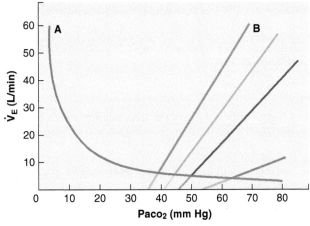

(From Tamul PC, Ault ML. Respiratory function in anesthesia. In: Barash PG, Cullen BF, Stoelting RK, et al, eds. *Clinical Anesthesia.* 7th ed. Philadelphia: Wolters Kluwer; 2013:263-286, with permission.)

Reference:
1. Tamul PC, Ault ML. Respiratory function in anesthesia. In: Barash PG, Cullen BF, Stoelting RK, et al, eds. *Clinical Anesthesia.*
7th ed. Philadelphia: Wolters Kluwer; 2013:263-286.

46. **Correct answer: C**

The slope of the carbon dioxide response curve represents carbon dioxide sensitivity. As the slope of the curve increases—such as when the Pao_2 is less than 65 mm Hg—it leads to increased ventilatory drive. The set point is where the carbon dioxide response curve and the metabolic hyperbola (curve A) intersect and represent normal resting $Paco_2$. The apneic threshold is where the carbon dioxide response curve intercepts that x-axis when extrapolated, usually near 32 mm Hg.

Reference:
1. Tamul PC, Ault ML. Respiratory function in anesthesia. In: Barash PG, Cullen BF, Stoelting RK, et al, eds. *Clinical Anesthesia.*
7th ed. Philadelphia: Wolters Kluwer; 2013:263-286.

47. **Correct answer: D**

Above 100 mm Hg, Pao_2 does not influence the carbon dioxide response curve. There is a small effect on the carbon dioxide response curve at levels between 65 and 100 mm Hg. Once Pao_2 falls below 65 mm Hg, it leads to a shift in the carbon dioxide response curve to the left with an increasing slope; this is coupled with an increased ventilatory drive.

Reference:
1. Tamul PC, Ault ML. Respiratory function in anesthesia. In: Barash PG, Cullen BF, Stoelting RK, et al, eds. *Clinical Anesthesia.* 7th ed. Philadelphia: Wolters Kluwer; 2013:263-286.

48. **Correct answer: D**

Any ventilatory depressants either move the carbon dioxide response curve to the right or decrease the slope. Normal sleep can lead to displacement of the curve to the right leading to an increase of $Paco_2$ of 10 mm Hg. Opioids cause a rightward shift and a decrease in the slope of the carbon dioxide response curve because of their impact on decreasing ventilatory rate with increasing TV. Inhaled anesthetics also displace the carbon dioxide response curve to the right, which leads to a higher $Paco_2$ steady state and apneic threshold.

Reference:
1. Tamul PC, Ault ML. Respiratory function in anesthesia. In: Barash PG, Cullen BF, Stoelting RK, et al, eds. *Clinical Anesthesia.* 7th ed. Philadelphia: Wolters Kluwer; 2013:263-286.

49. **Correct answer: B**

Conditions that shift the oxyhemoglobin dissociation curve to the left increase the affinity of hemoglobin for oxygen and include low 2-3 DPG, hypothermia, alkalosis, and fetal hemoglobin.

Reference:
1. Connor CW. Commonly used monitoring techniques. In: Barash PG, Cullen BF, Stoelting RK, et al, eds. *Clinical Anesthesia.* 7th ed. Philadelphia: Wolters Kluwer; 2013:699-722.

50. **Correct answer: A**

Fetal hemoglobin has higher affinity for oxygen than adult hemoglobin, thus shifting the hemoglobin dissociation curve to the left.

Reference:
1. Hall SC, Suresh S. Neonatal anesthesia. In: Barash PG, Cullen BF, Stoelting RK, et al, eds. *Clinical Anesthesia.* 7th ed. Philadelphia: Wolters Kluwer; 2013:1178-1215.

51. **Correct answer: D**

Smoking negatively impacts pulmonary function in a variety of ways. It causes decreased ciliary motility and increased sputum production leading to poor clearance of sputum. Normal carboxyhemoglobin concentration in nonsmokers is 1% compared with as high as 8%-10% in smokers. Initially, V/Q mismatch, bronchitis and airway hyperreactivity are present. Eventually these changes can lead to chronic obstructive pulmonary disease. Increased gas trapping leads to significant dead space ventilation. Smoking is one of the main risk factors associated with postoperative morbidity. These patients are at increased risk of postoperative pneumonia and their overall postoperative pulmonary complication rate is higher.

Reference:
1. Tamul PC, Ault ML. Respiratory function in anesthesia. In: Barash PG, Cullen BF, Stoelting RK, et al, eds. *Clinical Anesthesia.* 7th ed. Philadelphia: Wolters Kluwer; 2013:263-286.

52. **Correct answer: A**

In a study done by Warner et al, of 200 patients undergoing coronary artery bypass grafting, the patients who stopped smoking less than 8 weeks preoperatively had a 4-fold increase in complication rate compared with those who quit more than 8 weeks preoperatively. In general, smokers continue to acquire equal amounts of nicotine from fewer cigarettes by changing their technique of smoking when they are not using other nicotine replacement therapies. Smokers should be advised to stop smoking 2 months preoperatively to maximize the effect of cessation. For improved mucociliary function and reduction in postoperative pulmonary complications, smoking cessation needs to occur at least 4 weeks before the procedure.

References:
1. Warner MA, Divertie MB, Tinker JH. Preoperative cessation of smoking and pulmonary complications in coronary artery bypass patients. *Anesthesiology.* 1984;60(4):380-383.
2. Tamul PC, Ault ML. Respiratory function in anesthesia. In: Barash PG, Cullen BF, Stoelting RK, et al, eds. *Clinical Anesthesia.* 7th ed. Philadelphia: Wolters Kluwer; 2013:263-286.

53. Correct answer: D

Bronchodilators such as albuterol work by activating β2-adrenergic receptors in bronchial smooth muscle. Activation of these receptors activates adenyl cyclase and leads to increased conversion of ATP to cyclic adenosine-3',5'-monophosphate (cAMP). Stimulation leads to bronchial relaxation.

Reference:
1. Grecu L. Autonomic nervous system: physiology and pharmacology. In: Barash PG, Cullen BF, Stoelting RK, et al, eds. *Clinical Anesthesia.* 7th ed. Philadelphia: Wolters Kluwer; 2013:362-407.

54. Correct answer: B

Anticholinergics, such as ipratropium, block the formation of cyclic guanosine monophosphate, which promotes bronchodilation. They act as a muscarinic antagonist and have no action on nicotinic receptors.

References:
1. Grecu L. Autonomic nervous system: physiology and pharmacology. In: Barash PG, Cullen BF, Stoelting RK, et al, eds. *Clinical Anesthesia.* 7th ed. Philadelphia: Wolters Kluwer; 2013:362-407.
2. Eisenkraft JB, Cohen E, Neustein SM. Anesthesia for thoracic surgery. In: Barash PG, Cullen BF, Stoelting RK, et al, eds. *Clinical Anesthesia.* 7th ed. Philadelphia: Wolters Kluwer; 2013:1030-1075.

55. Correct answer: C

Activation of β2-adrenergic receptors on bronchial smooth muscle leads to the formation of cAMP. Anticholinergics such as ipratropium block the formation of cyclic guanosine monophosphate, which promotes bronchodilation.

Reference:
1. Eisenkraft JB, Cohen E, Neustein SM. Anesthesia for thoracic surgery. In: Barash PG, Cullen BF, Stoelting RK, et al, eds. *Clinical Anesthesia.* 7th ed. Philadelphia: Wolters Kluwer; 2013:1030-1075.

56. Correct answer: D

Leukotrienes are arachidonic acid metabolites. They cause bronchoconstriction, increased capillary permeability, vasodilation, coronary vasoconstriction, and myocardial depression. Leukotriene modifiers include medications such as zafirlukast, montelukast, and zileuton and are used for asthma. They act by antagonizing the leukotriene receptor.

References:
1. Krawiec ME, Wenzel SE. Use of leukotriene antagonists in childhood asthma. *Curr Opin Pediatr.* 1999;11(6):540-548.
2. Levy JH. The allergic response. In: Barash PG, Cullen BF, Stoelting RK, et al, eds. *Clinical Anesthesia.* 7th ed. Philadelphia: Wolters Kluwer; 2013:287-303.

57. Correct answer: D

IgE is a proinflammatory cytokine and primary contributor of allergic airway inflammation. Omalizumab is a monoclonal antibody that inhibits the binding of IgE to its receptor on the surface of mast cells and basophils. Omalizumab has been used in the treatment of moderate to severe asthma.

Reference:
1. Chipps BE, Marshik PL. Targeted IgE therapy for patients with moderate to severe asthma. *Biotechnol Healthc.* 2004;1(3):56-61.

58. Correct answer: B

Mast cell stabilizers such as cromolyn sodium work by stabilizing mast cells, which prevents release of chemical mediators following exposure to an allergen. They are used in the treatment of allergic disorders including asthma. Second-generation medications that target mast cells also possess antihistamine properties.

Reference:

1. Finn DF, Walsh JJ. Twenty-first century mast cell stabilizers. *Br J Pharmacol.* 2013;170(1):23-37.

59. Correct answer: D

Endogenous glucocorticoids are synthesized in the adrenal cortex. Exogenous glucocorticoids such as methylprednisolone, prednisone, fluticasone, and budesonide are commonly used steroid agents for inflammatory diseases such as asthma. Exogenous glucocorticoids exert their mechanism of action through binding of the endogenous glucocorticoid receptors, which leads to inhibition of inflammatory molecules such as cytokines, chemokines, and arachidonic acid metabolites. They also upregulate anti-inflammatory mediators.

Reference:

1. Van der Velden VH. Glucocorticoids: mechanisms of action and anti-inflammatory potential in asthma. *Mediators Inflamm.* 1998;7(4):229-237.

60. Correct answer: B

All glucocorticoid preparations have a degree of anti-inflammatory properties, but not all have mineralocorticoid properties. Dexamethasone has significantly more anti-inflammatory effect compared with hydrocortisone. Prednisone and methylprednisolone have similar levels of anti-inflammatory properties.

Reference:

1. Schwartz JJ, Akhtar S, Rosenbaum SH. Endocrine function. In: Barash PG, Cullen BF, Stoelting RK, et al, eds. *Clinical Anesthesia.* 7th ed. Philadelphia: Wolters Kluwer; 2013:1326-1355.

5

CARDIOVASCULAR AND VASCULAR SYSTEMS

Michael Fitzsimons and Alexandra Plichta

1. **Which portion of the cardiac cycle has the highest myocardial oxygen consumption?**

   A. Isovolumic relaxation period
   B. Ejection
   C. Diastasis
   D. Isovolumic contraction period

2. **Which of the following defines the Frank-Starling relationship?**

   A. The relationship between preload (resting myocardial length) and contractile performance
   B. The relationship between the left ventricle (LV) pressure and wall stress
   C. The relationship between pressure, flow, and resistance
   D. The balance between hydrostatic pressure and oncotic pressure gradients across a membrane

3. **Which of the following is the *earliest indicator* of myocardial ischemia?**

   A. Increased left ventricle end-diastolic volume (LVEDV) and decreased compliance
   B. ECG abnormalities
   C. Wall motion abnormalities
   D. Congestive heart failure

4. **Which of the following contribute(s) to cardiac output?**

   A. Heart rate
   B. Stroke volume
   C. Preload
   D. Afterload
   E. All of the above

5. **Which of the following factors will *increase* venous oxygen saturation measured in the pulmonary artery?**

   A. Decreases in cardiac output
   B. Increases in oxygen consumption
   C. Decreased temperature
   D. Lower hemoglobin concentration

6. **Which of the following indicate(s) impaired diastolic function of the LV?**

   A. Prolonged isovolumic relaxation time
   B. "E" wave to "A" wave ratio less than 1 (E/A <1)
   C. Prolonged time constant for LV relaxation measured at cardiac catheterization
   D. All of the above

7. **Which of the following statements is false concerning baroreceptor function?**

   A. Pressure-sensitive stretch receptors are located in the carotid sinus and aortic arch.
   B. The effects of such stretch are to reduce heart rate at the sinoatrial node, as well as the atrioventricular node.
   C. The vagus nerve is the only nerve involved in the afferent limb of the baroreceptor response.
   D. Massage of the carotid artery will increase parasympathetic stimuli and can slow narrow complex supraventricular tachycardia.

8. **Which of the following statements is true regarding blood pressure in the arterial vascular tree?**

   A. Pulse pressure is the difference between the systolic blood pressure (SBP) in the ventricle and the diastolic blood pressure (DBP) measured within the ventricle.
   B. Mean arterial blood pressure (MAP) = DBP + (0.33 * pulse pressure).
   C. The SBP measured in the femoral artery is lower than that measured in the aorta.
   D. The DBP is higher in the femoral artery than in the aorta.

9. **Spontaneous respiration facilitates venous return primarily due to which of the following conditions?**

   A. Thoracic expansion creates a slightly positive pressure in the chest.
   B. Mean intrathoracic pressure during spontaneous ventilation is slightly negative, facilitating venous return.
   C. Downward movement of the diaphragm reduces intra-abdominal pressure.
   D. Muscle contraction moves blood from the vasculature into muscles.

10. **Distribution of blood throughout the circulatory system is not uniform. Which of the following components of the tree has the largest blood volume?**

    A. Venous system
    B. Arterial system
    C. Pulmonary vasculature
    D. Heart

11. **Which of the following statements is true?**

    A. The arterial system has higher compliance than the venous system.
    B. The compliance of the venous system is 10-20 times greater than the arterial system.
    C. Small changes of blood within the venous system result in large changes in pressure.
    D. The cross-sectional area of the small and large arteries is larger than that of the corresponding veins.

12. **Which of the following does NOT contribute to reduced cardiac output and blood pressure in the setting of acute massive pulmonary embolism?**

    A. Tricuspid regurgitation
    B. Occlusion of the pulmonary arterial vasculature by thrombotic material
    C. Shift of the interventricular septum toward the left
    D. Hypokinesis of the LV

13. **Which of the following is/are the primate determinant(s) of capillary blood flow?**

    A. Transmural pressure
    B. Oncotic pressure
    C. Contraction and relaxation of the precapillary and postcapillary sphincters
    D. A and C

14. **Blood flow through a tube is determined by several factors and explained by the Poiseuille equation. Which of the following statements is true?**

    A. Blood flow is inversely proportional to the pressure gradient.
    B. Blood flow is proportional to the radius of the tube to the second power.
    C. Blood flow is proportional to the length of the tube.
    D. Blood flow is inversely proportional to the viscosity of the fluid.

15. **Which of the following tissues has the greatest capillary density?**

    A. Fat
    B. Cartilage
    C. Bone
    D. Skeletal muscle

16. **Myocardial tissue has the highest oxygen extraction of any tissue. Which of the following statements is false concerning myocardial metabolism?**

    A. Normal coronary blood flow is approximately 250 mL/min or 5% of cardiac output.
    B. Myocardial oxygen consumption is affected by heart rate, contractility, and wall stress.
    C. Coronary blood flow to both the right and left ventricles occurs exclusively during diastole.
    D. Venous oxygen saturation is higher in the right atrium than in the pulmonary artery.

17. **All of the following concerning cerebral perfusion are true EXCEPT which one?**

    A. Cerebral perfusion pressure is the difference between the MAP and the intracranial pressure or central venous pressure (CVP), whichever is higher.
    B. Cerebral blood flow (CBF) always varies consistently depending on the blood pressure.
    C. Blood carbon dioxide tension ($Paco_2$) plays a more important role in determining CBF than oxygen tension (Pao_2).
    D. CBF remains constant if the MAP is between 60 and 160 mm Hg.

18. **Which of the following statements is false?**

    A. There are 3 mechanisms whereby renal blood flow and glomerulofiltration rate are regulated: myogenic response, tubuloglomerular feedback, and sympathetic nervous system input.
    B. The renal system does not exhibit autoregulation.
    C. Sympathetic nervous system input results in constriction of all renal vessels.
    D. The myogenic response is an intrinsic action of vascular smooth muscle in response to increased transmural pressure.

19. **Approximately what percentage of cardiac output goes to the liver?**

    A. 5%
    B. 10%
    C. 15%
    D. 25%

20. **Which of the following statements describes coronary perfusion pressure?**

    A. The difference between the pressures in the aorta during systole and diastole
    B. The difference between the pressure in the aorta and the mean arterial pressure
    C. The difference between the aortic root pressure and the left or right ventricular pressure
    D. The difference between the mean pulmonary pressure and the left atrial pressure (LAP)

21. A 73-year-old man complains of weakness and then falls to the ground. Cardiopulmonary resuscitation (CPR) including chest compressions is initiated. A monitor reveals that the patient is in ventricular fibrillation (VF). Defibrillation is performed, and the monitor reveals a wide complex rhythm at 90 beats per minute. Which of the following is appropriate?

   A. Continue CPR for 2 minutes.
   B. Cease CPR immediately.
   C. Administer sodium bicarbonate.
   D. Administer vasopressin.

22. Which of the following indicates adequacy of CPR during resuscitation?

   A. PETco$_2$ more than 10 mm Hg during CPR
   B. DBP less than 20 mm Hg
   C. PETco$_2$ less than 10 mm Hg
   D. Peripheral cyanosis

23. A patient is found to be in cardiac arrest, and asystole is noted on the ECG. CPR is initiated, and venous access is established. Which of the following is the first medication indicated?

   A. Vasopressin 40 units
   B. Epinephrine 1 mg
   C. Amiodarone 300 mg
   D. Sodium bicarbonate 50 mEq

24. A young man is found lying down on the street unresponsive. He appears to be gasping for air intermittently. Which of the following actions is/are reasonable?

   A. Initiate CPR and continue for 2 minutes.
   B. After 2 minutes of CPR if necessary, leave the patient and call 9-1-1.
   C. Administer naloxone.
   D. All of the above.

25. A patient is noted to have altered mental status and hypotension and complains of chest pain. The heart monitor shows a hear rate of 27 beats per minute. Blood pressure is 60/30 mm Hg. After administration of oxygen and lying the patient flat, atropine 0.5 mg is administered every 5 minutes for a total of 3 mg. No response is noted. Which of the following actions is next indicated?

   A. Amiodarone 300 mg IV (intravenous) over 10 minutes
   B. Additional atropine
   C. Vasopressin 40 units
   D. Dopamine infusion at 2-20 µg/kg/min

26. A patient is found to be in cardiac arrest. CPR is initiated, and IV access is established. After 2 minutes of CPR, VF is noted on the heart monitor. Epinephrine is administered, and CPR is resumed. VF is still noted. Which of the following is the next medication to be administered?

   A. Amiodarone 150 mg IV
   B. Amiodarone 300 mg IV
   C. Atropine 0.5 mg
   D. Vasopressin 40 units

27. Which of the following is true concerning alternative routes of drug administration?

   A. Interosseous (IO) access should not be attempted in children.
   B. The same drug dose should be administered via the endotracheal tube as via IV/IO.
   C. CPR does not need to be stopped when a medication is administered via the endotracheal route.
   D. When administering lidocaine, epinephrine, or vasopressin via the endotracheal tube, the dose should be diluted in 10 mL or normal saline or sterile water.

28. **A patient presents with complaints of slight light-headedness as well as palpitations. ECG is obtained, and it is noted that he has a narrow complex (QRS <0.12 s), monomorphic, regular rhythm. Which of the following is/are indicated?**

    A. Vagal maneuver
    B. β-Blocker or calcium channel blocker
    C. Adenosine
    D. All of the above

29. **All of the following are considered goals for in the management of acute coronary syndrome in the setting of ST-segment elevation myocardial infarction (STEMI) EXCEPT?**

    A. Door-to-balloon time of 90 minutes for percutaneous coronary intervention (PCI)
    B. Door-to-needle time of 30 minutes when fibrinolysis is utilized
    C. Emergency room assessment of 10 minutes or less
    D. Complete stabilization within the emergency department before catheterization

30. **Which of the following statements is false regarding airway management during CPR?**

    A. Cricoid pressure should always be applied throughout chest compressions.
    B. The oral pharyngeal size should be approximately the same as the distance from the tip of the patient's nose to the earlobe.
    C. An excessively long oropharyngeal airway (OPA) may enter the esophagus and may result in gastric distention with air during bag-mask ventilation.
    D. Ventilations during CPR should occur every 5-6 seconds.

31. **Which of the following coronary arteries is located in the posterior interventricular groove?**

    A. Left anterior descending coronary artery
    B. Right coronary artery
    C. Posterior interventricular (descending) coronary artery (PDA)
    D. Left circumflex coronary artery

32. **The aortic valve is composed of which of the following 3 leaflets?**

    A. Right, left, and anterior
    B. Right, left, and noncoronary
    C. Anterior, posterior, and septal
    D. Anterolateral, posteromedial, and septal

33. **A patient presents with acute severe pulmonary edema and cardiogenic shock. Transesophageal echocardiography (TEE) demonstrates a ruptured papillary muscle. Which papillary muscle is most commonly affected?**

    A. Posteromedial
    B. Septal
    C. Noncoronary
    D. Anterolateral

34. **A 55-year-old man is undergoing coronary artery bypass grafting. The TEE shows an enlarged coronary sinus. When saline is injected into an IV line in the left upper extremity, bubbles are noted, entering the left atrium (LA) near the inferior vena cava. Which of the following conditions most likely explains the findings?**

    A. An aberrant right coronary artery
    B. Anomalous pulmonary venous return
    C. A left-sided superior vena cava (SVC)
    D. A patent foramen ovale

35. **Which of the following structures is responsible for the conduction of impulses from the right atrium to the LA?**

    A. Purkinje fibers
    B. Bundle of His
    C. Left bundle branch
    D. Bachmann bundle

36. **Which of the following structures is depicted in the image below and annotated with a "Y"?**

    A. The left atrium
    B. The superior vena cava
    C. The right atrium
    D. The left ventricle

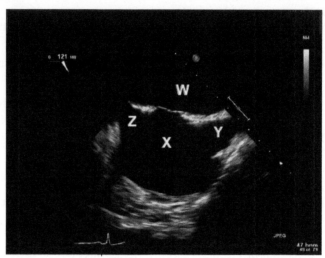

37. **Which of the following is depicted in the image below?**

    A. Transgastric midpapillary view
    B. Midesophageal 4 chamber view
    C. Transgastric long axis view
    D. Transgastric right ventricle (RV) view

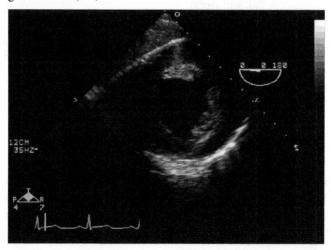

38. **Which of the following is depicted in the image below?**

    A. Midesophageal 3 chamber view
    B. Midesophageal commissural view
    C. Midesophageal RV view
    D. Midesophageal inflow-outflow view

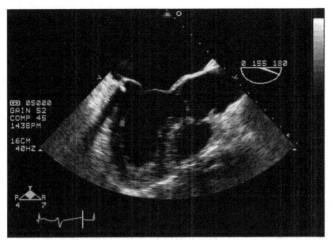

39. **Which of the following statements is/are true based on the image below, which is obtained across the aortic valve?**

    A. The image demonstrates Doppler flow.
    B. The <u>peak</u> gradient across the valve is approximately 64 mm Hg.
    C. The maximum blood velocity across the valve is approximately 400 cm/s.
    D. All of the above.

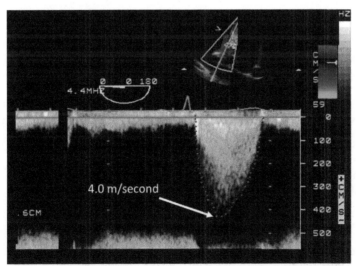

40. **A 79-year-old man is scheduled to undergo lumbar laminectomy for spinal stenosis. His medical history is significant for aortic stenosis, with a valve area of 0.9 cm² and a mean gradient of 45 mm Hg. Which of the following vasoactive agents would be most beneficial to this patient?**

    A. Dopamine
    B. Phenylephrine
    C. Hydralazine
    D. Nitroglycerin

41. Which of the following is the MOST accurate description of perfusion of the left and right sides of the heart in a normal healthy adult?

    A. Both the left and right sides of the heart are perfused during both systole and diastole.
    B. Both the left and right sides of the heart are perfused during diastole only.
    C. The left side of the heart is perfused during both systole and diastole; the right side of the heart is perfused during systole only.
    D. The left side of the heart is perfused during diastole only; the right side of the heart is perfused during both systole and diastole.

42. In a patient with severe pulmonary hypertension (HTN), use of which of the following agents would *best* preserve perfusion to the right side of the heart during induction of anesthesia?

    A. Milrinone
    B. Vasopressin
    C. Dobutamine
    D. Phenylephrine

43. On a preoperative evaluation, the American College of Cardiology/American Heart Association (ACC/AHA) guidelines do NOT help direct your decision-making process with regard to which of the following ECG abnormalities?

    A. Left bundle branch block
    B. Atrial fibrillation with rapid ventricular response
    C. Mobitz type II block
    D. ST-elevation myocardial infarction

44. Which of the following components of the cardiac conduction system has the FASTEST conduction velocity?

    A. SA node
    B. AV node
    C. His-Purkinje system
    D. Ventricular myocardium

45. A patient who received a heart transplant 2 years ago presents for laparoscopic appendectomy. Which of the following medications should be avoided during this planned general anesthetic?

    A. Cisatracurium
    B. Vecuronium
    C. Neostigmine
    D. Glycopyrrolate

46. In a normal CVP tracing, where does the tricuspid valve close?

    A. Between the a-wave and c-wave
    B. At the peak of the c-wave
    C. Between the c-wave and x-descent
    D. Between the x-descent and v-wave

47. **In the figure below, which of the following processes does the arrow indicating movement of line 1 to line 2 depict?**

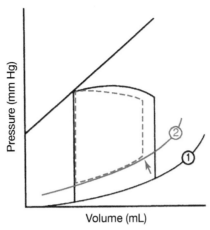

Volume (mL)

(From Chatterjee NA, Fifer MA. Heart failure. In: Lilly LS, ed. *Pathophysiology of Heart Disease*. Philadelphia: Wolters Kluwer Health; 2010:216-243.)

    A. Nitroglycerin therapy
    B. Cocaine withdrawal
    C. Systolic dysfunction
    D. Diastolic dysfunction

48. **The V5 ECG lead is MOST SENSITIVE for detecting which of the following?**

    A. Atrial fibrillation
    B. Anteroseptal ischemia
    C. Lateral wall ischemia
    D. Conduction abnormalities

49. **Which of the following cardiac abnormalities would be MOST LIKELY to benefit from relative tachycardia?**

    A. Aortic stenosis
    B. Mitral regurgitation
    C. Hypertrophic obstructive cardiomyopathy (HOCM)
    D. Unstable angina

50. **Which of the following is the "agent of choice" for treatment of tachyarrhythmias associated with Wolff-Parkinson-White?**

    A. Metoprolol
    B. Verapamil
    C. Carvedilol
    D. Procainamide

51. **Which of the following is NOT considered a "cyanotic" heart lesion?**

    A. Truncus arteriosus
    B. Pulmonic stenosis
    C. Tricuspid atresia
    D. Total anomalous pulmonary venous return

52. Which of the following is LEAST LIKELY to be a complication of a transcatheter aortic valve replacement?

    A. Complete heart block
    B. Pneumothorax
    C. Cardiac tamponade
    D. Embolic stroke

53. A patient with long-standing HTN and normally well-managed congestive heart failure is also found to have bilateral coarse rales on lung examination. He admits that he went to a wedding and had a dietary indiscretion, which is very rare for him. Which of the following is most likely true?

    If heard, an S3 gallop is most likely associated with _____(1)_____ and is most likely to be _____ (2)_____, whereas an S4 gallop is most likely associated with ____(3)____ and is most likely to be _____(4) _____.

1	2	3	4
A. Volume overload	Transient	Noncompliant ventricle	Permanent
B. Volume overload	Permanent	Noncompliant ventricle	Transient
C. Noncompliant ventricle	Transient	Volume overload	Transient
D. Noncompliant ventricle	Permanent	Volume overload	Permanent

54. Which of the following is the MOST UNLIKELY cause of myocardial ischemia?

    A. Severe tachycardia
    B. Severe hypotension
    C. Severe anemia
    D. Severe hypokalemia

55. Which of the following is false regarding heart failure with preserved ejection fraction (HFpEF)?

    A. The most sensitive test of adequacy of tissue perfusion is mixed venous O_2 saturation at rest.
    B. The most common causes of HFpEF in the United Sates are chronic HTN and aortic stenosis .
    C. Diagnosis of HFpEF requires echocardiography with Doppler.
    D. Atrial systole contributes relatively more to the left ventricular end diastolic volume (LVEDV) in patients with HFpEF than it does to those with normal ventricular function.

56. Which of the following is false regarding heart rate in normal healthy adults?

    A. Cholinergic slowing of heart rate occurs via M2 muscarinic receptors.
    B. Factors that decrease the rate of SA node depolarization increase the likelihood that the pacemaker of the heart will become located at the AV junction.
    C. The normal intrinsic rate of the SA node increases over time.
    D. β1-Adrenergic stimulation increases the rate of phase 4 depolarization.

57. When the surgeon requests for the patient be placed in the "reverse Trendelenburg" position, which of the following is the PRIMARY parameter initially affected?

    A. Systemic afterload
    B. Venous return
    C. Myocardial inotropy
    D. Cerebral perfusion

58. You are about to induce anesthesia in a 38-year-old man with HOCM. Which of the following options should be your goals with regard to preload, afterload, rate, rhythm, and contractility?

	PRELOAD	AFTERLOAD	RATE	RHYTHM	CONTRACTILITY
A.	Increased	Increased	Normal	Sinus	Depressed
B.	Increased	Decreased	Decreased	Sinus	Increased
C.	Decreased	Increased	Decreased	Sinus	Depressed
D.	Decreased	Decreased	Increased	Sinus	Increased

59. Which of the following conditions is MOST sensitive to loss of the "atrial kick"?

A. Mitral regurgitation
B. Aortic insufficiency
C. Mitral stenosis
D. Diastolic dysfunction

60. Which of the following is false regarding mitral stenosis?

A. Hyperdynamic states, such as sepsis, can lead to pulmonary edema.
B. Pulmonary capillary wedge pressure approximates left ventricular end-diastolic pressure (LVEDP).
C. The progression of disease includes right ventricular hypertrophy and dysfunction.
D. Medical management of mitral stenosis includes use of β-blockers and calcium channel blockers.

Chapter 5 ▪ Answers

1. Correct answer: D

The most energy consuming event in the cardiac cycle is isovolumic contraction. This is the brief period when the ventricle contracts against closed valves without a change in overall volume.

Reference:

1. Sharar SR, von Homeyer. Cardiovascular anatomy and physiology. In: Barash PG, Cullen BF, Stoelting RK, et al, eds. *Clinical Anesthesia Fundamentals*. Philadelphia: Wolters Kluwer Health; 2015:47-49.

2. Correct answer: A

The relationship between preload (resting myocardial length) and contractile performance defines the Frank-Starling relationship. The relationship between the LV pressure and wall stress is the Laplace law. The Ohm law related pressure to flow and resistance (pressure = flow × resistance). The Starling hypothesis refers to the phenomenon that flow across a porous membrane is determined by the hydrostatic and oncotic pressures across that membrane.

Reference:

1. Sharar SR, von Homeyer. Cardiovascular anatomy and physiology. In: Barash PG, Cullen BF, Stoelting RK, et al, eds. *Clinical Anesthesia Fundamentals*. Philadelphia: Wolters Kluwer Health; 2015:52-57.

3. Correct answer: A

The earliest indicators of myocardial ischemia are an increased LVEDV and decreased compliance. Wall motion abnormalities, ECG abnormalities, and clinical symptoms of heart failure are late findings.

Reference:

1. Sharar SR, von Homeyer. Cardiovascular anatomy and physiology. In: Barash PG, Cullen BF, Stoelting RK, et al, eds. *Clinical Anesthesia Fundamentals*. Philadelphia: Wolters Kluwer Health; 2015:52-57.

4. Correct answer: E

Cardiac output is the amount of blood flow generated by the heart over an interval of time, generally 1 minute. Heart rate is the number of contractions per minute. Stroke volume is the difference between EDV and end-systolic volume. Preload is the amount of blood filling the ventricle before ejection and on a cellular level is the amount of sarcomere stretch before ejection. Afterload is the resistance that the ventricle must overcome when contracting. Resistance is generally at the vascular level but may also be due to stenotic valvular lesions.

Reference:

1. Sharar SR, von Homeyer. Cardiovascular anatomy and physiology. In: Barash PG, Cullen BF, Stoelting RK, et al, eds. *Clinical Anesthesia Fundamentals*. Philadelphia: Wolters Kluwer Health; 2015:52-57.

5. Correct answer: C

The Fick principle states that the oxygen utilization by tissues is a factor of the oxygen delivery that tissue and the arterial-venous concentration difference across the organ. The mixed venous saturation (SVo_2) measured in the pulmonary artery reflects overall oxygen utilization by the body. Factors such as increased hemoglobin, increased cardiac output, and increased hemoglobin saturation will increase the SVo_2, whereas conditions such as cardiogenic shock and hyperthermia will increase oxygen utilization and decrease SVo_2.

Reference:

1. Sharar SR, von Homeyer. Cardiovascular anatomy and physiology. In: Barash PG, Cullen BF, Stoelting RK, et al, eds. *Clinical Anesthesia Fundamentals*. Philadelphia: Wolters Kluwer Health; 2015:57-58.

6. Correct answer: D

Impaired relaxation of the LV is referred to as diastolic dysfunction. Direct hemodynamic measures include the maximum rate of LV pressure reduction (−dP/dT) and the time constant for LV relaxation. Echocardiography allows measurement of the isovolumic relaxation time and measurement of the flow velocity across the mitral valve. Flow across the mitral valve during early diastole generates an "E" wave, whereas flow during atrial contraction generates an "A" wave. The normal diastolic function is indicated by an "E" to "A" ration more than 1. With impaired diastolic dysfunction, the deceleration time of the "E" wave is prolonged and the "A" velocity increases. The ratio of the "E" to "A" reverses with the "A" becoming more prominent.

Reference:
1. Sharar SR, von Homeyer. Cardiovascular anatomy and physiology. In: Barash PG, Cullen BF, Stoelting RK, et al, eds. *Clinical Anesthesia Fundamentals*. Philadelphia: Wolters Kluwer Health; 2015:50-51.

7. Correct answer: C

Pressure-sensitive receptors are located in the carotid sinus and the aortic arch. When these sensors are stimulated, the vagus nerve and the glossopharyngeal nerve mediate information to the medullary vaso-motor center in the brain. Efferent stimuli are mediated via the vagus nerve to the sinoatrial and atrio-ventricular nodes to decrease both the heart rate and vascular tone, which in turn decrease the blood pressure.

Reference:
1. Sharar SR, von Homeyer. Cardiovascular anatomy and physiology. In: Barash PG, Cullen BF, Stoelting RK, et al, eds. *Clinical Anesthesia Fundamentals*. Philadelphia: Wolters Kluwer Health; 2015:58-62.

8. Correct answer: B

The pulse pressure is the difference between the SBP and the DBP; it is not measured within the ventricles of the heart. MAP is calculated as the DBP plus one-third of the pulse pressure. The measured blood pressure changes as one proceeds from the aortic root to more peripheral arterial vessels. The SBP is higher in the femoral artery, whereas the DBP is lower.

Reference:
1. Sharar SR, von Homeyer. Cardiovascular anatomy and physiology. In: Barash PG, Cullen BF, Stoelting RK, et al, eds. *Clinical Anesthesia Fundamentals*. Philadelphia: Wolters Kluwer Health; 2015:58-62.

9. Correct answer: B

Spontaneous ventilation facilitates venous return to the heart through several mechanisms. Descent of the diaphragm drops intrathoracic pressure and increases pressure in the abdomen. This action increases the pressure gradient between the extrathoracic vasculature and the intrathoracic cavity, which facilitates venous return. The pressure within the thoracic venous system and the right atrium also drops, further enhancing venous return.

Reference:
1. Sharar SR, von Homeyer. Cardiovascular anatomy and physiology. In: Barash PG, Cullen BF, Stoelting RK, et al, eds. *Clinical Anesthesia Fundamentals*. Philadelphia: Wolters Kluwer Health; 2015:52-57.

10. Correct answer: A

The largest volume of blood in the vasculature lies in the venous system (65%) with lesser amounts in the arterial system (15%) and the pulmonary tree (10%).

Reference:
1. Sharar SR, von Homeyer. Cardiovascular anatomy and physiology. In: Barash PG, Cullen BF, Stoelting RK, et al, eds. *Clinical Anesthesia Fundamentals*. Philadelphia: Wolters Kluwer Health; 2015:62-63.

11. Correct answer: B

Veins are thinner and slightly larger than arteries, and the compliance of veins is 10-20 times higher as compared with that of arteries. The increased capacitance allows the veins to accommodate large changes in volume without a significant increase in pressure. Sympathetic innervation to the veins in times of stress will increase venous compliance and thus increase venous return to the thoracic cavity and the heart.

Reference:
1. Sharar SR, von Homeyer. Cardiovascular anatomy and physiology. In: Barash PG, Cullen BF, Stoelting RK, et al, eds. *Clinical Anesthesia Fundamentals*. Philadelphia: Wolters Kluwer Health; 2015:62-63.

12. **Correct answer: D**

Acute massive pulmonary embolism is associated with decreased cardiac output and blood pressure, often leading to cardiogenic shock for several reasons. Acute massive embolism causes an immediate pressure overload in the RV. The RV is thin walled and not able to compensate for the blockage and dilates, which may contribute to tricuspid regurgitation. The reduced filling of the LV along with dilation of the right results in a shift of the septum further to the left side, resulting in even less filling. The LV is generally hyperkinetic because of tachycardia and hypovolemia.

13. **Correct answer: D**

Capillary blood flow is determined by the transmural pressure (intravascular minus extravascular pressure) and the tone of the precapillary and postcapillary sphincters. The postcapillary sphincter is affected by both neural and humoral factors. Intense precapillary vasoconstriction may completely abolish blood flow to a capillary bed and divert blood to local arteriovenous shunts.

Reference:

1. Sharar SR, von Homeyer. Cardiovascular anatomy and physiology. In: Barash PG, Cullen BF, Stoelting RK, et al, eds. *Clinical Anesthesia Fundamentals*. Philadelphia: Wolters Kluwer Health; 2015:63-66.

14. **Correct answer: D**

Blood flow through a tube is described according to the Poiseuille equation.

Flow = (pressure gradient X π X r^4)/8 X L X viscosity)

Flow is proportional to the pressure gradient and the radius to the fourth power and inversely proportional to the length and viscosity.

Reference:

1. Sharar SR, von Homeyer. Cardiovascular anatomy and physiology. In: Barash PG, Cullen BF, Stoelting RK, et al, eds. *Clinical Anesthesia Fundamentals*. Philadelphia: Wolters Kluwer Health; 2015:63-66.

15. **Correct answer: D**

Tissues with the highest metabolic rate or those that must function across a wide variety of rates have the highest capillary density. Such tissue includes the heart and skeletal muscle, whereas cartilage and fat have lower-density beds.

Reference:

1. Sharar SR, von Homeyer. Cardiovascular anatomy and physiology. In: Barash PG, Cullen BF, Stoelting RK, et al, eds. *Clinical Anesthesia Fundamentals*. Philadelphia: Wolters Kluwer Health; 2015:63-66.

16. **Correct answer: C**

Myocardial tissue has the highest oxygen extraction of any organ (approximately 70%). When the metabolic rate of the heart increases in times of stress, oxygen supply must increase. This occurs via local coronary vasodilation associated with mediators as well as β2-adrenergic stimulation.

Reference:

1. Sharar SR, von Homeyer. Cardiovascular anatomy and physiology. In: Barash PG, Cullen BF, Stoelting RK, et al, eds. *Clinical Anesthesia Fundamentals*. Philadelphia: Wolters Kluwer Health; 2015:50-51.

17. **Correct answer: B**

The brain needs continuous delivery of both oxygen and glucose, and the lack of such substrate can result in damage in approximately 5 minutes. CBF is constant between a mean arterial pressure of 60 and 160 mm Hg because of the phenomenon of autoregulation. CBF is linearly associated with the partial pressure of carbon dioxide ($Paco_2$), whereas oxygen (Pao_2) plays less of a role. The driving pressure for perfusion is the difference between the mean arterial pressure and either the intracranial pressure or the CVP, whichever is higher.

Reference:

1. Bebawy JF, Koht A. Anesthesia for neurosurgery. In: Barash PG, Cullen BF, Stoelting RK, et al, eds. *Clinical Anesthesia Fundamentals*. Philadelphia: Wolters Kluwer Health; 2015:557-560.

18. Correct answer: B

There are 3 mechanisms through which renal blood flow and glomerular filtration rate are regulated: the myogenic response, tubuloglomerular feedback, and input from the sympathetic nervous system. These mechanisms control renal blood flow within a range referred to as autoregulation, much like the cerebral vasculature. The myogenic response occurs when increased transmural pressure results in renal arteriole constriction to allow constant blood flow.

Reference:
1. Garwood S. The renal system. In: Barash PG, Cullen BF, Stoelting RK, et al, eds. *Clinical Anesthesia Fundamentals*. Philadelphia: Wolters Kluwer Health; 2015:87-93.

19. Correct answer: D

Nearly 25% of the cardiac output goes to the liver, which also accounts for about 20% of the resting oxygen consumption. When the liver and the splanchnic system are considered together, the organs contain about 10%-15% of the blood volume of the body.

Reference:
1. Chapman N. Liver anatomy and physiology. In: Barash PG, Cullen BF, Stoelting RK, et al, eds. *Clinical Anesthesia Fundamentals*. Philadelphia: Wolters Kluwer Health; 2015:112.

20. Correct answer: C

Coronary prefusion pressure is the difference between the pressure in the aortic root (aorta) and that within the ventricle. This is the driving pressure for coronary perfusion. Perfusion to the LV is variable, highest during early diastole and lowest during early systole at the time that the coronary vessels are compressed by ventricular contraction. Perfusion to the RV is more constant throughout the cardiac cycle because of lower ventricular pressures.

Reference:
1. Sharar SR, von Homeyer. Cardiovascular anatomy and physiology. In: Barash PG, Cullen BF, Stoelting RK, et al, eds. *Clinical Anesthesia Fundamentals*. Philadelphia: Wolters Kluwer Health; 2015:50-51.

21. Correct answer: A

The 2016 Advanced Cardiovascular Life Support Guidelines from the American Heart Association recommend that CPR continue at least 2 minutes after return of spontaneous circulation (CPR) after defibrillation.

References:
1. *Part 5 The ACLS Cases Advanced Cardiovascular Life Support Provider Manual*. American Heart Association; 2016:95-109.

22. Correct answer: A

Chest compressions during CPR should occur at a rate of 100-120 compressions/min to a depth of 2.0-2.4 inches (5-6 cm). Compression beyond 2.4 inches may cause injury. CPR should be improved when PETco$_2$ is less than 10 mm Hg and DBP measured via an arterial line is less than 20 mm Hg.

Reference:
1. *Part 5 The ACLS Cases Advanced Cardiovascular Life Support Provider Manual*. America Heart Association; 2016:101.

23. Correct answer: B

When asystole is diagnosed, CPR should be initiated immediately. After IV access is established, the first medication to be administered is epinephrine 1 mg either IV or IO. Epinephrine should be continued every 3-5 minutes. If there is no heart rhythm that is amenable to defibrillation, then CPR should be continued and reversible causes should be considered and treated (such as hypovolemia, hypoxemia, potassium abnormalities, hypothermia, tamponade or tension pneumothorax, toxins, or thrombosis [either coronary or pulmonary]).

Reference:
1. *Part 5 The ACLS Cases Advanced Cardiovascular Life Support Provider Manual*. American Heart Association; 2016:116.

24. **Correct answer: D**

New to the ACLS guidelines is the Opioid-Associated Life-Threatening Emergency (Adult) Algorithm. When an individual is found unresponsive, CPR should be initiated. If there are no breaths or only gasping, CPR should be continued for 2 minutes before leaving to call 9-1-1, or an automated external defibrillator (AED) and naloxone should be obtained. Then, naloxone should be administered (2 mg intranasal or 0.4 mg intramuscular). If no improvement is noted, CPR should be continued. If the patient becomes responsive, then monitoring and reassessment is continued until help arrives.

Reference:
1. *Part 5 The ACLS Cases Advanced Cardiovascular Life Support Provider Manual.* American Heart Association; 2016:108.

25. **Correct answer: D**

The initial steps in the management of symptomatic bradycardia are to maintain the airway, administer oxygen, establish IV access, and obtain a 12-lead ECG to diagnose rhythm. Atropine 0.5 mg IV every 3-5 minutes to a total dose of 3 mg is indicated. If bradycardia persists, other options include transcutaneous pacing, epinephrine 2-10 µg/min, or dopamine 2-20 µg/kg/min.

Reference:
1. *Part 5 The ACLS Cases Advanced Cardiovascular Life Support Provider Manual.* American Heart Association; 2016:123.

26. **Correct answer: B**

VF and pulseless ventricular tachycardia are treated in the same fashion. CPR is initiated and continued for 2 minutes and IV/IO access is established. Epinephrine 1 mg is given every 3-5 minutes. If VF/pulseless ventricular tachycardia continued, amiodarone 300 mg IV is administered as the initial dose (150 mg for a subsequent dose). Amiodarone is a class III antiarrhythmic drug that blocks sodium channels. Some providers will administer lidocaine 1-1.5 mg IV if amiodarone is not available. Magnesium sulfate may be considered for torsades de pointes.

Reference:
1. *Part 5 The ACLS Cases Advanced Cardiovascular Life Support Provider Manual.* American Heart Association; 2016:123.

27. **Correct answer: D**

Drugs administered via the endotracheal tube should be diluted in 10 mL normal saline to facilitate absorption. Adequate IV access may not be easy to establish in cardiopulmonary arrest, and alternative routes may need to be considered. IO is quick and easy to establish in all age groups, and all drugs may be administered via this route. The endotracheal route has limitations such as administering unknown optimal drug doses and the need to stop CPR while drugs are administered.

Reference:
1. *Part 5 The ACLS Cases Advanced Cardiovascular Life Support Provider Manual.* American Heart Association; 2016:104-106.

28. **Correct answer: D**

In addition to hemodynamic stability, the major factor to consider in the management of tachycardia is whether the rhythm is narrow (QRS <0.12 s) or wide (QRS ≥0.12 s). Wide complex tachycardia has a propensity to deteriorate into VF. Narrow complex rhythms are unlikely to progress to VF. The primary initial treatment is a vagal maneuver (Valsalva or carotid sinus massage). Vagal maneuvers are successful in about 25% of cases. If the rhythm does not respond, then adenosine 6 mg may be administered. A second dose of 12 mg may be given if the first is not successful.

Reference:
1. *Part 5 The ACLS Cases Advanced Cardiovascular Life Support Provider Manual.* American Heart Association; 2016:132-135.

29. **Correct answer: D**

Acute coronary syndrome includes STEMI, non-STEMI, and unstable angina. When a patient exhibits symptoms suggestive of ischemia or infarction, time is critical. Quick emergency department assessment (10 min) is followed by movement to the catheterization for PCI (goal 90 min) or treatment with fibrinolysis (goal 30 min). Complete stabilization may delay critical PCI.

Reference:

1. *Part 5 The ACLS Cases Advanced Cardiovascular Life Support Provider Manual*. American Heart Association; 2016:59-62.

30. Correct answer: A

Several complications can occur if airway management during CPR is not appropriate. An appropriately sized OPA can improve the effectiveness of bag-mask ventilation by opening the airway by lifting the tongue off the back of the throat. The appropriate length is approximately the distance from the tip of the nose to the earlobe. An OPA that is too long may enter the esophagus and allow air to enter the stomach, which could displace fluid or solid material into the mouth and then the lungs. Cricoid pressure is not recommended during CPR because it may interfere with airway management.

Reference:

1. *Part 5 The ACLS Cases Advanced Cardiovascular Life Support Provider Manual*. American Heart Association; 2016:47-54.

31. Correct answer: C

The posterior interventricular (descending) coronary artery is located in the inferior interventricular groove. The origin of this artery determines the coronary artery dominance and the blood supply to the inferior wall of the heart.

Reference:

1. Sharar SR, von Homeyer. Cardiovascular anatomy and physiology. In: Barash PG, Cullen BF, Stoelting RK, et al, eds. *Clinical Anesthesia Fundamentals*. Philadelphia: Wolters Kluwer Health; 2015:41-47.

32. Correct answer: B

The aortic valve is made up of 3 leaflets, the left, right, and noncoronary artery. The right coronary leaflet is the most anterior and furthest away from the TEE probe when an examination is being performed. The tricuspid valve is composed of the anterior, posterior, and septal leaflets, whereas the pulmonary valve has the left, right, and anterior leaflets. The mitral valve has only 2 leaflets named the anterolateral and posteromedial.

Reference:

1. Sharar SR, von Homeyer. Cardiovascular anatomy and physiology. In: Barash PG, Cullen BF, Stoelting RK, et al, eds. *Clinical Anesthesia Fundamentals*. Philadelphia: Wolters Kluwer Health; 2015:41-47.

33. Correct answer: A

The posteromedial papillary muscle is most likely to rupture in association with a myocardial infarction. The posteromedial papillary muscle has a single blood supply from the posterior descending papillary muscle. The anterolateral papillary muscle has a dual blood supply by branches of the left circumflex coronary artery and branches of the left anterior descending coronary artery.

Reference:

1. Sharar SR, von Homeyer. Cardiovascular anatomy and physiology. In: Barash PG, Cullen BF, Stoelting RK, et al, eds. *Clinical Anesthesia Fundamentals*. Philadelphia: Wolters Kluwer Health; 2015:41-47.

34. Correct answer: C

The coronary sinus drains into the right atrium medial to the inferior vena cava. Normally, blood from the upper extremities and head will drain through the SVC, but when a left-sided SVC is present, drainage from the left will return through the coronary sinus and then into the right atrium rather than the SVC.

35. Correct answer: D

Bachmann bundle is responsible for conduction of impulses from the right to the LA, while the conduction terminates in the Purkinje fibers. The Bundle of His is responsible for conducting impulses from the AV node (to the Purkinje fibers) but splits into both the left and right bundle branches. All conduction terminates in the Purkinje fibers.

36. **Correct answer: B**

The image is referred to as a "bicaval view." The view is obtained at an omniplane of approximately 120°. The structure annotated in the image by the "Y" is the SVC. The "W" notes the LA, the "X" the right atrium, and the "Z" the inferior vena cava.

37. **Correct answer: A**

The image depicted is the transgastric midpapillary view. The view allows visualization of the wall motion of 6 segments (inferior, anterior, anterolateral, inferolateral, anteroseptal, and inferoseptal).

38. **Correct answer: A**

The image depicted is the midesophageal 3 chamber view. Structures visualized include the LA, LV, mitral valve, aortic valve, and aortic root.

39. **Correct answer: D**

The image depicted is the continuous Doppler imaging across the aortic valve. The maximum blood flow velocity across the valve is 400 cm/s or 4 m/s. Using the modified Bernoulli equation (gradient = 4 * [maximum velocity]^2), the peak gradient is 64 mm Hg.

40. **Correct answer: B**

By definition, this patient has severe aortic stenosis. Specific anesthetic considerations for this population include maintenance of a moderately elevated systemic vascular resistance (SVR) to maintain forward flow and "slower" heart rates (<60 is ideal; however, 60-80 is the goal), optimizing preload, and avoiding arrhythmias. Phenylephrine is a peripherally acting α-agonist, which will cause vasoconstriction, increase SVR, and does not cause tachycardia. Although dopamine has the ability to cause vasoconstriction, it is arrythmogenic and should be avoided. Hydralazine should be avoided because it is a direct arterial vasodilator, which will drop SVR. It can also lead to tachycardia via activation of the baroreceptor reflex. Nitroglycerin will vasodilate the arteries, decrease SVR, and decrease preload via vasodilatation of the venous system and hence should be avoided.

41. **Correct answer: D**

Blood flows down pressure gradients. The aortic blood pressure is always (in both systole and diastole) higher than right-sided heart pressures, with blood flowing from the higher-pressure aorta to the lower-pressure right coronary artery. However, on the left side of the heart, LV pressure approximates aortic pressure during systole. The aortic pressure is only higher than left main coronary artery (and left anterior descending + left circumflex arteries) pressure during diastole, which is the main period during which left side of the heart is perfused.

Reference:

1. Skubas NJ, Lichtman AD, Sharma A, Thomas SJ. Anesthesia for cardiac surgery. In: Barash PG, Cullen BF, Stoelting RK, et al, eds. *Clinical Anesthesia*. Philadelphia: Wolters Kluwer Health; 2013:1077.

42. **Correct answer: B**

The right side of the heart is USUALLY perfused during systole and diastole. However, with severe pulmonary HTN, the right ventricular systolic pressure may rise to approximate the systemic pressure, leaving the right side of the heart to be perfused only during systole. Preserving right-sided heart perfusion can be accomplished by (1) increasing SVR and/or (2) decreasing pulmonary vascular resistance (PVR) and (3) increasing inotropy.

Dobutamine would not be an ideal agent because it decreases SVR without a decrease in PVR.

Milrinone could be used because it increases inotropy and increases forward flow of a sluggish right side of the heart. However, because it is in the class of agents of "ino-vasodilators," it has the potential of decreasing SVR. It may be administered peripherally if central access is not available.

Vasopressin is an ideal agent for patients with severe pulmonary HTN because it increases SVR without affecting PVR.

Phenylephrine will increase both SVR and PVR but should be used with caution because increases in PVR are generally poorly tolerated in those with pulmonary HTN and can lead to right-sided heart failure.

Reference:

1. Grecu L. Autonomic nervous system: physiology and pharmacology. In: Barash PG, Cullen BF, Stoelting RK, et al, eds. *Clinical Anesthesia*. Philadelphia: Wolters Kluwer Health; 2013:362-407.

43. Correct answer: A

Although the 2014 ACC/AHA guidelines outline recommendations for a number of structural and electrophysiological cardiac pathologies, there is no guidance regarding the preoperative management of patients found to have the ECG finding of a left bundle branch block.

Reference:

1. Fleisher LA, Kirsten E, Fleischmann KE, et al. 2014 ACC/AHA Guideline on Perioperative Cardiovascular Evaluation and Management of Patients Undergoing Noncardiac Surgery. *JACC*. 2014;64:e77-e137.

44. Correct answer: C

The conduction velocity through the His-Purkinje system—which includes the Bundle of His as well as the left and right bundle branches, and the Purkinje fibers—is the fastest in the heart. This ensures that both the lateral and septal walls of both ventricles will be depolarized together and contract together.

Reference:

1. Pagel PS, Kampine JP, Stowe DF. Cardiac anatomy and physiology. In: Barash PG, Cullen BF, Stoelting RK, et al, eds. *Clinical Anesthesia*. Philadelphia: Wolters Kluwer Health; 2013:239-262.

45. Correct answer: C

As the transplanted heart is denervated and therefore has no vagal input, many falsely believe acetylcholinesterase inhibitors such as neostigmine to have no effect on the heart rate of these patients. However, as early as 6 months after transplant, innervation begins to be reestablished. Likewise, the cardiac transplant patient's response to neostigmine has been found to produce a dose-dependent bradycardia that is atropine sensitive. (Edrophonium also evokes a bradycardic response in cardiac transplants, although the magnitude of the HR decrease is smaller and less variable.) Furthermore, several case reports describe cardiac arrest as a result of neostigmine administration. The mechanism by which this occurs is not completely understood; however, it is thought to be due to variable vagal reinnervation, as well as denervation hypersensitivity at the level of postganglionic neurons and cardiac muscarinic receptors to acetylcholinesterase inhibitors.

To avoid such a devastating outcome, many advise various strategies to avoid a situation in which administration of neostigmine is necessary, for example, (1) avoidance of long-acting neuromuscular blockers (NMBs), (2) reversal of NMBs with sugammadex where available, and (3) maintenance of muscle relaxation with agents such as remifentanil. Whenever administration of neostigmine is deemed necessary, it should always be coadministered with an antimuscarinic agent (such as glycopyrrolate) to (1) *attempt* to avoid this bradycardic/asystolic response and (2) block the muscarinic receptors elsewhere in the body to avoid other potentially lethal consequences such as bronchorrhea and bronchoconstriction.

All the other medications listed are considered "safe" in transplanted patients.

References:

1. Kostopanagiotou G. Anticholinesterases and the transplanted heart. *Anesth Analg*. 2000;90:1000-1008.
2. Gomez-Rios MA. Anaesthesia for non-cardiac surgery in a cardiac transplant recipient. *Indian J Anaesth*. 2012;56(1):88-89.
3. Kostopanagiotou G, Smyrniotis V, Arkadopoulos N, et al. Anesthetic and perioperative management of adult transplant recipients in nontransplant surgery. *Anesth Analg*. 1999;89:613-622.
4. Bjerke RJ, Mangione MP. Asystole after intravenous neostigmine in a heart transplant recipient. *Can J Anaesth*. 2001;48:305-307.

46. Correct answer: A

CVP TRACING COMPONENT	EVENT	CARDIAC CYCLE	TRICUSPID VALVE
a-wave	Atrial contraction ("kick")	Diastole	Open
c-wave	Isovolumetric ventricular contraction	Systole	Closed
x-descent	Ventricular ejection	Systole	Closed
v-wave	Passive atrial filling	Systole	Closed
y-descent	Passive ventricular filling	Diastole	Open

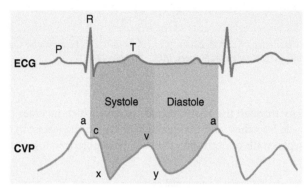

(Redrawn from Mark JB. Central venous pressure monitoring: clinical insights beyond the numbers. *J Cardiothorac Vasc Anesth.* 1991;5:163-173.)

The tricuspid valve closes after atrial contraction (a-wave), and before ventricular contraction (which has 2 components, the c-wave and x-descent). Thus, it occurs between the a- and c-waves.

Reference:
1. Pagel PS, Kampine JP, Stowe DF. Cardiac anatomy and physiology. In: Barash PG, Cullen BF, Stoelting RK, et al, eds. *Clinical Anesthesia.* Philadelphia: Wolters Kluwer Health; 2013:239-262.

47. Correct answer: D

A normal pressure-volume (PV) loop is shown along line 1. The tracing of a PV loop of someone with diastolic dysfunction compared with normal PV loop is indicated in blue with a dashed line. The lines 1 and 2 correspond to passive diastolic filling of the LV during the cardiac cycle. With diastolic dysfunction, there is increased stiffness of the ventricle, and this ventricle would have a higher pressure for any given volume compared with a normal LV. Because of reduced filling of a less compliant ventricle at an increased end-diastolic pressure, a heart with diastolic dysfunction also has a decreased EDV.

Reference:
1. Chatterjee NA, Fifer MA. Heart failure. In: Lilly LS, ed. *Pathophysiology of Heart Disease.* Philadelphia: Wolters Kluwer Health; 2010:216-243.

48. Correct answer: C

Lateral wall ischemia, which corresponds to the vascular territory of the left circumflex artery, will readily be seen as ST elevation in lead V5. Other lateral leads include I, aVL, and V6. Lead II is also monitored intraoperatively, which is primarily used for detecting rhythm and conduction disturbances, as the P wave is most readily apparent in leads II and V1. Inferior wall ischemia can also be observed with ST- and T-wave abnormalities in lead II.

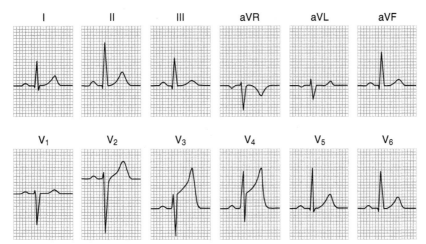

(From Badescu GC, Sherman B, Zaidan JR, Barash PG. Atlas of electrocardiography. In: Barash PG, Cullen BF, Stoelting RK, et al, eds. *Clinical Anesthesia*. Philadelphia: Wolters Kluwer Health; 2010:1701-1720, with permission.)

Reference:
1. Badescu GC, Sherman B, Zaidan JR, Barash PG. Atlas of electrocardiography. In: Barash PG, Cullen BF, Stoelting RK, et al, eds. *Clinical Anesthesia*. Philadelphia: Wolters Kluwer Health; 2010:1701-1720.

49. Correct answer: B

An increase in heart rate is effective in decreasing the regurgitation of blood from the LV to the LA.

	PRELOAD	AFTERLOAD	CONTRACTILITY	HR	DIASTOLIC FUNCTION
Aortic stenosis	Increased	Increased	No change	Decreased	Impaired relaxation
Aortic regurgitation	Increased	Decreased	No change	Increased	Restrictive
Mitral stenosis	Increased	No change	No change	Decreased	Normal
Mitral regurgitation	Decreased or no change	Decreased	No change	Increased	Restrictive
HOCM	Increased	Increased	Decreased	Decreased	Impaired relaxation
Tricuspid stenosis	Increased	Increased or no change	No change	Decreased or no change	Normal
Tricuspid regurgitation	Increased	No change	No change	Increased or no change	Normal
Pulmonic stenosis	Increased	No change	No change	Increased or no change	Normal
Pulmonic regurgitation	Increased	No change	No change	Increased or no change	Normal

a—Typical transmitral Doppler flow velocity profile pattern.
b—Augmentation of preload usually is required to maintain forward stroke volume. However, excessive preload can induce further LV dilation and exacerbate mitral regurgitation and LA HTN.
Adapted from Chaney MA, Cheung AT, Troianos CA, et al. Cardiac anesthesia. In: Longnecker DE, Brown DL, Newman MF, Zapol WM, eds. Anesthesiology. New York: McGraw-Hill Education; 2012:898-926.

Reference:
1. Chaney MA, Cheung AT, Troianos CA, et al. Cardiac anesthesia. In: Longnecker DE, Brown DL, Newman MF, Zapol WM, eds. *Anesthesiology*. New York: McGraw-Hill Education; 2012:898-926.

50. Correct answer: D

AV nodal blocking agents such as metoprolol (β-blockers, class II antiarrhythmics) and verapamil (calcium channel blockers, class IV antiarrhythmics) should be avoided as a treatment for tachydysrhythmias in those with accessory pathways such as Wolff-Parkinson-White patients. Slowing or blocking conduction at the AV node instead channels atrial impulses to the ventricles via the accessory pathway, which has no "filter," and is capable of impulse conduction at a much faster rate as compared to the AV node.

References:

1. Grecu L. Autonomic nervous system: physiology and pharmacology. In: Barash PG, Cullen BF, Stoelting RK, et al, eds. *Clinical Anesthesia*. Philadelphia: Wolters Kluwer Health; 2013:362-407.
2. Butterworth JF, Mackey DC. Anesthesia for patients with cardiovascular disease. In: *Morgan and Mikhail's Clinical Anesthesiology*. 5th ed. Philadelphia: McGraw Hill; 2013:375-434.
3. Hu R, Stevenson WG, Strichartz GR, Lilly LS. Mechanisms of cardiac arrhythmias. In: Lilly LS, ed. *Pathophysiology of Heart Disease*. Philadelphia: Wolters Kluwer Health; 2010:261-278.

51. Correct answer: B

Congenital heart defects can be broadly classified into 2 groups: acyanotic and cyanotic lesions. Acyanotic lesions include atrial septal defects, ventricular setpal defects, pulmonic stenosis, and coarctation of the aorta. Cyanotic lesions are thus named because they involve shunting of deoxygenated blood from the right to left. They can be remembered by the popular mnemonic of the "5 T's"

1. Truncus arteriosus (1 vessel)
2. Transposition (2 switched vessels)
3. Tricuspid atresia (Tri = 3)
4. Tetralogy of Fallot (Tetra = 4)
5. TAPVR (total anomalous pulmonary venous return = 5 words)

References:

1. Berg DD, Brown DW. Congenital heart disease. In: Lilly LS, ed. *Pathophysiology of Heart Disease*. Philadelphia: Wolters Kluwer Health; 2010:361-385.
2. Le T, Bhushan V. *First Aid for the USMLE Step 1 2014*. New York: McGraw-Hill Education; 2014.

52. Correct answer: B

Many complications are possible when performing a transcatheter aortic valve replacement, both in the intraoperative and postoperative periods. A hematoma/hemorrhage is possible at the site of arterial cannulation, most commonly the groin (femoral artery). Femoral artery or aortic dissection is also possible. As catheters travel up toward the heart from this site, showering of emboli is possible, resulting in embolic stroke, myocardial infarction, or other embolic phenomenon. Frequently, valvuloplasty will be performed before valve deployment. It is not uncommon to see new conduction abnormalities such as left bundle branch blocks or complete heart block after valvuloplasty. A feared complication of valve deployment is aortic root rupture, which if not contained leads to catastrophic hemodynamic collapse. If contained, this aortic root rupture can present as would cardiac tamponade or hemothorax. If the valve is malpositioned too close to the AV node, complete heart block may again be observed. If the valve is deployed slightly too high, it may occlude one of the coronary ostia, essentially causing a myocardial infarction, which would present as regional wall motion abnormalities on TEE.

Reference:

1. Jaffe RA, Schmiesing CA, Golanu B. Cardiovascular surgery. In: *Anesthesiologist's Manual of Surgical Procedures*. 5th ed. Philidelphia: Wolters Kluwer; 2014:345-478.

53. Correct answer: A

It seems as though the patient above is having an acute CHF exacerbation because of eating a (presumably) high-salt content meal at the wedding reception. An S3 usually indicates volume overload owing to CHF, but is transient, and will no longer be heard if the patient above is diuresed appropriately. However, an S4 gallop indicates a stiff ventricle (ie, from chronic uncontrolled HTN) and is a permanent finding even if the patient's blood pressure is adequately controlled with antihypertensive agents.

Reference:

1. Jung H, Lilly LS. The cardiac cycle: mechanisms of heart sounds and murmurs. In: Lilly LS, ed. *Pathophysiology of Heart Disease*. Philadelphia: Wolters Kluwer Health; 2010:28-43.

54. Correct answer: D

Severe tachycardia, hypotension, and anemia are all factors in determining myocardial oxygen balance, whereas potassium balance does not play a role. Tachycardia both increases demand directly and decreases supply by decreasing diastolic time. Hypotension directly decreases coronary blood flow. Severe anemia decreases the amount of oxygen delivered to the myocardium by affecting the hemoglobin factor on the supply side.

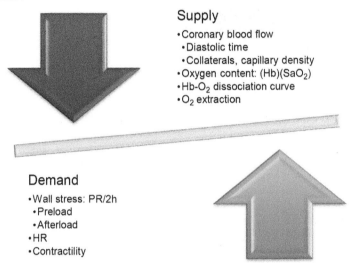

(Adapted from Skubas NJ, Lichtman AD, Sharma A, Thomas SJ. Anesthesia for cardiac surgery. In: Barash PG, Cullen BF, Stoelting RK, et al, eds. *Clinical Anesthesia*. Philadelphia: Wolters Kluwer Health; 2013:1077, with permission.)

Reference:
1. Skubas NJ, Lichtman AD, Sharma A, Thomas SJ. Anesthesia for cardiac surgery. In: Barash PG, Cullen BF, Stoelting RK, et al, eds. *Clinical Anesthesia*. Philadelphia: Wolters Kluwer Health; 2013:1077.

55. Correct answer: A

Oftentimes the mixed venous O_2 saturation (Svo_2) at rest will be normal in HFpEF. The most sensitive test to assess the adequacy of tissue perfusion would actually be to measure the Svo_2 at exertion.

References:
1. Skubas NJ, Lichtman AD, Sharma A, Thomas SJ. Anesthesia for cardiac surgery. In: Barash PG, Cullen BF, Stoelting RK, et al, eds. *Clinical Anesthesia*. Philadelphia: Wolters Kluwer Health; 2013:1076-1111.
2. Butterworth JF, Mackey DC. Anesthesia for patients with cardiovascular disease. In: *Morgan and Mikhail's Clinical Anesthesiology*. 5th ed. Philadelphia: McGraw Hill; 2013:375-434.

56. Correct answer: C

The vagus nerve secretes acetylcholine, which acts on M2 receptors to slow heart rate. Muting of the SA node, which has an intrinsic pacemaker activity of 60-100 beats per minute, makes it more likely for junctional rhythms (40-60 bpm) to predominate. The normal intrinsic rate of the SA node in young adults is about 90-100 beats per minute and **decreases** with age. Phase 4 is the "funny current," which is always leaking, and β1-adrenergic stimulation increases the rate of depolarization, therefore increasing the heart rate.

References:
1. Pagel PS, Kampine JP, Stowe DF. Cardiac anatomy and physiology. In: Barash PG, Cullen BF, Stoelting RK, et al, eds. *Clinical Anesthesia*. Philadelphia: Wolters Kluwer Health; 2013:239-262.
2. Butterworth JF, Mackey DC. Anesthesia for patients with cardiovascular disease. In: *Morgan and Mikhail's Clinical Anesthesiology*. 5th ed. Philadelphia: McGraw Hill; 2013:375-434.

57. Correct answer: B

Reverse Trendelenburg puts patients with their lower extremities down and head up, which pools their blood volume in their lower extremities (by gravity), decreasing venous return to the heart. The patients may become profoundly hypotensive, especially if they are volume depleted (ie, bowel prep) or if a neuraxial anesthetic is being used, resulting in sympatholysis. Cerebral perfusion may drop as a result of decreased venous return (if the heart is not able to compensate and cardiac output is low). One would expect afterload to increase and inotropy to increase as compensatory mechanisms in a normal healthy patient.

Reference:

1. Pagel PS, Kampine JP, Stowe DF. Cardiac anatomy and physiology. In: Barash PG, Cullen BF, Stoelting RK, et al, eds. *Clinical Anesthesia*. Philadelphia: Wolters Kluwer Health; 2013:239-262.

58. Correct answer: A

With HOCM, the asymmetrically hypertrophied interventricular septum bulges into the left ventricular outflow tract (LVOT) from one side, and by Venturi forces, the anterior leaflet of the mitral valve gets drawn into the LVOT during systole from the other side and obstructs outflow in this manner (dynamic obstruction). Anything that decreases the size of the LV (ie, increased contractility or HR, or decreased preload or afterload) increases this gradient that favors obstruction. The anesthetic management of patients with HOCM is aimed at maintaining ventricular filling and avoiding factors predisposing to LVOT obstruction.

Reference:

1. Skubas NJ, Lichtman AD, Sharma A, Thomas SJ. Anesthesia for cardiac surgery. In: Barash PG, Cullen BF, Stoelting RK, et al, eds. *Clinical Anesthesia*. Philadelphia: Wolters Kluwer Health; 2013:1076-1111.

59. Correct answer: D

Stiff ventricles (ie, diastolic dysfunction) are most sensitive to loss of atrial kick because they lose a significant amount of preload during passive ventricular filling. Blood is prematurely arrested flowing down its pressure gradient from LA to LV because the pressure on the LV side is higher from the stiffened ventricle/increased LVEDP. This stiffened ventricle is unable to accommodate extra volume via this passive mechanism and therefore needs the "atrial kick."

Patients with mitral regurgitation are not affected by the loss of an "atrial kick" because a large portion of the regurgitant blood flows back into the atrium with each ventricular systole.

The resulting hemodynamic collapse that can be seen in patients with mitral stenosis and atrial fibrillation with rapid ventricular response is usually secondary to tachycardia in itself and not directly related to the absence of the "atrial kick."

Reference:

1. Skubas NJ, Lichtman AD, Sharma A, Thomas SJ. Anesthesia for cardiac surgery. In: Barash PG, Cullen BF, Stoelting RK, et al, eds. *Clinical Anesthesia*. Philadelphia: Wolters Kluwer Health; 2013:1076-1111.

60. Correct answer: B

In a patient with mitral stenosis, the pulmonary capillary wedge pressure is *greater than* the LVEDP, and the difference is at least the amount, that is, the transmitral pressure gradient. Pulmonary edema can indeed be precipitated by states of increased forward flow (tachycardia) such as sepsis, pregnancy, and hyperthyroidism. This is more formally related in the equation

$$LAP = LVDP + \left[\frac{flow}{(K)(MVA)} \right]^2$$

where LAP = left atrial pressure, LVDP = left ventricular diastolic pressure, K = hydraulic pressure constant, and MVA = mitral valve area.

LAP increases with increased flow.

Persistently elevated LAP is reflected back through pulmonary vasculature, causing pulmonary HTN and ultimately right ventricular hypertrophy. Once the patient develops pulmonary HTN, the operative risk is now increased.

Mitral stenosis is a pathology that should ultimately be surgically treated with a valve replacement, but if being medically managed, the hemodynamic goal is to decrease the heart rate via β-blockade.

Reference:

1. Skubas NJ, Lichtman AD, Sharma A, Thomas SJ. Anesthesia for cardiac surgery. In: Barash PG, Cullen BF, Stoelting RK, et al, eds. *Clinical Anesthesia*. Philadelphia: Wolters Kluwer Health; 2013:1076-1111.

6

GI AND HEPATIC SYSTEMS

Qing Yang

1. **What percentage of *hepatic blood flow* comes from the portal vein?**

   A. 25%
   B. 50%
   C. 75%
   D. 90%

2. **What percentage of *oxygen delivery* to the liver comes from the hepatic artery?**

   A. 25%
   B. 50%
   C. 75%
   D. 90%

3. **Hepatomegaly may be observed in all of the following conditions EXCEPT which one?**

   A. Congestive heart failure
   B. Hypovolemic shock
   C. Leukemia
   D. Renal failure

4. **The round ligament separates which 2 hepatic segments?**

   A. 1 and 2
   B. 2 and 3
   C. 3 and 4
   D. 4 and 5

5. **Which of the following signaling factors is *decreased* in a cirrhotic liver?**

   A. Nitric oxide
   B. Endothelin
   C. Norepinephrine
   D. Thromboxane A2

6. Compared with the hepatic artery, which statement about portal vein is true?

   A. Portal vein supplies 50% of the liver's overall blood flow.
   B. Portal vein is a low-pressure/low-resistance system.
   C. Portal vein blood is richly oxygenated.
   D. Portal vein supplies 75% of the liver's overall oxygen delivery.

7. *Increase* in the serum level of which of the following may be observed in liver failure?

   A. IgG
   B. Factor VII
   C. Albumin
   D. Ammonia

8. Glucose is synthesized in the liver as the result of all of the following processes EXCEPT which one?

   A. Glycogenolysis
   B. Gluconeogenesis
   C. Tricarboxylic acid cycle
   D. Oxidation of lactate

9. In the assessment of patient with liver failure, which parameter is used in the MELD (model for end-stage liver disease) scoring system but NOT the Child-Pugh scoring system?

   A. Creatinine
   B. International normalized ratio (INR)
   C. Bilirubin
   D. Albumin

10. *Elevation* in the serum level of which factor is a specific marker of acute liver injury?

   A. Aspartate aminotransferase (AST)
   B. Alanine aminotransferase (ALT)
   C. Alkaline phosphatase
   D. Lactate dehydrogenase (LDH)

11. Which laboratory test is a sensitive indicator for decreased synthetic function of the liver?

   A. Aspartate aminotransferase
   B. Albumin
   C. International normalized ratio
   D. γ-Glutamyl transpeptidase (GGT)

12. A liver failure patient may show all of the following clinical signs EXCEPT which one?

   A. Jaundice
   B. Easy bruising
   C. Confusion
   D. Hyperglycemia

13. The level of which coagulation factor may not be affected by advanced liver disease?

   A. II
   B. V
   C. VII
   D. VIII

14. **A patient with an elevated total serum bilirubin and an elevated indirect serum bilirubin may have which of the following conditions?**

    A. Gilbert syndrome
    B. Primary biliary cirrhosis
    C. Primary sclerosing cholangitis
    D. Wilson disease

15. **Which of the following is the mechanism by which lactulose relieves symptoms of hepatic encephalopathy?**

    A. Inhibition of hepatic ammonia production
    B. Increasing the conversion of ammonia to urea
    C. Acidification of the colon
    D. Diuresis to decrease intracranial pressure

16. **Metabolism and clearance of morphine may be *increased* in which of the following situations?**

    A. Congestive heart failure
    B. Inhaled anesthetics
    C. Intra-abdominal surgery
    D. Sepsis

17. **The clearance of which of the following drugs through the liver is NOT dependent on liver blood flow?**

    A. Propofol
    B. Morphine
    C. Fentanyl
    D. Midazolam

18. **Inducers of cytochrome P450 system include all of the following EXCEPT which one?**

    A. Ethanol
    B. Phenytoin
    C. Isoniazid
    D. Rifampin

19. **A 60-year-old man who has just been listed for a liver transplant remains overly sedated for 24 hours after being administered midazolam 4 mg IV. What other medication might he be taking at the same time?**

    A. Erythromycin
    B. Penicillin
    C. Gentamicin
    D. Vancomycin

20. **A patient with deactivating mutation in the cytochrome P450 2D6 gene may have *ineffective* analgesia from which of the following opioids?**

    A. Morphine
    B. Codeine
    C. Fentanyl
    D. Methadone

Chapter 6 ▪ Answers

1. Correct answer: C

The liver has dual blood supply consisting of 75% from portal vein and 25% from hepatic artery. Although portal blood is deoxygenated, its higher flow rate results in equivalent oxygen delivery as compared with the hepatic artery. Portal blood flows into the hepatic sinusoids from portal venules through inlet sphincters. Hepatic arterioles enter the sinusoids through arteriosinus twigs (portal venules). The portal vein, hepatic artery, and bile duct together form the portal triad. Unlike other organs the liver regulates its blood flow independent of autonomic or systemic factors. If portal blood flow decreases, arterial blood supply can be increased through paracrine vasodilators, such as adenosine and nitric oxide.

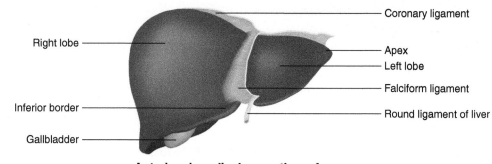

A **Anterior view, diaphragmatic surface**

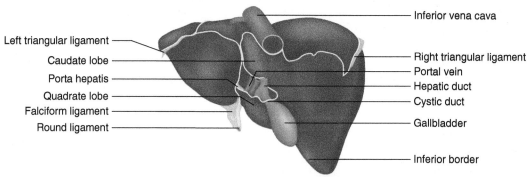

B **Posterior-inferior view, visceral surface**

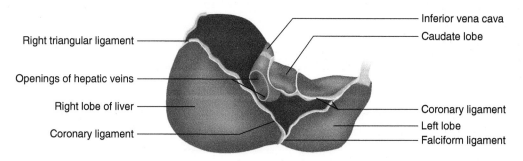

C **Superior view**

(From Moore KL, Agur AMR, Dalley AF. *Clinically Oriented Anatomy.* 7th ed. Philadelphia: Wolters Kluwer; 2013, with permission.)

Reference:
1. Chapman N. Liver anatomy and physiology. In: Barash PG, Cullen BF, Stoelting RK, et al, eds. *Clinical Anesthesia Fundamentals.* Philadelphia: Lippincott; 2015:109-118.

2. **Correct answer: B**

The liver has dual blood supply. The flow ratio is 75% from portal vein, which provides blood from the intestines and spleen, and 25% from the hepatic artery, which provides arterial blood directly. Although the portal blood is deoxygenated, the higher flow results in equivalent oxygen delivery (50%) compared with hepatic artery.

The reason for this distribution is that that oxygen delivery depends on both the oxygen content of blood and tissue blood flow:

$$\text{Delivery O}_2 = \text{content O}_2 \times \text{blood flow}$$

Oxygen content is calculated by the following equation:

$$\text{Content O}_2 = \left(\text{Hb} \times 1.39 \times \text{sat O}_2\right) + \left(\text{pressure O}_2 \times 0.003\right)$$

References:

1. Chapman N. Liver anatomy and physiology. In: Barash PG, Cullen BF, Stoelting RK, et al, eds. *Clinical Anesthesia Fundamentals*. Philadelphia: Lippincott; 2015:109-118.
2. Pierce ET, Wiklund RA. Evaluation of patients with hepatic disease. In: Longnecker DE, Brown DL, Newman MF, et al, eds. *Anesthesiology*. 2nd ed. New York: McGraw Hill; 2012:180-195.
3. Barash PG, Cullen BF, Stoelting RK, et al. Formulas. In: *Clinical Anesthesia Fundamentals*. Philadelphia: Lippincott; 2015: 825-828.

3. **Correct answer: B**

Because of its sinusoidal nature, the liver functions as an autologous reservoir for blood and is thus able to store blood during high blood volume states. In low blood volume states, these stores are readily mobilized. Several conditions associated with high volume states are known to cause hepatomegaly. With congestive heart failure, especially right-sided heart failure, excess fluid backs up into the liver through the vena cava and hepatic veins, leading to hepatomegaly. In renal failure, protein loss and impaired filtration of the kidneys lead to fluid accumulation, and increased volume is absorbed into the liver, leading to enlargement. The liver is also part of the mononuclear phagocyte system (aka reticuloendothelial system), which contributes to coordinated immune function. Hepatosplenomegaly is a common symptom of leukemia and other blood malignancies. Conversely, in hypovolemia, the liver "squeezes" blood out into the systemic circulation to augment low blood volume; thus it is not enlarged.

Reference:

1. Chapman N. Liver anatomy and physiology. In: Barash PG, Cullen BF, Stoelting RK, et al, eds. *Clinical Anesthesia Fundamentals*. Philadelphia: Lippincott; 2015:109-118.

4. **Correct answer: C**

Conventionally, the liver is divided into 8 segments based on the branching pattern of the portal vein and hepatic veins, a pattern that was first noted by the French surgeon Claude Couinaud. The left portal vein supplies segments 2, 3, and 4, whereas the right branches into segments 5, 6, 7, and 8. Segment 1 is considered part of the caudate lobe and supplied by small branches near the portal bifurcation. The boundary between the segments is not clearly defined by surface anatomy when looking at an intact liver, with the exception of round ligament dividing segments 3 and 4 and the gallbladder fossa dividing segments 4 and 5.

Extended right hepatectomy (right trisegmentectomy)

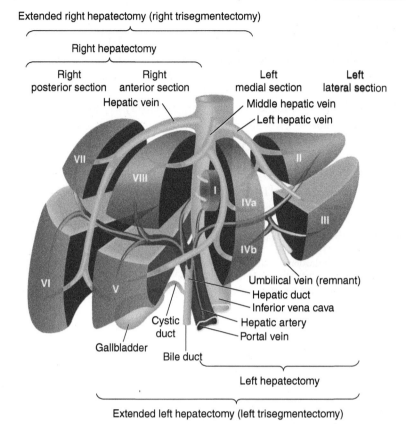

(From Chapman N. Liver anatomy and physiology. In: Barash PG, Cullen BF, Stoelting RK, et al, eds. *Clinical Anesthesia Fundamentals*. Philadelphia: Lippincott; 2015:109-118, with permission.)

References:
1. Pierce ET, Wiklund RA. Evaluation of patients with hepatic disease. In: Longnecker DE, Brown DL, Newman MF, et al, eds. *Anesthesiology*. 2nd ed. New York: McGraw Hill; 2012:180-195.
2. Majno P, Mentha G, Toso C, et al. Anatomy of the liver: an outline with three levels of complexity – a further step towards tailored territorial liver resections. *J Hepatol*. 2014;60:654-662.

5. **Correct answer: A**

Liver cirrhosis occurs via remodeling of liver cells, including sinusoidal endothelial cells, hepatic stellate cells, and Kuffer cells. The dysfunctional cells acquire a vasoconstrictor phenotype and increase release of endogenous vasoconstrictors, including endothelin, thromboxane A2, and norepinephrine, leading to increase in hepatic vascular resistance and portal hypertension. Nitric oxide (NO) is the most important vasodilator regulating the hepatic vascular tone. NO production is reduced in cirrhosis, likely secondary to decreased endothelial nitric oxide synthase (eNOS) activity and increased NO scavenging, further aggravating portal hypertension.

References:
1. Chapman N. Liver anatomy and physiology. In: Barash PG, Cullen BF, Stoelting RK, et al, eds. *Clinical Anesthesia Fundamentals*. Philadelphia: Lippincott; 2015:109-118.
2. Garcia-Pagan JC, Gracia-Sancho J, Bosch J. Functional aspects on the pathophysiology of portal hypertension in cirrhosis. *J Hepatol*. 2012;57:458-461.

6. **Correct answer: B**

The liver has dual blood supply, 75% from the portal vein and 25% from the hepatic artery, each of which account for half of the oxygen delivered to the liver. The valveless portal vein is a low-pressure/low-resistance, or capacitance, system, whereas the hepatic artery is a high-pressure/high-resistance system. The hepatic artery pressure is similar to that in the aorta. Portal vein pressure is reported to be 6-10 mm Hg in normal subjects. Portal pressure depends on constriction or dilation of the mesenteric and splanchnic vascular beds and intrahepatic resistance. With liver cirrhosis, intrahepatic resistance increases, leading to portal hypertension.

References:
1. Chapman N. Liver anatomy and physiology. In: Barash PG, Cullen BF, Stoelting RK, et al, eds. *Clinical Anesthesia Fundamentals*. Philadelphia: Lippincott; 2015:109-118.
2. Eipel C, Abshagen K, Vollmar B. Regulation of hepatic blood flow: the hepatic arterial buffer response revisited. *World J Gastroenterol*. 2010;16:6046-6057.

7. Correct answer: D

The liver is responsible for the synthesis of the majority of blood proteins, including albumin, vitamin K–dependent coagulation factors (II, VII, IX, and X), and vitamin K–independent coagulation factors (V, XI, XII, and XIII and fibrinogen). A decrease in albumin production during liver failure can lead to fluid accumulation and ascites. A decrease in factor VII production during liver failure can lead to coagulation defects and elevated PT/INR.

The liver also functions to detoxify drugs and other substances produced endogenously. Ammonia is the breakdown product of amino acid metabolism and converted to urea in the liver. Following breakdown, urea is then secreted via the urine. In liver failure, ammonia accumulates, which can in turn lead to hepatic encephalopathy.

One class of serum proteins that are not manufactured by the liver are antibodies. IgG is an antibody produced by B cells in lymphoid tissue. IgG levels are not affected by liver function.

Reference:
1. Chapman N. Liver anatomy and physiology. In: Barash PG, Cullen BF, Stoelting RK, et al, eds. *Clinical Anesthesia Fundamentals*. Philadelphia: Lippincott; 2015:109-118.

8. Correct answer: C

In the fasting state, the liver breaks down glycogen stored in hepatocytes. This process is stimulated by glucagon from the pancreatic α cells and catecholamines from the adrenal medulla. These hormones activate glycogen phosphorylase, which hydrolyzes glycogen into glucose. In prolonged starvation, glycogen stores are depleted secondary to glycogenolysis, and hepatocytes produce glucose through gluconeogenesis using lactate, pyruvate, glycerol, and amino acids. During this process, lactate is oxidized by LDH to generate pyruvate, which is converted to glucose after multiple biochemical reactions. In comparison, the tricarboxylic acid cycle, aka citric acid cycle or Krebs cycle, is a catabolic process through which acetyl-CoA is consumed to produce ATP and is involved in the breakdown of glucose when it is readily available in the fed state.

References:
1. Chapman N. Liver anatomy and physiology. In: Barash PG, Cullen BF, Stoelting RK, et al, eds. *Clinical Anesthesia Fundamentals*. Philadelphia: Lippincott; 2015:109-118.
2. Rui L. Energy metabolism in the liver. *Comp Physiol*. 2014;4:177-197.

9. Correct answer: A

Two commonly used tools for assessing patients with liver failure are the MELD and the Child-Pugh scoring systems. The MELD score uses 3 laboratory values, INR, creatinine, and bilirubin, in a logarithmic calculation and correlates linearly with predicted 30-day mortality. A MELD <8 confers a mortality of 6%, whereas a MELD >20 is associated with >50% mortality.

The Child-Pugh score utilizes both laboratory and clinical factors to classify patients. Laboratory values required to calculate this score are PT, INR, albumin, and bilirubin. Clinical features that also play a role in the score are degree of ascites and encephalopathy. Child-Pugh class A has 10% perioperative mortality, class B has 30%, and class C has 70%.

Modified Child-Pugh Score

	POINTS[a]		
Presentation	1	2	3
Albumin (g/dL)	>3.5	2.8-3.5	<2.8
Prothrombin time			
Seconds prolonged	<4	4-6	>6
International normalized ratio	<1.7	1.7-2.3	>2.3
Bilirubin (mg/dL)[b]	<2	2-3	>3
Ascites	Absent	Slight to moderate	Tense
Encephalopathy	None	Grades I-II	Grades III-IV

[a]Class A = 5-6 points; B = 7-9 points, C = 10-15 points. Perioperative mortality: Class A: 10%, B: 30%, C: >80%.
[b]For cholestatic diseases, assign 1, 2, and 3 points for bilirubin <4, 4-10, and >10 mg/dL, respectively.
From Kamath PS. Clinical approach to the patient with abnormal liver test results. Mayo Clin Proc. 1996;71:1089, with permission.

Reference:

1. Krishnan S. Anesthetic considers in patients with obesity, hepatic disease, and other gastrointestinal diseases. In: Barash PG, Cullen BF, Stoelting RK, et al, eds. *Clinical Anesthesia Fundamentals*. Philadelphia: Lippincott; 2013:519-538.

10. Correct answer: B

Standard laboratory tests can provide information on hepatocellular integrity, synthetic function of the liver, cholestasis, and systemic effects of organ dysfunction. During liver injury, enzymes that normally reside in hepatocytes may leak out into the blood because of cellular damage. These enzymes include AST, ALT, AP (alkaline phosphatase), and GGT.

ALT and GGT are both almost exclusively found in the liver; however, GGT is generally elevated with biliary tract disease. ALT thus represents the most specific markers of livery injury. In comparison, AST, which although is also found in hepatocytes, is present in muscle and other nonhepatic tissue. Additionally, alkaline phosphatase is found in bone, intestines, and the placenta and is not specific to hepatic injury. LDH is a nonspecific marker that is increased with hemolysis, rhabdomyolysis, tumor necrosis, and myocardial infarction and is not specifically associated with liver damage.

References:

1. Chapman N. Liver anatomy and physiology. In: Barash PG, Cullen BF, Stoelting RK, et al, eds. *Clinical Anesthesia Fundamentals*. Philadelphia: Lippincott; 2015:109-118.
2. Rui L. Energy metabolism in the liver. *Comp Physiol.* 2014;4:177-197.

11. Correct answer: C

The liver synthesizes vitamin K–dependent coagulation factors (II, VII, IX, and X), which are necessary to maintain normal PT/INR values. The short half-life of factor VII (4-6 h) makes INR the most sensitive indicator for acute changes in liver's synthetic function. Albumin, which is also synthesized by the liver, has a relatively long half-life (2-3 wk), and decreases in serum albumin level may be attributed to loss through kidneys and the GI tract in addition to decreased synthesis in the liver. AST can be a marker for hepatocellular injury (ie, hepatocyte integrity) but not the synthetic function of the liver. GGT is an enzyme whose levels are a sensitive marker for biliary tract disease (ie, excretory function).

Liver Function Tests

FUNCTION	TEST	REMARKS
Hepatocyte integrity	AST	Formerly, SGOT. Produced in the liver, heart, skeletal muscle, kidney, brain, and red blood cells.
	ALT	Formerly, SGPT. Produced in the liver.
	LDH	Also increased with hemolysis, rhabdomyolysis, tumor necrosis, myocardial infarction.
	GST	Released from cells in the centrilobular region (zone 3). Sensitive marker of centrilobular necrosis in the early stages. Short plasma half-life (30 min).
Synthetic function	Albumin	Protein loss through the gastrointestinal tract and kidneys and increased catabolism can also cause hypoalbuminemia. Long half-life (2-3 wk).
	PT/INR	Both bile salt–mediated vitamin K absorption and hepatic synthesis of coagulation factors are necessary to maintain normal PT/INR. Short half-life of factor VII (4-6 h) makes PT/INR a sensitive indicator of acute liver disease.
	Ammonia	Markedly elevated in patients with hepatic encephalopathy, when hepatic urea synthesis is disrupted.
Excretory function	Alkaline phosphatase	Present in biliary canaliculi, bone, intestine, liver, and placenta. Lacks specificity for hepatobiliary disease.
	GGT	Elevated in hepatobiliary disease, closely tracks alkaline phosphatase in timeline. Most sensitive laboratory marker of biliary tract disease, but not specific.
	5′ NT	Elevations are specific to hepatobiliary obstruction.
	Bilirubin	Product of heme catabolism. Indirect (unconjugated) hyperbilirubinemia happens in prehepatic disease, whereas direct (conjugated) hyperbilirubinemia is present in intrahepatic or extrahepatic bile duct obstruction. Hepatic disease causes elevation of both kinds of bilirubin.

5′ NT, 5′-nucleotidase; ALT, alanine aminotransferase; AST, aspartate aminotransferase; GGT, γ-glutamyl transferase; GST, glutathione S-transferase; LDH, lactate dehydrogenase; PT/INR, prothrombin time/international normalized ratio; SGOT, serum glutamic-oxaloacetic transaminase; SGPT, serum glutamic-pyruvic transaminase.
From Krishnan S. Anesthetic considerations for patients with obesity, hepatic diseas, and other gastrointestinal issues. In: Barash PG, Cullen BF, Stoelting RK, et al, eds. Clinical Anesthesia Fundamentals. Philadelphia: Wolters Kluwer; 2015:528, with permission.

References:
1. Krishnan S. Anesthetic considers in patients with obesity, hepatic disease, and other gastrointestinal diseases. In: Barash PG, Cullen BF, Stoelting RK, et al, eds. *Clinical Anesthesia Fundamentals*. Philadelphia: Lippincott; 2013:519-538.
2. Chapman N. Liver anatomy and physiology. In: Barash PG, Cullen BF, Stoelting RK, et al, eds. *Clinical Anesthesia Fundamentals*. Philadelphia: Lippincott; 2015:109-118.

12. **Correct answer: D**

The liver converts excess blood glucose into glycogen and releases glucose back into the blood through glycogenosis and gluconeogenesis during starvation. This process is regulated by insulin, glucagon, and catecholamines. The liver also plays a crucial role in the metabolism of insulin. Liver failure is associated with hyperinsulinemia and hypoglycemia, not hyperglycemia.

Jaundice arises from excess bilirubin. Easy bruising results from decreased coagulation factor production. Confusion may be manifestation of haptic encephalopathy from high ammonia levels. All 3 of which can be seen in liver failure.

Clinical Manifestations of Cirrhosis and Portal Hypertension

Cardiovascular	Hyperdynamic circulation
	Low systemic vascular resistance
	Low systemic systolic blood pressure
	Systolic and diastolic dysfunction
	Reduced effective circulating volume
Pulmonary	Decreased functional residual capacity
	Restrictive ventilation due to ascites and pleural effusion
	Hepatopulmonary syndrome
	Portopulmonary hypertension
Gastrointestinal	Ascites
	Esophageal varices
	Hemorrhoids
	Gastrointestinal bleeding
Renal	Salt and water retention
	Decreased renal function
	Hepatorenal syndrome
Hematologic	Anemia
	Coagulopathy
	Thrombocytopenia
	Spontaneous bacterial peritonitis
Metabolic	Sodium, potassium, calcium, and magnesium abnormalities
	Hypoalbuminemia
	Hypoglycemia
Neurologic	Hepatic encephalopathy

From Krishnan S. Anesthetic considerations for patients with obesity, hepatic diseas, and other gastrointestinal issues. In: Barash PG, Cullen BF, Stoelting RK, et al, eds. Clinical Anesthesia Fundamentals. *Philadelphia: Wolters Kluwer; 2015:529, with permission.*

References:

1. Chapman N. Liver anatomy and physiology. In: Barash PG, Cullen BF, Stoelting RK, et al, eds. *Clinical Anesthesia Fundamentals*. Philadelphia: Lippincott; 2015:109-118.
2. Krishnan S. Anesthetic considers in patients with obesity, hepatic disease, and other gastrointestinal diseases. In: Barash PG, Cullen BF, Stoelting RK, et al, eds. *Clinical Anesthesia Fundamentals*. Philadelphia: Lippincott; 2013:519-538.

---

13. **Correct answer: D**

The liver produces all vitamin K–dependent factors, which are II, VII, IX, and X, and some vitamin K–independent factors, including factors V, XI, XII, and XIII. The liver also produces fibrinogen (factor I) and proteins C and S. Factor VIII is produced by both the liver and endothelial cells throughout the body. For this reason, factor VIII levels will likely be normal even in advanced liver disease.

References:

1. Chapman N. Liver anatomy and physiology. In: Barash PG, Cullen BF, Stoelting RK, et al, eds. *Clinical Anesthesia Fundamentals*. Philadelphia: Lippincott; 2015:109-118.
2. Carabini LM, Ramsey G. Blood therapy. In: Barash PG, Cullen BF, Stoelting RK, et al, eds. *Clinical Anesthesia Fundamentals*. Philadelphia: Lippincott; 2013:451-468.

14. **Correct answer: A**

The liver conjugates bilirubin with glucuronic acid to produce water-soluble bilirubin that is excreted in the bile. Gilbert syndrome is an inherited disorder of bilirubin metabolism. It is caused by mutation in the gene that codes for uridine diphosphate-glucuronosyltransferase, an enzyme that mediates the glucuronidation of bilirubin. Patients with Gilbert syndrome present with an unconjugated (indirect) hyperbilirubinemia triggered by physical stressors such as viral infections, dehydration, and physical exertion. Gilbert syndrome is a benign condition and does not lead to progressive liver disease. However, Crigler-Najjar syndrome is a severe variant of the same enzyme deficiency, necessitating intervention.

Other causes of unconjugated hyperbilirubinemia (elevated total bilirubin with normal direct bilirubin levels) include hemolysis, hematoma, and neonatal jaundice. Primary biliary cirrhosis and primary sclerosing cholangitis affect the bile ducts and result in conjugated hyperbilirubinemia. Wilson disease is an autosomal-recessive disorder of copper metabolism, which can lead to fulminant hepatic failure if treatment with penicillamine (a copper chelator) is not undertaken and there is an elevation in both conjugated and unconjugated bilirubin.

References:
1. Pierce ET, Wiklund RA. Evaluation of patients with hepatic disease. In: Longnecker DE, Brown DL, Newman MF, et al, eds. *Anesthesiology*. 2nd ed. New York: McGraw Hill; 2012:180-195.
2. Fargo MV, Grogan SP, Saguil A. Evaluation of jaundice in adults. *Am Fam Physician*. 2017;95(3):164-168.

15. **Correct answer: C**

Ammonia is produced by protein metabolism and readily crosses from the gut into blood. In the liver it is converted into urea, which is then excreted in the urine. In liver failure, excess blood levels of ammonia can lead to hepatic encephalopathy, and symptoms include confusion, agitation, and coma.

Lactulose is a synthetic sugar, which is converted into lactic acid by colonic bacteria, increasing the acidity of the colon. In the acidified colon, ammonia is converted to the ammonium ion, which is unable to pass from the gut into the blood and is then eliminated in stool. Lactulose does not affect the production or metabolism of ammonia. It also does not affect intracranial pressure. Other interventions for hepatic encephalopathy include neomycin, which decreases the ammonia-producing bacteria in the gut, and in severe cases, exchange transfusion or extracorporal organ perfusion can be utilized.

Reference:
1. Pierce ET, Wiklund RA. Evaluation of patients with hepatic disease. In: Longnecker DE, Brown DL, Newman MF, et al, eds. *Anesthesiology*. 2nd ed. New York: McGraw Hill; 2012:180-195.

16. **Correct Answer: D**

Morphine is a drug with a high extraction ratio whose clearance and metabolism through liver depends on liver blood flow. Drugs with high extraction ratios undergo significant first-pass metabolism and are often referred to as high clearance drugs. This contrasts with drugs with low extraction ratios, which require a prolonged period of time for biotransformation and are often protein bound.

Conditions that increase liver blood flow, such as sepsis (high cardiac output), can increase morphine clearance. On the other hand, conditions that decrease liver blood flow, such as congestive heart failure, will slow down morphine clearance. Inhaled anesthetic use and intra-abdominal surgery have been shown to decrease liver blood flow by more than 80% and thus would slow down morphine metabolism.

Examples of Hepatic Clearance Patterns of Common Pharmaceuticals

HIGH CLEARANCE (HIGH EXTRACTION RATIO THAT IS BLOOD FLOW DEPENDENT)	INTERMEDIATE CLEARANCE	LOW CLEARANCE (LOW EXTRACTION RATIO THAT IS BLOOD FLOW INDEPENDENT)
Morphine	Aspirin	Warfarin
Lidocaine	Quinine	Phenytoin
Propofol	Codeine	Rocuronium
Propranolol	Nortriptyline	Methadone
Fentanyl	Vecuronium	Diazepam
Sufentanil	Alfentanil	Lorazepam

From Chapman N. Liver anatomy and physiology. In: Barash PG, Cullen BF, Stoelting RK, et al, eds. Clinical Anesthesia Fundamentals. Philadelphia: Wolters Kluwer; 2015:116, with permission.

References:
1. Chapman N. Liver anatomy and physiology. In: Barash PG, Cullen BF, Stoelting RK, et al, eds. *Clinical Anesthesia Fundamentals*. Philadelphia: Lippincott; 2015:109-118.
2. Pierce ET, Wiklund RA. Evaluation of patients with hepatic disease. In: Longnecker DE, Brown DL, Newman MF, et al, eds. *Anesthesiology*. 2nd ed. New York: McGraw Hill; 2012:180-195.

17. Correct answer: D

Hepatic metabolism and clearance of drugs depends on 3 factors: intrinsic ability of liver cells to metabolize the drug (presence of appropriate enzymes), hepatic blood flow, and the extent of drug bound to blood components (ie, albumin). Drugs that are cleared rapidly, essentially on the first pass through the liver, are usually lipophilic, have a low fraction of protein binding, and are quickly processed by liver enzymes. These drugs are said to have a high extraction ratio. They include propofol, some opioids, propranolol, and some local anesthetics such as lidocaine. The clearance of the high extraction ratio drugs depends mainly on hepatic blood flow.

Other drugs, which require a prolonged time for processing in the liver, are more hydrophilic, or highly protein bound, are said to have a low extraction ratio. Their clearance is independent of hepatic blood flow. They include benzodiazepines, methadone, phenytoin, warfarin, and some muscle relaxants such as rocuronium.

Reference:
1. Chapman N. Liver anatomy and physiology. In: Barash PG, Cullen BF, Stoelting RK, et al, eds. *Clinical Anesthesia Fundamentals*. Philadelphia: Lippincott; 2015:109-118.

18. Correct answer: C

The majority of drugs utilized in anesthesia practice are either biotransformed or eliminated via the liver. To be transformed into more lipophilic or water-soluble substances, and subsequently excreted, drugs are transformed via 1 of 2 enzyme systems, phase I or phase II. The cytochrome P450 group are phase I enzymes that utilize oxidation, hydrolysis, and reduction to convert the compound or drug into a polar metabolite. In comparison, phase II enzymes conjugate drugs with water-soluble ligands, such as glucuronide or sulfate.

Chronic or high doses of drugs can cause an increase in P450 enzyme levels as an adaptive response for the body to avoid accumulation of toxic intermediate metabolites. Some drugs are capable of inducing P450 enzymes even at therapeutic levels. These include ethanol, tobacco smoke, rifampin, barbiturates, and antiepileptics.

Other drugs can inhibit P450 enzymes by forming a complex with the enzyme and deactivate it. These include macrolide antibiotics, fluoroquinolones, isoniazid, azole antifungals, calcium channel blockers, omeprazole, cimetidine, and grapefruit juice. Inducers of P450 will shorten or lessen the effect of other drugs metabolized by the same pathway. Conversely, inhibitors of P450 will prolong the effect of other drugs.

References:
1. Chapman N. Liver anatomy and physiology. In: Barash PG, Cullen BF, Stoelting RK, et al, eds. *Clinical Anesthesia Fundamentals*. Philadelphia: Lippincott; 2015:109-118.
2. Boville JG. Adverse drug interactions in anesthesia. *J Clin Anesth*. 1997;9:3S-13S.
3. Pierce ET, Wiklund RA. Evaluation of patients with hepatic disease. In: Longnecker DE, Brown DL, Newman MF, et al, eds. *Anesthesiology*. 2nd ed. New York: McGraw Hill; 2012:180-195.

19. Correct answer: A

Macrolide antibiotics are potent inducers of the P450 isoform 3A4, which is also responsible for the biotransformation of midazolam. Deep unconsciousness and prolonged sedation have been reported in patients treated simultaneously with erythromycin and midazolam. The other antibiotics listed do not have any known significant interactions with the cytochrome P450 enzymes.

Reference:
1. Boville JG. Adverse drug interactions in anesthesia. *J Clin Anesth*. 1997;9:3S-13S.

20. Correct answer: B

Codeine is a prodrug, which requires metabolism by the cytochrome P450 2D6 isozyme to exert its analgesic effect. Large amounts of population variability in the 2D6 alleles exist with approximately 10% of Caucasian populations lacking this enzyme altogether. In comparison, 1%-2% of the population possesses multiple copies of the active 2D6 genes and can rapidly convert codeine to morphine, resulting in higher risk of complications such as sedation and respiratory depression. As a result a black box warning was issued by the FDA in 2013 against the use of codeine in children undergoing tonsillectomy. In comparison with codeine, morphine, fentanyl, and methadone are all active drugs that do not require in vivo conversion to exert their analgesic effects.

Reference:
1. Thackeray EM, Egan TD. Analgesics. In: Barash PG, Cullen BF, Stoelting RK, et al, eds. *Clinical Anesthesia Fundamentals*. Philadelphia: Lippincott; 2015:165-184.

7

RENAL SYSTEM

Jamie L. Sparling

1. **What is the approximate glomerular filtration rate (GFR) in a patient with normal renal function?**

   A. 10 mL/min
   B. 125 mL/min
   C. 500 mL/min
   D. 1000 mL/min

2. **Which of the following tissues has the highest oxygen extraction ratio in the body?**

   A. Renal medulla
   B. Cardiac myocytes
   C. Neurons
   D. Hepatocytes

3. **Which of the following factors will increase sodium resorption in the proximal tubule?**

   A. Increased blood pressure
   B. Increased extracellular volume
   C. High salt intake
   D. Angiotensin II

4. **Sodium reabsorption in the distal nephron (connecting the segment and collecting duct) is mediated directly by which substance?**

   A. Aldosterone
   B. Angiotensin II
   C. Vasopressin
   D. Renin

5. **An increase in which of the following will decrease the GFR?**

   A. Renal blood flow (RBF)
   B. Afferent arteriolar pressure
   C. Efferent arteriolar pressure
   D. Plasma osmotic pressure

6. **Sympathetic stimulation increases sodium and water retention through which of the following mechanisms?**

    A. Increased Na^+/H_2O reabsorption in the nephron
    B. Vasoconstriction leading to decreased net filtration
    C. Activation of the renin-angiotensin-aldosterone system (RAAS)
    D. All of the above

7. **Which of the following statements is true of renal function and aging?**

    A. Production of vitamin D is preserved in the aging kidney.
    B. Progressive decline in renal function begins to occur at 30-40 years of age.
    C. Serum creatinine tends to rise with age.
    D. GFR is preserved in healthy adults at the age of 80 years.

8. **Which of the following situations meets criteria for stage 3 acute kidney injury (AKI) according to the Acute Kidney Injury Network (AKIN) classifications?**

    A. Creatinine rise from 0.8 to 1.5
    B. Creatinine rise from 4.1 to 4.3
    C. Commencement of renal replacement therapy
    D. Urine output of 40 mL/h for a 70-kg man

9. **RBF represents what fraction of cardiac output?**

    A. 10%
    B. 25%
    C. 40%
    D. 50%

10. **Which of the following classes of drugs is known to raise serum creatinine by decreasing tubular secretion?**

    A. Cimetidine
    B. Cephalosporins
    C. Vitamin D
    D. Aminoglycosides

11. **A patient is admitted to the surgical ICU following a motor vehicle accident and is now status post an open splenectomy with massive hemorrhage. Which of the following sets of laboratory indices is most consistent with a diagnosis of prerenal AKI, assuming a serum sodium of 140 mEq/L and a urine creatinine of 50 mg/dL?**

CR (mg/dL)	BLOOD UREA NITROGEN (mg/dL)	URINE Na+(mEq/L)	URINE OSMOLALITY (mOsm/L)
A. 2.1	30	40	300
B. 2.1	45	40	200
C. 2.1	30	14	400
D. 2.1	45	14	800

12. **What percentage of the kidney's nephrons must be affected to see a rise in serum creatinine?**

    A. 25%
    B. 50%
    C. 75%
    D. 90%

13. **Where is angiotensinogen produced?**

    A. Kidney
    B. Lung
    C. Liver
    D. Muscle

14. **Which of the following substances is principally responsible for renal vasodilation in the face of surgical stress?**

    A. Nitric oxide
    B. Prostaglandins
    C. Endothelial-derived hyperpolarizing factor
    D. Atrial natriuretic peptide (ANP)

15. **Release of which of the following substances is most likely to lead to postoperative hyponatremia?**

    A. Angiotensin II
    B. Aldosterone
    C. Renin
    D. Vasopressin

16. **What is the net effect of angiotensin II on the glomerular arterioles and RBF?**

	AFFERENT ARTERIOLE	EFFERENT ARTERIOLE	RENAL BLOOD FLOW
A.	Vasodilation	Vasodilation	Increased
B.	Vasodilation	Vasoconstriction	Increased
C.	Vasoconstriction	Vasodilation	Decreased
D.	Vasoconstriction	Vasoconstriction	Decreased

17. **What is the net effect of ANP on the glomerular arterioles, RBF, and GFR?**

	AFFERENT ARTERIOLE	EFFERENT ARTERIOLE	RENAL BLOOD FLOW	GFR
A.	Vasodilation	Vasodilation	Increased	Unchanged
B.	Vasodilation	Vasoconstriction	Increased	Increased
C.	Vasoconstriction	Vasodilation	Decreased	Decreased
D.	Vasoconstriction	Vasoconstriction	Decreased	Unchanged

18. **Which of the following is the treatment of choice for a patient who has acutely developed hypernatremia with a urine output of 600 cc/h in the postanesthesia care unit following transphenoidal resection of a pituitary adenoma?**

    A. Normal saline
    B. Desmopressin
    C. Spironolactone
    D. Hydrocortisone

19. **Which of the following mechanisms primarily accounts for the normalization of arterial pH after prolonged hyperventilation in a patient with head injury?**

    A. Increased renal excretion of bicarbonate ions
    B. Decreased RBF
    C. Decreased renal absorption of hydrogen ions
    D. Increased renal resorption of bicarbonate ions

20. **The following laboratory values are most consistent with which of the following acid-base disturbances?**

pH	7.29
$Paco_2$	35 mm Hg
Pao_2	112 mm Hg
Sodium	139 mEq/L
Potassium	4.3 mEq/L
Chloride	105 mEq/L
Bicarbonate	17 mEq/L
Albumin	4.6 g/dL

    A. Anion gap acidosis
    B. Respiratory alkalosis with metabolic compensation
    C. Mixed anion gap and nonanion gap metabolic acidosis
    D. Combined metabolic and respiratory acidosis

21. **Which of the following is a cause of metabolic alkalosis?**

    A. Prolonged suction on nasogastric tube
    B. Administration of acetazolamide
    C. Diarrhea
    D. Ethylene glycol administration

22. **An increase in which of the following ions will decrease the strong ion difference (SID)?**

    A. Calcium
    B. Sodium
    C. Chloride
    D. Magnesium

23. **An anion gap metabolic acidosis with a normal osmolar gap is seen with ingestion of which of the following substances?**

    A. Methanol
    B. Ethanol
    C. Ethylene glycol
    D. Aspirin

24. **Which of the following best describes the acid-base disturbances seen with salicylate overdose?**

    A. Anion gap metabolic acidosis with respiratory compensation
    B. Respiratory alkalosis with renal compensation
    C. Combined metabolic acidosis and respiratory alkalosis
    D. Combined metabolic and respiratory acidosis

25. **Excretion of which of the following intravenous anesthetics is unaffected in patients with end-stage renal disease (ESRD)?**

    A. Propofol
    B. Ketamine
    C. Etomidate
    D. Thiopental

26. **Increased levels of normeperidine, seen in patients with renal failure, are associated with what symptoms?**

    A. Emesis
    B. Seizures
    C. Bradycardia
    D. Hypotension

27. **Which of the following classes of drugs must be dosage-adjusted in patients with renal impairment?**

    A. Phenothiazines (eg, promethazine)
    B. Antidopaminergics (eg, droperidol)
    C. H_2-receptor antagonists
    D. 5-HT_3 antagonists

28. **Which inhalation agent can react with barium hydroxide lime or soda lime to form compound A?**

    A. Isoflurane
    B. Desflurane
    C. Sevoflurane
    D. Nitrous oxide

29. **Approximately how much is potassium concentration elevated following administration of succinylcholine in patients with ESRD?**

    A. 0-0.2 mEq/L
    B. 0.5-1 mEq/L
    C. 1.0-1.5 mEq/L
    D. 1.5-2 mEq/L

30. **What is the primary form of elimination of vecuronium?**

    A. Renal excretion
    B. Biliary excretion
    C. Degradation by nonspecific esterases
    D. Hoffman elimination

31. **Cisatracurium is often used in patients with renal impairment. What is the primary mode of metabolism of cisatracurium?**

    A. Renal excretion
    B. Biliary excretion
    C. Degradation by nonspecific esterases
    D. Hoffman elimination

32. **Which of the following morphine metabolites can be responsible for delayed respiratory depression in patients with renal impairment?**

    A. Morphine-3-glucuronide
    B. Morphine-6-glucuronide
    C. Normorphine
    D. Codeine

33. **In what population has mannitol been shown to be protective against AKI?**

    A. Patients undergoing laparoscopic partial nephrectomies
    B. Patients undergoing infrarenal abdominal aortic aneurysm repair
    C. Cadaveric kidney transplant recipients
    D. Patients with traumatic rhabdomyolysis

34. **Which of the following statements is true of eplerenone?**

    A. It may cause gynecomastia in males.
    B. Hypokalemia is a common side effect.
    C. It acts in the distal convoluted tubule.
    D. It is indicated in patients with ascites due to end-stage liver disease.

35. **Nonsteroidal anti-inflammatory drugs (NSAIDs) most commonly contribute to what type of kidney injury?**

    A. Prerenal
    B. Acute tubular necrosis
    C. Glomerulonephritis
    D. Postrenal obstruction

36. **Which of the following is true of fenoldopam?**

    A. Rebound hypertension may occur when an infusion is discontinued.
    B. It is a nonselective α- and β-agonist.
    C. It is equipotent with dopamine.
    D. It is a selective DA1 receptor agonist.

37. **On which part of the nephron do loop diuretics work?**

    A. Proximal tubule
    B. Thick ascending limb
    C. Distal convoluted tubule
    D. Collecting duct

38. **Which of the following is the mechanism of action of acetazolamide?**

    A. Inhibition of carbonic anhydrase
    B. Blockade of NaCl cotransporter in the distal convoluted tubule
    C. Increasing the oncotic pressure in tubular filtrate
    D. Inhibition of the Na-K-2Cl cotransporter in the thick ascending loop

39. **Which of the following electrolyte abnormalities is most likely to be seen with uremia?**

    A. Hypokalemia
    B. Hypernatremia
    C. Hyperphosphatemia
    D. Hypomagnesemia

40. **In a patient with a blood urea nitrogen (BUN) of 80 mg/dL, which of the following elements meets criteria for a diagnosis of uremia?**

    A. Potassium of 6.1 mEq/L
    B. Serum creatinine of 4.5 mg/dL
    C. Urine output of 100 cc over a 24-hour period
    D. Asterixis and hiccups

Chapter 7 ▪ Answers

1. Correct answer: B

The GFR is the volume of filtrate formed by both kidneys per minute and is the product of the RBF and the filtration fraction. The GFR amounts to approximately 125 mL/min in patients with normal renal function. Both the RBF and the GFR are autoregulated through a combination of vascular smooth muscle contraction of the arterioles, tubuloglomerular feedback, and the sympathetic nervous system (SNS).

Reference:

1. Garwood S. The renal system. In: Barash PG, Cullen BF, Stoelting RK, et al, eds. *Clinical Anesthesia Fundamentals*. Philadelphia: Wolters Kluwer Health; 2015:87-108.

2. Correct answer: A

Normal oxygen extraction in the renal medulla is the highest in the body at 79%, compared with 65% in the heart. This extraction ratio is a consequence of both the high metabolic demands and the relatively poor oxygen delivery, only 5%-10% of total cardiac output. In the face of decreased renal perfusion, metabolic requirements are increased because of the drive to actively resorb more solutes from the tubular fluid, compounded by the decreased delivery of oxygen supply. The medulla is also susceptible to a number of nephrotoxins, heightening the risk for AKI.

Reference:

1. Stafford-Smith M, Raja A, Shaw AD. Evaluation of the patient with renal disease. In: Longnecker DE, Brown DL, Newman MF, Zapol WM, eds. *Anesthesiology*. 2nd ed. New York: McGraw Hill; 2012:166-179.

3. Correct answer: D

Sodium moves from the glomerulus into the Bowman capsule at the same concentration of the plasma. Of the filtrate that travels to the proximal tubule, approximately two-thirds is resorbed. This portion is affected by a number of factors, listed in the table below. Water reabsorption occurs via osmosis (passively) and is coupled with sodium transport through the cells.

FACTORS THAT INCREASE (↑) Na+ REABSORPTION	FACTORS THAT DECREASE (↓) Na+ REABSORPTION
Reduced blood pressure	Increased blood pressure
Hypovolemia/hemorrhage	High salt intake
Low salt intake	Increased extracellular volume
Sympathetic stimulation	Angiotensin-converting enzyme inhibitors
Angiotensin II	Angiotensin II receptor antagonists

Adapted from Table 5-2 in Garwood S. The renal system. In: Barash PG, Cullen BF, Stoelting RK, et al, eds. Clinical Anesthesia Fundamentals. *Philadelphia: Wolters Kluwer Health; 2015:87-108.*

Reference:

1. Garwood S. The renal system. In: Barash PG, Cullen BF, Stoelting RK, et al, eds. *Clinical Anesthesia Fundamentals*. Philadelphia: Wolters Kluwer Health; 2015:87-108.

4. Correct answer: A

Sodium reabsorption in the distal nephron is mediated by hormone-sensitive apical epithelial sodium channels, which are stimulated by aldosterone and are found in connecting cells and principal cells. Renin is secreted by the kidney in response to low perfusion of the afferent arteriole and catalyzes the conversion of angiotensinogen to angiotensin I. This substance is then converted to angiotensin II in the lungs by the angiotensin-converting enzyme (ACE). Thus, these two substances play a role in the RAAS, but it is aldosterone that directly acts in the distal nephron to mediate sodium reabsorption.

Vasopressin, or antidiuretic hormone (ADH), is released by the posterior pituitary in response to increased plasma osmolarity. It acts separately in the collecting duct to increase the permeability to water.

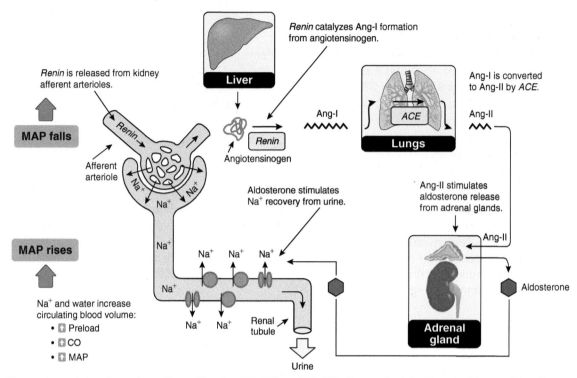

The renin angiotensin system. (From Preston RR, Wilson TE. Filtration and micturition. In: Harvey RA, ed. *Physiology*. Philadelphia: Lippincott Williams & Wilkins; 2013, with permission.)

References:
1. Garwood S. The renal system. In: Barash PG, Cullen BF, Stoelting RK, et al, eds. *Clinical Anesthesia Fundamentals*. Philadelphia: Wolters Kluwer Health; 2015:87-108.
2. Linn KA, Pagel PS. Cardiovascular pharmacology. In: Barash PG, Cullen BF, Stoelting RK, et al, eds. *Clinical Anesthesia Fundamentals*. Philadelphia: Wolters Kluwer Health; 2015:229-254.

5. Correct answer: C

Glomerular filtration occurs via bulk flow proportional to the difference in hydrostatic pressure between the afferent and efferent arterioles. Thus, an increase in afferent arteriolar pressure will increase the GFR, whereas an increase in efferent arteriolar pressure will decrease the GFR. This is opposed by the capsular hydrostatic pressure, which is approximately 15 mm Hg. RBF will increase the volume of filtrate. An increase in plasma osmotic pressure will favor a decrease in filtration because large molecules do not pass through the filtration membrane and thus high osmotic pressure will oppose filtration.

Reference:
1. Garwood S. The renal system. In: Barash PG, Cullen BF, Stoelting RK, et al, eds. *Clinical Anesthesia Fundamentals*. Philadelphia: Wolters Kluwer Health; 2015:87-108.

6. Correct answer: D

All of the above are mechanisms by which SNS activation results in retention of sodium and water. During times of stress, whether secondary to hypovolemia, surgical stress, or other causes, the SNS produces an intense vasoconstriction of all the renal vessels, which decreases the GFR. Additionally, the fraction of sodium, and secondarily water, reabsorbed in the proximal tubule will increase, and activation of the RAAS will produce aldosterone, which further increases sodium reabsorption in the distal nephron.

Reference:
1. Garwood S. The renal system. In: Barash PG, Cullen BF, Stoelting RK, et al, eds. *Clinical Anesthesia Fundamentals*. Philadelphia: Wolters Kluwer Health; 2015:87-108.

7. Correct answer: B

All renal functions, including GFR, tubular active transport, urine concentration and dilution, and acidification, decline with age, beginning around the age of 30-40 years. The RAAS, vitamin D metabolism, and ADH response are similarly affected. Both creatinine production and clearance each decrease approximately 1% per year, so the serum creatinine levels tend to remain flat. Despite this, the GFR has declined by about half to a third by the end of the eighth decade. This is the reason why formulas for calculating GFR and creatinine clearance take into account a patient's age.

Reference:

1. Stafford-Smith M, Raja A, Shaw AD. Evaluation of the patient with renal disease. In: Longnecker DE, Brown DL, Newman MF, Zapol WM, eds. *Anesthesiology.* 2nd ed. New York: McGraw Hill; 2012:166-179.

8. Correct answer: C

The AKIN classifications for AKI were published in 2007 and are widely accepted. AKI is divided into three stages, which replaced earlier classifications (in RIFLE) of risk, injury, and failure. The change in creatinine is measured over a 48-hour period. Stage 1 is diagnosed when creatinine increases by 50% or at least 0.3 mg/dL or when urine output is less than 0.5 mL/kg/h for 6 hours. Stage 2 is diagnosed when creatinine doubles or when urine output less than 0.5 mL/kg/h persists for 12 hours. Stage 3 is diagnosed when creatinine rises greater than 3-fold or is above 4.0 mg/dL and an increase of 0.5 mg/dL or greater is noted to occur acutely. Urine output criteria include anuria equal to or greater than 12 hours, and urine output is less than 0.3 mL/kg/h over 24 hours. Stage 3 also includes the new initiation of renal replacement therapy. Only answer choice C above meets these criteria. These criteria are outlined in the figure below.

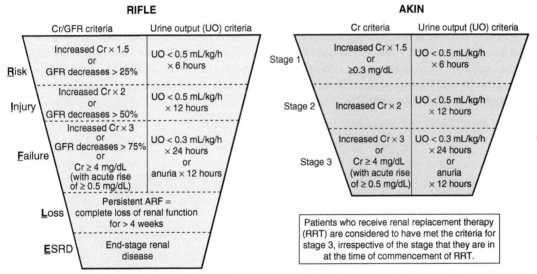

(From Cruz DN, Ricci Z, Ronco C. Clinical review RIFLE AKIN – time for reappraisal. *Crit Care.* 2009;13(3):211-219, with permission.)

References:

1. Garwood S. The renal system. In: Barash PG, Cullen BF, Stoelting RK, et al, eds. *Clinical Anesthesia Fundamentals.* Philadelphia: Wolters Kluwer Health; 2015:87-108.
2. Cruz DN, Ricci Z, Ronco C. Clinical review: RIFLE AKIN – time for reappraisal. *Crit Care.* 2009;13(3):211-219.

9. Correct answer: B

RBF represents approximately 25% of the total cardiac output, which is the highest on a per-gram basis, of any core organ in the body. The RBF amounts to approximately 309 mL/min/100 g, compared with 54 mL/min/100 g to the brain and 70 mL/min/100 g. Of all the organs, the liver has the highest absolute blood flow, but on a per-weight basis it is second to the kidneys with only 96 mL/min/100 g.

References:
1. Garwood S. The renal system. In: Barash PG, Cullen BF, Stoelting RK, et al, eds. *Clinical Anesthesia Fundamentals*. Philadelphia: Wolters Kluwer Health; 2015:87-108.
2. Stafford-Smith M, Raja A, Shaw AD. Evaluation of the patient with renal disease. In: Longnecker DE, Brown DL, Newman MF, Zapol WM, eds. *Anesthesiology*. 2nd ed. New York: McGraw Hill; 2012:166-179.
3. Smith JJ, Kampine JP. *Circulatory Physiology-The Essentials*, 2nd ed. Baltimore: Lippincott, Williams & Wilkins; 1984:1-352.

10. Correct answer: A

Several drugs can affect serum creatinine levels. Cimetidine (answer choice A) is an H_2-antagonist that is known to decrease tubular secretion of creatinine. Trimethoprim-sulfamethoxazole has a similar effect. Cephalosporins (answer choice B) can interfere with the assay for serum creatinine, thus falsely elevating the readings and implying a lower renal function. Aminoglycosides (answer choice D) are known nephrotoxic agents; however, at therapeutic doses, they do not interfere with the creatinine assay commonly used in laboratory analysis.

References:
1. Garwood S. The renal system. In: Barash PG, Cullen BF, Stoelting RK, et al, eds. *Clinical Anesthesia Fundamentals*. Philadelphia: Wolters Kluwer Health; 2015:87-108.
2. Syal K, Banerjee D, Srinivasan A. Creatinine estimation and interference. *Indian J Clin Biochem*. 2013;28(2):210-211.

11. Correct answer: D

AKI can be classified according to prerenal, intrinsic renal, or postrenal etiologies. Answer choice D is consistent with a diagnosis of prerenal AKI. In prerenal failure, the BUN is often elevated out of proportion to the creatinine because of maximal tubular resorption. A BUN/Cr ratio >20 is consistent with prerenal etiologies. Additionally, urine sodium is low (<20 mEq/L) in prerenal etiologies, whereas sodium is lost in intrinsic renal disease and is therefore elevated (>40 mEq/L). Similarly, a low fractional excretion of sodium (Fe_{Na}) favors prerenal disease (<1%), whereas a high Fe_{Na} favors intrinsic renal or postrenal etiologies. Conversely, urine osmolality is elevated (>500 mOsm/L) in prerenal etiologies, whereas it is lowered in intrinsic renal disease (<400 mOsm/L) because of impaired concentrating abilities.

The fractional excretion of sodium is calculated as follows:

$$Fe_{Na}(\%) = (\text{urine Na/serum Na})/(\text{urine Cr/serum Cr}) \times 100$$

$$Fe_{Na}(\%) = (14/140)/(50/2.1) \times 100 = 0.4\% < 1\%$$

To summarize:

INDICES	PRERENAL	RENAL	POSTRENAL
Creatinine (mg/dL)	↑	↑	↑
BUN (mg/dL)	↑↑	↑	↑
BUN/Cr	>20	<10	10-20
Urine Na+ (mEq/L)	<20	>40	>20
Urine osmolality (mOsm/L)	>500	<400	<350
Fe_{Na} (%)	<1	>2	>2

BUN, blood urea nitrogen; FE_{Na}, fraction sodium excreted in urine; Na, sodium.
Adapted from Table 5-5 (p. 98) in Garwood S. The renal system. In: Barash PG, Cullen BF, Stoelting RK, et al, eds. Clinical Anesthesia Fundamentals. *Philadelphia: Wolters Kluwer Health; 2015:87-108.*

Reference:
1. Garwood S. The renal system. In: Barash PG, Cullen BF, Stoelting RK, et al, eds. *Clinical Anesthesia Fundamentals*. Philadelphia: Wolters Kluwer Health; 2015:87-108.

12. Correct answer: B

Approximately half the kidney's nephrons must be damaged to see a rise in the serum creatinine. Thus, when used alone, creatinine levels may not detect subtle fluctuations in renal function. Additionally, the rise in creatinine may lag behind clinical injury.

Reference:

1. Garwood S. The renal system. In: Barash PG, Cullen BF, Stoelting RK, et al, eds. *Clinical Anesthesia Fundamentals*. Philadelphia: Wolters Kluwer Health; 2015:87-108.

13. Correct answer: C

Angiotensinogen is produced by the liver and then cleaved by renin into angiotensin I. ACE in the lungs converts angiotensin I into angiotensin II, which is the active form. Its actions include stimulating the release of aldosterone from the adrenal glands, causing generalized vasoconstriction, an increase in blood pressure, and sodium retention from the collecting duct.

Reference:

1. Garwood S. The renal system. In: Barash PG, Cullen BF, Stoelting RK, et al, eds. *Clinical Anesthesia Fundamentals*. Philadelphia: Wolters Kluwer Health; 2015:87-108.

14. Correct answer: A

Several endogenous substances are responsible for protecting the kidney via local vasodilation in response to the vasoconstriction seen during surgical stress. Nitric oxide contributes 50%-70% of renal vasodilation. It primarily counteracts sympathetic stimulation and works via stimulation of guanylate cyclase, increasing formation of cyclic guanosine monophosphate and ultimately producing smooth muscle relaxation. Prostaglandins counteract angiotensin II and vasopressin and contribute 20%-40% of renal vasodilation. Endothelial-derived hyperpolarizing factor refers to a number of metabolites grouped together, which counteract the renin angiotensin system and contribute less than 20% of renal vasodilation.

RENAL VASODILATORS

Factor	Site of Action	Mainly Counteracts	Time Course	Contribution to Vasodilation
Nitric oxide	Medulla +++ Cortex ++	Renal sympathetic nerve stimulation	Later prolonged effect	50%-70%
Prostaglandins	Medulla +++ Cortex +/−	Angiotensin II Vasopressin	Later prolonged effect	20%-40%
EDHF	Medulla +++ Cortex 0	RAS	Initial response, short-lived	<20%

EDHF, endothelial-derived hyperpolarizing factor; RAS, renin angiotensin system.
From Garwood S. The renal system. In: Barash PG, Cullen BF, Stoelting RK, et al, eds. Clinical Anesthesia Fundamentals. Philadelphia: Wolters Kluwer Health; 2015:87-108.

Reference:

1. Garwood S. The renal system. In: Barash PG, Cullen BF, Stoelting RK, et al, eds. *Clinical Anesthesia Fundamentals*. Philadelphia: Wolters Kluwer Health; 2015:87-108.

15. Correct answer: D

Nonosmotic release of vasopressin (ADH) during surgery can trigger hyponatremia, especially in conjunction with the administration of hypotonic fluids (eg, 5% or 10% dextrose). Activation of the renin angiotensin system would increase levels of angiotensin II, aldosterone, and renin but would result in decreased RBF and increased absorption of both sodium and free water. Vasopressin, on the other hand, increases free water reabsorption without affecting sodium absorption, resulting in an imbalance and subsequent hyponatremia.

References:
1. Butterworth JF, Mackey DC, Wasnick JD. Renal physiology & anesthesia. In: *Morgan and Mikhail's Clinical Anesthesiology.* 5th ed. New York: McGraw Hill Education; 2014:631-652.
2. Chung HM, Kluge R, Schrier RW, Anderson RJ. Postoperative hyponatremia. A prospective study. *Arch Intern Med.* 1986;146(2):333-336.

16. Correct answer: D

Angiotensin II causes both afferent and efferent arteriolar vasoconstriction, and the net result is decreased RBF. However, the efferent arteriole is smaller, so the same degree of vasoconstriction results in a greater increase in resistance. Thus, the pressure gradient of afferent to efferent arterioles is maintained, and GFR is largely preserved.

Reference:
1. Butterworth JF, Mackey DC, Wasnick JD. Renal physiology & anesthesia. In: *Morgan and Mikhail's Clinical Anesthesiology.* 5th ed. New York: McGraw Hill Education; 2014:631-652.

17. Correct answer: B

ANP is released by the atrial myocytes in response to atrial distension. It acts by directly dilating smooth muscle, and it opposes both norepinephrine and angiotensin II, preferentially dilating the afferent arteriole while constricting the efferent arteriole. The net result is an increase in both RBF and GFR.

Reference:
1. Butterworth JF, Mackey DC, Wasnick JD. Renal physiology & anesthesia. In: *Morgan and Mikhail's Clinical Anesthesiology.* 5th ed. New York: McGraw Hill Education; 2014:631-652.

18. Correct answer: B

Central diabetes insipidus (DI) may develop following head trauma or neurosurgical procedures; it is characterized by polydipsia and polyuria in the absence of hyperglycemia. In an unconscious patient under general anesthesia (or a sedated patient recovering from general anesthesia), the absence of thirst or the inability to take in oral fluids can rapidly produce hypovolemia and hypernatremia. The diagnosis is confirmed and treated with administration of desmopressin (DDAVP), which is a synthetic analogue of vasopressin. Although it is important to provide adequate hydration, normal saline (A) will not correct the underlying deficit. Spironolactone (C) is an aldosterone receptor antagonist and plays no role in the treatment of DI. Steroids (D) are not used to treat central DI.

Reference:
1. Butterworth JF, Mackey DC, Wasnick JD. Management of patients with fluid & electrolyte abnormalities. In: *Morgan and Mikhail's Clinical Anesthesiology.* 5th ed. New York: McGraw Hill Education; 2014:1107-1140.

19. Correct answer: A

The kidneys have the ability to control the amount of bicarbonate reabsorbed from the filtered tubular fluid, as well as eliminate hydrogen ions in the form of titratable ions and ammonium ions. These compensatory mechanisms can counter both metabolic and respiratory acid-base disturbances. In the case of an induced respiratory alkalosis, as above, the kidneys can increase renal excretion of bicarbonate. In general, renal compensation is able to protect against alkalosis except in cases of concurrent sodium deficiency or mineralocorticoid excess. These compensatory mechanisms begin to take effect at the time of the disturbance, but clinical effects are generally not appreciable until 12-24 hours and not maximal until up to 5 days.

Reference:
1. Butterworth JF, Mackey DC, Wasnick JD. Acid-base management. In: *Morgan and Mikhail's Clinical Anesthesiology.* 5th ed. New York: McGraw Hill Education; 2014:1141-1160.

20. Correct answer: C

To determine the acid-base disturbance in this clinical scenario, begin by determining the primary disturbance, which in this case is an acidosis. Both the bicarbonate and $Paco_2$ are reduced, indicating that there is a metabolic acidosis. Next, calculate the anion gap:

$$\text{Anion gap (AG)} = \left[Na^+ \right] - \left(\left[Cl^- \right] \right) + \left[HCO_3^{\ -} \right]$$

$$AG = 139 - (105 + 17) = 17$$

The anion gap is elevated (normal value is approximately 8-12 mmol/L), indicating the presence of an anion gap acidosis. Now, we must evaluate whether a second process is involved by calculating the delta ratio.

$$\text{Delta ratio} = \Delta AG / \Delta \left[HCO_3^{\ -} \right] = \left(AG - \text{normal AG} \right) \Big/ \left(24 - \left[HCO_3^{\ -} \right] \right)$$

$$\text{Delta ratio} = (17 - 12)/(24 - 17) = 5/7$$

$$\text{Delta ratio} < 1$$

A delta ratio below 1 indicates a fall in the bicarbonate greater than that explained by the anion gap. Thus, both an anion gap and nonanion gap metabolic acidosis are present in this patient. Causes of anion gap metabolic acidosis include lactic acidosis, diabetic ketoacidosis, and uremia. Causes of a nonanion gap metabolic acidosis include diarrhea, renal tubular acidosis, acetazolamide, spironolactone, and hyperalimentation.

Reference:

1. Hess DR, Kacmarek RM. Monitoring respiratory function. In: Longnecker DE, Brown DL, Newman MF, Zapol WM, eds. *Anesthesiology*. 2nd ed. New York: McGraw Hill, 2012:458-474.

21. Correct answer: A

Metabolic alkalosis can develop because of loss of acid from the upper gastrointestinal tract, such as in prolonged vomiting or suction on a gastric tube. Other causes of metabolic alkalosis include bicarbonate administration and hypokalemia. The other answer choices (B-D) are causes of metabolic acidosis. Anion gap metabolic acidosis can develop because of elevated lactic acid, ketoacidosis (eg, diabetic, alcoholic), uremic acidosis, and several poison ingestions (eg, methanol, ethylene glycol, aspirin). Nonanion gap metabolic acidosis can develop because of loss of base from either the lower gastrointestinal tract (eg, diarrhea) or the kidneys, as occurs with the administration of acetazolamide or in renal tubular acidosis.

Reference:

1. Hess DR, Kacmarek RM. Monitoring respiratory function. In: Longnecker DE, Brown DL, Newman MF, Zapol WM, eds. *Anesthesiology*. 2nd ed. New York: McGraw Hill; 2012:458-474.

22. Correct answer: C

The SID represents the difference between the charge carried by strong cations and that carried by strong anions. The formula for calculating SID is as follows:

$$SID = \left(\left[Na^+ \right] + \left[K^+ \right] + \left[Ca^{2+} \right] + \left[Mg^{2+} \right] \right) - \left(\left[Cl^- \right] \right) + \left[\text{other strong anions} : A^- \right]$$

A normal SID is 40-44 mEq/L; this represents the excess positive charge, which is balanced by an equal amount of unmeasured buffers, including phosphate, albumin, and bicarbonate. If these buffers are kept constant, an increase in SID will cause a decrease in [H⁺] and a resultant metabolic alkalosis, whereas a decrease in SID will cause an increase in [H⁺] and a resultant metabolic acidosis.

From the formula above, one can see that an increase in chloride concentration will decrease the SID and thus cause a hyperchloremic metabolic acidosis (answer choice C).

ACID-BASE ABNORMALITY	CAUSE
Respiratory acidosis	Increased P_{CO_2}
Respiratory alkalosis	Decreased P_{CO_2}, increased SID
Metabolic acidosis	Decreased SID, increased Cl^- (hyperchloremic), decreased Na^{+2} (dilutional)
Metabolic alkalosis	Increased SID, decreased Cl^-, increased Na^{+2} (contraction)

Adapted from Neligan PJ. Monitoring and managing perioperative electrolyte abnormalities, acid-base disorders, and fluid replacement. In: Longnecker DE, Brown DL, Newman MF, Zapol WM, eds. Anesthesiology. *2nd ed. New York: McGraw Hill; 2012:507-545.*

Reference:

1. Neligan PJ. Monitoring and managing perioperative electrolyte abnormalities, acid-base disorders, and fluid replacement. In: Longnecker DE, Brown DL, Newman MF, Zapol WM, eds. *Anesthesiology.* 2nd ed. New York: McGraw Hill; 2012:507-545.

23. Correct answer: D

The anion gap is calculated as follows:

$$AG = \left[Na^+\right] - \left(\left[Cl^-\right] + \left[HCO_3^{\;-}\right]\right)$$

A normal anion gap is 8-12 mmol/L. All of the answer choices above can cause an anion gap metabolic acidosis. To further elucidate a cause of metabolic acidosis, calculation of the osmolar gap can be useful. The osmolar gap represents the difference between the measured and the calculated osmolarities. To calculate the expected osmolarity, the following formula can be used:

$$\text{Calculated osmolarity} = 2\left[Na^+\right] + [\text{glucose}]/18 + [\text{BUN}]/2.8 + [\text{Ethanol}]/4.6$$

Osmolar gap = measured osmolarity - calculated osmolarity

If the osmolar gap is greater than 10 mOsm/L, this represents osmotically active particles, which are not measured differently. An elevated osmolar gap is consistent with methanol, ethanol, and ethylene glycol ingestions (answer choices A-C).

CAUSES OF METABOLIC ACIDOSIS

High Anion Gap

- **K**etones—diabetic, starvation

- **U**remia

- **L**actate—sepsis, hypovolemia, congestive heart failure

- **T**oxins—methanol, ethylene glycol, paraldehydes, salicylates, isoniazid

Nonanion Gap

- Hyperchloremia (excessive administration)

- Renal tubular acidosis

- Gastrointestinal losses (diarrhea, ileostomy)

From Hankinson EE, Joffe AM. Fluids and electrolytes. In: Barash PG, Cullen BF, Stoelting RK, et al, eds. Clinical Anesthesia Fundamentals. *Philadelphia: Wolters Kluwer Health; 2015:87-108.*

References:

1. Hess DR, Kacmarek RM. Monitoring respiratory function. In: Longnecker DE, Brown DL, Newman MF, Zapol WM, eds. *Anesthesiology.* 2nd ed. New York: McGraw Hill; 2012:458-474.
2. Hankinson EE, Joffe AM. Fluids and electrolytes. In: Barash PG, Cullen BF, Stoelting RK, et al, eds. *Clinical Anesthesia Fundamentals.* Philadelphia: Wolters Kluwer Health; 2015:87-108.

24. Correct answer: C

Salicylate overdose is manifested first by respiratory alkalosis resulting from stimulation of the respiratory center of the brain, causing hyperpnea and resultant hypocarbia. Subsequently, oxidative phosphorylation is uncoupled, leading to increased oxygen and glucose demand with parallel inhibition of the Krebs cycle enzymes, which in turn leads to increased organic acids. Finally, alterations in lipid and amino acid metabolisms contribute to the developing anion gap metabolic acidosis as well.

Reference:
1. Temple AR. Pathophysiology of aspirin overdosage toxicity, with implications for management. *Pediatrics*. 1978;62 (5 Pt 2 Suppl):873-876.

25. Correct answer: A

Thiopental is extensively protein bound; thus the free fraction is increased in chronic kidney disease. Uremic acidosis may also increase the nonionized fraction of drug and thus favor a more rapid entry of these agents into the brain. Ketamine and etomidate are affected to a lesser degree. Propofol, however, is transformed into inactive metabolites in the liver, which are then excreted unchanged by the kidney. Benzodiazepines are also highly protein bound and thus have increased availability in the free fraction; several benzodiazepines (including midazolam, lorazepam, and alprazolam) also have active metabolites that are excreted by the kidney.

References:
1. Garwood S. The renal system. In: Barash PG, Cullen BF, Stoelting RK, et al, eds. *Clinical Anesthesia Fundamentals*. Philadelphia: Wolters Kluwer Health; 2015:87-108.
2. Butterworth JF, Mackey DC, Wasnick JD. Anesthesia for patients with kidney disease. In: *Morgan and Mokhail's Clinical Anesthesiology*. 5th ed. New York: McGraw Hill Education; 2014:653-670.

26. Correct answer: B

Normeperidine is an active metabolite of meperidine and accumulates in patients with renal failure. It may prolong respiratory depression and is associated with central nervous system excitability, including anxiety, tremulousness, myoclonus, and seizures. This effect is not reversed by naloxone.

References:
1. Barash PG, Cullen BF, Stoelting RK, et al. Analgesics. In: *Clinical Anesthesia Fundamentals*. Philadelphia: Wolters Kluwer Health; 2015:165-184.
2. Butterworth JF, Mackey DC, Wasnick JD. Analgesic agents. In: *Morgan and Mikhail's Clinical Anesthesiology*. 2nd ed. New York: McGraw Hill Education; 2014:189-198.
3. Butterworth JF, Mackey DC, Wasnick JD. Anesthesia for patients with kidney disease. In: *Morgan and Mikhail's Clinical Anesthesiology*. 2nd ed. New York: McGraw Hill Education; 2014:653-670.

27. Correct answer: C

H_2-receptor antagonists are excreted by the kidney, and thus their dosage should be reduced in patients with renal impairment. Most phenothiazines are hepatically metabolized to inactive compounds. Antidopaminergic drugs may be partly dependent on the kidneys, but their pharmacokinetics is not appreciably changed in patients with renal impairment and those drugs do not require dose adjustment. $5\text{-}HT_3$ antagonists also do not require dose adjustment, despite nearly 50% excretion in the urine.

Reference:
1. Butterworth JF, Mackey DC, Wasnick JD. Anesthesia for patients with kidney disease. In: *Morgan and Mikhail's Clinical Anesthesiology*. 5th ed. New York: McGraw Hill Education; 2014:653-670.

28. Correct answer: C

When sevoflurane contacts a strong base, including the carbon dioxide absorbents barium hydroxide lime and soda lime, it is degraded to form compound A (fluromethyl-2-2-difluoro-1-[trifluoromethyl] vinyl ether). This product has been shown to be nephrotoxic and even fatal at high doses in rats, but it has never been proven to cause any significant renal injury in humans. In studies of healthy volunteers, even high doses (300 ppm-hours) failed to produce any elevation of BUN or creatinine. Factors that increase the accumulation of compound A include increased temperatures, low fresh gas flows, dry barium hydroxide absorbent, high sevoflurane concentrations, and long duration. Despite the lack of evidence showing any renal impairment attributable to sevoflurane in humans, many clinicians use fresh gas flows of at least 2 L/min when administering sevoflurane. In the package insert for sevoflurane, the manufacturers specifically recommend against fresh gas flows <1 L/min.

References:
1. Butterworth JF, Mackey DC, Wasnick JD. Renal physiology & anesthesia. In: *Morgan and Mikhail's Clinical Anesthesiology.* 5th ed. New York: McGraw Hill Education; 2014:631-652.
2. Butterworth JF, Mackey DC, Wasnick JD. Inhalation anesthetics. In: *Morgan and Mkhail's Clinical Anesthesiology.* 5th ed. New York: McGraw Hill Education; 2014:153-174.
3. Forman SA, Benkwitz C. Pharmacology of inhalational anesthetics. In: Longnecker DE, Brown DL, Newman MF, Zapol WM, eds. *Anesthesiology.* 2nd ed. New York: McGraw Hill; 2012:596-616.

29. Correct answer: B

Administration of succinylcholine in healthy patients transiently increases the potassium concentration approximately 0.5-1 mEq/L. Despite an elevated baseline potassium, the magnitude of increase is unchanged in ESRD. Thus, succinylcholine may be safely used in patients with ESRD in the absence of hyperkalemia at the time of induction. The increase in potassium seen with succinylcholine, however, may be higher in patients with burns, massive trauma, disuse atrophy, paresis, spinal cord injury, and other neuromuscular disease because of the increase in extrajunctional acetylcholine receptors. Thus, succinylcholine administration is contraindicated in these populations but not in ESRD.

References:
1. Butterworth JF, Mackey DC, Wasnick JD. Renal physiology & anesthesia. In: *Morgan and Mikhail's Clinical Anesthesiology.* 5th ed. New York: McGraw Hill Education; 2014:631-652.
2. Pino RM, Ali HH. Monitoring and managing neuromuscular blockade. In: Longnecker DE, Brown DL, Newman MF, Zapol WM, eds. *Anesthesiology.* 2nd ed. New York: McGraw Hill; 2012:492-507.

30. Correct answer: B

Vecuronium is a monoquarternary steroidal nondepolarizing neuromuscular blocker. It is primarily eliminated by biliary clearance and approximately 20%-25% by renal clearance. The effects of large doses of vecuronium are only slightly prolonged in patients with renal impairment. However, continuous infusions of vecuronium in the ICU may produce a significantly prolonged blockade, particularly in females, renal failure, steroid therapy, and sepsis.

Similarly, rocuronium is largely hepatically metabolized, but prolonged duration in the setting of severe renal impairment has been reported. With appropriate monitoring and minor dose reduction, however, both vecuronium and rocuronium may be safely used as intermittent boluses in patients with renal impairment.

References:
1. Butterworth JF, Mackey DC, Wasnick JD. Renal physiology & anesthesia. In: *Morgan and Mikhail's Clinical Anesthesiology.* 5th ed. New York: McGraw Hill Education; 2014:631-652.
2. Butterworth JF, Mackey DC, Wasnick JD. Neuromuscular blocking agents. In: *Morgan and Mikhail's Clinical Anesthesiology.* 5th ed. New York: McGraw Hill Education; 2014:199-222.
3. Pino RM, Ali HH. Monitoring and managing neuromuscular blockade. In: Longnecker DE, Brown DL, Newman MF, Zapol WM, eds. *Anesthesiology.* 2nd ed. New York: McGraw Hill; 2012:492-507.

31. Correct answer: D

Cisatracurium is degraded by organ-independent Hoffman elimination, yielding inactive metabolites. Thus, metabolism and elimination are independent of both liver and kidney functions. One of the metabolites produced by Hoffman elimination, laudanosine, is neuroexcitatory and raises the minimum alveolar concentration and may precipitate seizures. Because laudanosine is metabolized by the liver, patients with hepatic failure are at higher risk of toxicity but only with exceptionally large total doses. Moreover, because of the greater potency of cisatracurium compared with atracurium, the amount of laudanosine produced for an equal clinical effect and duration is much less. Nonspecific esterases (C) are involved in metabolism of atracurium but not the stereoisomer cisatracurium.

References:
1. Butterworth JF, Mackey DC, Wasnick JD. Renal physiology & anesthesia. In: *Morgan and Mikhail's Clinical Anesthesiology.* 5th ed. New York: McGraw Hill Education; 2014:631-652.
2. Butterworth JF, Mackey DC, Wasnick JD. Neuromuscular blocking agents. In: *Morgan and Mikhail's Clinical Anesthesiology.* 5th ed. New York: McGraw Hill Education; 2014:199-222.

32. Correct answer: B

Morphine is biotransformed in the liver to morphine-3-glucuronide and morphine-6-glucuronide, and a small amount is *N*-demethylated to form normorphine. Conversely, codeine is a prodrug of morphine and is converted to morphine via CYP2A6. Accumulation of morphine-6-glucuronide in patients with renal impairment can contribute to respiratory depression, sedation, nausea, and vomiting.

References:

1. Smith HS. Opioid metabolism. *Mayo Clin Proc.* 2009;84(7):613-624.
2. Thorn CF, Klein TE, Altman RB. Codeine and morphine pathway. *Pharmacogenet Genom.* 2009;19(7):556-558.
3. Rosow C, Dershwitz M. Pharmacology of opioid analgesics. In: Longnecker DE, Brown DL, Newman MF, Zapol WM, eds. *Anesthesiology.* 2nd ed. New York: McGraw Hill; 2012:703-724.
4. Butterworth JF, Mackey DC, Wasnick JD. Analgesic agents. In: *Morgan and Mikhail's Clinical Anesthesiology.* 5th ed. New York: McGraw Hill Education; 2014:189-198.

33. Correct answer: C

Mannitol is an osmotic diuretic, which is filtered at the glomerulus but is poorly reabsorbed. Thus, the osmotic pressure in the tubular fluid prevents further reabsorption of water from the tubules and additionally draws water from cells into the plasma, effectively increasing RBF. It is often used for renal protection in a variety of clinical scenarios; however, evidence to support these practices is lacking. In patients undergoing infrarenal abdominal aortic aneurysm repairs, mannitol alone or in conjunction with dopamine did not prevent a decline in GFR (B); similarly it did not improve kidney function in patients with acute rhabdomyolysis (D). Mannitol use did not improve renal function at any point in the first 6 months of follow-up for patients undergoing partial nephrectomies (A). Conversely, early studies showed a decrease in the rate of acute tubular necrosis following cadaveric kidney transplants in recipients receiving mannitol (C).

References:

1. Butterworth JF, Mackey DC, Wasnick JD. Renal physiology & anesthesia. In: *Morgan and Mikhail's Clinical Anesthesiology.* 5th ed. New York: McGraw Hill Education; 2014:631-652.
2. Stafford-Smith M, Raja A, Shaw AD. Evaluation of the patient with renal disease. In: Longnecker DE, Brown DL, Newman MF, Zapol WM, eds. *Anesthesiology.* 2nd ed. New York: McGraw Hill; 2012:166-179.
3. Fleisher LA. *Evidence-Based Practice of Anesthesiology: What is the Best Means of Preventing Perioperative Renal Injury?* Vol 241. Philadelphia: Elsevier Health Sciences; 2013.
4. Power NE, Maschino AC, Savage C, et al. Intraoperative mannitol use does not improve long-term renal function outcomes after minimally invasive partial nephrectomy. *Urology.* 2012;79(4):821-825.
5. Tiggeler RG, Berden JH, Hoitsma AJ, Koene RA. Prevention of acute tubular necrosis in cadaveric kidney transplantation by the combined use of mannitol and moderate hydration. *Ann Surg.* 1985;201(2):246-251.

34. Correct answer: D

Eplerenone is a direct-acting aldosterone antagonist, which inhibits aldosterone-mediated Na^+ reabsorption and K^+ secretion in the collecting tubules (C); thus hyperkalemia (not hypokalemia) can be a side effect (B). Coadministration with a β-blocker or ACE inhibitor increases the risk of hyperkalemia. Aldosterone antagonists are shown to improve survival in heart failure patients. They are also known to be efficacious in treating ascites in patients with end-stage liver disease, when secondary hyperaldosteronism can occur (D). Unlike spironolactone, eplerenone lacks the side effects of gynecomastia and sexual dysfunction (A).

References:

1. Butterworth JF, Mackey DC, Wasnick JD. Renal physiology & anesthesia. In: *Morgan nd Mikhail's Clinical Anesthesiology.* 5th ed. New York: McGraw Hill Education; 2014:631-652.
2. Stafford-Smith M, Raja A, Shaw AD. Evaluation of the patient with renal disease. In: Longnecker DE, Brown DL, Newman MF, Zapol WM, eds. *Anesthesiology.* 2nd ed. New York: McGraw Hill; 2012:166-179.

35. Correct answer: A

NSAIDs influence renal perfusion, as they inhibit prostaglandin synthesis via the COX-1 and COX-2 pathways, which are responsible for promoting vasodilation of the afferent and efferent arterioles. Thus, NSAIDs increase the risk of prerenal azotemia in susceptible patients. Those at higher risk of AKI with administration of NSAIDs include the elderly and patients with congestive heart failure, atherosclerotic vascular disease, or chronic kidney disease. This risk is compounded with concomitant use of ACE inhibitors and angiotensin II receptor blockers because of their ability to alter autoregulation of glomerular filtration. Generally, NSAID-induced renal injury is reversible but may become permanent with prolonged exposure.

NSAIDs may also cause an acute tubulointerstitial nephropathy, but this is much less common. This entity is characterized by an acute drop in GFR that persists for days to weeks.

Reference:

1. Stafford-Smith M, Raja A, Shaw AD. Evaluation of the patient with renal disease. In: Longnecker DE, Brown DL, Newman MF, Zapol WM, eds. *Anesthesiology*. 2nd ed. New York: McGraw Hill; 2012:166-179.

36. Correct answer: D

Fenoldopam is a selective DA1 receptor agonist, 10 times more potent than dopamine (C), which is used to decrease blood pressure without an increase in heart rate or contractility. It does not exert an effect at DA1, α, or β receptor (B). It is unique in that it does not cause rebound hypertension when an infusion is discontinued. Fenoldopam dilates coronary arteries, afferent and efferent arterioles of the kidney, and mesenteric arteries. It is often used for renal protection, particularly for patients undergoing cardiac, vascular, and transplant surgical procedures. A recent meta-analysis showed that fenoldopam significantly reduces the rate of AKI but has no impact on the rate of renal replacement therapy or mortality.

References:

1. Bronheim D, Nicoara A, Abel M. Cardiovascular drugs. In: Longnecker DE, Brown DL, Newman MF, Zapol WM, eds. *Anesthesiology*. 2nd ed. New York: McGraw Hill; 2012:742-766.
2. Gillies MA, Kakar V, Parker RJ, Honoré PM, Ostermann M. Fenoldopam to prevent acute kidney injury after major surgery—a systematic review and meta-analysis. *Crit Care*. 2015;19:449.

37. Correct answer: B

Loop diuretics work by inhibiting the Na^+-K^+-$2Cl^-$ cotransporter in the thick ascending limb of the loop of Henle. These molecules bind at the Cl^- binding site and thus reduce both Na^+ and Cl^- reabsorption. The result is that a greater sodium load is delivered to the distal nephron, overwhelming its reabsorptive capacity. Side effects include hypokalemia and metabolic alkalosis because the increased delivery of Na^+ to the distal tubule promotes K^+ and H^+ secretion. Calcium and magnesium excretion is also increased with loop diuretics, which can result in both hypocalcemia and hypomagnesemia, as well as urinary stone formation.

Carbonic anhydrase inhibitors act at the proximal tubule (A). Thiazide diuretics work at the distal convoluted tubule (C). Aldosterone antagonists act in the collecting duct (D).

References:

1. Butterworth JF, Mackey DC, Wasnick JD. Renal physiology & anesthesia. In: *Morgan and Mikhail's Clinical Anesthesiology*. 5th ed. New York: McGraw Hill Education; 2014:631-652.
2. Stafford-Smith M, Raja A, Shaw AD. Evaluation of the patient with renal disease. In: Longnecker DE, Brown DL, Newman MF, Zapol WM, eds. *Anesthesiology*. 2nd ed. New York: McGraw Hill; 2012:166-179.

38. Correct answer: A

Acetazolamide inhibits carbonic anhydrase, which catalyzes the conversion of carbonic acid to water and carbon dioxide:

$$H_2CO_3 \rightarrow H_2O + CO_2$$

The net effect in the proximal tubule is that sodium and bicarbonate are not reabsorbed, leading to an alkaline diuresis. However, its diuretic effects are limited because of compensatory resorption in the most distal segments of the nephron. Because it alkalinizes the urine, acetazolamide is also used to augment the excretion of weakly acidic compounds such as uric acid. In addition to its use as a diuretic, acetazolamide may also be used to reduce the intraocular pressure in open-angle glaucoma and to increase the $Paco_2$ to improve respiratory drive in patients with central sleep apnea. It may be used as prophylaxis against altitude sickness.

Thiazide diuretics, such as hydroclorothiazide and metolazone, act by blocking the NaCl cotransporter in the distal convoluted tubule (B). Osmotic diuretics, such as mannitol, act by increasing the oncotic pressure in the tubular fluid, inhibiting fluid reabsorption (C). Loop diuretics, such as furosemide, inhibit the Na^+-K^+-$2Cl^-$ cotransporter in the thick ascending loop of Henle. As a result, a larger salt load is delivered to the distal convoluted tubule and overwhelms the reabsorbing capacity there (D). For this reason, loop diuretics and thiazide diuretics are often used in conjunction to maximize diuresis.

References:
1. Butterworth JF, Mackey DC, Wasnick JD. Renal physiology & anesthesia. In: *Morgan and Mikhail's Clinical Anesthesiology*. 5th ed. New York: McGraw Hill Education; 2014:631-652.
2. Stafford-Smith M, Raja A, Shaw AD. Evaluation of the patient with renal disease. In: Longnecker DE, Brown DL, Newman MF, Zapol WM, eds. *Anesthesiology*. 2nd ed. New York: McGraw Hill; 2012:166-179.

39. Correct answer: C

The clinical syndrome of uremia is associated with numerous metabolic abnormalities. Metabolic acidosis occurs due to the inability to excrete anionic acids, including phosphates and sulfates. Hyperkalemia, hypermagnesemia, and hyperphosphatemia occur due to failure of the kidneys to excrete these ions, respectively. Hyponatremia occurs secondary to the development of total body fluid overload. Hypocalcemia can occur due to abnormal renal loss of calcium and decreased renal conversion of vitamin D to active 1,25(OH)2D.

References:
1. Butterworth JF, Mackey DC, Wasnick JD. Renal physiology & anesthesia. In: *Morgan and Mikhail's Clinical Anesthesiology*. 5th ed. New York: McGraw Hill Education; 2014:631-652.
2. Stafford-Smith M, Raja A, Shaw AD. Evaluation of the patient with renal disease. In: Longnecker DE, Brown DL, Newman MF, Zapol WM, eds. *Anesthesiology*. 2nd ed. New York: McGraw Hill; 2012:166-179.

40. Correct answer: D

Uremia literally means "urine in the blood" and is a clinical diagnosis characterized by the accumulation of urea in the blood, along with clinical symptoms. Symptoms may include lethargy, fatigue, nausea, anorexia, asterixis, and hiccups. The term "azotemia" may be used to describe accumulation of nitrogenous by-products without symptoms. BUN is often used as a proxy for severity, but the threshold above which symptoms develop varies by patient. BUN values below 70 mg/dL rarely cause symptoms, whereas values above 100 mg/dL nearly always have accompanying symptoms. The presence of uremic symptoms is an indication for dialysis.

Reference:
1. Stafford-Smith M, Raja A, Shaw AD. Evaluation of the patient with renal disease. In: Longnecker DE, Brown DL, Newman MF, Zapol WM, eds. *Anesthesiology*. 2nd ed. New York: McGraw Hill; 2012:166-179.

8

HEMATOLOGY

Matthieu A. Newton

1. **Clinical effects of unfractionated heparin (UFH) are best monitored by which of the following?**

   A. Partial thromboplastin time (PTT)
   B. Prothrombin time (PT)
   C. International normalized ratio (INR)
   D. Antithrombin III (ATIII)

2. **With respect to reversal with protamine, which of the following statements is true when comparing UFH and low-molecular-weight heparin (LMWH)?**

   A. UFH results in less predictable reversibility.
   B. UFH results in more predictable reversibility.
   C. Hypotension is less likely with UFH.
   D. Hypotension is more likely with UFH.

3. **Heparin-induced thrombocytopenia type 2 (HIT2) is mediated by which of the following?**

   A. IgG antibodies binding to heparin-PF-4 complexes on the surface of red blood cells (RBCs)
   B. IgG antibodies binding to ATIII on the surface of RBCs
   C. IgG antibodies binding to heparin-PF-4 complexes on the surface of platelets
   D. IgG antibodies binding to ATIII on the surface of platelets

4. **HIT typically presents in what period after the initiation of therapy?**

   A. 1-3 days
   B. 3-5 days
   C. 5-10 days
   D. 10-15 days

5. **The mechanism of action of *hirudin-derived* compounds involves which of the following?**

   A. Inhibition of vitamin K–derived clotting factors
   B. Inhibition of thrombin in its free and fibrin-bound states
   C. Potentiation of vitamin K–derived clotting factors
   D. Potentiation of thrombin in its free and fibrin-bound states

6. **Warfarin's primary mechanism of action is inhibition of the synthesis of vitamin K–dependent clotting factors. These factors include which of the following?**

   A. Factors II, VII, VIII, and X and protein C
   B. Factors II, VII, VIII, and XII and proteins C and S
   C. Factors VII, IX, X, and XII and protein S
   D. Factors II, VII, IX, and X and proteins C and S

7. **Before undergoing a trigger finger release under local anesthesia at an orthopedic surgeon's office, a patient's dabigatran should be discontinued for what length of time?**

   A. 12 hours
   B. 24 hours
   C. 36 hours
   D. 48 hours

8. **Tranexamic acid, a lysine analogue, acts by which of the following mechanisms?**

   A. Reversibly binds to plasminogen, thereby preventing the degradation of fibrin
   B. Inhibition of COX-1 and COX-2
   C. Inhibition of vitamin K–dependent clotting factors
   D. Inhibition of glycoprotein (GP) IIb/IIIa expression on the surface of activated platelets

9. **When comparing prothrombin complex concentrates (PCCs) with fresh frozen plasma (FFP), which of the following is true?**

   A. PCCs have a faster correction of coagulopathy.
   B. PCCs have a higher risk of infection.
   C. PCCs require a larger volume for administration.
   D. PCCs require a type and cross before administration.

10. **Fondaparinux exerts its effects by which of the following?**

    A. Acting as an antagonist to free factor VII
    B. Acting as an antagonist to free factor IX
    C. Acting as an antagonist to free factor Xa
    D. Acting as an antagonist to the expression of GP IIb/IIIa

11. **The effects of aspirin therapy can be reversed by infusing which of the following products?**

    A. Vitamin K
    B. Platelets
    C. Protamine
    D. von Willebrand factor

12. **The effects of aspirin therapy rely primarily on the direct inhibition of which of the following?**

    A. COX-1, TxA2
    B. COX-2, TxA1
    C. COX-1, COX-2
    D. COX-1 only

13. **For patients on aspirin therapy at a high risk of cardiac events in the perioperative period, which of the following should be performed?**

    A. Aspirin should be discontinued 24 hours before surgery and resumed after 6 weeks.
    B. Aspirin should be continued throughout the perioperative period.
    C. Aspirin should be discontinued at least 5 days (preferably 10 days) before surgery and resumed after 24 hours.
    D. Aspirin should be continued until surgery and discontinued for 6 weeks postoperatively.

14. **Which of the following is the mechanism of action of ADP receptor antagonists such as clopidogrel?**

    A. Inhibition of GP IIb/IIIa expression on the surface of activated platelets
    B. Inhibition of the action of GP Ib
    C. Promotion of GP IIb/IIIa expression on the surface of activated platelets
    D. Promotion of the action of GP Ib

15. **Eptifibatide (integrellin) is an inhibitor of which of the following?**

    A. Cyclooxygenase
    B. Phosphodiesterase
    C. ADP receptors
    D. GP IIb/IIIa receptors

16. **Autologous blood transfusion involves which 3 methods?**

    A. Preoperative autologous blood donation, acute normovolemic hemodilution, and perioperative blood cell salvage
    B. Preoperative allogenic blood donation, acute normovolemic hemodilution, and perioperative blood cell salvage
    C. Preoperative autologous blood donation, acute hypervolemic hemodilution, and perioperative blood cell salvage
    D. Preoperative allogenic blood donation, acute hypovolemic hemodilution, and perioperative blood cell salvage

17. **To increase the amount of times one may safely donate his/her own blood (autologous blood donation) for a future surgical procedure, which of the following may be administered to the patient before donation?**

    A. Intravenous iron
    B. Oral iron
    C. Factor VIII concentrate
    D. Erythropoietin

18. **Which of the following examples could be an indication for using the process known as "acute normovolemic hemodilution"?**

    A. Congenital heart disease
    B. Refusal of allogenic blood products
    C. Anticipated blood loss of one-third of the patient's volume
    D. Preoperative anemia

19. **A primary concern with intraoperative blood cell salvage includes which of the following?**

    A. Lack of validated evidence
    B. Increased rates of infection compared with allogenic blood products
    C. Dilutional coagulopathy
    D. Decreased stimulation of erythropoiesis

20. **Perioperative blood salvage can be considered if the estimated blood loss will likely exceed which of the following?**

    A. 500 mL
    B. 1000 mL
    C. 1500 mL
    D. 2000 mL

21. **Jehovah's Witnesses are a population whose beliefs lead to a refusal to accept blood products. Which of the following represents the best management of a conscious Jehovah's Witness patient who presents for emergency surgery with a high likelihood of significant blood loss?**

    A. Transfuse blood products as clinically indicated.
    B. Refuse to transfuse blood products.
    C. Have a discussion with patients about their beliefs about blood products.
    D. Meet with hospital ethics team and legal counsel before surgery.

22. **When an individual's hematocrit falls below a certain value, erythropoietin is released. Which of the following % is the "critical" value for its release?**

    A. 25%
    B. 30%
    C. 35%
    D. 40%

23. **A 66-year-old man is scheduled to undergo a right total hip replacement and prefers a neuraxial technique. You note that he has a history of thrombocytopenia. Which of the following is the platelet transfusion threshold for patients undergoing neuraxial anesthesia?**

    A. 10 000
    B. 50 000
    C. 75 000
    D. 100 000

24. **Routine transfusion of packed red cells in a (stable) critically ill patient is NOT necessary unless the hemoglobin concentration is below which of the following?**

    A. 5.8 g/dL
    B. 6.5 g/dL
    C. 7 g/dL
    D. 8.6 g/dL

25. **What is the most appropriate storage parameters for packed RBCs that LACK an additive solution?**

    A. 1°C-6°C for 21-35 days
    B. <−65°C for 10 years
    C. 20°C-24°C for 5 days
    D. <−18°C for 1 year

26. **Blood donors in the United States are required to have a minimum hemoglobin level of which of the following?**

    A. 7
    B. 9.5
    C. 11
    D. 12.5

27. **Which of the following statements is true with regard to transfusing FFP?**

    A. It contains all factors involved in hemostasis.
    B. It does not need to be ABO-compatible.
    C. It must be used within 1 year of collection.
    D. It carries no risk of transfusion-related acute lung injury (TRALI).

28. Cryoprecipitate contains all of the following factors EXCEPT which one?

   A. von Willebrand factor
   B. Factor VIII
   C. Factor IX
   D. Factor XIII

29. The most common reaction observed during transfusions of blood products is which of the following?

   A. An anaphylactoid reaction
   B. Febrile nonhemolytic transfusion reaction (FNHTR)
   C. Acute hemolytic transfusion reaction (AHTR)
   D. Delayed hemolytic transfusion reaction (DHTR)

30. Immediately following a blood transfusion in the PACU, a patient becomes tachycardic, hypotensive, and febrile, and his nurse notes that he appears to have blood leaking from his incision. After stopping the transfusion and administering IV fluids, which of the following is the most appropriate test to conduct?

   A. Tryptase
   B. Direct Coombs test
   C. Indirect Coombs test
   D. Caffeine-halothane contracture test

31. Seven days following embolization for an occult gastrointestinal (GI) bleed, a patient is noted to be jaundiced, in addition to having a mild fever and hematuria. Which of the following is the best initial course of action?

   A. Liver biopsy
   B. Aspartate aminotransferase/alanine aminotransferase
   C. Prothrombin time/international normalized ratio
   D. IV fluids

32. Allergic reactions to blood products in patients with a known IgA deficiency can be avoided by which of the following?

   A. Leukoreduction
   B. Washing
   C. Irradiation
   D. Premedication with acetaminophen

33. Which of the following is true about anaphylactoid responses to blood product tranfusions?

   A. They show evidence of anti-IgA antibodies.
   B. They are type I hypersensitivity IgE-mediated reactions.
   C. The majority occur secondary to IgM-mediated antibody-antigen complexes.
   D. They show evidence of IgG alloantibodies to Rh.

34. To decrease the risk of transfusion-related graft-versus-host disease (GVHD), cellular components of blood should undergo which of the following?

   A. Leukoreduction
   B. Washing
   C. Irradiation
   D. Preservation using citrate phosphate dextrose adenine (CDPA) solution

35. Following exploratory laparotomy for trauma in which a patient underwent a massive transfusion, the patient is noted to have twitching of the ipsilateral facial muscles when tapping on the face just below the zygomatic bone, as well as wrist flexion and hyperextension of the fingers when a blood pressure cuff is inflated above systolic blood pressure. Which of the following is the most likely cause for these symptoms?

    A. Hyperkalemia
    B. Hypokalemia
    C. Citrate toxicity
    D. Hypothermia

36. A patient received several units of blood products because of a massive GI hemorrhage. Which of the following sets of parameters is most concerning for TRALI?

    A. Onset of shortness of breath 3 days after transfusion with chest X-ray (CXR) showing focal infiltrates in the right lower lobe
    B. Decreased lung compliance after induction of anesthesia with CXR showing no acute changes
    C. CXR showing pulmonary edema, elevated B-type natriuretic peptide, and transthoracic echocardiogram showing left atrial enlargement
    D. CXR showing pulmonary edema with acute bilateral infiltrates, Pao_2/Fio_2 <300, Sao_2, 90% on room air, no evidence of left atrial hypertension

37. A patient received several units of blood products because of a massive GI hemorrhage. Which of the following sets of parameters is most concerning for transfusion-related acute cardiovascular overload (TACO)?

    A. Onset of shortness of breath 3 days after transfusion with CXR showing focal infiltrates in the right lower lobe
    B. Decreased lung compliance after induction of anesthesia with CXR showing no acute changes
    C. CXR showing bilateral pulmonary edema, elevated B-type natriuretic peptide, and transthoracic echocardiogram showing left atrial hypertension
    D. CXR showing pulmonary edema with acute bilateral infiltrates, Pao_2/Fio_2 <300, Sao_2, 90% on room air, no evidence of left atrial hypertension

38. Which of the following infections carries the highest residual risk post blood product transfusion in the United States?

    A. Human immunodeficiency virus (HIV)
    B. Hepatitis C virus
    C. Hepatitis B virus
    D. Cytomegalovirus (CMV)

39. Transfusion of which of the following blood products has the highest rate of infection?

    A. Red blood cells
    B. Platelets
    C. Fresh frozen plasma
    D. Cryoprecipitate

40. Transfusion of blood products has been associated with which of the following?

    A. Increased flares in patients afflicted with Crohn disease
    B. Decreased rate of miscarriages in women with history of recurrent spontaneous abortion
    C. Decreased reactivation of latent tuberculosis
    D. Decreased rates of recurrent malignancies

Chapter 8 ▪ Answers

1. Correct answer: A

Two forms of heparin are used clinically, UFH and LMWH. UFH binds to ATIII causing a conformational change in the molecule, thus inhibiting thrombin and factor Xa. The clinical effects of UFH are best monitored by the PTT and ACT. In patients with a congenital deficiency of ATIII, heparin may be a poor choice for anticoagulation. Heparin can be fully reversed with the administration of protamine. LMWH is fractionated heparin that specifically inhibits factor Xa. It is preferred to UFH because there are no laboratory monitoring requirements except in the obese and patients with renal disease. In these patients, LMWH is monitored via factor Xa levels. Reversal of LMWH with protamine is less predictable than that of UFH and is less likely to completely resolve a bleeding diathesis.

Reference:

1. Carabini LM, Ramsey G. Hemostasis and transfusion medicine. In: Barash PG, Cullen BF, Stoelting RK, et al, eds. *Clinical Anesthesia.* 7th ed. Philadelphia: Wolters Kluwer Health; 2013:408-444.

2. Correct answer: B

See answer explanation given for question 1.

Two forms of heparin are used clinically, UFH and LMWH. UFH binds to ATIII causing a conformational change in the molecule, thus inhibiting thrombin and factor Xa. The clinical effects of UFH are best monitored by the PTT and ACT. In patients with a congenital deficiency of ATIII, heparin may be a poor choice for anticoagulation. Heparin can be fully reversed with the administration of protamine. LMWH is fractionated heparin that specifically inhibits factor Xa. It is preferred to UFH because there are no laboratory monitoring requirements except in the obese and patients with renal disease. In these patients, LMWH is monitored via factor Xa levels. Reversal of LMWH with protamine is less predictable than that with UFH and is less likely to completely resolve a bleeding diathesis.

Reference:

1. Carabini LM, Ramsey G. Hemostasis and transfusion medicine. In: Barash PG, Cullen BF, Stoelting RK, et al, eds. *Clinical Anesthesia.* 7th ed. Philadelphia: Wolters Kluwer Health; 2013:408-444.

3. Correct answer: C

HIT is the development of thrombocytopenia within 5-10 days of initiating therapy with heparin. The disorder develops in 1%-5% of patients and leads to thromboembolic phenomena. UFH and LMWH can both cause HIT; however, HIT is more common with the use of UFH. Two forms of HIT exist; HIT1 is milder and involves only a mild thrombocytopenia, whereas HIT2 is a complex immune-mediated response causing hypercoagulability. In HIT2, IgG antibodies bind to heparin-PF-4 complexes on the surface of platelets, inhibiting hemostasis and thrombin generation.

HIT should be considered in patients who have recently begun an anticoagulation regimen with heparin and show a fall in platelets to less than 150 000 or greater than 50% from baseline. Diagnosis is confirmed with either an ELISA or serotonin release assay. Treatment then consists of immediately stopping all forms of heparin and necessitates anticoagulation with another agent (except warfarin).

Reference:

1. Carabini LM, Ramsey G. Hemostasis and transfusion medicine. In: Barash PG, Cullen BF, Stoelting RK, et al, eds. *Clinical Anesthesia.* 7th ed. Philadelphia: Wolters Kluwer Health; 2013:408-444.

4. Correct answer: C

See answer explanation given for question 3.

HIT is the development of thrombocytopenia within 5-10 days of initiating therapy with heparin. The disorder develops in 1%-5% of patients and leads to thromboembolic phenomena. UFH and LMWH can both cause HIT; however, HIT is more common with the use of UFH. Two forms of HIT exist; HIT1 is milder and involves only a mild thrombocytopenia, whereas HIT2 is a complex immune-mediated response causing hypercoagulability. In HIT2, IgG antibodies bind to heparin-PF-4 complexes on the surface of platelets, inhibiting hemostasis and thrombin generation.

HIT should be considered in patients who have recently begun an anticoagulation regimen with heparin and show a fall in platelets to less than 150 000 or greater than 50% from baseline. Diagnosis is confirmed with either an ELISA or serotonin release assay. Treatment then consists of immediately stopping all forms of heparin and necessitates anticoagulation with another agent (except warfarin).

Reference:
1. Carabini LM, Ramsey G. Hemostasis and transfusion medicine. In: Barash PG, Cullen BF, Stoelting RK, et al, eds. *Clinical Anesthesia*. 7th ed. Philadelphia: Wolters Kluwer Health; 2013:408-444.

5. Correct answer: B

Lepirudin, desirudin, argatroban, and bivalirudin are parenteral direct thrombin inhibitors derived from hirudin. These drugs act to directly inhibit thrombin in both its free and fibrin-bound states. They are commonly used for anticoagulation in the setting of a diagnosis of HIT because they are not immunogenic. There are no antidotes to these therapies; thus reversal depends on the varying rates of clearance of each individual drug. Lepirudin and desirudin are metabolized by the kidney, argatroban is metabolized by the liver, and bivalirudin is metabolized by plasma proteases. Drug effects are monitored via PTT or ACT.

Reference:
1. Carabini LM, Ramsey G. Hemostasis and transfusion medicine. In: Barash PG, Cullen BF, Stoelting RK, et al, eds. *Clinical Anesthesia*. 7th ed. Philadelphia: Wolters Kluwer Health; 2013:408-444.

6. Correct answer: D

Warfarin is an anticoagulant agent that exerts its effect by competing with vitamin K for carboxylation-binding sites and inhibits the synthesis of vitamin K–dependent clotting factors, factors II, VII, IX, and X and proteins C and S. Given that proteins C and S both have a shorter half-life than the other factors, patients may become hypercoagulable during the initial phase of therapy, thus necessitating bridging with another anticoagulant. Warfarin therapy is monitored via INR for a target range usually between 2 and 3.

Warfarin is metabolized by the liver and P450 CYP2 enzymes and can therefore interact with many other medications that are also metabolized by this system. In addition, the clinical effect will vary depending on the amount of vitamin K in a person's diet. Daily intake of vitamin K should remain as stable as possible during the patients' treatment course with warfarin to avoid fluctuations in their INR, necessitating adjustment of warfarin dosing.

Reversal of warfarin depends on the clinical situation and the value of the measured INR. In stable patients with an INR above 5, warfarin should be held for 1 to 2 doses. Supplemental oral vitamin K should be administered if the INR is above 8. If a patient cannot take oral medication, vitamin K can be given intravenously or subcutaneously. In patients with major bleeding or those requiring emergency surgery, 4-factor (factors II, VII, IX, and X) PCCs and vitamin K or FFP if 4-factor PCCs are not available, should be given.

Reference:
1. Carabini LM, Ramsey G. Hemostasis and transfusion medicine. In: Barash PG, Cullen BF, Stoelting RK, et al, eds. *Clinical Anesthesia*. 7th ed. Philadelphia: Wolters Kluwer Health; 2013:408-444.

7. Correct answer: B

Dabigatran is a renally excreted direct thrombin inhibitor approved for stroke prophylaxis and therapeutic anticoagulation in patients with a history of thromboembolism. It has few drug interactions and a wide therapeutic window. To date, there lacks a reliable coagulation test to study the effects of therapy nor is there a reliable reversal regimen. However, PCCs are commonly used, and there are reports of dialysis removing dabigatran. Before minor surgery and diagnostic procedures, dabigatran should be stopped for 24 hours, and in the case of major surgery or procedures involving the eye, brain, or spine, it should be stopped for 48 hours.

Reference:
1. Carabini LM, Ramsey G. Hemostasis and transfusion medicine. In: Barash PG, Cullen BF, Stoelting RK, et al, eds. *Clinical Anesthesia*. 7th ed. Philadelphia: Wolters Kluwer Health; 2013:408-444.

8. Correct answer: A

Tranexamic acid (TXA) is a synthetic derivative of lysine that competitively inhibits the binding site of plasminogen, preventing cleavage to plasmin that results in fibrinolysis. TXA decreases bleeding in cardiac surgery, liver transplant, and orthopedic procedures. It has recently been shown to decrease bleeding and all-cause mortality in trauma and has been shown to be effective in prevention and treatment for postpartum hemorrhage. TXA is renally excreted, and there have been few reported side effects.

Reference:

1. Carabini LM, Ramsey G. Hemostasis and transfusion medicine. In: Barash PG, Cullen BF, Stoelting RK, et al, eds. *Clinical Anesthesia*. 7th ed. Philadelphia: Wolters Kluwer Health; 2013:408-444.

9. Correct answer: A

PCCs are formulations of 3 (factors II, IX, and X) or 4 (factors II, VII, IX, and X) coagulation factors and an anticoagulant (heparin, antithrombin, or proteins C and S). PCCs are indicated for the reversal of vitamin K antagonists and critical bleeding associated with major surgery, trauma, or liver failure. PCCs have become the drug of choice for reversing the effects of oral anticoagulants over FFP because of their faster correction of coagulopathy, smaller volume of the product itself, decreased risk of infection, and transfusion reactions.

Reference:

1. Carabini LM, Ramsey G. Hemostasis and transfusion medicine. In: Barash PG, Cullen BF, Stoelting RK, et al, eds. *Clinical Anesthesia*. 7th ed. Philadelphia: Wolters Kluwer Health; 2013:408-444.

10. Correct answer: C

Fondaparinux can be used for both prophylaxis and treatment of deep venous thromboses (DVTs). It is a highly specific antagonist for free factor Xa and also binds ATIII. Fondaparinux is renally eliminated, and coagulation monitoring is not necessary because of its long half-life, unless it is used in patients with renal impairment, in which case it would require monitoring of factor Xa levels. At this time, there is no reversal agent for fondaparinux.

Reference:

1. Carabini LM, Ramsey G. Hemostasis and transfusion medicine. In: Barash PG, Cullen BF, Stoelting RK, et al, eds. *Clinical Anesthesia*. 7th ed. Philadelphia: Wolters Kluwer Health; 2013:408-444.

11. Correct answer: B

Aspirin is a noncompetitive inhibitor of cyclooxygenase (COX)-1 and COX-2. COX-1 helps to maintain the gastric lining and renal blood flow and initiates the formation of TxA2. COX-2 mediates the synthesis of prostaglandins responsible for pain and inflammation. Because of the noncompetitive nature of aspirin, platelets in circulation during treatment are irreversibly impaired, and its effects can only be reversed with platelet transfusion. Once aspirin therapy has been discontinued, the newly transfused platelets are not subject to its effects; however, the patient's native platelets remain affected and therefore are deemed "nonfunctional."

Perioperative management of patients on antiplatelet therapy depends on both individual patient factors and the procedure being performed. In patients with coronary stents, elective surgery should be postponed for 4-6 weeks in those with bare metal stents and for 12 months in those with drug-eluting stents. In patients at high risk of cardiac events (exclusive of coronary stents), aspirin should be continued throughout the perioperative period. Finally, in patients at low risk of cardiac events, aspirin should be stopped 7-10 days before surgery and can be resumed 24 hours postoperatively.

References:

1. Carabini LM, Ramsey G. Hemostasis and transfusion medicine. In: Barash PG, Cullen BF, Stoelting RK, et al, eds. *Clinical Anesthesia*. 7th ed. Philadelphia: Wolters Kluwer Health; 2013:408-444.
2. Horlocker TT, Wedel DJ, Rowlingson JC, et al. Regional anesthesia in the patient receiving antithrombotic or thrombolytic therapy: American Society of Regional Anesthesia and Pain Medicine Evidence-Based Guidelines. 3rd ed. *Reg Anesth Pain Med*. 2010;35(1):64-101.

12. **Correct answer: C**

See answer explanation given for question 11.

Aspirin is a noncompetitive inhibitor of cyclooxygenase (COX)-1 and COX-2. COX-1 helps to maintain the gastric lining and renal blood flow and initiates the formation of TxA2. COX-2 mediates the synthesis of prostaglandins responsible for pain and inflammation. Because of the noncompetitive nature of aspirin, platelets in circulation during treatment are irreversibly impaired, and its effects can only be reversed with platelet transfusion. Once aspirin therapy has been discontinued, the newly transfused platelets are not subject to its effects; however, the patient's native platelets remain affected and therefore are deemed "nonfunctional."

Perioperative management of patients on antiplatelet therapy depends on both individual patient factors and the procedure being performed. In patients with coronary stents, elective surgery should be postponed for 4-6 weeks in those with bare metal stents and for 12 months in those with drug-eluting stents. In patients at high risk of cardiac events (exclusive of coronary stents), aspirin should be continued throughout the perioperative period. Finally, in patients at low risk of cardiac events, aspirin should be stopped 7-10 days before surgery and can be resumed 24 hours postoperatively.

References:

1. Carabini LM, Ramsey G. Hemostasis and transfusion medicine. In: Barash PG, Cullen BF, Stoelting RK, et al, eds. *Clinical Anesthesia*. 7th ed. Philadelphia: Wolters Kluwer Health; 2013:408-444.
2. Horlocker TT, Wedel DJ, Rowlingson JC, et al. Regional anesthesia in the patient receiving antithrombotic or thrombolytic therapy: American Society of Regional Anesthesia and Pain Medicine Evidence-Based Guidelines. 3rd ed. *Reg Anesth Pain Med*. 2010;35(1):64-101.

13. **Correct answer: B**

See answer explanation given for question 11.

Aspirin is a noncompetitive inhibitor of cyclooxygenase (COX)-1 and COX-2. COX-1 helps to maintain the gastric lining and renal blood flow and initiates the formation of TxA2. COX-2 mediates the synthesis of prostaglandins responsible for pain and inflammation. Because of the noncompetitive nature of aspirin, platelets in circulation during treatment are irreversibly impaired, and its effects can only be reversed with platelet transfusion. Once aspirin therapy has been discontinued, the newly transfused platelets are not subject to its effects; however, the patient's native platelets remain affected and therefore are deemed "nonfunctional."

Perioperative management of patients on antiplatelet therapy depends on both individual patient factors and the procedure being performed. In patients with coronary stents, elective surgery should be postponed for 4-6 weeks in those with bare metal stents and for 12 months in those with drug-eluting stents. In patients at high risk of cardiac events (exclusive of coronary stents), aspirin should be continued throughout the perioperative period. Finally, in patients at low risk of cardiac events, aspirin should be stopped 7-10 days before surgery and can be resumed 24 hours postoperatively.

References:

1. Carabini LM, Ramsey G. Hemostasis and transfusion medicine. In: Barash PG, Cullen BF, Stoelting RK, et al, eds. *Clinical Anesthesia*. 7th ed. Philadelphia: Wolters Kluwer Health; 2013:408-444.
2. Horlocker TT, Wedel DJ, Rowlingson JC, et al. Regional anesthesia in the patient receiving antithrombotic or thrombolytic therapy: American Society of Regional Anesthesia and Pain Medicine Evidence-Based Guidelines. 3rd ed. *Reg Anesth Pain Med*. 2010;35(1):64-101.

14. **Correct answer: A**

Clopidogrel is a noncompetitive and irreversible P2Y12 ADP receptor antagonist, which prevents the expression of GP IIb/IIIa on the surface of activated platelets, inhibiting platelet adhesion and aggregation. ADP receptor antagonists are used clinically to inhibit thromboembolism, prevent myocardial infarction (MI), and prevent in-stent thrombosis. Clopidogrel is a "prodrug," meaning that it must be oxidized to its active form.

Reference:

1. Carabini LM, Ramsey G. Hemostasis and transfusion medicine. In: Barash PG, Cullen BF, Stoelting RK, et al, eds. *Clinical Anesthesia*. 7th ed. Philadelphia: Wolters Kluwer Health; 2013:408-444.

15. Correct answer: D

Eptifibatide belongs to the class of drugs known as GP IIb/IIIa receptor blockers, which inhibit the cross-linkage of fibrinogen. These medications are used for the management of acute coronary syndrome (ACS), and effects are monitored via serial activated clotting times (ACTs). Eptifibatide is renally excreted and thus has a prolonged mechanism of action in those with renal impairment. Currently, there are not any reversal agents available; thus reversal depends on clearance of the drugs, which have a half-life of approximately 2.5 hours.

Reference:
1. Carabini LM, Ramsey G. Hemostasis and transfusion medicine. In: Barash PG, Cullen BF, Stoelting RK, et al, eds. *Clinical Anesthesia*. 7th ed. Philadelphia: Wolters Kluwer Health; 2013:408-444.

16. Correct answer: A

Autologous blood transfusion is a process that involves harvesting one's own blood for use in the perioperative arena. Three distinct methods are available: preoperative autologous blood donation, acute normovolemic hemodilution, and perioperative blood cell salvage. Benefits of autologous transfusion include elimination of risks of viral pathogens and alloimmunization, as well as providing a mechanism for those with limited donors secondary to multiple and/or rare antibodies. These procedures should be avoided in those with active infections, aortic stenosis, recent MI, cerebrovascular accident, or uncontrolled hypertension.

In preoperative autologous blood donation, patients' whole blood is extracted for storage weekly, until 72 hours before a planned procedure. This blood is then utilized for the patient in the event a blood transfusion is required during the planned procedure.

In acute normovolemic hemodilution, the patient's blood is extracted immediately preoperatively, and the volume is replaced with crystalloid and colloid intravenous fluid at a ratio of either 3:1 (crystalloid) or 1:1 (colloid). Acute normovolemic hemodilution is indicated when blood loss is expected to be greater than 50% of the circulating blood volume, is difficult to cross match, or patients refuse allogenic blood. During the procedure, the blood that is lost is lower in hemoglobin and clotting factors. Patients who are otherwise healthy can tolerate this state of "anemia" by increasing their cardiac output. However, one should advise against this in patients with a history of angina or other cardiac problems where they could sustain permanent injury/death resulting from tachycardia or decreased oxygen delivery. Postoperatively, patients are reinfused with their previously extracted units, which replace hemoglobin and clotting factors.

Perioperative blood cell salvage includes the use of intraoperative and postoperative cell salvage. "Intraoperative salvage" is a blood-saving technique that uses suction to withdraw blood from the surgical site into a machine that will anticoagulate the recovered blood using heparin or citrate and then employ filtration, centrifugation, and washing mechanisms before reinfusing red cells back to the patient. Perioperative blood salvage is best indicated for orthopedic and off-pump cardiac surgical procedures with expected blood loss of >1000 mL or ~20% of one's circulating volume. One must always be cognizant of the certain pitfalls that are associated with intraoperative salvage, including, but not limited to, hemolysis, contamination with other various substances in the surgical field both from the patient and related to the procedure, and dilutional coagulopathy because the washed red cells lack clotting factors. Postoperative blood salvage includes a similar process; however, the red cells are collected from external draining devices instead of the surgical field. The primary danger of postoperative salvage is that externally collected blood can contain inflammatory mediators, leading to coagulopathy, lung, and renal damage.

Reference:
1. Carabini LM, Ramsey G. Hemostasis and transfusion medicine. In: Barash PG, Cullen BF, Stoelting RK, et al, eds. *Clinical Anesthesia*. 7th ed. Philadelphia: Wolters Kluwer Health; 2013:408-444.

17. Correct answer: D

See answer explanation given for question 16.

Autologous blood transfusion is a process that involves harvesting one's own blood for use in the perioperative arena. Three distinct methods are available: preoperative autologous blood donation, acute normovolemic hemodilution, and perioperative blood cell salvage. Benefits of autologous transfusion include elimination of risks of viral pathogens and alloimmunization, as well as providing a mechanism for those with limited donors secondary to multiple and/or rare antibodies. These procedures should be avoided in those with active infections, aortic stenosis, recent MI, cerebrovascular accident, or uncontrolled hypertension.

In preoperative autologous blood donation, patients' whole blood is extracted for storage weekly, until 72 hours before a planned procedure. This blood is then utilized for the patient in the event a blood transfusion is required during the planned procedure.

In acute normovolemic hemodilution, the patient's blood is extracted immediately preoperatively, and the volume is replaced with crystalloid and colloid intravenous fluid at a ratio of either 3:1 (crystalloid) or 1:1 (colloid). Acute normovolemic hemodilution is indicated when blood loss is expected to be greater than 50% of the circulating blood volume, is difficult to cross match, or patients refuse allogenic blood. During the procedure, the blood that is lost is lower in hemoglobin and clotting factors. Patients who are otherwise healthy can tolerate this state of "anemia" by increasing their cardiac output. However, one should advise against this in patients with a history of angina or other cardiac problems where they could sustain permanent injury/death resulting from tachycardia or decreased oxygen delivery. Postoperatively, patients are reinfused with their previously extracted units, which replace hemoglobin and clotting factors.

Perioperative blood cell salvage includes the use of intraoperative and postoperative cell salvage. "Intraoperative salvage" is a blood-saving technique that uses suction to withdraw blood from the surgical site into a machine that will anticoagulate the recovered blood using heparin or citrate and then employ filtration, centrifugation, and washing mechanisms before reinfusing red cells back to the patient. Perioperative blood salvage is best indicated for orthopedic and off-pump cardiac surgical procedures with expected blood loss of >1000 mL or ~20% of one's circulating volume. One must always be cognizant of the certain pitfalls that are associated with intraoperative salvage, including, but not limited to, hemolysis, contamination with other various substances in the surgical field both from the patient and related to the procedure, and dilutional coagulopathy because the washed red cells lack clotting factors. Postoperative blood salvage includes a similar process; however, the red cells are collected from external draining devices instead of the surgical field. The primary danger of postoperative salvage is that externally collected blood can contain inflammatory mediators, leading to coagulopathy, lung, and renal damage.

Reference:
1. Carabini LM, Ramsey G. Hemostasis and transfusion medicine. In: Barash PG, Cullen BF, Stoelting RK, et al, eds. *Clinical Anesthesia*. 7th ed. Philadelphia: Wolters Kluwer Health; 2013:408-444.

18. Correct answer: B

See answer explanation given for question 16.

Reference:
1. Carabini LM, Ramsey G. Hemostasis and transfusion medicine. In: Barash PG, Cullen BF, Stoelting RK, et al, eds. *Clinical Anesthesia*. 7th ed. Philadelphia: Wolters Kluwer Health; 2013:408-444.

19. Correct answer: C

See answer explanation given for question 16.

Reference:
1. Carabini LM, Ramsey G. Hemostasis and transfusion medicine. In: Barash PG, Cullen BF, Stoelting RK, et al, eds. *Clinical Anesthesia*. 7th ed. Philadelphia: Wolters Kluwer Health; 2013:408-444.

20. Correct answer: B

See answer explanation given for question 16.

Reference:
1. Carabini LM, Ramsey G. Hemostasis and transfusion medicine. In: Barash PG, Cullen BF, Stoelting RK, et al, eds. *Clinical Anesthesia*. 7th ed. Philadelphia: Wolters Kluwer Health; 2013:408-444.

21. Correct answer: C

Jehovah's Witnesses are a religious group that adheres to literal translations of the Bible and have particular beliefs about the use of blood products that often lead to their refusal of blood products. Individuals may vary with regard to the specifics of accepting and refusing "blood" products. Oftentimes, they will carry a card to inform medical providers of their wishes. When possible, the medical team should have a discussion with patients about their beliefs regarding blood products to provide optimal medical management of patients in accordance with their belief system. As always, if a person is unconscious, his/her belief system is unknown, and it is an emergent situation, the medical professional should obviously provide all lifesaving measures, including transfusion of blood products.

Reference:

1. Carabini LM, Ramsey G. Hemostasis and transfusion medicine. In: Barash PG, Cullen BF, Stoelting RK, et al, eds. *Clinical Anesthesia*. 7th ed. Philadelphia: Wolters Kluwer Health; 2013:408-444.

22. Correct answer: B

Erythropoietin's release is stimulated by hematocrit levels below 30% or hypoxia. Classically, erythropoietin is used for cases of refractory anemia, especially in patients with renal failure. Currently, erythropoietin is becoming well known in other arenas because perioperative autologous blood donation continues to grow.

Reference:

1. Carabini LM, Ramsey G. Hemostasis and transfusion medicine. In: Barash PG, Cullen BF, Stoelting RK, et al, eds. *Clinical Anesthesia*. 7th ed. Philadelphia: Wolters Kluwer Health; 2013:408-444.

23. Correct answer: B

The platelet transfusion threshold depends primarily on the clinical setting in which a procedure is taking place.

Guidelines for platelet transfusions:

1. Stable patients without evidence of bleeding: <10 000
2. Prophylaxis for invasive procedures such as lumbar puncture, neuraxial anesthesia, central venous catheterization, endoscopy with biopsy, liver biopsy, or major surgery: <50 000
3. Stable patients with clinical evidence of bleeding or coagulopathy: <50 000
4. Patients with disseminated intravascular coagulation (DIC) and signs of ongoing bleeding: <50 000
5. Patients undergoing massive transfusions with other blood products: <75 000
6. Patients having surgery of the eye or central nervous system: <100 000

Reference:

1. Carabini LM, Ramsey G. Hemostasis and transfusion medicine. In: Barash PG, Cullen BF, Stoelting RK, et al, eds. *Clinical Anesthesia*. 7th ed. Philadelphia: Wolters Kluwer Health; 2013:408-444.

24. Correct answer: C

Transfusion thresholds in the treatment of the critically ill have been well studied. Most recently, the Transfusion Requirements in Critical Care (TRICC) study compared the 30-day mortality of a restrictive threshold of 7 g/dL with a conventional threshold of 10 g/dL and found that there was no significant difference between the two, but the trend favored the restrictive group in many subgroups. Since this trial, there has been a concerted effort to use the more restrictive strategy; however, it has been found that the mean transfusion threshold remains much higher at 8.6 g/dL.

One must always take into account whether or not the patient has had a recent MI, has ongoing ischemia, or is actively hemorrhaging.

References:

1. Hallman MR, Treggiari MM, Deem S. Critical care medicine. In: Barash PG, Cullen BF, Stoelting RK, et al, eds. *Clinical Anesthesia*. 7th ed. Philadelphia: Wolters Kluwer Health; 2013:1580-1610.
2. Herbert P, Wells G, Blajchman M, et al. A multicenter, randomized, controlled clinical trial of transfusion requirements in critical care. *N Engl J Med*. 1999;340:409-417.

25. Correct answer: A

The following parameters are typically utilized for the safe storage of blood components:

- Packed red blood cells: 1°C-6°C for 21-35 days **without** an additive solution
- Packed red blood cells: 1°C-6°C for 42 days **with** an additive solution
- Red blood cells, frozen: <−65°C for 10 years
- Platelets, whole blood derived: 20°C-24°C for 5 days
- Platelets, apheresis: 20°C-24°C for 5 days
- Plasma, fresh frozen: <−18°C for 1 year OR <−65°C for 7 years
- Plasma, frozen within 24 hours: <−18°C for 1 year
- Cryoprecipitate: <−18°C for 1 year

Reference:
1. Carabini LM, Ramsey G. Hemostasis and transfusion medicine. In: Barash PG, Cullen BF, Stoelting RK, et al, eds. *Clinical Anesthesia*. 7th ed. Philadelphia: Wolters Kluwer Health; 2013:408-444.

26. Correct answer: D

In the United States, blood donors are screened via confidential interviews for specific exposure before donating blood. If they pass this initial screening, they can donate at which point their blood is tested for a variety of pathogens and diseases, including hepatitis B and C and HIV. Blood donors are required to have a hemoglobin and hematocrit above 12.5 g/dL and 38%, respectively. Donors are limited to donating once every 8 weeks to avoid becoming anemic.

Reference:
1. Carabini LM, Ramsey G. Hemostasis and transfusion medicine. In: Barash PG, Cullen BF, Stoelting RK, et al, eds. *Clinical Anesthesia*. 7th ed. Philadelphia: Wolters Kluwer Health; 2013:408-444.

27. Correct answer: A

FFP contains all the factors involved in hemostasis. Indication for the use of FFP includes, but is not limited to, the following:
- Correction of inherited factor deficiencies when there is no available or existing factor concentrate **and** the PT or PTT is >1.5× normal
- Correction of acquired multifactor deficiencies **with** evidence of critical bleeding **or** in anticipation of a major surgery or invasive procedure with PT or PTT >1.5× normal
- Liver dysfunction, DIC, or microvascular bleeding associated with massive transfusion, reversal of warfarin, heparin resistance, treatment of thrombotic microangiopathies
- Treatment of hereditary angioedema when C1-esterase is unavailable

Reference:
1. Carabini LM, Ramsey G. Hemostasis and transfusion medicine. In: Barash PG, Cullen BF, Stoelting RK, et al, eds. *Clinical Anesthesia*. 7th ed. Philadelphia: Wolters Kluwer Health; 2013:408-444.

28. Correct answer: C

Cryoprecipitate is formulated as FFP thaws, which allows for precipitation of large molecules that are centrifuged with fibrinogen, fibronectin, von Willebrand factor, factor VIII, and factor XIII. Compared with FFP, cryoprecipitate has a higher percentage of fibrinogen and functions as a low-volume fibrinogen replacement.

Indications for cryoprecipitate infusion include the following:
- Microvascular bleeding with hyperfibrinogenemia
- DIC with fibrinogen levels of <80-100 mg/dL
- Hemorrhage or massive transfusion with fibrinogen levels of <100-150 mg/dL
- Prophylaxis in patients with hemophilia A and von Willebrand disease
- Prophylaxis for patients with congenital dysfibrinogenemias

Reference:
1. Carabini LM, Ramsey G. Hemostasis and transfusion medicine. In: Barash PG, Cullen BF, Stoelting RK, et al, eds. *Clinical Anesthesia*. 7th ed. Philadelphia: Wolters Kluwer Health; 2013:408-444.

29. Correct answer: B

FNHTR is the most common complication/reaction associated with blood product transfusion. FNHTRs are a result of recipient alloimmunization to human leukocyte antigens (HLAs) from donor white blood cell (WBC), in addition to cytokines released during storage of blood products. The risk of developing a FNHTR increases successively with each additional/multiple transfusion. FNHTR classically presents within the first 4 hours of receiving a blood transfusion.

Signs and symptoms associated with a FNHTR include the following:
- Increase in body temperature (at least 1°C)
- Chills
- Rigors
- Anxiety
- Headache

FNHTRs are usually self-limiting and are easily managed with antipyretic and anti-inflammatory medications. The incidence of developing a FNHTR has decreased from 30% to 0.03%-2.18% with the use of leukoreduced products.

AHTRs are one of the leading causes of mortality secondary to transfusions. AHTR can not only result from transfusion of incompatible blood products, often ABO incompatibility, but it can also be due to incompatible plasma and RBC antigens, including Kidd, Kell, and Duffy. AHTR causes hemolysis, release of bradykinin, and histamine, leading to hemodynamic instability, bronchospasm, urticaria, dyspnea, flushing, anxiety, renal failure, DIC, and death in 50% of patients. Treatment includes immediately stopping the transfusion, starting aggressive hydration with IV fluids, and generalized supportive care, namely vasopressors to counteract the hemodynamic instability. Diagnosis involves confirmation via laboratory testing, showing increased free hemoglobin, low haptoglobin, increased bilirubin, hematuria, and a positive direct Coombs test.

DHTRs are due to alloantibodies to minor red blood cell antigens in Rh, Kidd, Kell, and Duffy groups. The symptoms are significantly milder than an acute hemolytic reaction and typically present 3-10 days post transfusion. Signs and symptoms include jaundice, hematuria, low haptoglobin, decreasing hemoglobin, and a positive direct Coombs test. The mainstay of treatment is aggressive hydration to limit damage to the renal tubules.

Anaphylactoid reactions due to blood transfusions are rare but can be fatal if not recognized. Most commonly, these reactions occur in IgA-deficient patients with IgA antibodies and present with hypotension, bronchospasm, and hemodynamic instability. These reactions can be minimized by washing blood in patients who are IgA deficient or by using blood obtained from IgA-deficient individuals.

Reference:

1. Carabini LM, Ramsey G. Hemostasis and transfusion medicine. In: Barash PG, Cullen BF, Stoelting RK, et al, eds. *Clinical Anesthesia.* 7th ed. Philadelphia: Wolters Kluwer Health; 2013:408-444.

---

30. **Correct answer: B**

This patient is suffering from an **AHTR**, which is one of the leading causes of mortality secondary to transfusions. AHTR can not only result from transfusion of incompatible blood products, often ABO incompatibility, but it can also be due to incompatible plasma and RBC antigens, including Kidd, Kell, and Duffy. AHTR causes hemolysis, release of bradykinin, and histamine, leading to hemodynamic instability, bronchospasm, urticaria, dyspnea, flushing, anxiety, renal failure, DIC, and death in 50% of patients. Treatment includes immediately stopping the transfusion, starting aggressive hydration with IV fluids, and generalized supportive care, namely vasopressors to counteract the hemodynamic instability. Diagnosis involves confirmation via laboratory testing, showing increased free hemoglobin, low haptoglobin, increased bilirubin, hematuria, and a positive direct Coombs test.

Reference:

1. Carabini LM, Ramsey G. Hemostasis and transfusion medicine. In: Barash PG, Cullen BF, Stoelting RK, et al, eds. *Clinical Anesthesia.* 7th ed. Philadelphia: Wolters Kluwer Health; 2013:408-444.

---

31. **Correct answer: D**

This patient is suffering from a **DHTR**. Development of DHTRs is due to alloantibodies to minor RBS antigens in Rh, Kidd, Kell, and Duffy groups. The symptoms are significantly milder than an acute hemolytic reaction and typically present 3-10 days post transfusion. Signs and symptoms include jaundice, hematuria, low haptoglobin, decreasing hemoglobin, and a positive direct Coombs test. The mainstay of treatment is aggressive hydration to limit damage to the renal tubules.

Reference:

1. Carabini LM, Ramsey G. Hemostasis and transfusion medicine. In: Barash PG, Cullen BF, Stoelting RK, et al, eds. *Clinical Anesthesia.* 7th ed. Philadelphia: Wolters Kluwer Health; 2013:408-444.

---

32. **Correct answer: B**

Blood component processing helps to alleviate many of the concerns with blood transfusion incompatibility and infections and includes screening for pathogens as well as certain treatments. **Leukoreduction** removes WBCs from RBCs and platelets and reduces the risk of HLA alloimmunization, FNHTRs, and CMV transmission. **Washing** removes plasma for patients with allergic transfusion reactions, including those with IgA deficiency; however, it does not prevent GVHD or HLA alloimmunization. **Irradiation** of cellular components is used to prevent GVHD in those who are immunosuppressed, including those with leukemia, lymphoma, post–stem cell transplants, and congenital immunodeficiencies. Premedicating a patient with acetaminophen would not aid in avoiding any specific reaction to blood products.

Reference:

1. Carabini LM, Ramsey G. Hemostasis and transfusion medicine. In: Barash PG, Cullen BF, Stoelting RK, et al, eds. *Clinical Anesthesia*. 7th ed. Philadelphia: Wolters Kluwer Health; 2013:408-444.

33. Correct answer: A

Anaphylactoid reactions due to blood transfusion are rare but can be fatal if not recognized. Most commonly, these reactions occur in IgA-deficient patients with IgA antibodies and present with hypotension, bronchospasm, and hemodynamic instability. These reactions can be minimized by washing blood in patients who are IgA deficient or by using blood obtained from IgA-deficient individuals.

Reference:

1. Carabini LM, Ramsey G. Hemostasis and transfusion medicine. In: Barash PG, Cullen BF, Stoelting RK, et al, eds. *Clinical Anesthesia*. 7th ed. Philadelphia: Wolters Kluwer Health; 2013:408-444.

34. Correct answer: C

Blood component processing helps to alleviate many of the concerns with blood transfusion incompatibility and infections and includes screening for pathogens as well as certain treatments. **Leukoreduction** removes WBCs from RBCs and platelets and reduces the risk of HLA alloimmunization, FNHTRs, and CMV transmission. **Washing** removes plasma for patients with allergic transfusion reactions, including those with IgA deficiency; however, it does not prevent GVHD or HLA alloimmunization. **Irradiation** of cellular components is used to prevent GVHD in those who are immunosuppressed, including those with leukemia, lymphoma, post–stem cell transplants, and congenital immunodeficiencies. Specific preservatives do not protect against GVHD.

Reference:

1. Carabini LM, Ramsey G. Hemostasis and transfusion medicine. In: Barash PG, Cullen BF, Stoelting RK, et al, eds. *Clinical Anesthesia*. 7th ed. Philadelphia: Wolters Kluwer Health; 2013:408-444.

35. Correct answer: C

Citrate is an anticoagulant added to stored blood to prevent clotting during storage. During transfusion of large quantities of blood, such as during trauma resuscitation, the liver is unable to completely clear the citrate and it begins to accumulate and chelate calcium, resulting in hypocalcemia, which when severe can cause muscle weakness, tetany, arrhythmias, myocardial dysfunction, and coagulopathies.

Reference:

1. Carabini LM, Ramsey G. Hemostasis and transfusion medicine. In: Barash PG, Cullen BF, Stoelting RK, et al, eds. *Clinical Anesthesia*. 7th ed. Philadelphia: Wolters Kluwer Health; 2013:408-444.

36. Correct answer: D

TRALI, the leading cause of transfusion-related mortality, is defined as a reaction that occurs within 6 hours of blood component therapy and includes noncardiogenic pulmonary edema with acute bilateral infiltrates and hypoxemia with a Pao_2/Fio_2 <300 mm Hg or oxygen saturation <90% on room air with no evidence of left atrial hypertension. Those most at risk population for TRALI include critical care patients, those receiving massive transfusion, and those with a predisposition to ALI such as sepsis, burns, and aspirations. The pathophysiology of TRALI has yet to be fully elucidated; however, it likely involves a vulnerable immune system, as well as immunogenic components of stored blood products. Treatment of TRALI is primarily supportive and includes measures to limit lung injury, such as positive end-expiratory pressure and low tidal volumes, as well as treating the underlying cause, thus limiting the need for further transfusions.

Reference:

1. Carabini LM, Ramsey G. Hemostasis and transfusion medicine. In: Barash PG, Cullen BF, Stoelting RK, et al, eds. *Clinical Anesthesia*. 7th ed. Philadelphia: Wolters Kluwer Health; 2013:408-444.

37. Correct answer: C

TACO is the acute episode of hydrostatic pulmonary edema following blood component transfusion. Diagnosis can be difficult and relies on clinical evidence of volume overload with left atrial hypertension after transfusion. Risk factors for TACO include high rates and volumes of transfusion. TACO responds well to diuresis and afterload reduction.

Reference:

1. Carabini LM, Ramsey G. Hemostasis and transfusion medicine. In: Barash PG, Cullen BF, Stoelting RK, et al, eds. *Clinical Anesthesia*. 7th ed. Philadelphia: Wolters Kluwer Health; 2013:408-444.

38. Correct answer: D

All blood component products are tested for residual risk of viral infections. The incidence of infection has decreased significantly over the past several decades. CMV is the most common disease transmitted by blood component transfusion, with an incidence of 1%-3%. Hepatitis B virus is the next most common with a residual risk of 1/366 500, followed by hepatitis C virus (1/1 657 700), HIV (1/1 860 800), and human T-cell lymphotropic virus (1/3 394 000).

Reference:

1. Carabini LM, Ramsey G. Hemostasis and transfusion medicine. In: Barash PG, Cullen BF, Stoelting RK, et al, eds. *Clinical Anesthesia*. 7th ed. Philadelphia: Wolters Kluwer Health; 2013:408-444.

39. Correct answer: B

Platelets are stored at room temperature to preserve clotting function at 20°C-24°C for up to 5 days. This results in a higher risk of bacterial growth compared with other blood products that are refrigerated. The risk of bacterial contamination of platelets is 1/15 000 compared with the risk of bacterial contamination of packed RBCs at 1/35 000.

Reference:

1. Carabini LM, Ramsey G. Hemostasis and transfusion medicine. In: Barash PG, Cullen BF, Stoelting RK, et al, eds. *Clinical Anesthesia*. 7th ed. Philadelphia: Wolters Kluwer Health; 2013:408-444.

40. Correct answer: B

Transfusion-related immunomodulation is the brief depression of the immune system following blood product transfusion and was initially discovered when patients undergoing renal allografts who had received a transfusion pretransplant were shown to have improved survival. Since then, the immunosuppression associated with blood transfusion has shown a decreased rate of miscarriage for women with a history of recurrent spontaneous abortion and a reduced risk of recurrent Crohn disease in patients who have received transfusions. However, the immunosuppression has caused increased rates of malignancies and reactivation of latent TB, CMV, and HIV. Transfusion-related immunomodulation is thought to be from 2-fold: (1) the "first hit" is the specific condition that the patient is requiring a transfusion, eg, trauma, critical illness, anemia, and (2) the "second hit" is the transfusion of blood products, including WBCs, HLAs, and cytokines.

Reference:

1. Carabini LM, Ramsey G. Hemostasis and transfusion medicine. In: Barash PG, Cullen BF, Stoelting RK, et al, eds. *Clinical Anesthesia*. 7th ed. Philadelphia: Wolters Kluwer Health; 2013:408-444.

9

ENDOCRINE AND METABOLIC SYSTEMS

Jamie L. Sparling

1. **While performing a preoperative assessment on a patient with acromegaly, you note that his home medication list includes octreotide. Which of the following is the mechanism of action of octreotide?**

    A. Competitive inhibition at the growth hormone (GH) receptor
    B. Inhibition of GH and IGF-1 secretion
    C. Stimulation of insulin secretion
    D. Agonism at the dopamine receptor

2. **Which of the following hormones is released from the posterior pituitary gland?**

    A. Thyroid-stimulating hormone (TSH)
    B. Vasopressin (antidiuretic hormone [ADH])
    C. Corticotropin (adrenocorticotropic hormone [ACTH])
    D. Growth hormone

3. **Which of the following statements is true of the syndrome of inappropriate antidiuretic hormone (SIADH)?**

    A. Chronic hyponatremia from SIADH should be corrected with hypertonic saline.
    B. Peripheral edema is a common physical exam finding.
    C. Most cases of SIADH are due to an intrinsic pituitary disorder.
    D. Demeclocycline may be used to treat SIADH.

4. **Which of the following statements is true with regard to diabetes insipidus (DI)?**

    A. Desmopressin administration can distinguish central versus nephrogenic DI.
    B. Patients with nephrogenic DI will increase urine osmolality in response to desmopressin.
    C. Thiazide diuretics may be used to treat central DI.
    D. Patients with central DI will fail to respond to exogenous desmopressin administration.

5. **Which of the following features is more consistent with a diagnosis of a pituitary macroadenoma than that of a pituitary microadenoma?**

    A. Galactorrhea
    B. Visual field deficit
    C. Thyrotoxicosis
    D. Cushing disease

6. Which of the following sets of laboratory values is consistent with a diagnosis of subclinical hypothyroidism?

TSH	FREE T$_4$
A. Decreased	Increased
B. Increased	Decreased
C. Decreased	Decreased
D. Increased	Normal

7. Which of the following statements pertaining to thyroid storm is true?

   A. Atrial fibrillation is required for diagnosis.
   B. Mortality rate may exceed 20%.
   C. TSH levels are elevated.
   D. Hyperthermia is rare.

8. Which of the following is likely to be seen when a patient with hypothyroidism is under general anesthesia?

   A. Hypotension
   B. Prolongation of nondepolarizing neuromuscular blockers
   C. Bradycardia
   D. Hyperglycemia

9. Which of the following statements is true with regard to potential complications associated with thyroid surgery?

   A. Unilateral recurrent laryngeal nerve damage will cause aphonia.
   B. Unanticipated difficult airway is present in 5%-8% of thyroid cases.
   C. Retrosternal thyroid may cause airway obstruction with prone positioning.
   D. Postoperative hypocalcemia typically manifests immediately in the postanesthesia care unit.

10. Which of the following diagnostic results is consistent with a diagnosis of Grave disease?

    A. Elevated TSH
    B. Normal free T$_4$
    C. Diffusely increased radioactive iodine uptake
    D. Decreased free T$_3$

11. Which statement correctly describes one of the actions of parathyroid hormone (PTH)?

    A. PTH increases Ca^{2+} resorption in the ascending loop of Henle, distal tubule, and collecting tubule of the kidney.
    B. PTH inhibits 1α-hydroxylase gene in renal cells.
    C. PTH promotes uptake of calcium by osteocytes.
    D. PTH increases the reabsorption of phosphate and bicarbonate in the nephron.

12. Which of the following is the *primary* mechanism by which calcitonin reduces serum Ca^{2+} levels?

    A. Increasing the renal excretion of phosphate
    B. Decreasing the intestinal absorption of calcium
    C. Promotion of osteoblastic activity to increase bone formation
    D. Inhibition of osteoclast activity to decrease bone resorption

13. **What is the initial step in the management of a patient with *symptomatic* hypercalcemia?**

   A. Calcitonin
   B. Furosemide
   C. Normal saline
   D. Pamidronate

14. **What is the adjusted plasma calcium for a patient with end-stage liver disease who is hypoalbuminemic with the following laboratory values?**

Plasma calcium	7.6 mg/dL
Plasma albumin	1.6 g/dL

   A. 5.7 mg/dL
   B. 7.6 mg/dL
   C. 9.5 mg/dL
   D. 10 mg/dL

15. **Which of the following causes an *increase* in the ionized calcium concentration?**

   A. Increased serum albumin
   B. Alkalosis
   C. Transfusion of fresh frozen plasma
   D. Acidosis

16. **Which of the following sets of values would you expect to observe in a patient with primary adrenal insufficiency?**

	CRH	ACTH	CORTISOL	ALDOSTERONE
A.	Elevated	Elevated	Decreased	Decreased
B.	Elevated	Elevated	Decreased	Normal
C.	Elevated	Decreased	Decreased	Decreased
D.	Decreased	Elevated	Decreased	Normal

17. **Which of the following statements is true regarding the preoperative preparation for a patient with pheochromocytoma?**

   A. Selective α_1-blockers have a longer duration of action compared with phenoxybenzamine.
   B. β-Blockade should be initiated before α-blockade.
   C. Calcium channel blockers are contraindicated in patients with pheochromocytoma.
   D. The primary side effect of phenoxybenzamine is orthostatic hypotension.

18. **Which of the following steroids *lacks* mineralocorticoid activity?**

   A. Hydrocortisone
   B. Dexamethasone
   C. Methylprednisolone
   D. Prednisone

19. **In which of the following patients is stress dose steroid administration indicated?**

    A. A 67-year-old man on prednisone 10 mg daily for 5 days for chronic obstructive pulmonary disease exacerbation presenting for laparoscopic cholecystectomy

    B. A 40-year-old woman on prednisone 2.5 mg daily for 6 years for systemic lupus erythematosus presenting for total knee arthroplasty

    C. A 23-year-old man on prednisone 20 mg daily for ulcerative colitis presenting for subtotal colectomy

    D. A 56-year-old woman on prednisone 40 mg daily for rheumatoid arthritis presenting for superficial lymph node biopsy

20. **Which of the following correctly describes a physiologic effect of glucocorticoids?**

    A. Increase in eosinophils and basophils

    B. Decreased protein catabolism

    C. Sensitization to insulin

    D. Promotion of gluconeogenesis

21. **Which of the following characteristics is *most consistent* with nonketotic hyperosmolar coma?**

    A. Metabolic acidosis

    B. Hypokalemia

    C. Skeletal muscle weakness

    D. Profound hyperglycemia >600 mg/dL

22. **Long-term type 1 diabetes is associated with which of the following anesthetic complications?**

    A. Malignant hyperthermia

    B. Difficult airway

    C. Pseudocholinesterase deficiency

    D. Anaphylaxis to local anesthetics

23. **Which of the following statements is true of glucose metabolism in the perioperative period?**

    A. Glucagon levels are decreased.

    B. Blood glucose levels in nondiabetic patients may rise as much as 60 mg/dL.

    C. Catecholamines inhibit gluconeogenesis.

    D. ACTH levels are decreased.

24. **In which of the following scenarios is it acceptable to administer metformin therapy?**

    A. The night before elective surgery

    B. In the presence of NYHA class II heart failure

    C. The morning a patient will undergo CT scan with IV contrast

    D. In a patient with pyelonephritis who remains normotensive

25. **Which of the following statements is true regarding the cardiac risk in patients with diabetes mellitus?**

    A. Diabetic patients reliably present with classic angina symptoms in the setting of acute myocardial infarction.

    B. Aspirin therapy is recommended for diabetic patients in the absence of known coronary disease.

    C. Routine stress testing is indicated for all diabetic patients to identify silent ischemia.

    D. ACE inhibitors should be avoided in diabetes because they are at risk of diabetic nephropathy.

26. **The process of glycolysis converts glucose into what molecule?**

    A. NADPH

    B. Acetyl-CoA

    C. Pyruvate

    D. Lactate

27. Which molecule is common to carbohydrate, lipid, and amino acid metabolism and does directly enter the Krebs cycle for further metabolism?

    A. Acetyl-CoA
    B. Pyruvate
    C. Citrate
    D. Succinyl-CoA

28. Which of the following molecules accelerates the Krebs cycle via activation of pyruvate dehydrogenase phosphatase?

    A. Citrate
    B. ATP
    C. NADH
    D. Calcium

29. Which of the following is the final acceptor of electrons in the electron transport chain?

    A. NADH
    B. NAD+
    C. Oxygen
    D. FADH+

30. Which of the following organs is/are responsible for gluconeogenesis?

    A. Liver only
    B. Kidney only
    C. Brain
    D. Liver and kidney

31. Which of the following is the mechanism of action of simvastatin in lowering lipid levels?

    A. Prevention of intestinal absorption of triacylglycerides (TAGs)
    B. HMG-CoA reductase inhibition
    C. PCSK9 inhibition
    D. Upregulation of β-oxidation of fatty acids

32. Which of the following is true of lipid digestion?

    A. Cholecystokinin speeds gastric motility.
    B. TAGs are absorbed unchanged in the small intestine.
    C. Emulsification of lipids occurs primarily in the small intestine.
    D. Lipids diffuse into enterocytes unchanged because of their water solubility.

33. Patients with pancreatic exocrine insufficiency are at risk for which vitamin deficiency?

    A. Thiamine
    B. Pyridoxine
    C. Vitamin B_{12}
    D. Vitamin D

34. Which of the following statements is true with regard to lipid metabolism in the liver?

    A. The liver may package TAGs into very-low-density lipoproteins for transport to other tissues.
    B. The liver can extract energy from ketones via ketoacyl-CoA transferase.
    C. Insulin activates β-oxidation of fatty acids in the liver.
    D. When there is a deficiency in glycogen, the liver converts glucose to TAGs for storage.

35. Which organ is unable to utilize fatty acid oxidation in times of starvation and thus relies primarily on ketone metabolism?

A. Heart
B. Liver
C. Brain
D. Muscle

36. Which of the following statements is true regarding cholesterol metabolism?

A. Bile salts are recirculated through enterohepatic circulation several times a day.
B. Cholesterol is converted into bile salts in the gall bladder.
C. Bile salts are excreted into the colon.
D. Cholesterols are hydrophilic molecules.

37. Which of the following is the mechanism of action of ezetimibe in lowering lipid levels?

A. Prevention of intestinal absorption of TAGs
B. HMG-CoA reductase inhibition
C. PCSK9 inhibition
D. Upregulating β-oxidation of fatty acids

38. Inhaled nitric oxide (NO) produces pulmonary vasodilation via increased concentration of which of the following substances?

A. Calcium
B. Atrial natriuretic peptide
C. Cyclic adenosine monophosphate (cAMP)
D. Cyclic guanosine monophosphate (cGMP)

39. Phosphodiesterase-5 inhibitors, such as sildenafil, will have which of the following effects?

A. Increase the intracellular level of cAMP
B. Increase the intracellular level of cGMP
C. Decrease the intracellular level of cAMP
D. Decrease the intracellular level of cGMP

40. Activation of the β_1-adrenergic receptor will increase the concentration of which of the following secondary messengers?

A. Cyclic guanosine monophosphate
B. Cyclic adenosine monophosphate
C. Ca^{2+}
D. Inositol triphosphate (IP_3)

Chapter 9 ▪ Answers

1. Correct answer: B

Acromegaly is caused by GH hypersecretion in adults, almost always because of a **pituitary adenoma.** Untreated, acromegaly leads to physical deformity, as well as a 2- to 3-fold increase in **mortality** because of cardiovascular disease, cancer, and respiratory compromise. Anesthesiologists treating these patients should be aware that acromegaly is also associated with macroglossia, prognathism, hypertension, diabetes, and cardiomegaly.

Upon diagnosis, 70% of patients with acromegaly have macroadenomas, whereas the other 30% have microadenomas. Surgery provides a relatively low cure rate for macroadenomas; radiation therapy is preferred and often provides a greater chance of definitive therapy. Other treatments include medication to control GH secretion and tumor growth.

Acromegaly can be treated with octreotide, which is a synthetic, more potent analogue of the endogenous hormone somatostatin. It inhibits the release of GH from the anterior pituitary through a negative feedback loop. There is also evidence that octreotide directly inhibits IGF-1 expression in hepatocytes, thus inhibiting insulin secretion. Bromocriptine is a dopamine agonist that may also be used in the treatment of pituitary tumors.

ORGAN SYSTEM EFFECTED BY ACROMEGALY	MANIFESTATION
Cardiovascular	Hypertension, cardiac enlargement, congestive heart failure
Musculoskeletal	Prognathism (jaw protrusion), arthritis
Respiratory	Tongue enlargement, sleep apnea
Neurologic	Paresthesia
Metabolic	Diabetes mellitus, hyperlipidemia, hypercalcemia

Adapted from Table 60-17 Manifestation of Acromegaly in Peterfreund RA, Lee SL. Endocrine surgery and intraoperative management of endocrine conditions. In: Longnecker DE, Brown DL, Newman MF, Zapol WM, eds. Anesthesiology. 2nd ed. New York: McGraw Hill; 2012:1112-1133.

References:
1. John AD. Evaluation of the patient with endocrine disease or diabetes. In: Longnecker DE, Brown DL, Newman MF, Zapol WM, eds. *Anesthesiology*. 2nd ed. New York: McGraw Hill; 2012:150-166.
2. Peterfreund RA, Lee SL. Endocrine surgery and intraoperative management of endocrine conditions. In: Longnecker DE, Brown DL, Newman MF, Zapol WM, eds. *Anesthesiology*. 2nd ed. New York: McGraw Hill; 2012:1112-1133.
3. Serri O, Brazeau P, Kachra Z, Posner B. Octreotide inhibits insulin-like growth factor-i hepatic gene expression in the hypophysectomized rat: evidence for a direct and indirect mechanism of action. *Endocrinology*. 1992;130(4):1816-1821.

2. Correct answer: B

The pituitary gland consists of the adenohypophysis (anterior pituitary) and the neurohypophysis (posterior pituitary). The production and release of hormones by the adenohypophysis is dependent on the release of hormones produced by the hypothalamus. The neurohypophysis is considered an extension of the hypothalamus and does not require releasing hormones. The adenohypophysis secretes TSH, ACTH, follicle-stimulating hormone, luteinizing hormone, GH, and prolactin. The neurohypophysis secretes ADH and oxytocin. The actions of the pituitary hormones are summarized in the figure below.

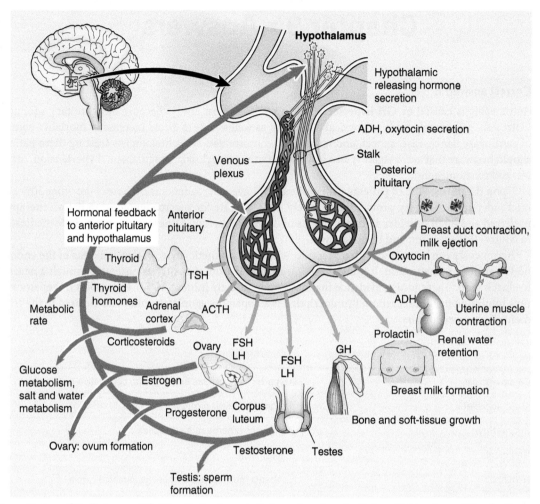

(From Turbow SD, Patterson BC. Hypothalamic and pituitary disorders. In: Felner EI, Umpierez GF, eds. *Endocrine Pathophysiology*. Philadelphia: Wolters Kluwer Health/Lippincott Williams & Wilkins; 2014:17, with permission.)

References:
1. John AD. Evaluation of the patient with endocrine disease or diabetes. In: Longnecker DE, Brown DL, Newman MF, Zapol WM, eds. *Anesthesiology*. 2nd ed. New York: McGraw Hill; 2012:150-166.
2. Akhtar S. Endocrine function. In: Barash PG, Cullen BF, Stoelting RK, et al, eds. *Clinical Anesthesia Fundamentals*. Philadelphia: Wolters Kluwer Health; 2015:335-356.

3. **Correct answer: D**

SIADH secretion is a common cause of euvolemic hyponatremia. It is most often NOT associated with a primary pituitary pathology. On the contrary, SIADH may occur in the setting of a number of tumors, pulmonary diseases, and CNS disorders and as a side effect from many drugs (eg, phenothiazines, tricyclic antidepressants, carbamazepine, selective serotonin reuptake inhibitors).

CRITERIA FOR DIAGNOSIS OF SIADH

Hyponatremia with plasma hypo-osmolality

Inappropriately increased urine osmolality

Increased renal sodium excretion

Normovolemia (absence of edema or volume depletion)

Other causes for hyponatremia ruled out

Adapted from Table 13-18 Criteria of Syndrome of Inappropriate Secretion of Antidiuretic Hormone in John AD. Evaluation of the patient with endocrine disease or diabetes. In: Longnecker DE, Brown DL, Newman MF, Zapol WM, eds. Anesthesiology. 2nd ed. New York: McGraw Hill; 2012:150-166.

Treatment of SIADH depends on the severity of hyponatremia and the time course over which it has developed. For chronic hyponatremia, fluid restriction is the treatment of choice. If patients are demonstrating the neurologic symptoms associated with symptomatic hyponatremia (such as irritability or nausea and vomiting), hypertonic saline should be administered with a target correction of no more than 0.5 mmol/L/h to prevent neurologic complications. Demeclocycline is a tetracycline that causes nephrogenic diabetes and may also be used in treatment of SIADH. Vasopressin receptor antagonists have also recently become available for the treatment of SIADH.

Reference:

1. John AD. Evaluation of the patient with endocrine disease or diabetes. In: Longnecker DE, Brown DL, Newman MF, Zapol WM, eds. *Anesthesiology*. 2nd ed. New York: McGraw Hill; 2012:150-166.

4. Correct answer: A

DI may occur secondary to a deficiency of vasopressin secretion (central DI) or resistance of the kidneys to the effects of vasopressin (nephrogenic DI). Central DI is more common and may occur secondary to or as a result of head trauma, hypothalamic tumors, infiltrative processes, cerebral aneurysms, ischemia, or neurosurgery. Both forms are characterized by polyuria with an intact thirst mechanism, which appears to autoregulate volume status. A water deprivation test can be used to diagnose DI and distinguish this disease process: central versus nephrogenic etiologies. In healthy individuals, urine will become maximally concentrated (≥700 mOsm/L) within 8 hours of water deprivation, whereas patients with either type of DI will continue to have dilute urine. In patients with central DI, administration of desmopressin at that point will prompt concentration of the urine, whereas in patients with nephrogenic DI, desmopressin will have no effect. Desmopressin can be used therapeutically in central DI, whereas nephrogenic DI is treated with oral hydration, decreased sodium intake, thiazide diuretics, amiloride, and NSAIDs (eg, indomethacin).

Reference:

1. John AD. Evaluation of the patient with endocrine disease or diabetes. In: Longnecker DE, Brown DL, Newman MF, Zapol WM, eds. *Anesthesiology*. 2nd ed. New York: McGraw Hill; 2012:150-166.

5. Correct answer: B

Pituitary adenomas are classified as microadenomas, if they are ≤1 cm in diameter, and macroadenomas, if they are >1 cm in diameter. Microadenomas tend to present with hypersecretion syndromes, such as galactorrhea from prolactin excess, infertility from follicle-stimulating hormone luteinizing hormone excess, thyrotoxicosis from TSH excess, and Cushing disease from ACTH excess. Macroadenomas present with symptoms of mass effect, including visual field deficits (classically, bitemporal hemianopia), headaches, cranial nerve III palsy and, in rare cases, even hydrocephalus.

TYPE OF PITUITARY ADENOMA	SYMPTOMS/SIGNS
Prolactinoma	Amenorrhea, impotence
Somatotroph adenoma	Gigantism (children), acromegaly (adults), cardiovascular disease, colon cancer, respiratory impairment
Corticotroph adenoma	Cushing disease, proximal myopathy, glucose intolerance, truncal obesity, hypokalemia, hypercoagulability
Thyrotroph adenoma	Thyrotoxicosis, goiter
Nonsecreting adenoma	Mass effect, hypopituitarism

References:

1. John AD. Evaluation of the patient with endocrine disease or diabetes. In: Longnecker DE, Brown DL, Newman MF, Zapol WM, eds. *Anesthesiology*. 2nd ed. New York: McGraw Hill; 2012:150-166.
2. Peterfreund RA, Lee SL. Endocrine surgery and intraoperative management of endocrine conditions. In: Longnecker DE, Brown DL, Newman MF, Zapol WM, eds. *Anesthesiology*. 2nd ed. New York: McGraw Hill; 2012:1112-1133.
3. Hannon V, Appleby I. Pituitary disease and anaesthesia. *Anaesth Intensive Care Med*. 2017;18(5):255-258.

6. **Correct answer: D**

Thyroid disease must be diagnosed through a combination of both laboratory values and clinical presentation. Laboratory measurements are often used to support diagnosis and include TSH and free thyroxine (FT_4). Hyperthyroidism is characterized by a low TSH (<0.05 μU/mL) and a high FT_4 (>1.8 ng/dL). Primary hypothyroidism is caused by failure of the thyroid gland to respond to TSH and is thus characterized by high TSH (>10 mU/L) and a low FT_4 (<0.7 ng/dL). Secondary hypothyroidism is quite rare and is due to a deficiency of TSH because of pituitary or hypothalamic dysfunction; it is thus characterized by a low TSH and low FT_4 (choice C). Subclinical hypothyroidism is a common entity, affecting up to 20% of women older than 50 years. It is characterized by an elevated TSH (>4.5 mU/L) and normal FT_4. Despite a normal FT_4, it is still recommended to treat patients with a TSH level >10 mU/L to normalize TSH levels. Treatment consists of once-a-day dosing of thyroxine, a medication with a long half-life of approximately 1 week.

Reference:

1. John AD. Evaluation of the patient with endocrine disease or diabetes. In: Longnecker DE, Brown DL, Newman MF, Zapol WM, eds. *Anesthesiology*. 2nd ed. New York: McGraw Hill; 2012:150-166.

7. **Correct answer: B**

Thyroid storm is a severe, life-threatening form of hyperthyroidism. The diagnosis is mainly clinical and the criteria are outlined below.

CRITERIA FOR THYROID STORM

1. Hyperthermia with diaphoresis

2. Tachycardia disproportionate to the level of hyperthermia

3. Cerebral dysfunction

4. Gastrointestinal disturbance

*Jaundice is a poor prognostic sign

Some precipitants of thyroid storm include infection, surgery (particularly those involving manipulation of the thyroid gland), radioactive iodine administration, iodinated contrast administration, amiodarone, and other acute stressors. Treatment includes supportive care, antiadrenergic drugs (eg, propranolol or esmolol), thionamide drugs to block further synthesis of thyroid hormone (and to block peripheral conversion of T_4 to T_3, in the case of propylthiouracil), and treatment of the underlying cause. In some cases, high-dose iodine is given to prevent further release of thyroid hormone. Corticosteroids may also be considered to prevent the release of and peripheral conversion of T_4 to T_3, as well as to avoid adrenal suppression, which may coexist. Finally, cholestyramine may be administered to prevent enterohepatic recirculation of thyroid hormone.

Reference:

1. John AD. Evaluation of the patient with endocrine disease or diabetes. In: Longnecker DE, Brown DL, Newman MF, Zapol WM, eds. *Anesthesiology*. 2nd ed. New York: McGraw Hill; 2012:150-166.

8. **Correct answer: C**

Hypothyroidism is a general hypometabolic state, characterized by symptoms including fatigue, cold intolerance, depression, and impaired concentration. These symptoms are accompanied by clinical signs including bradycardia, diastolic hypertension, ileus, urinary retention, carpal tunnel syndrome, and even myxedema coma. Even in the absence of myalgias or muscle cramps, hypothyroid patients may exhibit an elevated creatinine phosphokinase; however, hypothyroidism does not affect the duration of action of neuromuscular blockers. Other abnormalities seen intraoperatively may include increased bleeding, hyponatremia, hypoglycemia, and hypothermia from a decreased basal metabolic rate.

References:

1. John AD. Evaluation of the patient with endocrine disease or diabetes. In: Longnecker DE, Brown DL, Newman MF, Zapol WM, eds. *Anesthesiology*. 2nd ed. New York: McGraw Hill; 2012:150-166.

2. Peterfreund RA, Lee SL. Endocrine surgery and intraoperative management of endocrine conditions. In: Longnecker DE, Brown DL, Newman MF, Zapol WM, eds. *Anesthesiology*. 2nd ed. New York: McGraw Hill; 2012:1112-1133.

9. **Correct answer: B**

Thyroid surgery is typically performed under general endotracheal anesthesia. Given the proximity of the pathology and the surgical procedure to the airway, it is important to recognize several potential surgical, as well as airway, complications. Enlarged thyroid glands may result in airway obstruction or tracheal deviation, leading to unanticipated difficult airway in 5%-8% of cases. Recurrent laryngeal nerve damage is a common surgical complication; unilateral nerve damage results in hoarseness, whereas bilateral damage results in aphonia. Retrosternal thyroids may behave clinically as an anterior mediastinal mass, possessing the potential to cause airway obstruction with supine positioning. Postoperative hypocalcemia, secondary to removal of the parathyroid glands, typically presents within 24-48 hours post procedure and can manifest as stridor or laryngospasm. Other complications include bleeding, which should be treated immediately with opening of the surgical incision to prevent or reverse airway compromise from compression.

COMPLICATIONS OF THYROID SURGERY

Thyroid storm: It should be distinguished from malignant hyperthermia, pheochromocytoma, and inadequate anesthesia; it most often develops in undiagnosed or untreated hyperthyroid patients because of the stress of surgery.

Airway obstruction: Hematoma in the neck or tracheomalacia causing airway obstruction.

Recurrent laryngeal nerve damage: Hoarseness may be present if the damage is unilateral, and aphonia may be present if the damage is bilateral.

Hypoparathyroidism: Symptoms of hypocalcemia develop within 24-48 h and include laryngospasm.

From Barash PG, Cullen BF, Stoelting RK, et al, eds. Handbook of Clinical Anesthesia. *7th ed. Philaelphia: Wolters Kluwer/Lippincott Williams & Wilkins; 2013.*

Reference:
1. Akhtar S. Endocrine function. In: Barash PG, Cullen BF, Stoelting RK, et al, eds. *Clinical Anesthesia Fundamentals.* Philadelphia: Wolters Kluwer Health; 2015:335-356.

10. **Correct answer: C**

Grave disease is a cause of hyperthyroidism in which the body produces antibodies against the TSH receptor. Goiter and exophthalmos may be present on examination. Thyroid function tests are consistent with hyperthyroidism, including decreased TSH and elevated free T_4 and free T_3. Radioactive iodine studies show diffusely increased uptake, as compared with focally increased uptake that can be seen with a toxic adenoma, or decreased uptake because of thyroiditis or factitious hyperthyroidism.

Reference:
1. John AD. Evaluation of the patient with endocrine disease or diabetes. In: Longnecker DE, Brown DL, Newman MF, Zapol WM, eds. *Anesthesiology.* 2nd ed. New York: McGraw Hill; 2012:150-166.

11. **Correct answer: A**

PTH, together with vitamin D and calcitonin, is responsible for maintaining calcium homeostasis within the body. PTH is secreted by the parathyroid glands and acts via several mechanisms to increase the available level of Ca^{2+} in the body:
1. PTH activates osteoclasts to promote bone resorption.
2. PTH increases renal calcium resorption in the ascending loop of Henle, distal tubule, and collecting tubule.
3. PTH increases expression of 1α-hydroxylase, which converts inactive 25-OH-vitamin D to active $1,25\text{-}(OH)_2$-vitamin D.

PTH also increases the *excretion* of phosphate, bicarbonate, potassium, sodium, and certain amino acids. These actions are summarized in the figure below.

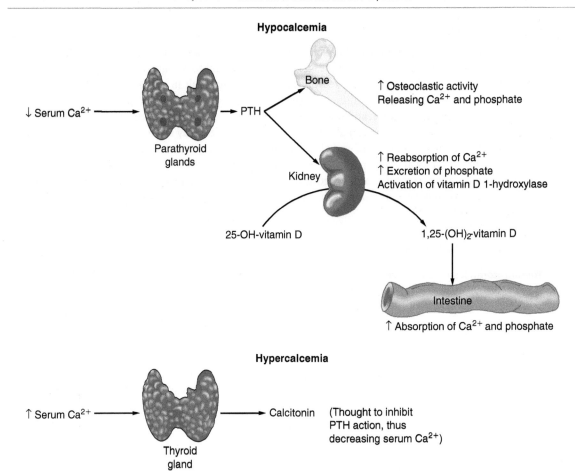

Hypocalcemia

↓ Serum Ca²⁺ ⟶ Parathyroid glands ⟶ PTH

Bone
↑ Osteoclastic activity
Releasing Ca²⁺ and phosphate

Kidney
↑ Reabsorption of Ca²⁺
↑ Excretion of phosphate
Activation of vitamin D 1-hydroxylase

25-OH-vitamin D

1,25-(OH)₂-vitamin D

Intestine
↑ Absorption of Ca²⁺ and phosphate

Hypercalcemia

↑ Serum Ca²⁺ ⟶ Thyroid gland ⟶ Calcitonin   (Thought to inhibit PTH action, thus decreasing serum Ca²⁺)

(From Schwartz JJ, Akhtar S, Rosenbaum SH. Endocrine function. In: Barash PG, Cullen BF, Stoelting RK, et al, eds. *Clinical Anesthesia.* 7th ed. Philadelphia: Wolters Kluwer Health/Lippincott Williams & Wilkins; 2013:1327, with permission.)

References:
1. John AD. Evaluation of the patient with endocrine disease or diabetes. In: Longnecker DE, Brown DL, Newman MF, Zapol WM, eds. *Anesthesiology.* 2nd ed. New York: McGraw Hill; 2012:150-166.
2. Akhtar S. Endocrine function. In: Barash PG, Cullen BF, Stoelting RK, et al, eds. *Clinical Anesthesia Fundamentals.* Philadelphia: Wolters Kluwer Health; 2015:335-356.

12. Correct answer: D

Calcitonin is excreted by parafollicular C cells of the thyroid in response to high serum Ca²⁺ levels. The primary mechanism to decrease the serum calcium levels is by the inhibition of osteoclastic activity, which subsequently decreases bone resorption. This is in opposition to the action of PTH, which activates osteoclasts. As a secondary role, calcitonin also reduces the resorption of calcium, phosphate, sodium, and potassium in the kidney. Calcitonin does not affect intestinal absorption of calcium, which is instead promoted by vitamin D. There is no direct effect of calcitonin on the osteoblasts. In severe cases of hypercalcemia, exogenous calcitonin may be used to reduce PTH secretion for several days, after which tachyphylaxis can develop.

References:
1. John AD. Evaluation of the patient with endocrine disease or diabetes. In: Longnecker DE, Brown DL, Newman MF, Zapol WM, eds. *Anesthesiology.* 2nd ed. New York: McGraw Hill; 2012:150-166.
2. Butterworth JF, Mackey DC, Wasnick JD. Anesthesia for patients with endocrine disease. In: *Clinical Anesthesiology.* 5th ed. New York: McGraw Hill Education; 2014:727-745.

13. **Correct answer: C**

Hypercalcemia generally becomes symptomatic at levels above 12 mg/dL and may become life-threatening at levels above 14 mg/dL. Symptoms include gastrointestinal upset, nephrolithiasis and polyuria, dehydration, hypertension, altered mental status, weakness, and pruritus. Hypercalcemia may be accompanied by ECG changes, including bradyarrhythmias, bundle-branch blocks, and complete heart block. In these patients, it is imperative to correct the hypercalcemia before proceeding with general anesthesia. As patients become dehydrated because of hypercalciuria and impaired Na^+ reabsorption, one must correct patients' fluid deficit first. Once fluid replete, the continued intravenous administration of normal saline together with a loop diuretic can produce a reduction in serum Ca^{2+} levels by 2-3 mg/dL. Further lowering of the calcium level may be accomplished by exogenous calcitonin, which will inhibit osteoclast activity to limit bone resorption. The onset of calcitonin is very rapid (within 1-2 h); however, its use is limited by tachyphylaxis, which can be seen after the first 48 hours of administration. Bisphosphonates may also be administered to inhibit bone resorption; however, they require approximately 2 days before an effect is seen. Steroids may be used in conjunction with calcitonin to enhance its effect.

Reference:
1. John AD. Evaluation of the patient with endocrine disease or diabetes. In: Longnecker DE, Brown DL, Newman MF, Zapol WM, eds. *Anesthesiology*. 2nd ed. New York: McGraw Hill; 2012:150-166.

14. **Correct answer: C**

Normal calcium homeostasis maintains the plasma calcium level between 8.5 and 10.5 mg/dL. However, serum protein concentrations can affect the proportion of bound calcium. Thus, the plasma calcium level should be adjusted if the plasma albumin level is abnormal. If albumin levels are low, then the levels of plasma calcium level should be upwardly adjusted, whereas the opposite is true if albumin levels are high.

To adjust for plasma albumin level, the following formula is used:

$$\text{Adjusted calcium} = [Ca^{2+}] + 0.8 \, (4.0 - [\text{albumin}])$$
$$\text{Adjusted calcium} = 7.6 + 0.8 \, (4.0 - 1.6) = 9.5 \text{ mg/dL}$$

Acid-base status will also affect the level of calcium protein binding. Acidosis will increase the circulating levels of ionized calcium, potentially provoking hypercalcemia. Alkalosis, on the other hand, will increase protein binding and thus may lead to hypocalcemia.

Reference:
1. John AD. Evaluation of the patient with endocrine disease or diabetes. In: Longnecker DE, Brown DL, Newman MF, Zapol WM, eds. *Anesthesiology*. 2nd ed. New York: McGraw Hill; 2012:150-166.

15. **Correct answer: D**

Calcium in the body is either bound to albumin, phosphate, bicarbonate, or citrate or it exists in an ionized state. It is the ionized form that plays a large role in muscle contraction, neurotransmitter release, and intracellular functions. For this reason, calcium homeostasis is closely dependent on protein binding and, in particular, serum albumin levels. Much of the serum calcium is bound to albumin (approximately 50%); thus an increase in serum albumin may shift some ionized calcium to the bound form. Alkalosis increases the amount of calcium bound to the protein and similarly decreases the proportion of ionized calcium. Acidosis, on the other hand, can decrease protein binding and even lead to hypercalcemia. Blood products, specifically fresh frozen plasma and platelets, contain citrate, which chelates calcium and can decrease the ionized calcium concentration.

References:
1. John AD. Evaluation of the patient with endocrine disease or diabetes. In: Longnecker DE, Brown DL, Newman MF, Zapol WM, eds. *Anesthesiology*. 2nd ed. New York: McGraw Hill; 2012:150-166.
2. Peterfreund RA, Lee SL. Endocrine surgery and intraoperative management of endocrine conditions. In: Longnecker DE, Brown DL, Newman MF, Zapol WM, eds. *Anesthesiology*. 2nd ed. New York: McGraw Hill; 2012:1112-1133.
3. Akhtar S. Endocrine function. In: Barash PG, Cullen BF, Stoelting RK, et al, eds. *Clinical Anesthesia Fundamentals*. Philadelphia: Wolters Kluwer Health; 2015:335-356.

16. **Correct answer: A**

Adrenal insufficiency is classified as primary or secondary. Primary adrenal insufficiency is caused by adrenal gland destruction, such as surgical removal, autoimmune disease, tuberculosis, hemorrhage, or infiltrative disease. Secondary adrenal insufficiency refers to suppression of the hypothalamic-pituitary axis. In primary adrenal insufficiency, low cortisol will cause upregulation of corticotropin-releasing hormone (CRH) and ACTH to compensate for the irregularity. However, the damaged adrenal gland is unable to provide cortisol in response to ACTH. Mineralocorticoid (aldosterone) deficiency also occurs due to the absence of the zona glomerulosa. In patients with secondary adrenal insufficiency, mineralocorticoid function is preserved because only a small portion of mineralocorticoid release is regulated by ACTH.

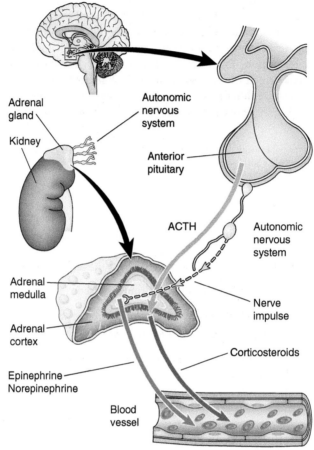

(From Hammel JA, Umpierrez GE. Adrenal gland disorders. In: Felner EI, Umpierez GF, eds. *Endocrine Pathophysiology*. Philadelphia: Wolters Kluwer Health/Lippincott Williams & Wilkins; 2014:480, with permission.)

References:
1. John AD. Evaluation of the patient with endocrine disease or diabetes. In: Longnecker DE, Brown DL, Newman MF, Zapol WM, eds. *Anesthesiology*. 2nd ed. New York: McGraw Hill; 2012:150-166.
2. Akhtar S. Endocrine function. In: Barash PG, Cullen BF, Stoelting RK, et al, eds. *Clinical Anesthesia Fundamentals*. Philadelphia: Wolters Kluwer Health; 2015:335-356.

17. **Correct answer: D**

Preoperative optimization of a patient with pheochromocytoma is critical to avoid the potentially catastrophic perioperative cardiovascular morbidity and requires close coordination between the anesthesiologist, surgeon, and endocrinologist. The goal is to preoperatively decrease catecholamine production and blunt the adrenergic response. Phenoxybenzamine is a nonselective α-adrenergic blocker, which is often used as it offers a long half-life (12 h). The dose is increased until symptoms of catecholamine excess are resolved or until its use is limited by side effects, most often orthostatic hypotension. Other side effects include reflex tachycardia, nasal congestion, and dehydration requiring intravascular fluid replacement. Alternative options for pretreating these patients include selective α_1-blockers, such as doxazosin or prazosin, which have a shorter half-life versus phenoxybenzamine and whose effects may be more titratable after surgery. The lack of α_2 action limits the amount of reflex tachycardia. Finally, calcium channel blockers may also be initiated preoperatively, even with as a little as 24 hours remaining before surgery. Calcium channel blockers do not cause orthostatic hypotension unlike other treatment modalities.

Reference:
1. John AD. Evaluation of the patient with endocrine disease or diabetes. In: Longnecker DE, Brown DL, Newman MF, Zapol WM, eds. *Anesthesiology*. 2nd ed. New York: McGraw Hill; 2012:150-166.

18. Correct answer: B

It is important to understand steroids' relative glucocorticoid and mineralocorticoid potencies because in primary adrenal insufficiency, there is a deficiency of both glucocorticoids and mineralocorticoids. In secondary adrenal insufficiency, only glucocorticoid deficiency exists because of lack of ACTH stimulation. For instance, in patients receiving chronic steroid therapy, hypothalamic-pituitary-adrenal axis suppression may occur, leading to low CRH and ACTH levels and the resultant atrophy of the zona fasciculata and a decrease in endogenous cortisol production.

Mineralocorticoids cause fluid retention, edema, and hypokalemia; thus, it is important to make a rational choice when selecting a steroid when stress dosing is indicated. Dexamethasone is unique in that it lacks mineralocorticoid activity. Hydrocortisone is the same molecule as endogenous cortisol and has both glucocorticoid and mineralocorticoid effects. Prednisone has approximately 5× the glucocorticoid activity as mineralocorticoid activity, whereas methylprednisolone has approximately 10× the glucocorticoid activity as mineralocorticoid activity.

Reference:
1. Liu MM, Reidy AB, Saatee S, Collard CD. Perioperative steroid management: approaches based on current evidence. *Anesthesiology*. 2017;127(1):166-172.

19. Correct answer: C

Common practice is to administer stress dose steroids in all patients presenting for surgery who are at a reasonable risk of hypothalamic-pituitary-adrenal axis suppression because of chronic steroid administration. Recent data suggest this practice may not be necessary in many cases, but nonetheless, the administration of stress dose steroids carries minimal risk compared with the potential for perioperative adrenal insufficiency. Most sources agree that patients meeting the following criteria would benefit from stress dose steroid administration:

- Receiving the equivalent of ≥20 mg daily prednisone for ≥3 weeks OR those with clinical features of Cushing syndrome
- Patients undergoing more than superficial procedures (eg, dental surgery or biopsy)

Reference:
1. Liu MM, Reidy AB, Saatee S, Collard CD. Perioperative steroid management: approaches based on current evidence. *Anesthesiology*. 2017;127(1):166-172.

20. Correct answer: D

Glucocorticoids are involved in a wide spectrum of metabolic activities and exert an overall anti-inflammatory and anti-insulin effect. They increase serum glucose by promoting glycogenolysis and gluconeogenesis. Glucocorticoids increase protein catabolism, explaining the muscle wasting seen in Cushing disease. Additionally, glucocorticoids increase neutrophils, platelets, and erythrocytes, while decreasing eosinophils and basophils. Glucocorticoids are also required for glucagon and catecholamines to exert their effects.

References:
1. Akhtar S. Endocrine function. In: Barash PG, Cullen BF, Stoelting RK, et al, eds. *Clinical Anesthesia Fundamentals*. Philadelphia: Wolters Kluwer Health; 2015:335-356.
2. John AD. Evaluation of the patient with endocrine disease or diabetes. In: Longnecker DE, Brown DL, Newman MF, Zapol WM, eds. *Anesthesiology*. 2nd ed. New York: McGraw Hill; 2012:150-166.

21. Correct answer: D

Severe hyperglycemia is associated with 2 life-threatening emergencies in diabetic patients, diabetic ketoacidosis (DKA) and nonketotic hyperosmolar coma.

In DKA, lack of insulin prevents tissues from adequately utilizing glucose, necessitating the generation of ketoacids for energy and the development of hyperglycemia. DKA is seen more frequently in type 1 diabetics and may be precipitated by an acute stressor, such as infection, or often by noncompliance with insulin therapy. Treatment is with aggressive intravenous fluids, electrolyte repletion, and insulin therapy.

Nonketotic hyperosmolar coma is manifested by extreme hyperglycemia in the absence of ketoacidosis. This entity is more commonly seen in type 2 diabetes, especially elderly patients with impaired thirst mechanisms. Endogenous insulin remains present in these patients, therefore blunting lipid metabolism. Hence, this does not result in the formation of ketones.

Clinical Characteristics of DKA and Nonketotic Hyperosmolar Coma

DIABETIC KETOACIDOSIS	NONKETOTIC HYPEROSMOLAR COMA
Typically affects type 1 diabetics	Typically affects type 2 diabetics; may be mild to moderate diabetics
Hyperglycemia (300-500 mg/dL)	Profound hyperglycemia (>600 mg/dL)
Presence of ketoacidosis	Absence of ketoacidosis
Accompanied by hypokalemia (exaggerated once acidosis is corrected)	Symptoms of hyperosmolarity (seizures, coma, venous thrombosis)
Dehydration	Dehydration
Skeletal muscle weakness	May have impaired thirst mechanisms

References:
1. John AD. Evaluation of the patient with endocrine disease or diabetes. In: Longnecker DE, Brown DL, Newman MF, Zapol WM, eds. *Anesthesiology*. 2nd ed. New York: McGraw Hill; 2012:150-166.
2. Akhtar S. Endocrine function. In: Barash PG, Cullen BF, Stoelting RK, et al, eds. *Clinical Anesthesia Fundamentals*. Philadelphia: Wolters Kluwer Health; 2015:335-356.

22. Correct answer: B

Numerous studies have demonstrated long-standing diabetes as a predictor of difficult intubation, with the incidence reported as high as 30%-40%. New intubating techniques have reduced this rate significantly in more recent studies, however. Difficult intubation is thought to be attributable to tissue glycosylation, resulting in reduced mobility of the cervical spine and the temporomandibular joints. A bedside test used to assess for joint stiffness is the "prayer test," in which the patient is asked to oppose the interphalangeal joints; the inability to do so is a positive prayer sign and associated with difficult direct laryngoscopy.

References:
1. John AD. Evaluation of the patient with endocrine disease or diabetes. In: Longnecker DE, Brown DL, Newman MF, Zapol WM, eds. *Anesthesiology*. 2nd ed. New York: McGraw Hill; 2012:150-166.
2. Warner ME, Contreras MG, Warner MA, et al. Diabetes mellitus and difficult laryngoscopy on renal and pancreatic transplant patients. *Anesth Analg*. 1998;86(3):516-519.
3. Hogan K, Rusy D, Springman SR, et al. Difficult laryngoscopy and diabetes mellitus. *Anesth Analg*. 1988;67(12):1162-1165.
4. Reissell E, Orko R, Manunuksela EL, et al. Predictability of difficult laryngoscopy in patients with long-term diabetes mellitus. *Anaesthesia*. 1990;45(12):1024-1027.

23. Correct answer: B

Surgery provokes a physiologic stress response characterized by increased sympathetic tone and hyperglycemia and mediated through increased glucagon, ACTH, and GH. Catecholamines stimulate glycogenolysis and gluconeogenesis in the liver and inhibit glucose uptake in insulin-dependent tissues. α- and β-receptors have differing effects on pancreatic function; α-receptors inhibit the release of insulin, whereas β-receptors enhance insulin and glucagon release. During the intraoperative and immediate postoperative period, effects of α-receptors predominate. The net result of each of these processes is a dramatic increase in serum glucose, even in nondiabetic patients, as much as 60 mg/dL above preoperative levels.

References:
1. John AD. Evaluation of the patient with endocrine disease or diabetes. In: Longnecker DE, Brown DL, Newman MF, Zapol WM, eds. *Anesthesiology*. 2nd ed. New York: McGraw Hill; 2012:150-166.
2. Bagry HS, Raghavendran S, Carli F. Metabolic syndrome and insulin resistance: perioperative considerations. *Anesthesiology*. 2008;108(3):506-523.

24. **Correct answer: A**

Metformin is a biguanide oral antihyperglycemic agent that suppresses hepatic gluconeogenesis and glycogenolysis and increases insulin sensitivity and synthesis of glucagonlike peptide-1. There are several important side effects of metformin, the most common of which is gastrointestinal distress. More serious side effects include lactic acidosis, which occurs more frequently in patients with heart failure as well as those with impaired renal function. Metformin is similarly contraindicated in patients who have liver disease, alcoholism, sepsis, and hypoxemia and in patients with administration of IV contrast.

Metformin is often held the morning of elective surgery. There is evidence for its safety up until the evening before presentation, however. A retrospective study of patients taking metformin at baseline and presenting for elective cardiac surgery showed that patients receiving metformin the night before surgery and those who resumed it early postoperatively did not have a greater cardiac morbidity, neurologic morbidity, or inhospital mortality. Additionally, metformin-treated patients required a shorter duration of intubation and had a lower rate of infections and overall morbidity.

References:

1. John AD. Evaluation of the patient with endocrine disease or diabetes. In: Longnecker DE, Brown DL, Newman MF, Zapol WM, eds. *Anesthesiology*. 2nd ed. New York: McGraw Hill; 2012:150-166.
2. Bagry HS, Raghavendran S, Carli F. Metabolic syndrome and insulin resistance: perioperative considerations. *Anesthesiology*. 2008;108(3):506-523.
3. Duncan AI, Koch CG, Xu M, et al. Recent metformin ingestion does not increase in-hospital morbidity or mortality after cardiac surgery. *Anesth Analg*. 2007;104(1):42-50.

25. **Correct answer: B**

Diabetic patients are at increased risk for coronary artery disease, and those who develop a myocardial infarction have a higher risk of both prehospital and inhospital mortality compared with nondiabetic patients. It is well recognized that diabetics may present without symptoms or with atypical symptoms, such as nausea and jaw or arm pain, rather than classic substernal chest pain. Despite this, studies fail to show well-established data to recommend routine preoperative stress testing in asymptomatic patients. Aspirin is shown to decrease the risk of myocardial infarction in diabetics. Although diabetics are at risk for nephropathy, ACE inhibitors have a protective effect in microalbuminuria and are appropriate for use in diabetics with hypertension.

Reference:

1. John AD. Evaluation of the patient with endocrine disease or diabetes. In: Longnecker DE, Brown DL, Newman MF, Zapol WM, eds. *Anesthesiology*. 2nd ed. New York: McGraw Hill; 2012:150-166.

26. **Correct answer: C**

Glycolysis is a process used by the body to break down 1 molecule of glucose (6-carbons) into 2 molecules of pyruvate (3-carbons), which then enter the Krebs cycle to produce large amounts of energy for cellular utilization. Additionally, 2 molecules of ATP are released for each molecule of glucose broken down by glycolysis. This process is anaerobic and takes place within the cytosol of the cell. Alternatively, glucose can undergo glycogen synthesis in the liver.

In aerobic metabolism, once pyruvate is produced by glycolysis, it is converted via decarboxylation into acetyl-CoA, which is the common molecule of carbohydrate, lipid, and amino acid metabolism. Acetyl-CoA then enters the Krebs cycle. Under anaerobic conditions, pyruvate can be reduced to lactate.

Reference:

1. Shulman GI, Petersen KF. Metabolism. In: Boron WF, Boulpep EL, eds. *Medical Physiology*. 3rd ed. Philadelphia: Elsevier Health; 2017:1170-1192.

27. **Correct answer: A**

Acetyl-CoA is the common molecule that enters the Krebs cycle from carbohydrate, lipid, and amino acid metabolism. Glucose is broken down by glycolysis into pyruvate, which is then converted to acetyl-CoA via decarboxylation. Fatty acids are broken down via β-oxidation into smaller fatty acids with acetyl-CoA as a by-product. Finally, branched chain ketogenic amino acids are converted to α-ketoacids and eventually into acetyl-CoA and acetoacetate. From each of these pathways, acetyl-CoA can then enter the Krebs cycle, where energy is extracted in the form of electrons for subsequent oxidative phosphorylation.

Reference:

1. Shulman GI, Petersen KF. Metabolism. In: Boron WF, Boulpep EL, eds. *Medical Physiology*. 3rd ed. Philadelphia: Elsevier Health; 2017:1170-1192.

28. Correct answer: D

To prevent overproduction and underutilization of energy, the Krebs cycle is regulated by both substrate availability and inhibition feedback. For example, the substrate NADH inhibits pyruvate dehydrogenase, isocitrate dehydrogenase, α-ketoglutarate dehydrogenase, and citrate synthase. ATP inhibits citrate synthase and α-ketoglutarate dehydrogenase. Mitochondrial calcium activates pyruvate dehydrogenase phosphatase, isocitrate dehydrogenase, and α-ketoglutarate dehydrogenase, increasing the rate of several steps of the cycle and thus increasing the downstream flux into the electron transport chain.

Reference:
1. Shulman GI, Petersen KF. Metabolism. In: Boron WF, Boulpep EL, eds. *Medical Physiology*. 3rd ed. Philadelphia: Elsevier Health; 2017:1170-1192.

29. Correct answer: C

During oxidative phosphorylation, electrons are passed along a series of protein complexes and electron carriers along the inner mitochondrial membrane, which undergo successive oxidation and reduction reactions. NADH and $FADH_2$ formed from the Krebs cycle begin the process by donating electrons. This process is coupled to the pumping of electrons across their concentration gradient, increasing the gradient. The final electron recipient is oxygen, which is reduced to water. Thus, oxidative phosphorylation is an aerobic process. Finally, with the large ionic gradient that has been created, ATP synthase couples ADP and P_i to form ATP. NADH and is an electron donor. NAD+ and FADH+ are electron recipients, but neither is the final recipient in oxidative phosphorylation.

Reference:
1. Shulman GI, Petersen KF. Metabolism. In: Boron WF, Boulpep EL, eds. *Medical Physiology*. 3rd ed. Philadelphia: Elsevier Health; 2017:1170-1192.

30. Correct answer: D

Gluconeogenesis is a pathway of 11 enzyme-catalyzed steps, which results in the production of glucose from glycerol, glucogenic amino acids, lipids, and other intermediaries in carbohydrate metabolism, including pyruvate and lactate. In humans, gluconeogenesis occurs in the liver and, to a lesser extent, the kidney and small intestine. Like glycolysis, gluconeogenesis is largely regulated by substrate availability and feedback inhibition. These processes act on many of the same substrates in reverse, which allows for reciprocal control and therefore prevents a futile cycle of synthesizing and subsequently breaking down glucose in excess of a cell's metabolic requirements.

Reference:
1. Shulman GI, Petersen KF. Metabolism. In: Boron WF, Boulpep EL, eds. *Medical Physiology*. 3rd ed. Philadelphia: Elsevier Health; 2017:1170-1192.

31. Correct answer: B

Lipid metabolism includes a number of complex metabolic pathways intertwining with the metabolism of other compounds, including carbohydrates. Pharmacologic agents are available and act at targeting many different steps in these pathways. Statins, such as simvastatin, work through inhibiting the enzyme HMG-CoA reductase, which plays a key role in synthesizing new cholesterol in the liver. Ezetimibe is a unique drug that inhibits intestinal absorption of TAGs via a complex mechanism. Similarly, bile acid sequestrants or resins, such as cholestyramine, inhibit the enterohepatic recirculation of cholesterol by binding these compounds in the intestinal lumen. PCSK9 inhibitors are a new class of drugs that increase the expression of the LDL receptor on drug membranes, leading to decreased concentrations in the extracellular fluid. Fibrates, such as gemfibrozil, stimulate β-oxidation of fatty acids in peroxisomes and the mitochondria.

References:
1. Suchy FJ. Hepatobiliary function. In: Boron WF, Boulpep EL, eds. *Medical Physiology*. 3rd ed. Philadelphia: Elsevier Health; 2017:944-971.
2. Binder HJ, Mansbach II CM. Nutrient digestion and absorption. In: Boron WF, Boulpep EL, eds. *Medical Physiology*. 3rd ed. Philadelphia: Elsevier Health; 2017:914-943.
3. Fairman KA, Davis LE, Sclar DA. Real-world use of PCSK-9 inhibitors by early adopters: cardiovascular risk factors, statin co-treatment, and short-term adherence in routine clinical practice. *Ther Clin Risk Manag*. 2017;13:957-965.

32. **Correct answer: C**

Lipids are large, water-insoluble molecules and cannot be absorbed directly (answer choice D). Digestion of lipids consists of 3 steps: emulsification, enzymatic hydrolysis, and the creation of water-soluble products, which allows lipids to be absorbed. In the stomach, hydrochloric acid (HCl) combines with food, and lipase is subsequently released, thus initiating the process of enzymatic breakdown. Only short-chain fatty acids can be absorbed in the stomach. Cholecystokinin is released in response to a lipid load in the small bowel, and it functions to slow, not speed, gastric motility and emptying (answer choice A). In the small bowel, emulsification occurs (answer choice C) where fatty acids are assembled into chylomicrons with bile salts and phosphatidylcholine. Lipases, released from the pancreas, act on TAG to form free fatty acids and 2-monoacylglycerol, which can be absorbed across the brush border on the surface of intestinal epithelial cells.

Reference:

1. Miller RD. Gastrointestinal physiology and pathophysiology. In: *Miller's Anesthesia*. Philadelphia: Saunders Elsevier; 2015: 492-519.

33. **Correct answer: D**

The exocrine pancreas secretes amylase, lipase, and protease, which play roles in digestion of carbohydrates, lipids, and proteins, respectively. Fat-soluble vitamins must be solubilized into micelles before they can be passively absorbed by intestinal endothelial cells. Without lipase, this process is impaired, leading to deficiency of the fat-soluble vitamins: A, D, E, and K. Vitamin A deficiency can lead to night blindness, hyperkeratosis, and keratomalacia. Vitamin D deficiency can lead to rickets and osteomalacia. Vitamin E deficiency can cause hemolytic anemia in neonates and sterility or spontaneous abortions in adults.

Reference:

1. Miller RD. Gastrointestinal physiology and pathophysiology. In: *Miller's Anesthesia*. Philadelphia: Saunders Elsevier; 2015:492-519.

34. **Correct answer: A**

The liver plays a complex role in the production, uptake, release, and oxidation of fatty acids. The liver receives dietary fatty acids primarily in the form of chylomicrons but may also synthesize fatty acids de novo or uptake them from blood-borne lipoproteins. When the liver is glycogen-replete, *not* deficient, the liver will convert glucose to TAG for storage. TAG may be packaged into very-low-density lipoproteins or other lipoproteins for transport to other tissues. Glucagon activates β-oxidation of fatty acids, whereas insulin inhibits β-oxidation. When the production of acetyl-CoA overwhelms the capacity of the Krebs cycle, acetyl-CoA is metabolized to ketones, which may be used by tissues other than the liver. The liver is unable to utilize ketones because of the lack of ketoacyl-CoA transferase.

Reference:

1. Miller RD. Hepatic physiology and pathophysiology. In: *Miller's Anesthesia*. Philadelphia: Saunders Elsevier; 2015:520-544.

35. **Correct answer: C**

In times of starvation, when glucose is not readily available, most tissues in the human body can utilize β-oxidation of fatty acids to supply metabolic requirements. The brain, however, is unable to metabolize fatty acids and is thus dependent on ketone bodies. This is possible because the enzymes responsible for ketone metabolism are present in brain tissue in sufficient quantities to produce acetyl-CoA to enter the Krebs cycle at an adequate rate to satisfy the high metabolic requirements of the brain.

References:

1. Siegel GJ, Agranoff BW, Albers RW, et al. Circulation and energy metabolism of the brain. In: *Basic Neurochemistry: Molecular, Cellular and Medical Aspects*. 6th ed. Philadelphia: Lippincott-Raven; 1999:637-670.
2. Owen OE. Ketone bodies as a fuel for the brain during starvation. *Biochem Mol Biol Educ*. 2005;33(4):246-251.

36. **Correct answer: A**

The liver converts cholesterol into bile salts, which are drained via the biliary tree through the ampulla of Vater into the duodenum. In the intestinal lumen, bile salts form micelles, which facilitate emulsification and absorption of dietary lipids and fat-soluble vitamins. Bile salts are reabsorbed in the distal ileum to complete the process of enterohepatic recirculation, which occurs multiple times a day.

Reference:
1. Miller RD. Hepatic physiology and pathophysiology. In: *Miller's Anesthesia*. Philadelphia: Saunders Elsevier; 2015:520-544.

37. Correct answer: A

See answer explanation given for question 31.

Lipid metabolism includes a number of complex metabolic pathways intertwining with the metabolism of other compounds including carbohydrates. Pharmacologic agents are available, targeting many different steps in these pathways. Ezetimibe is a unique drug that inhibits intestinal absorption of TAGs via a complex mechanism. Similarly, bile acid sequestrants or resins, such as cholestyramine, inhibit the enterohepatic recirculation of cholesterol by binding these compounds in the intestinal lumen. Statins work through inhibiting the enzyme HMG-CoA reductase, which is responsible for synthesizing new cholesterol in the liver. PCSK9 inhibitors are a new class of drugs that increase the expression of the LDL receptor on drug membranes, leading to decreased concentrations of LDL in the extracellular fluid. Fibrates, such as gemfibrozil, stimulate β-oxidation of fatty acids in peroxisomes and the mitochondria.

References:
1. Suchy FJ. Hepatobiliary function. In: Boron WF, Boulpep EL, eds. *Medical Physiology*. 3rd ed. Philadelphia: Elsevier Health; 2017:944-971.
2. Binder HJ, Mansbach II CM. Nutrient digestion and absorption. In: Boron WF, Boulpep EL, eds. *Medical Physiology*. 3rd ed. Philadelphia: Elsevier Health; 2017:914-943.
3. Fairman KA, Davis LE, Sclar DA. Real-world use of PCSK-9 inhibitors by early adopters: cardiovascular risk factors, statin co-treatment, and short-term adherence in routine clinical practice. *Ther Clin Risk Manag*. 2017;13:957-965.

38. Correct answer: D

NO is synthesized endogenously by NO synthases. NO has a number of physiologic roles, largely mediated by its activation of guanylate cyclase, which catalyzes the conversion of guanosine-5′-triphosphate to cGMP. cGMP activates cGMP-dependent protein kinase G to produce vascular relaxation. NO binds tightly to hemoglobin once it is absorbed in the lung, so it is no longer in its free form, and thus its vasodilation effects are limited to the pulmonary vasculature.

Reference:
1. Miller RD. Nitric oxide and other inhaled pulmonary vasodilators. In: *Miller's Anesthesia*. Philadelphia: Saunders Elsevier; 2015:3084-3087.

39. Correct answer: B

cGMP and cAMP are both secondary messengers that are triggered by G protein–coupled receptors (GPCRs). Although some phosphodiesterases degrade both cAMP and cGMP, phosphodiesterase-5 selectively converts cGMP into 5′-GMP. Increased levels of cGMP lead to vasodilation, which is of therapeutic benefit in pulmonary hypertension.

Reference:
1. Maurice DH, Ke H, Ahmad F, Chung J, Manganiello VC. Advances in targeting cyclic nucleotide phosphodiesterases. *Nat Rev Drug Discov*. 2014;13(4):290-314.

40. Correct answer: B

GPCRs are transmembrane proteins that have extracellular domains for ligand binding. When a ligand binds, the cytoplasmic aspect of the GPCR undergoes a conformational change that activates a guanine nucleotide–binding protein. Types of G proteins include stimulatory (G_s), inhibitory (G_i), pertussis toxin sensitive and insensitive (G_o and G_{Bq}), and transducin (G_t). The $\beta1$-adrenergic receptor is of the G_s subtype, activating adenylate cyclase, which catalyzes the conversion of ATP to cAMP. Increased cAMP leads to the downstream effects of the β_1-adrenergic receptor.

References:
1. Grecu L. Central and autonomic nervous systems. In: Barash PG, Cullen BF, Stoelting RK, et al, eds. *Clinical Anesthesia Fundamentals*. Philadelphia: Wolters Kluwer Health; 2015:69-85.
2. Gartner LP, Hiatt JL. Cytoplasm. In: *Concise Histology*. Philadelphia: Saunders Elsevier; 2011:8-25.

10

NEUROMUSCULAR JUNCTION DISEASES

Qing Yang

1. **Acetylcholine (Ach) binds to which subunit of the nicotinic acetylcholine receptor (nAchR) on the skeletal muscle?**

   A. α
   B. β
   C. γ
   D. δ

2. **Which of the following is the correct sequence of signals, leading to skeletal muscle contraction?**

   A. Release of Ach → ligand-gated Na^+ channels → motor nerve depolarization → voltage-gated Ca^{++} channels → muscle depolarization
   B. Motor nerve depolarization → voltage-gated Ca^{++} channels → release of Ach → ligand-gated Na^+ channels → muscle depolarization
   C. Motor nerve depolarization → ligand-gated Na^+ channels → release of Ach → voltage-gated Ca^{++} channels → muscle depolarization
   D. Ligand-gated Na^+ channels → voltage-gated Ca^{++} channels → release of Ach → motor nerve depolarization → muscle depolarization

3. **All of the following conditions may increase extrajunctional acetylcholine receptors (AchRs), EXCEPT which one?**

   A. Severe burn
   B. Prolonged ICU stay
   C. Stroke
   D. Renal failure

4. **The effect of Ach at the neuromuscular junction (NMJ) is terminated by which of the following mechanisms?**

   A. Break down by acetylcholinesterase
   B. Break down by pseudocholinesterase
   C. Degradation by tissue esterase
   D. Reuptake into the nerve terminal

5. **How many Ach molecules must bind to each postsynaptic receptor on muscle cells to induce conformational change?**

   A. 1
   B. 2
   C. 3
   D. 4

6. **All of the following drugs inhibit nAchRs EXCEPT which one?**

   A. α-Bungarotoxin
   B. Curare
   C. Pancuronium
   D. Atropine

7. **Ca^{+2} binding to which component of the NMJ induces muscle contraction?**

   A. Actin
   B. Thin filaments
   C. Troponin
   D. Nicotinic acetylcholine receptor

8. **Which of the following structures of the skeletal muscle does not change in length as the muscle contracts?**

   A. A band
   B. I band
   C. H zone
   D. Z line

9. **Which subunit of the nAchR is present in receptors located at the endplate NMJ but NOT in extrajunctional receptors?**

   A. β
   B. γ
   C. δ
   D. ε

10. **Which of the following is the resting potential of the skeletal muscle cell?**

    A. −90 mV
    B. −70 mV
    C. −50 mV
    D. 0 mV

11. **Which of the following agents leads to an *increase* of Ach release from motor neuron terminals?**

    A. Calcium channel blockers
    B. Magnesium
    C. Tetanus toxin
    D. Botulinum toxin

12. **Synthesis of Ach is facilitated by which enzyme?**

    A. Acetylcholinesterase
    B. Choline acetyltransferase
    C. Choline kinase
    D. Choline transporter

13. Which of the following is the *correct* configuration of voltage-gated sodium channels in the repolarization phase *immediately* after the peak of an action potential?

    A. Activation and inactivation gates both open
    B. Activation gate open, inactivation gate closed
    C. Activation gate closed, inactivation gate open
    D. Activation and inactivation gates both closed

14. Tetanic fade following administration of nondepolarizing neuromuscular blockers (NMBs) indicates the *inhibition* of which group of receptors?

    A. Presynaptic nAchR
    B. Postsynaptic nAchR
    C. Presynaptic calcium channels
    D. Postsynaptic calcium channels

15. Potential adverse effects of succinylcholine include all of the following EXCEPT which one?

    A. Myalgia
    B. Aspiration
    C. Increased intraocular pressure
    D. Anaphylaxis

16. Which of the following statements provides the most accurate explanation behind the "faster onset" of rocuronium as compared with cisatracurium?

    A. Rocuronium is less potent.
    B. Rocuronium is more potent.
    C. Rocuronium is ultrashort acting.
    D. Rocuronium is long acting.

17. Which of the following agents belongs to the group of benzylisoquinolinium NMBs?

    A. Rocuronium
    B. Cisatracurium
    C. Vecuronium
    D. Succinylcholine

18. Compared with its precursor atracurium, what is the main advantage of cisatracurium?

    A. Rapid, organ-independent degradation
    B. Faster onset
    C. Longer duration because of active metabolites
    D. Decreased histamine release

19. When a long-duration depolarizing NMB (eg, pancuronium) is added at the end of an intermediate-duration NMB (eg, rocuronium) block, how will the recovery pattern change?

    A. Recovery will be similar to rocuronium.
    B. Recovery will be similar to pancuronium.
    C. Recovery will be synergistically prolonged, significantly longer than pancuronium.
    D. Recovery will be antagonistically shortened, significantly shorter than rocuronium.

20. Compared with the phase I block elicited by succinylcholine, the phase II block has which of the following characteristics?

    A. Same twitch strength with repetitive stimulation
    B. Posttetanic potentiation
    C. Similarity with depolarizing block
    D. Posttetanic depression

21. **Which statement regarding the phase II block that can be associated with succinylcholine administration is true?**

    A. Phase II block occurs only after prolonged exposure to succinylcholine.
    B. Receptor desensitization is a mechanism responsible for phase II block.
    C. Inhalation anesthetics delay the onset of phase II block.
    D. Phase II block results in train-of-four (TOF) fade but not tetanic fade.

22. **A patient was maintained on a succinylcholine infusion for 8 hours during surgery and does not regain spontaneous ventilation 30 minutes after the infusion was discontinued. TOF yields 1 twitch. Which of the following is the best course of action?**

    A. Give neostigmine.
    B. Send pseudocholinesterase activity test.
    C. Give naloxone.
    D. Wait for spontaneous recovery.

23. **Which mechanism best explains the fasciculations often seen preceding a phase I block by succinylcholine?**

    A. Activation of presynaptic nAchR
    B. Activation of postsynaptic nAchR
    C. Prolonged muscle depolarization
    D. Prolonged muscle repolarization

24. **A patient on succinylcholine infusion has a TOF ratio of 0.3. What does this tell about the patient's degree of paralysis?**

    A. Patient is in phase I block.
    B. Patient is in phase II block.
    C. Patient is recovering from block.
    D. Cannot tell from given information.

25. **Monitoring the TOF to assess the quality of a neuromuscular blockade offers what advantage over single twitch monitoring?**

    A. TOF offers objective assessment of fade.
    B. TOF ratio correlates with the amount of stimulating current applied.
    C. TOF does not require baseline measurement.
    D. TOF is best at detecting the onset of neuromuscular blockade.

26. **When the TOF ratio is 0.7, what portion of the AchRs is still blocked?**

    A. 25%
    B. 50%
    C. 75%
    D. 95%

27. **A TOF yields 0 twitch. Repeated 1 Hz stimulation following a 5-second 50 Hz tetanus produces 1 twitch. Assuming the patient was given an intermediate-acting NMB, how much time is expected until recovery to TOF twitch count of 1?**

    A. 1-2 minutes
    B. 5-10 minutes
    C. 20-30 minutes
    D. >1 hour

28. **Compared with TOF, what is an advantage of double-burst stimulation (DBS) for monitoring of neuromuscular blockade?**

    A. Easier to detect fade
    B. Does not use tetanic stimuli
    C. Ability to immediately apply a repeat stimulus
    D. Smaller current

29. **Side effects of neostigmine include all of the following EXCEPT which one?**

    A. Salivation
    B. Tachycardia
    C. Nausea/vomiting
    D. Bowel motility

30. **How long would a patient with a dibucaine number of 20 be expected to remain paralyzed after an intubating dose of succinylcholine?**

    A. 4 minutes
    B. 40 minutes
    C. 4 hours
    D. 4 days

31. **What differentiates Lambert-Eaton myasthenic syndrome (LEMS) from myasthenia gravis?**

    A. Patients with LEMS often have autonomic dysfunction.
    B. LEMS results from autoantibodies to the postsynaptic AchRs.
    C. Patients with LEMS feel more proximal than distal weakness.
    D. Patients with LEMS get progressively fatigued with repetitive use of muscles.

32. **In patients with myasthenia gravis, which factor best predicts the risk of requiring prolonged intubation and mechanical ventilator support?**

    A. Age of illness onset
    B. Involvement of muscle groups
    C. Dosage of acetylcholinesterase inhibitor at home
    D. Circulating autoantibody level

33. **How do patients with myasthenia gravis react to depolarizing NMBs and nondepolarizing NMBs?**

    A. Sensitive to depolarizing, but insensitive to nondepolarizing NMBs
    B. Insensitive to depolarizing, but sensitive to nondepolarizing NMBs
    C. Sensitive to both depolarizing and nondepolarizing NMBs
    D. Insensitive to both depolarizing and nondepolarizing NMBs

34. **A patient with myasthenia gravis presents with muscle weakness and respiratory failure. What is the best way to differentiate a myasthenia crisis from a cholinergic crisis?**

    A. Presence or absence of GI symptoms
    B. Pupillary exam
    C. Tensilon test
    D. Excessive sweating

35. **What is the inheritance pattern of Duchenne muscular dystrophy (DMD)?**

    A. Autosomal dominant
    B. Autosomal recessive
    C. X-linked dominant
    D. X-linked recessive

36. For patients with myotonic dystrophy, prolonged muscle contraction (myotonia) can be triggered by exposure to all of the following agents EXCEPT which one?

A. Succinylcholine
B. Rocuronium
C. Potassium
D. Neostigmine

37. Which intravenous anesthetic agent should be avoided in patients with mitochondrial myopathy?

A. Propofol
B. Etomidate
C. Ketamine
D. Dexmedetomidine

38. Malignant hyperthermia is a known risk for patients with the following conditions EXCEPT which one?

A. King Denborough syndrome
B. Multiminicore disease
C. Central core disease
D. Central cord syndrome

39. Which intravenous fluid should be avoided in patients with mitochondrial disorder?

A. Normal saline
B. Lactated Ringer (LR)
C. Dextrose
D. Albumin

40. Psuedocholinesterase activity is *increased* in which of the following conditions?

A. Pregnancy
B. Liver failure
C. Obesity
D. Malignancy

Chapter 10 ▪ Answers

1. **Correct answer: A**

The nAchR is a transmembrane protein with 5 subunits, 2 α subunits, and 1 each of β, ε (or γ in the case of the fetal isoform), and δ. Binding of Ach at the α subunits causes conformational changes that result in the opening of the central channel, allowing influx of Na^+ and efflux of K^+ ions, thereby depolarizing the muscle cell. At the NMJ there are around 5 million of these receptors; however, only a few hundred thousands are required for muscle contraction.

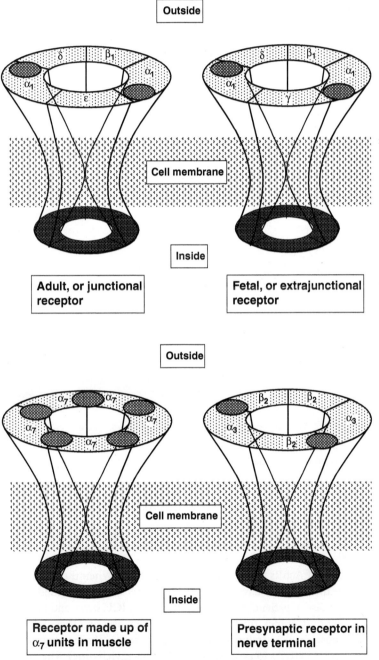

(From Donati F. Neuromuscular blocking agents. In: Barash PG, Cullen BF, Stoelting RK, et al, eds. *Clinical Anesthesia*. 7th ed. Philadelphia: Lippincott; 2013:528, with permission.)

References:
1. Brull SJ, Claudius C. Neuromuscular blocking agents. In: Barash PG, Cullen BF, Stoelting RK, et al, eds. *Clinical Anesthesia Fundamentals*. Philadelphia: Lippincott; 2013:185-208.
2. Butterworth JF, Mackey DC, Wasnick JD. Neuromuscular blocking agents. In: *Clinical Anesthesiology*. 5th ed. New York: McGraw Hill Education; 2014:199-222.

2. **Correct answer: B**

Skeletal muscle contraction occurs through the conversion of the electrical signals from the motor nerve into chemical signals, which in turn triggers an electrical event and motor response at the level of the muscle. First, arrival of the action potential at the motor nerve terminal synapse causes local depolarization of the nerve and opens voltage-gated Ca^{+2} channels. Influx of Ca^{+2} enables exocytosis of vesicles containing Ach. Ach diffuses across the synaptic cleft and binds to nAchR on muscle endplate. nAchRs are ligand-gated ion channels allowing influx of Na^+ and efflux of K^+, producing muscle depolarization.

Depolarization of the skeletal muscle then leads to release of Ca^{+2} from the sarcoplasmic reticulum as well as entry of extracellular Ca^{+2}. Ca^{+2} binds to and induces a conformational change in troponin, allowing formation of actin-myosin cross-bridge and activation of the myosin motor, thereby producing mechanical contraction.

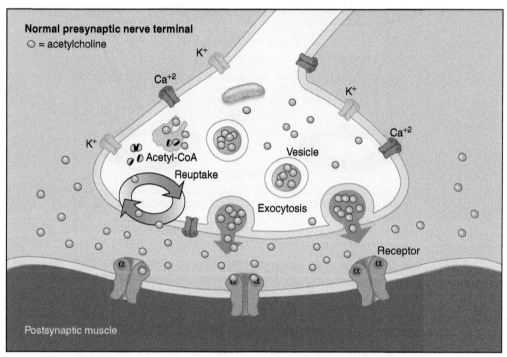

(From Brull SJ, Claudius C. Neuromuscular blocking agents. In: Barash PG, Cullen BF, Stoelting RK, et al, eds. *Clinical Anesthesia Fundamentals*. Philadelphia: Lippincott; 2013:186.)

Reference:
1. Brull SJ, Claudius C. Neuromuscular blocking agents. In: Barash PG, Cullen BF, Stoelting RK, et al, eds. *Clinical Anesthesia Fundamentals*. Philadelphia: Lippincott; 2013:185-208.

3. **Correct answer: D**

Normally the majority of AchRs are concentrated at the NMJ. When the frequency of stimulation at the NMJ decreases over the course of days or longer, usually because of extended periods of immobility and disuse, such as in the case of patients with severe burns, long ICU stays, and loss of limb function because of stroke or muscular dystrophies, the number of AchR increases and these extra receptors spread out to other areas of the muscle cell (extrajunctional receptor spread). These upregulated AchRs are immature and have heightened sensitivity to agonists (Ach and succinylcholine). The channel in these receptors also remains open for a longer period, risking release of large doses of K^+ into the systemic circulation if medications such as succinylcholine are utilized for muscle paralysis.

Renal failure can cause hyperkalemia, especially in patients who are dialysis dependent. However, renal failure is not associated with upregulation of extrajunctional AchR. In patients with normal muscle physiology, use of succinylcholine increases serum K^+ concentration by 0.5 mEq/L, which does not have significant clinical effects.

Reference:
1. Brull SJ, Claudius C. Neuromuscular blocking agents. In: Barash PG, Cullen BF, Stoelting RK, et al, eds. *Clinical Anesthesia Fundamentals*. Philadelphia: Lippincott; 2013:185-208.

4. Correct answer: A

After depolarization of the motor nerve and a rise in intracellular Ca^{+2} at the nerve terminal, vesicles containing Ach are released into the synaptic cleft. Binding of Ach to nAchRs on muscle cells induces muscle contraction. Ach is then rapidly hydrolyzed by acetylcholinesterase into choline and acetic acid in the synaptic cleft as well as at the basement membrane. Choline is subsequently reabsorbed at the presynaptic nerve terminal.

Pseudocholinesterase is an enzyme responsible for the degradation of succinylcholine, mivacurium, as well as ester local anesthetics. Similarly, tissue esterases are responsible for the degradation of other pharmacologic agents, such as remifentanil and atracurium. Neither of these enzymes plays a role in the degradation of Ach, resulting in termination of its action at the NMJ.

Reference:
1. Brull SJ, Claudius C. Neuromuscular blocking agents. In: Barash PG, Cullen BF, Stoelting RK, et al, eds. *Clinical Anesthesia Fundamentals*. Philadelphia: Lippincott; 2013:185-208.

5. Correct answer: B

nAchRs found on muscle cells contain 5 subunits. Two molecules of Ach bind to the 2 α subunits and induce a conformational change that opens up the central channel and allows Na^+ influx and K^+ efflux, depolarizing the muscle cell. If only 1 molecule of Ach is attached, the central pore will not open.

References:
1. Brull SJ, Claudius C. Neuromuscular blocking agents. In: Barash PG, Cullen BF, Stoelting RK, et al, eds. *Clinical Anesthesia Fundamentals*. Philadelphia: Lippincott; 2013:185-208.
2. Butterworth JF, Mackey DC, Wasnick JD. Neuromuscular blocking agents. In: *Clinical Anesthesiology*. 5th ed. New York: McGraw Hill Education; 2014:199-222.

6. Correct answer: D

nAchRs are 5-subunit ligand-gated channels found in the NMJ and central nervous system. Activation of muscle-type nAchR leads to muscle contraction and can be inhibited by binding of noncompetitive inhibitors such as curare, pancuronium, and α-bungarotoxin, a snake venom.

Atropine inhibits muscarinic acetylcholine receptors (mAchRs) are G protein–coupled receptors found in the end organs stimulated by postganglionic fibers of the parasympathetic nerve system.

References:
1. Brull SJ, Claudius C. Neuromuscular blocking agents. In: Barash PG, Cullen BF, Stoelting RK, et al, eds. *Clinical Anesthesia Fundamentals*. Philadelphia: Lippincott; 2013:185-208.
2. Grecu L. Central and autonomic nervous system. In: Barash PG, Cullen BF, Stoelting RK, et al, eds. *Clinical Anesthesia Fundamentals*. Philadelphia: Lippincott; 2013:69-86.

7. Correct answer: C

Binding of Ach to nAchRs causes a conformational change that lets Na^+ into the cell while K^+ out of the cell, depolarizing skeletal muscle. Depolarization leads to release of Ca^{+2} from the sarcoplasmic reticulum as well as entry of extracellular Ca^{+2}. Ca^{+2} binds to and induces a conformational change in troponin, allowing formation of actin-myosin cross-bridge and activation of the myosin motor, thereby producing mechanical contraction. Ca^{+2} does not directly bind to actin, also known as thin filaments.

Reference:
1. Brull SJ, Claudius C. Neuromuscular blocking agents. In: Barash PG, Cullen BF, Stoelting RK, et al, eds. *Clinical Anesthesia Fundamentals*. Philadelphia: Lippincott; 2013:185-208.

8. Correct answer: A

Skeletal muscle myofibril is composed of densely organized actin (thin) and myosin (thick) filaments. Histologically, A band contains overlapping actin and myosin, whereas I band contains actin only. The distance between 2 Z lines is defined as a sarcomere. When muscle cell is depolarized, rising intracellular Ca^{+2} leads to formation of actin-myosin cross-bridges in the A band and myosin motor activation pulls the actin filaments closer together. Thus, the spaces occupied by I band, H zone, and between the Z lines become shorter. The A band width remains unchanged.

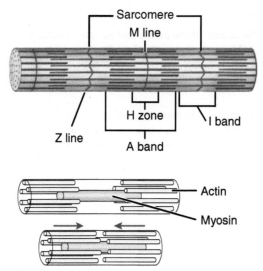

(From Grossman SC, Porth CM. *Porth's Pathophysiology*. 9th ed. Philadelphia: Wolters Kluwer Health/Lippincott Williams & Wilkins; 2014, with permission.)

Reference:
1. Rosendorff C. Molecular and cellular basis of myocardial contractility. In: *Essential Cardiology*. 3rd ed. Vol 1. New York: Springer; 2013:9-30.

9. Correct answer: D

nAchRs found on skeleton muscle are 5-subunit ligand-gated ion channels, consisting of 2 α subunits and 1 each of β, ε (or γ), and δ. ε subunit is found on mature receptors, which are normally located only in the NMJ (aka at the muscle endplate). With decreased stimulation from the neurons and muscle disuse, such as during periods of immobilization or with muscular dystrophy, stroke, or severe burn, immature, extrajunctional receptors develop, characterized by the substitution of γ for ε subunits.

Binding of Ach at the α subunits causes a conformational change that results in the opening of the central channel, allowing influx of Na^+ and efflux of K^+ ions and depolarizing the muscle cell. The immature receptors have relatively higher affinity for Ach, lower threshold of activation, and longer duration of staying open. Activation of the immature receptors thus leads to prolonged muscle depolarization and potassium efflux, placing patients at risk for systemic hyperkalemia.

Reference:
1. Brull SJ, Claudius C. Neuromuscular blocking agents. In: Barash PG, Cullen BF, Stoelting RK, et al, eds. *Clinical Anesthesia Fundamentals*. Philadelphia: Lippincott; 2013:185-208.

10. Correct answer: A

Resting potential of cells differs by type with skeletal and cardiac muscle cells typically around −90 mV. Resting potential for neurons is usually −70 mV, whereas resting potential for cardiac pacemaker cells is −60 to −50 mV.

Signal from the motor neuron causes depolarization by influx of positively charged Na^+ ions, achieving action potential of +40 mV. Voltage-gated potassium channels then open as the sodium channels close, causing repolarization, usually with hyperpolarization to slightly below the resting potential.

Reference:
1. Brull SJ, Claudius C. Neuromuscular blocking agents. In: Barash PG, Cullen BF, Stoelting RK, et al, eds. *Clinical Anesthesia Fundamentals*. Philadelphia: Lippincott; 2013:185-208.

11. **Correct answer: C**

Tetanus and botulinum toxins are both produced by the *Clostridium* species of bacteria and have similar molecular mechanisms of action; however, they act on different neuronal cell types. Tetanus neurotoxin binds to the presynaptic membrane of the NMJ, is internalized, and is then transported retroaxonally to the spinal cord. The spastic paralysis induced by the toxin is due to the blockade of neurotransmitter release from spinal inhibitory interneurons, which results in increased motor neuron activity and release of Ach into the NMJ. In contrast, botulinum neurotoxin exerts its effects peripherally via inducing a flaccid paralysis secondary to the inhibition of Ach release at the NMJ.

Calcium is responsible for vesicle fusion and Ach release. Inhibitors of voltage-gated calcium channels such as ω-agatoxin can prevent Ach release and abolish endplate potential. Magnesium also counteracts the effects of calcium. Hypermagnesemia can lead to weakness, hypotonia, and loss of skeletal muscle reflexes.

Reference:
1. Montecucco C, Schiavo G. Mechanism of action of tetanus and botulinum neurotoxins. *Mol Microbiol*. 1994;13(1):1-8.

12. **Correct answer: B**

Ach is synthesized from acetyl-CoA and choline in the motor neurons by the action of choline acetyltransferase. Acetylcholinesterase degrades Ach into acetic acid and choline in the synaptic cleft. Choline is reabsorbed into the neurons via choline transporter. Choline kinase is an enzyme involved in the synthesis of phosphatidylcholine.

Choline acetyltransferase deficiency is a congenital neuromuscular disease, characterized by apneic episodes and weakness.

Reference:
1. Brull SJ, Claudius C. Neuromuscular blocking agents. In: Barash PG, Cullen BF, Stoelting RK, et al, eds. *Clinical Anesthesia Fundamentals*. Philadelphia: Lippincott; 2013:185-208.

13. **Correct answer: B**

Voltage-gated sodium channels are responsible for propagation of action potentials in motor neurons. The channel has 2 gates: an activation gate that is voltage-sensitive and an inactivation gate that is time-dependent. In the resting state, the activation gate is closed and the inactivation gate is open. When an action potential arrives, depolarization of the membrane triggers a conformational change and the activation gate opens, allowing influx of Na^+ ions into the cell and thus bringing about further depolarization. The inactivation gate will then close, therefore terminating Na^+ influx. The refractory period comprises the period when the sodium channel remains inactive (ie, both during and immediately following the process of repolarization). Additionally, the process of repolarization and the fall in the membrane potential that ensues also lead to closing of the activation gate. As the inactivation gate eventually opens, the channel will return to its resting state.

Reference:
1. Armstrong AM. Na channel inactivation from open and closed states. *Proc Natl Acad Sci USA*. 2006;103(47):17991-17996.

14. **Correct answer: A**

Ach can bind to presynaptic nAchRs and induce positive feedback to increase its own release from motor neurons during high-frequency (>2 Hz) stimulation. These presynaptic receptors differ from postsynaptic receptors and autonomic ganglionic receptors (mAchRs). Nondepolarizing neuromuscular-blocking drugs block both presynaptic and postsynaptic receptors. Blockade of presynaptic nAchRs results in failure of mobilization of Ach, which adapts to the demands of high-stimulation frequency. Clinically, this is manifested as tetanic fade and TOF fade, in which there is a reduction in twitch height with successive stimuli. Ach, succinylcholine, and nondepolarizing NMBs do not bind to calcium channels.

Reference:
1. Appiah-Ankam J, Hunter JM. Pharmacology of neuromuscular blocking drugs. *Contin Educ Anaesth Crit Care Pain*. 2004;4(1):1-6.

15. Correct answer: B

Succinylcholine is a depolarizing NMB whose structure resembles 2 Ach molecules. When succinylcholine binds to nAchR, it produces prolonged depolarization and desensitization, leading to flaccid paralysis after an initial period of receptor activation (fasciculation).

Succinylcholine has multiple side effects, including bradycardia and asystole, myalgia, increased intraocular and intracranial pressure, hyperkalemia, rhabdomyolysis, malignant hypertension, allergic reactions, and anaphylaxis.

Although succinylcholine is known to increase intragastric pressure, it also increases the lower esophageal sphincter, and therefore, the risk of aspiration is not thought to be amplified. Succinylcholine is frequently used for rapid sequence inductions secondary to its fast onset of action and its ability to produce muscle paralysis suitable for intubation within 30 seconds to 1 minute.

Reference:
1. Brull SJ, Claudius C. Neuromuscular blocking agents. In: Barash PG, Cullen BF, Stoelting RK, et al, eds. *Clinical Anesthesia Fundamentals*. Philadelphia: Lippincott; 2013:185-208.

16. Correct answer: A

The rate of onset of nondepolarizing NMBs generally depends on their potency. Less potent agents, such as rocuronium (ED_{95} 0.3 mg/kg), have a faster onset of action as compared with more potent agents, such as cisatracurium (ED_{95} 0.05 mg/kg). Rocuronium and cisatracurium are both intermediate-acting NMBs and have a duration of action of approximately 30-50 minutes.

Reference:
1. Brull SJ, Claudius C. Neuromuscular blocking agents. In: Barash PG, Cullen BF, Stoelting RK, et al, eds. *Clinical Anesthesia Fundamentals*. Philadelphia: Lippincott; 2013:185-208.

17. Correct answer: B

Nondepolarizing NMBs are divided, based on their inherent molecular structure, into benzylisoquinolinium and aminosteroid groups. Benzylisoquinolinium NMBs include atracurium, cisatracurium, mivacurium, doxacurium, and tubocurarine, all of which can be degraded by esterases or the Hofmann reaction. They consist of 2 quaternary amine groups joined by a thin chain of methyl groups. They lack vagolytic effects but are more likely to cause histamine release, leading to hypotension.

Aminosteroid NMBs include pancuronium, rocuronium, vecuronium and pipecuronium. They are built on a steroid skeleton with Ach-like moieties on their rings. They depend on the liver and/or kidneys for both metabolism and excretion. The aminosteroid muscle relaxants may have a vagolytic effect, leading to tachycardia and catecholamine release, but do not tend to cause histamine release.

Reference:
1. Brull SJ, Claudius C. Neuromuscular blocking agents. In: Barash PG, Cullen BF, Stoelting RK, et al, eds. *Clinical Anesthesia Fundamentals*. Philadelphia: Lippincott; 2013:185-208.

18. Correct answer: D

Atracurium is a collection of various stereoisomers of the benzylisoquinolinium NMB. Cisatracurium is one of the stereoisomers obtained by purification. Compared with atracurium, cisatracurium is more potent, requiring a smaller dose for intubation, has a slower onset, and does not cause significant histamine release at clinically relevant doses. Both atracurium and cisatracurium are degraded by esterases and the Hofmann reaction and have a similar duration of action.

Dosing Regimens and Characteristics of Benzylisoquinolinium Nondepolarizing Neuromuscular Blocking Agents

AGENT[a]	ATRAC	CISATRAC
Type (duration)	Intermediate	Intermediate
Potency: ED$_{95}$ (mg/kg)	0.25	0.05
Intubation dose (mg/kg)	0.5	0.15
Onset time (min)	3-4	5-7
Clinical duration (min)	30-45	35-50
Recovery index (R$_{25-75}$) (min)	10-15	12-15
Maintenance dose (mg/kg)	0.1	0.01
Infusion dose (mg/kg/min)	10-20	1-3
Elimination route	Renal 10%; Hofmann 30%; ester hydrolysis 60%	Hofmann 30%; ester hydrolysis 60%
Active metabolites	No active metabolites	No active metabolites
Side effects	Histamine release; laudanosine and acrylates production	None; histamine release at high doses
Contraindications (other than specific allergy)	Hemodynamically unstable patients	None
Comments	Organ-independent elimination	Trivial histamine, laudanosine, and acrylate levels

Atrac, atracurium; Cisatrac, cisatracurium; ED$_{95}$, effective dose 95%.
[a]Agents in current clinical use in the United States. The data are averages obtained from published literature, assume there is no potentiation from other coadministered drugs (such as volatile inhalational anesthetics), and the effects are measured at the adductor pollicis muscle. Other factors, such as muscle temperature, mode of evoked response monitoring, and type or site of muscle monitoring, will affect the data.
From Brull SJ, Claudius C. Neuromuscular blocking agents. In: Barash PG, Cullen BF, Stoelting RK, et al, eds. Clinical Anesthesia Fundamentals. *Philadelphia: Wolters Kluwer Health; 2015:193, with permission.*

Reference:
1. Brull SJ, Claudius C. Neuromuscular blocking agents. In: Barash PG, Cullen BF, Stoelting RK, et al, eds. *Clinical Anesthesia Fundamentals*. Philadelphia: Lippincott; 2013:185-208.

---

19. Correct answer: A

When drugs with different durations of action are used for maintenance of neuromuscular blockade, **recovery will follow the pattern of the drug that was initially administered**. Recovery from a neuromuscular blockade will reflect the pharmacodynamics of the drug that blocked the majority (70%-90%) of the receptors. When a second NMB is administered, this "maintenance" drug only blocks a small proportion (10%-15%) of the receptors, which is the proportion of receptors that are free or unoccupied at that time.

Reference:
1. Brull SJ, Claudius C. Neuromuscular blocking agents. In: Barash PG, Cullen BF, Stoelting RK, et al, eds. *Clinical Anesthesia Fundamentals*. Philadelphia: Lippincott; 2013:185-208.

---

20. Correct answer: B

Usually, administration of intubating doses of succinylcholine produces a short, depolarizing neuromuscular blockade referred to as the phase I block. The force of muscle contractions is reduced; however, the twitch strength does not change in response to repetitive stimulation (eg, TOF or tetany).

Administration of large doses of succinylcholine (>3-5 mg/kg), prolonged exposure (>30 min), or the presence of abnormal/atypical plasma cholinesterases can lead to a phase II block, which resembles the level of paralysis generated by nondepolarizing NMBs. Fade of twitch strength is observed after repetitive stimulation and potentiation, or stronger twitches, is produced after a period of tetany.

Reference:

1. Brull SJ, Claudius C. Neuromuscular blocking agents. In: Barash PG, Cullen BF, Stoelting RK, et al, eds. *Clinical Anesthesia Fundamentals*. Philadelphia: Lippincott; 2013:185-208.

21. Correct answer: B

Phase II block occurs after repeated boluses or prolonged infusion of succinylcholine. It can also occur after a single bolus of succinylcholine in patients with pseudocholinesterase deficiency. Phase II block is characterized by fade of the TOF twitch response, tetanic fade, and posttetanic potentiation.

Several mechanisms have been proposed to explain the phase II block, including succinylcholine binding and inhibition of the presynaptic nAchR, postsynaptic receptor desensitization (locking of the receptor in an inactivated state unresponsive to further agonist binding), and membrane potential repolarization by activation of Na/K ATPase. Inhaled anesthetics accelerate, not delay, the onset of a phase II block.

References:

1. Brull SJ, Claudius C. Neuromuscular blocking agents. In: Barash PG, Cullen BF, Stoelting RK, et al, eds. *Clinical Anesthesia Fundamentals*. Philadelphia: Lippincott; 2013:185-208.
2. Appiah-Ankam J, Hunter JM. Pharmacology of neuromuscular blocking drugs. *Contin Educ Anaesth Crit Care Pain*. 2004;4(1): 1-6.

22. Correct answer: D

This patient likely has a phase II block as a result of a prolonged succinylcholine infusion. The recommended course of action at this time would be to continue sedation and mechanical ventilation until spontaneous recovery of muscle strength has occurred.

Although theoretically anticholinesterase drugs can antagonize phase II block by increasing the amount of Ach available in the synaptic cleft, the response is difficult to predict because those drugs will also prevent the degradation of succinylcholine and are therefore best avoided in this situation. Atypical pseudocholinesterase or pseudocholinesterase deficiency may be suspected if the patient developed a phase II block and prolonged paralysis after a single dose of succinylcholine. Naloxone is a reasonable choice if patient has full motor recovery (no fade on TOF) and still fails to initiate spontaneous ventilation, pointing to other causes of apnea, such as opioid overdose.

Reference:

1. Appiah-Ankam J, Hunter JM. Pharmacology of neuromuscular blocking drugs. *Contin Educ Anaesth Crit Care Pain*. 2004;4(1): 1-6.

23. Correct answer: A

Binding of succinylcholine to presynaptic nAchR activates those receptors, stimulating repetitive firing and Ach release from the motor nerve terminal, which are manifested as fasciculations. Succinylcholine competes with Ach for binding to the postsynaptic nAchR and is not metabolized by the acetylcholinesterase present at the synaptic cleft, producing prolonged activation of the nAchR and muscle depolarization. As the depolarized muscle membrane locks voltage-gated sodium channels in the inactivated confirmation, junctional neurotransmission is blocked and flaccid paralysis ensues. This is called a phase I, or accommodation, block. This block is terminated by unbinding and diffusion of succinylcholine away from the NMJ back into the plasma and subsequent hydrolysis by plasma cholinesterases.

Fasciculations can produce myalgia, and pretreatment with a small dose of nondepolarizing NMBs or NSAIDs has been shown to be effective for myalgia prophylaxis.

References:

1. Brull SJ, Claudius C. Neuromuscular blocking agents. In: Barash PG, Cullen BF, Stoelting RK, et al, eds. *Clinical Anesthesia Fundamentals*. Philadelphia: Lippincott; 2013:185-208.
2. Appiah-Ankam J, Hunter JM. Pharmacology of neuromuscular blocking drugs. *Contin Educ Anaesth Crit Care Pain*. 2004;4(1): 1-6.

24. **Correct answer: B**

Phase I, or accommodation, block is characterized by a uniform decrease in the amplitude of twitches compared with baseline. There is no fade with TOF on phase I block, and adequate recovery will demonstrate return of all 4 twitches. Phase II block is characterized by fade on TOF, tetanic fade, and posttetanus potentiation.

Reference:
1. Brull SJ, Claudius C. Neuromuscular blocking agents. In: Barash PG, Cullen BF, Stoelting RK, et al, eds. *Clinical Anesthesia Fundamentals*. Philadelphia: Lippincott; 2013:185-208.

25. **Correct answer: C**

Monitoring the TOF has several advantages over single twitch monitoring. At supramaximal stimulation, T_1 and single twitch amplitudes are the same, so TOF does not require a baseline measurement. All subsequent twitches are measured as a fraction of T_1. TOF allows the clinician to subjectively assess the degree of fade visually or tactilely or by counting the number of twitches elicited. TOF ratio remains the same over a range of stimulation currents, so lower current can be applied in recovering patients to maximize comfort. Single twitch is better at detecting the onset of blockade because it allows for comparison with a baseline value.

Reference:
1. Brull SJ, Claudius C. Neuromuscular blocking agents. In: Barash PG, Cullen BF, Stoelting RK, et al, eds. *Clinical Anesthesia Fundamentals*. Philadelphia: Lippincott; 2013:185-208.

26. **Correct answer: C**

The TOF ratio is used as an objective means to measure the degree of chemical paralysis on nondepolarizing NMB. The number of twitches detected on TOF correlates with the proportion of AchR occupied by the NMB.

Relationship Between % Receptor Occupancy and Train-of-Four Ratio During Nondepolarizing Block

PERCENT RECEPTOR OCCUPANCY (%)	FIRST TOF TWITCH (T_1) (% BASELINE)	FOURTH TWITCH (T_4) (% BASELINE)	TOF RATIO (T_1-T_4 RESPONSES)	TOF COUNT (TOFC)
100	0%	0%	0	TOFC = 0
90-95	0%	0%	0 (T_1 = 0)	TOFC = 0
85-90	10%	0%	0 (T_2 = 0)	TOFC = 1
	20%	0%	0 (T_3 = 0)	TOFC = 2
80-85	25%	0%	0 (T_4 = 0)	TOFC = 3
	80%-90%	48%-58%	0.60-0.70	TOFC = 4
	95%	69%-79%	0.70-0.75	TOFC = 4
70-75	100%	75%-100%	0.75-1.00	TOFC = 4
	100%	100%	0.9-1.0	TOFC = 4
50	100%	100%	1.0	TOFC = 4
25	100%	100%	1.0	TOFC = 4

TOF, train-of-four; T_1, first twitch of TOF; T_2, second twitch of TOF; T_3, third twitch of TOF; T_4, fourth twitch of TOF; TOFC, train-of-four count. From Brull SJ. Neuromuscular blocking agents. In: Barash PG, Cullen BF, Stoelting RK, et al, eds. Clinical Anesthesia. *8th ed. Philadelphia; 2017:544, with permission.*

Reference:
1. Brull SJ, Claudius C. Neuromuscular blocking agents. In: Barash PG, Cullen BF, Stoelting RK, et al, eds. *Clinical Anesthesia Fundamentals*. Philadelphia: Lippincott; 2013:185-208.

27. Correct answer: C

Posttetanic count (PTC) is used during periods of profound block when no twitch is elicited with TOF. Stimulation following the tetanus often produces twitches secondary to its potentiating effect in nondepolarizing blockade. The number of posttetanic twitches produced is inversely proportional to the depth of block. Generally, 20-30 minutes is expected between the PTC of 1 and TOF twitch count of 1. In clinical settings, PTC of 1-2 indicates level of block sufficient for surgeries that require diaphragmatic paralysis.

Reference:

1. Brull SJ, Claudius C. Neuromuscular blocking agents. In: Barash PG, Cullen BF, Stoelting RK, et al, eds. *Clinical Anesthesia Fundamentals*. Philadelphia: Lippincott; 2013:185-208.

28. Correct answer: A

In DBS, 2 sets of 3 stimuli at 50 Hz are given 750 ms apart. The relationship between the fade ratios in DBS and TOF is identical and linear between 0 and 1. Comparing 2 fused responses instead of T_1 and T_4 allows the provider to easily detect fade visually or by touching. The threshold of fade detection is improved from ratio of 0.4 in TOF to 0.6 in DBS.

The frequency at which the 3 stimuli of each burst are delivered is tetanic, so a longer recovery time is needed before applying subsequent stimulations. The same amount of current is used for DBS and TOF.

Reference:

1. Brull SJ, Claudius C. Neuromuscular blocking agents. In: Barash PG, Cullen BF, Stoelting RK, et al, eds. *Clinical Anesthesia Fundamentals*. Philadelphia: Lippincott; 2013:185-208.

29. Correct answer: B

Acetylcholinesterase inhibitors, such as neostigmine, physostigmine, pyridostigmine, and edrophonium, are used to reverse the effect of nondepolarizing NMBs. They act by increasing the amount of Ach available in the NMJ. Side effects are related to the increased Ach in neuronal junctions of the parasympathetic nerve system, where Ach binds to nAchR in the preganglionic to postganglionic transmission, and muscarinic receptors in the terminal organs. Side effects of anticholinesterases include bradycardia, hypotension, bronchospasm (and hypoxia), increased respiratory secretions, nausea/vomiting, increased GI motility and secretions, miosis, and decreased intraocular pressure.

Tachycardia is a side effect of glycopyrrolate and atropine, anticholinergic drugs that are often given in conjunction with neostigmine, inhibiting mAchR and blocking parasympathetic activity.

Reference:

1. Brull SJ, Claudius C. Neuromuscular blocking agents. In: Barash PG, Cullen BF, Stoelting RK, et al, eds. *Clinical Anesthesia Fundamentals*. Philadelphia: Lippincott; 2013:185-208.

30. Correct answer: C

Succinylcholine is degraded by plasma cholinesterase, also known as pseudocholinesterase. Patients with atypical forms of this enzyme due to genetic mutations exhibit impaired metabolism of succinylcholine, resulting in delayed recovery from the paralytic. In these patients there is either a decrease in the activity of pseudochlinesterase, as measured by the dibucaine number, or there is a deficiency in the amount of pseudocholinesterase produced. Dibucaine is a local anesthetic that can bind to and inhibit pseudocholinesterase, therefore reducing its activity. Dibucaine has a higher affinity and inhibitory effect for wild-type (normal) enzyme than atypical (decreased activity) enzyme. The dibucaine number indicates percentage of the enzyme inhibited by dibucaine. A dibucaine number of >70 indicates normal pseudocholinesterase, 30-60 indicates heterozygote atypical conveying a mild delay of recovery from succinylcholine paralysis, and <20 indicates homozygote atypical producing paralysis lasting 2-3 hours or more.

Reference:

1. Viby-Mogensen J, Hanel HK. Prolonged apnea after suxamethonium: an analysis of the first 225 cases reported to the Danish Cholinesterase Research Unit. *Acta Anaesthesiol Scand*. 1978;22(4):371-380.

31. Correct answer: A

Myasthenia gravis and Lambert-Eaton syndrome are autoimmune diseases affecting the NMJ, producing similar symptoms by distinct mechanisms. Comparison of the two conditions is as follows:

	LAMBERT-EATON SYNDROME	MYASTHENIA GRAVIS
Antibody against	Presynaptic voltage-gated calcium channels	Postsynaptic nAchR
Number of functional AchR	Normal	Fewer
Main symptoms	Proximal muscle weakness, autonomic involvement (gastroparesis, orthostatic hypotension, urinary retention)	Bulbar involvement (diplopia, ptosis), does not affect autonomic nervous system
Changes with activity	Weakness improves with repetitive effort	Weakness worsens, fatigue develops with repetitive effort
Associated conditions	Small cell lung cancer	Thymoma
Treatment	Aminopyridines	Acetylcholinesterase inhibitors
Reaction to Sux	Sensitive	Resistant
Reaction to nondepolarizing NMBs	Sensitive	Sensitive

Reference:

1. Spillane J, Beeson DJ, Kullman DM. Myasthenia and related disorders of the neuromuscular junction. *J Neurol Neurosurg Psychiatry.* 2010;81(8):850-857.

32. Correct answer: C

The factors that are shown to be predictive of an increased length of prolonged postoperative intubation and mechanical ventilation in patients with myasthenia gravis undergoing thymectomy include duration of disease greater than 6 years, history of chronic respiratory disease, pyridostigmine dose greater than 750 mg per day, and perioperative vital capacity less than 2.9 L. Age of illness onset, muscle groups involved, and circulating antibody level did not have significant correlation with postoperative intubation.

Patients with myasthenia gravis should be extubated when fully awake and close to their baseline neurologic status. Anticholinesterase medications should be continued in the perioperative period. Calcium channel blockers, magnesium, and aminoglycosides should be avoided because they can aggravate muscle weakness.

Reference:

1. Eisenkraft JB, Papatestas AE, Kahn CH, et al. Predicting the need for postoperative mechanical ventilation in myasthenia gravis. *Anesthesiology.* 1986;65(1):79-82.

33. Correct answer: B

Patients with myasthenia gravis have decreased nAchR on skeletal muscle, making them resistant to depolarizing NMBs and sensitive to nondepolarizing NMBs. In contrast, patients with Lambert-Eaton syndrome have an overall decrease in the amount of Ach released from motor neurons, making them more sensitive to both depolarizing and nondepolarizing NMBs.

Reference:

1. Spillane J, Beeson DJ, Kullman DM. Myasthenia and related disorders of the neuromuscular junction. *J Neurol Neurosurg Psychiatry.* 2010;81(8):850-857.

34. Correct answer: C

Muscle weakness and respiratory failure can result from either exacerbation of the myasthenia itself or an overdose of the anticholinesterase medications used to treat myasthenia gravis. The best way to distinguish between the 2 is to administer a small dose of a fast-acting cholinesterase inhibitor, such as edrophonium (tensilon test). A myasthenia crisis will improve with administration of edrophonium, whereas a cholinergic crisis will worsen.

Other differences between the 2 conditions are outlined as follows:

MYASTHENIA CRISIS	CHOLINERGIC CRISIS
Undermedication	Overmedication
Increased heart rate, blood pressure or respiratory rate	Decreased heart rate or blood pressure
Bowl and bladder incontinence	Abdominal cramps, nausea/vomitting, diarrhea
Decreased urine output	Blurred vision
Absent cough and swallow reflex	Miosis
Mydriasis	Fasciculations
Symptoms improve with cholinesterase inhibitors	Symptoms improve with anticholinergics (atropine)

Reference:

1. Tether JE. Management of myasthenic and cholinergic crises. *Am J Med*. 1955;19(5):740-742.

35. Correct answer: D

Muscular dystrophy is a group of hereditary diseases characterized by painless degeneration and atrophy of skeletal muscles. Duchenne muscular dystrophy and Becker muscular dystrophy are the most prevalent types, both caused by a recessive mutation on the X chromosome, leading to decreased dystrophin function and primarily affecting boys. Dystrophin stabilizes muscle cytoskeleton and plays a role in calcium homeostasis. Duchenne muscular dystrophy has an earlier onset and faster progression in children presenting with weakness and motor delay (difficulty walking, pseudohypertrophy of calves, frequent falls). The symptoms of Becker muscular dystrophy are classically milder and present in adolescence.

Reference:

1. Koenig M, Beggs AH, Moyer M, et al. The molecular basis for Duchenne versus Becker muscular dystrophy: correlation of severity with type of deletion. *Am J Hum Genet*. 1989;45(4):498.

36. Correct answer: B

Myotonic dystrophy is a group of muscular disorders characterized by prolonged contraction and muscle relaxation, progressive muscle weakness, and muscle wasting. Type 1 or classic myotonic dystrophy is caused by an expanding CTG repeat in chromosome 19 coding for myotonic dystrophy protein kinase. Patients can have involvement of the cardiac conduction system, leading to malignant dysrhythmias and sudden death. Other organ systems affected include the lungs leading to restrictive lung disease and impaired ventilation, GI system including weak pharyngeal muscles and high risk of aspiration, and endocrine system including diabetes, thyroid and adrenal dysfunction.

Succinylcholine should be avoided because it may trigger exacerbated contractions lasting several minutes and hyperkalemia. Similarly, drugs given to reverse a neuromuscular blockade can also trigger contractures and spasms. Other triggers include potassium hypothermia, shivering, and mechanical or electrical stimulation. If use of an NMB is truly needed for a procedure in these patients, short-acting, nondepolarizing agents, such as rocuronium and cisatracurium, are recommended.

Reference:

1. Campbell N, Brandom B, Day JW. Practical suggestions for the anesthetic management of a myotonic dystrophy patient. *Myotonic Dystrophy Foundation Toolkit*. 2012:73-82.

37. Correct answer: A

Mitochondrial disease is a common cause of hypotonia in infants and children, affecting 1 per 4000 live births. Defects in mitochondrial function manifest in the high energy–requiring organs, including the brain, heart, and skeletal muscles, as encephalopathy, seizure, deafness, ataxia, cardiomyopathy, myopathy, and gastrointestinal and hepatic diseases.

Propofol has been reported to be associated with multiorgan failure, rhabdomyolysis, and metabolic acidosis in patients with mitochondrial disease, especially after prolonged or high-dose infusions. The cause is thought to be direct mitochondrial toxicity, leading to respiratory chain dysfunction and impaired fatty acid metabolism. Children receiving concomitant catecholamines or steroids are at high risk of developing propofol infusion syndrome. Other anesthetics, including ketamine, etomidate, dexmedetomidine, and thiopental, do not have adverse events reported.

Reference:

1. Niezgoda J, Morphan PG. Anesthetic considerations in patients with mitochondrial defects. *Paediatr Anaesth*. 2013;23(9): 785-793.

38. Correct answer: D

To date, only a few diseases have definitive predisposition to malignant hyperthermia (MH). King Denborough syndrome, multiminicore disease, and central core disease are congenital myopathies with characteristically disorganized muscle fibrils and symptoms of weakness. Mutations in the ryanodine receptor gene are implicated in the pathogenesis of all 3 conditions.

Other diseases, including muscular dystrophies, certain inborn errors of metabolism such as McArdle disease, myoadenylate deaminase deficiency, and CPT-2 deficiency, and channelopathies, may produce malignant hyperthermialike reactions when these patients are exposed to triggering agents, with symptoms of rhabdomyolysis, hyperkalemia, muscle rigidity, and metabolic acidosis. However, the pathogenic mechanism is distinct from MH, and the patients are not in a hypermetabolic state. Central cord syndrome is a cervical spinal cord injury, resulting in loss of sensation and motor function in the upper extremities.

Reference:

1. Litman RS. MH-associated diseases: who really needs a non-triggering technique? *Semin Anesth Perioper Med Pain*. 2007;26: 133-119.

39. Correct answer: B

LR solution contains 30 mmol of sodium lactate, which is metabolized to bicarbonate in vivo. This conversion requires normal mitochondrial activity. In patients with mitochondrial disease, LR can lead to elevated serum lactate and metabolic acidosis.

Patients with mitochondrial disease have poor energy production and utilization. Many are TPN dependent because of decreased intestinal motility. Hypoglycemia should be avoided because these patients are not able to easily mobilize other energy substrates, such as fat. Preoperatively, a short NPO period is advised and patients are encouraged to take sugar-containing clear liquids up to 2 hours before their procedure. Once NPO, the patient should receive dextrose-containing IV fluids. Normal saline and albumin are not associated with adverse effects in patients with mitochondrial disease.

Reference:

1. Parikh S, Saneto R, Falk MJ, et al. A modern approach to the treatment of mitochondrial disease. *Curr Treat Options Neurol*. 2009;11(6):414-430.

40. Correct answer: C

Pseudocholinesterase degrades succinylcholine (SCh), mivacurium, and certain local anesthetics. Intrinsic levels can be affected by certain physiologic and pharmacologic factors, such as alcoholism or obesity, which both increase butyrylcholine (aka pseudocholinesterase) levels. Butyrylcholinesterase levels may decrease to 75% of normal during pregnancy and to 67% of normal during immediate postpartum period; this degree of decrease is not usually clinically significant, but occasional prolonged apnea from SCh administration may result. Similarly, significant decrease of synthetic liver function may also result in prolonged apnea. In addition, plasma butyrylcholinesterase may be inhibited by exogenous compounds, such as organophosphates (eg, insecticides, chemical warfare agents, and echothiophate, a topical glaucoma agent), anticholinesterase agents (eg, neostigmine, pyridostigmine, and edrophonium), and monoamine oxidase inhibitors (MAOIs).

Reference:

1. Sultan DL, Hopkins DA, Changiz G. Neurobiology of butyrylcholinesterase. *Nat Rev Neurosci*. 2003;4(2):131-138.

11

STATISTICS

Maricela Schnur

1. A researcher designs a study examining the relationship between the gender of patients and the development of phantom limb pain. In this example, "gender" is best described as which of the following types of variables?

    A. Continuous
    B. Dichotomous
    C. Ordinal and dichotomous
    D. Nominal and dichotomous

2. A researcher designs a study with the purpose of investigating postoperative analgesic and blood pressure effects when acetaminophen was administered preoperatively. One hundred patients are randomized to receive either acetaminophen or a placebo pill. Systolic blood pressure measurements are recorded in each group, both before their operative procedure and postoperatively. What type of statistical test would be best utilized to analyze data for this study?

    A. Paired t-test
    B. Unpaired (Student) t-test
    C. Chi-squared
    D. ANOVA

3. A researcher designs a study that examines the relationship between red hair and postoperative nausea and vomiting. Which of the following statistical tests is most appropriate to analyze the data from this study?

    A. Paired t-test
    B. Unpaired (Student) t-test
    C. Chi-squared
    D. ANOVA

4. A researcher performs a study comparing the average heart rate of 4 groups of patients receiving different doses of a new β-blocker. Which of the following statistical tests is most appropriate to analyze the data from this study?

    A. Paired t-test
    B. Unpaired (Student) t-test
    C. Chi-squared
    D. ANOVA

5. The probability of a newborn baby developing respiratory distress with a mother who is a smoker is 0.2
    What are the odds of a newborn baby developing respiratory distress with a mother who is a smoker ?

    A. 0.1
    B. 0.25
    C. 1
    D. 4

6. A researcher describes a group of data as being positively skewed. In this data set which of the
    following statements is true?

    A. Population values are normally distributed.
    B. The tail of the data distribution extends to the right.
    C. The mean and median are equal.
    D. The mode is greater than the mean.

7. A highly sensitive test is defined as which of the following?

    A. A test that correctly classifies those with the disease
    B. A test that correctly excludes those without the disease
    C. A test that if negative indicates the true absence of the disease
    D. A test that if positive indicates the true presence of the disease

8. A highly specific test is defined as which of the following?

    A. A test that correctly classifies those with the disease
    B. A test that correctly excludes those without the disease
    C. A test that if negative indicates the true absence of the disease
    D. A test that if positive indicates the true presence of the disease

9. A test with a high positive predictive value (PPV) is defined as which of the following?

    A. A test that correctly classifies those with the disease
    B. A test that correctly excludes those without the disease
    C. A test that if negative indicates the true absence of the disease
    D. A test that if positive indicates the true presence of the disease

10. A test with a high negative predictive value is best described as which of the following?

    A. A test that correctly classifies those with the disease
    B. A test that correctly excludes those without the disease
    C. A test that if negative indicates the true absence of the disease
    D. A test that if positive indicates the true presence of the disease

11. In which type of observational study are subjects chosen and followed over a period to observe the
    outcome of interest?

    A. Cohort
    B. Case-control studies
    C. Cross-sectional studies
    D. Case series

12. A survey is devised with the intent to compare patient satisfaction and anesthetic type (general or
    regional anesthesia). This inquiry is best described as which type of study design?

    A. Cohort
    B. Case-control
    C. Cross-sectional
    D. Randomized trial

13. **A type I error is defined as which of the following?**

    A. Incorrectly rejecting the null hypothesis
    B. Correctly rejecting the null hypothesis
    C. Incorrectly accepting the null hypothesis
    D. Incorrectly rejecting the alternative hypothesis

14. **A study is being designed to examine the impact of a new analgesic on postoperative pain. Patients will be randomized to receive either the new analgesic or placebo, and average postoperative pain scores will be compared in the 2 patient groups. An increase in sample size will be required if which of the following factors is increased?**

    A. Standard deviation
    B. α
    C. β
    D. Effect size

15. **The number needed to treat (NNT) is defined as which of the following?**

    A. The risk of the outcome in the experimental group
    B. The difference in risk in the treatment and control groups
    C. The number of patients who need to be treated to decrease the adverse outcome by 10%
    D. The number of patients who need to be treated to prevent 1 adverse outcome

16. **Which of the following statements regarding the null hypothesis (H_0) is most correct?**

    A. It represents the absence of a difference between groups.
    B. It hypothesizes that there is a difference between test groups.
    C. If incorrectly rejected, it is referred to as a type II error.
    D. It is represented by the Greek letter α.

17. **An investigator is interested in comparing the differences in survival over time for patients who receive general anesthesia versus regional anesthesia for prostatectomies. Which of the following statistics would be most appropriate to analyze these data?**

    A. Relative risk
    B. Hazard ratio (HR)
    C. Odds ratio
    D. Rate ratio

18. **In a randomized control trial, the term "crossover" refers to which of the following?**

    A. Patients who drop out of the trial
    B. Patients who do not receive treatment during the course of the trial
    C. Patients who receive a sequence of different treatments during the trial
    D. Patients who do not end up receiving an assigned treatment and instead are enrolled in another randomized control trial

19. **In a single-blinded randomized control trial, the individuals being blinded to receiving treatment are which of the following?**

    A. Subjects only
    B. Investigators only
    C. Statistician only
    D. Subjects and investigators

20. **In statistical tests the *P*-value is defined as which of the following?**

    A. The probability of rejecting the null hypothesis

    B. The probability of obtaining a test statistic value equal to or more extreme than the actual test statistics given the null hypothesis is true

    C. The probability of accepting the null hypothesis

    D. The probability of obtaining a test statistic value less extreme than the test statistics given the null hypothesis is true

Chapter 11 ▪ Answers

1. Correct answer: D

Gender is typically considered both a nominal and dichotomous variable. Dichotomous variables are variables in which there are only 2 categories available, whereas nominal variables are variables that involve 2 or more categories without any specific order. Other examples of variables that are both dichotomous and nominal variables include yes/no or infected/not infected. Ordinal variables have 2 or more categories and a distinct order such as small, medium, and large. Continuous variables can take on an infinite number of values such as weight or height. In contrast, data are considered to be discrete if they are a count such as the number of students in a class.

References:
1. Rosner B. Nonparametric methods. In: *Fundamentals of Biostatistics*. 7th ed. Boston: Brooks Cole; 2010:327-344.
2. Berg SM, Bittner EA, Zhao KH. Statistics and data. In: *Anesthesia Review: Blasting the Boards*. Philidelphia: Wolters Kluwer; 2016:301-306.

2. Correct answer: A

The best statistical test to analyze these data is a paired t-test, which compares the results of the intervention with all patients acting as their own control. In comparison, an unpaired t-test would be utilized if only postoperative blood pressures were compared between the 2 independent groups of patients. Comparatively, the chi-squared test compares the association between categorical variables. Analysis of variance (ANOVA) is a statistical test that compares more than 2 means in continuous data sets with normal distributions.

References:
1. Berg SM, Bittner EA, Zhao KH. Statistics and data. In: *Anesthesia Review: Blasting the Boards*. Philidelphia: Wolters Kluwer; 2016:301-306.
2. Pace NL. Experimental designs and statistics. In: Barash PG, Cullen BF, Stoelting RK, et al, eds. *Clinical Anesthesia*. 7th ed. Philadelphia: Lippincott Williams & Wilkins; 2013:219-238.

3. Correct answer: C

The chi-squared test is used to examine the association between 2 categorical variables.

References:
1. Berg SM, Bittner EA, Zhao KH. Statistics and data. In: *Anesthesia Review: Blasting the Boards*. Philidelphia: Wolters Kluwer; 2016:301-306.
2. Pace NL. Experimental designs and statistics. In: Barash PG, Cullen BF, Stoelting RK, et al, eds. *Clinical Anesthesia*. 7th ed. Philadelphia: Lippincott Williams & Wilkins; 2013:219-238.

4. Correct answer: D

ANOVA is used to compare the mean values of more than 2 groups.

References:
1. Berg SM, Bittner EA, Zhao KH. Statistics and data. In: *Anesthesia Review: Blasting the Boards*. Philidelphia: Wolters Kluwer; 2016:301-306..
2. Pace NL. Experimental designs and statistics. In: Barash PG, Cullen BF, Stoelting RK, et al, eds. *Clinical Anesthesia*. 7th ed. Philadelphia: Lippincott Williams & Wilkins; 2013:219-238.

5. Correct answer: B

Probability is a measure of the likelihood that an event will occur. Probabilities always range between 0 and 1. The odds are defined as the probability that the event will occur divided by the probability that the event will not occur. In this example, if the probability of the newborn baby developing respiratory distress with a mother who is a smoker = 0.2, then the odds are 0.20/(1−0.20) = 0.20/0.80 = 0.25.

Reference:
1. Berg SM, Bittner EA, Zhao KH. Statistics and data. In: *Anesthesia Review: Blasting the Boards*. Philidelphia: Wolters Kluwer; 2016:301-306.

6. **Correct answer: B**

When data values are not symmetrically distributed around the mean, the distribution of data is understood to be skewed. There are 2 types of skewed distributions: (1) positively skewed: if the scores fall toward the right side of the scale and (2) negatively skewed: if the scores fall toward the lower end of the scale.

The mode is the most commonly represented value in the data set, whereas the median is the value in which 50% of the data lie above and 50% lie below. In a set of data that is skewed to the right (positively skewed), the mean exceeds the median. In addition, without examining the actual data set, the location of the mode with respect to the mean cannot be determined.

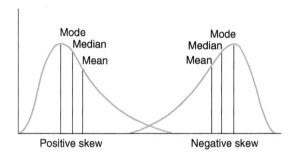

(From Polit DF, Beck CT. *Nursing Research: Generating and Assessing Evidence for Nursing Practice.* 10th ed. Philadelphia: Wolters Kluwer; 2017, with permission.)

Reference:
1. Glantz S. How to summarize data. In: Glantz SA, ed. *Primer of Biostatistics.* 7th ed. New York: McGraw-Hill; 2012:7-25.

7. **Correct answer: A**

Both sensitivity and specificity are 2 terms used to describe the performance of a binary statistical test. Sensitivity (also called the true positive rate) measures the proportion of individuals with the disease who are correctly identified by the test as having the disease. In the table below, the sensitivity is calculated by $[a/(a + c)]$.

	DISEASE	NO DISEASE
Positive test	a	b
Negative test	c	d

Reference:
1. Doucette JT, Krasnica S. Bedside statistical tools. In: Oropello JM, Pastores SM, Kvetan V, eds. *Critical Care.* New York: McGraw-Hill; 2017:1331-1338.

8. **Correct answer: B**

Specificity (also called the true negative rate) measures the proportion of individuals who do not have the disease and who are correctly identified by the test as such.

In the table below, the specificity is calculated as $d/(b + d)$.

	DISEASE	NO DISEASE
Positive test	a	b
Negative test	c	d

Reference:
1. Doucette JT, Krasnica S. Bedside statistical tools. In: Oropello JM, Pastores SM, Kvetan V, eds. *Critical Care.* New York: McGraw-Hill; 2017:1331-1338.

9. Correct answer: D

The PPV indicates whether a positive test actually represents the presence of a disease. In the table below, the PPV is calculated as [a/(a + b)]. The PPV depends on how prevalent the disease is in a given population. Using the same test in a population with higher prevalence increases PPV.

	DISEASE	NO DISEASE
Positive test	a	b
Negative test	c	d

Reference:
1. Doucette JT, Krasnica S. Bedside statistical tools. In: Oropello JM, Pastores SM, Kvetan V, eds. *Critical Care*. New York: McGraw-Hill; 2017:1331-1338.

10. Correct answer: C

Negative predictive value is the probability that subjects with a negative screening test truly do not have the disease. It is calculated by [d/(c + d)] and reflects those who test negative for the disease and do not have the disease.

	DISEASE	NO DISEASE
Positive test	a	b
Negative test	c	d

Reference:
1. Doucette JT, Krasnica S. Bedside statistical tools. In: Oropello JM, Pastores SM, Kvetan V, eds. *Critical Care*. New York: McGraw-Hill; 2017:1331-1338.

11. Correct answer: A

A cohort study follows a group of subjects (known as a cohort) over a period to observe exposure and the outcome of interest. Most cohorts are prospective studies. In a case-control study, the subjects are chosen after the outcome of interest has already occurred and compared with a control group who did not experience the outcome to determine whether past exposure or risk factors played a role in the outcomes. A cross-sectional study is a descriptive study in which the exposure status and outcome are measured simultaneously to provide a "snapshot" of the frequency and characteristics of a condition in a population at a particular point in time. A case report is a detailed report of the characteristics, diagnosis, treatment, and follow-up of an individual patient. A case series provides a description of a series of cases of a particular disease or condition.

Reference:
1. Doucette JT, Krasnica S. Bedside statistical tools. In: Oropello JM, Pastores SM, Kvetan V, eds. *Critical Care*. New York: McGraw-Hill; 2017:1331-1338.

12. Correct answer: C

A cross-sectional study is a descriptive study in which the exposure status and outcome are measured simultaneously in a given population. Cross-sectional studies can be thought of as providing a "snapshot" of the frequency and characteristics of a condition in a population at a particular point in time. A cohort study is a type of observational study in which individuals are followed up over time, and the individual's exposure and outcome are assessed during follow-up. Case-control studies are often used to identify factors that may contribute to a medical condition by comparing subjects who have that condition/disease (the "cases") with patients who do not have the condition/disease but are otherwise similar (the "controls").

Reference:
1. Doucette JT, Krasnica S. Bedside statistical tools. In: Oropello JM, Pastores SM, Kvetan V, eds. *Critical Care*. New York: McGraw-Hill; 2017:1331-1338.

13. Correct answer: A

A type I error is the incorrect rejection of a true null hypothesis (also known as a "false-positive" finding). A type II error is failing to reject a false null hypothesis (also known as a "false-negative" finding).

Reference:
1. Glantz S. What does "not significant" really mean? In: Glantz SA, ed. *Primer of Biostatistics*. 7th ed. New York, NY: McGraw-Hill; 2012:101-124.

14. Correct answer: A

Several factors must be considered in the calculation of an appropriate sample size. These include an estimate of the standard deviation of the data, the desired probabilities of making type I (α) and type II (β) errors, and the magnitude of the difference between groups to be detected (effect size). Increasing the variability will increase the sample size needed to detect a difference between groups, whereas increasing the effect size, α, or β will reduce the sample size.

Reference:
1. Rosner B. Hypothesis testing. In: *Fundamentals of Biostatistics*. 7th ed. Boston: Cengage Learning; 2010:204-256.

15. Correct answer: D

The NNT is the number of patients who need to be treated to prevent 1 adverse outcome. The ideal NNT is 1, where everyone improves with treatment and no one improves with control. The higher the NNT, the less effective is the treatment. The NNT is calculated as the inverse of the absolute risk reduction, where absolute risk reduction is the event rate in the control group minus the experimental event rate.

Reference:
1. Doucette JT, Krasnica S. Bedside statistical tools. In: Oropello JM, Pastores SM, Kvetan V, eds. *Critical Care*. New York: McGraw-Hill; 2017:1331-1338.

16. Correct answer: A

A "null hypothesis" is a general statement suggesting that there is no relationship between 2 measured groups. Rejecting the null hypothesis indicates that there *is* a relationship between 2 groups (eg, that a potential treatment has a measurable effect). The incorrect rejection of the null hypothesis is termed a "type I" error (also known as a "false-positive" finding). The probability of making a type I error is represented by the Greek letter α. A "type II" error is incorrectly retaining a false null hypothesis (also known as a "false-negative" finding).

Reference:
1. Doucette JT, Krasnica S. Bedside statistical tools. In: Oropello JM, Pastores SM, Kvetan V, eds. *Critical Care*. New York: McGraw-Hill; 2017:1331-1338.

17. Correct answer: B

Survival analysis is a collection of statistical technique used to compare the risks for death (or of some other event) associated with different treatments or groups, where the risk changes over time. In survival analysis, the HR is the ratio of the hazard rates corresponding to the risks of death being compared. The HR can be interpreted as the chance of an event occurring in the treatment arm divided by the chance of the event occurring in the control arm. HRs differ from relative risks and odds ratios in that relative risks and odds ratios are cumulative over an entire study, using a defined endpoint, while HRs represent instantaneous risk over the study time or some subset thereof.

Reference:
1. Doucette JT, Krasnica S. Bedside statistical tools. In: Oropello JM, Pastores SM, Kvetan V, eds. *Critical Care*. New York: McGraw-Hill; 2017:1331-1338.

18. **Correct answer: C**

In a crossover trial, subjects are randomly allocated to study arms, where each arm consists of a sequence of 2 or more treatments given consecutively. The simplest model is the AB/BA study. Subjects allocated to the AB study arm receive treatment A first, followed by treatment B, and vice versa in the BA arm. Crossover trials allow the response of a subject to treatment A to be contrasted with the same subject's response to treatment B.

Reference:

1. Doucette JT, Krasnica S. Bedside statistical tools. In: Oropello JM, Pastores SM, Kvetan V, eds. *Critical Care*. New York: McGraw-Hill; 2017:1331-1338.

19. **Correct answer: A**

Blinding in a study refers to keeping the knowledge of the treatment assignment hidden from at least one party involved in the study. The purpose of blinding is to minimize the amount of bias in the results. In a single-blinded study, the investigators, but not the subjects, know which treatment the subjects are receiving. In a double-blinded study, both the investigators and the study subjects are blinded.

Reference:

1. Doucette JT, Krasnica S. Bedside statistical tools. In: Oropello JM, Pastores SM, Kvetan V, eds. *Critical Care*. New York: McGraw-Hill; 2017:1331-1338.

20. **Correct answer: B**

The *P*-value is the probability of obtaining a test statistic value equal to or more extreme than the actual test statistics given the null hypothesis is true. Conventionally, a *P*-value of less than .05 is considered statistically significant.

References:

1. Kuroda MM. Principles of statistical methods for research in regional anesthesia. In: Hadzic A, ed. *NYSORA Textbook of Regional Anesthesia and Acute Pain Management*. New York: McGraw-Hill; 2007:1263-1288.
2. Biddison E, White DB. Interpreting and applying evidence in critical care medicine. In: Hall JB, Schmidt GA, Kress JP, eds. *Principles of Critical Care*. 4th ed. New York: McGraw-Hill; 2014:44-48.

ADVANCED SECTION

12

ADVANCED MONITORS

Abraham Sonny and Katarina Ruscic

1. **You perform thromboelastography for your hemorrhaging patient who has sustained massive abdominal trauma and it reveals a prolonged R time. Which of the following is an appropriate initial therapy to manage the patient's suspected coagulopathy?**

   A. Platelets
   B. Fresh frozen plasma
   C. Tranexamic acid
   D. Cryoprecipitate
   E. Packed red blood cells

2. **A 26-year-old patient with autoimmune thrombocytopenic purpura and a platelet count of 51 000 per microliter is scheduled for urgent appendectomy. Which thromboelastographic parameter do you expect to be altered in this patient?**

   A. Reaction (R) time
   B. Kinetic (K) time
   C. α angle
   D. Maximum amplitude (MA)
   E. Fibrinolysis (F)

3. **During the neohepatic phase of a liver transplant, the surgical team notices diffuse bleeding. Thromboelastography (TEG) reveals the following pattern. Based on this pattern, which intervention is the most appropriate for the patient's coagulopathy?**

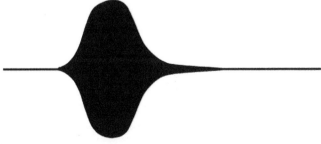

Image by Katarina Ruscic.

   A. Platelets
   B. Fresh frozen plasma
   C. Tranexamic acid
   D. Cryoprecipitate
   E. Packed red blood cells

4. TEG is performed and reveals an increased R time and decreased MA. These abnormalities are most suggestive of which of the following coagulation deficits?

   A. Decreased platelets
   B. Decreased clotting factors
   C. Decreased fibrinogen
   D. Increased fibrinolysis
   E. Both decreased platelets and decreased clotting factors

5. A patient is receiving blood product transfusions after undergoing aortic valve replacement. Despite the transfusions, the surgeons still note that their field is very "oozy." TEG is performed, which reveals a decreased α angle. Which blood product should be administered next?

   A. Platelets
   B. Fresh frozen plasma
   C. Tranexamic acid
   D. Cryoprecipitate
   E. Packed red blood cells

6. The complication rate (vascular complications and nerve injuries) associated with insertion of arterial lines closest to which of the following?

   A. 3-18 per 10 patients
   B. 3-18 per 100 patients
   C. 3-18 per 1000 patients
   D. 3-18 per 10 000 patients
   E. 3-18 per 100 000 patients

7. Which nerve is at greatest risk of suffering an injury during arterial catheter insertion into the brachial artery?

   A. Median nerve
   B. Radial nerve
   C. Ulnar nerve
   D. Musculocutaneous nerve
   E. Axillary nerve

8. A "flush test" is performed to assess damping of an arterial line pressure-monitoring system. A system with an appropriate dynamic response will have which of the following responses to rapid flushing?

   A. One large oscillation before a return to baseline
   B. One large and 1 small oscillation before a return to baseline
   C. One large and 3 small oscillations before a return to baseline
   D. Several large and several small oscillations before a return to baseline
   E. A square wave

9. Which of the following is most likely to produce underdamping in an arterial pressure monitoring system?

   A. Excessive tubing length
   B. Bubbles in the tubing system
   C. Kink in the arterial catheter
   D. Thrombus at the tip of the arterial catheter

10. **How does the systolic pressure measured in the dorsalis pedis artery differ from that measured in the aorta?**

    A. 5 mm Hg lower than the aorta
    B. 5 mm Hg higher than the aorta
    C. 20 mm Hg higher than the aorta
    D. 20 mm Hg lower than the aorta
    E. The same systolic pressure as the aorta

11. **Which component of a central venous pressure (CVP) waveform is most likely to be absent in a patient with a junctional rhythm?**

    A. a-wave
    B. x-descent
    C. c-wave
    D. Diastole descent
    E. v-wave

12. **A patient with severe tricuspid regurgitation would be expected to have which of the following CVP tracing abnormalities?**

    A. Cannon a-wave
    B. Tall c-v wave, diastole
    C. Exaggerated x-descent
    D. Exaggerated y-descent

13. **Where is the right internal jugular vein typically located in relation to the right carotid artery in the lower neck?**

    A. Posterior and medial
    B. Anterior and medial
    C. Posterior and lateral
    D. Anterior and lateral

14. **For insertion of a peripherally inserted central catheter, which vein is preferred, matched with its anatomical location?**

    A. Cephalic vein, lateral
    B. Cephalic vein, medial
    C. Basilic vein, lateral
    D. Basilic vein, medial

15. **Which of the following is the most common cause of death associated with iatrogenic pulmonary artery rupture (PAR)?**

    A. Anoxia
    B. Hemorrhagic shock
    C. Cardiac tamponade
    D. Myocardial infarction

16. **Which of the following ventilator parameters have been shown to prevent postoperative pulmonary complications among patients undergoing surgery? Choose all that apply.**

    A. 6-8 cc/kg ideal body weight
    B. 8-12 cc/kg ideal body weight
    C. ≥5 cm H_2O positive end-expiratory pressure (PEEP)
    D. ≤5 cm H_2O PEEP
    E. ≥16 cm H_2O plateau pressure
    F. ≤16 cm H_2O plateau pressure

17. A 65-kg patient is receiving volume-controlled ventilation with a tidal volume of 400 mL and frequency of 14 breaths per minute. The measured peak airway pressure is 18 cm H_2O, with a plateau pressure of 12 cm H_2O, and the PEEP is 2 cm H_2O. What is the static compliance of the patient's lung compliance?

   A. 40 mL/cm H_2O
   B. 67 mL/cm H_2O
   C. 25 mL/cm H_2O
   D. 25 cm H_2O/L
   E. 15 cm H_2O/L
   F. 40 cm H_2O/L

18. Which of the following ventilator pressure waveforms is most likely to be pressure support?

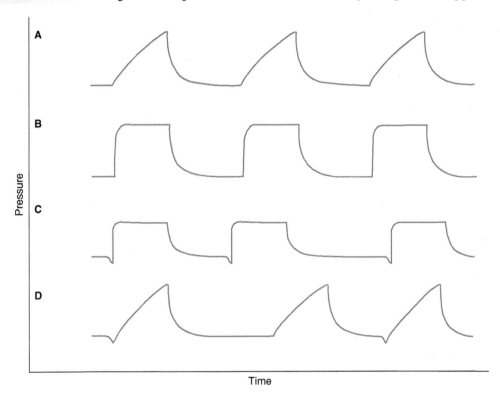

19. Optimization of PEEP to a level that promotes recruitment of alveoli and prevents alveolar overdistension would be expected to have which of the following pulmonary effects? Choose all that are correct:

   A. Pulmonary compliance will decrease.
   B. Pulmonary compliance will increase.
   C. The airway closing pressure will decrease.
   D. The airway closing pressure will increase.
   E. The functional residual capacity will decrease.
   F. The functional residual capacity will increase.

20. For a euvolemic patient with normal lung compliance and cardiac function, delivery of positive pressure ventilation (PPV) would be most likely to have which of the following hemodynamic effects?

   A. Decreased preload, decreased afterload, and increased cardiac output
   B. Decreased preload, increased afterload, and decreased cardiac output
   C. Decreased preload, increased afterload, and increased cardiac output
   D. Increased preload, decreased afterload, and decreased cardiac output
   E. Increased preload, decreased afterload, and increased cardiac output
   F. Increased preload, increased afterload, and decreased cardiac output

21. A patient is breathing steadily at a minute ventilation of 10 L/min while receiving supplemental oxygen via nasal cannula at a rate of 6 L/min. What is the approximate Fio_2 delivered to the patient during inspiration?

    A. 0.15-0.21
    B. 0.21-0.28
    C. 0.28-0.38
    D. 0.38-0.46
    E. 0.46-0.52

22. Which of the following statements about the differences between a partial rebreather and a nonrebreather oxygen delivery mask is most correct?

    A. A nonrebreather can theoretically reach an Fio_2 of 1.0, whereas a partial rebreather can reach an Fio_2 of 0.7-0.8.
    B. A nonrebreather utilizes a large reservoir bag of 600-1000 mL, whereas a partial rebreather utilizes a smaller reservoir bag.
    C. A nonrebreather allows expired gases to enter the reservoir bag, whereas a partial rebreather has a 1-way valve that inhibits expired gases from entering the reservoir bag.
    D. A nonrebreather allows inhaled nebulized bronchodilator therapy to be delivered, whereas a partial rebreather does not.

23. Which of the following statements is most correct regarding oxygen delivery to a patient wearing a Venturi mask?

    A. A variable Fio_2 is delivered depending on the patient's minute ventilation.
    B. A fixed Fio_2 is delivered based on the entrainment port size on the mask, independent of the patient's minute ventilation.
    C. A fixed Fio_2 is delivered to the patient based on the oxygen flow rate to the mask, independent of the patient's minute ventilation.
    D. A variable Fio_2 is delivered to the patient depending on the oxygen flow rate to the mask.

24. Which of the following statements regarding the benefit of high-flow nasal cannula (HFNC) is/are most correct?

    A. HFNC can provide PEEP.
    B. HFNC can improve CO_2 exchange.
    C. HFNC can achieve an Fio_2 between 0.21 and 1.0 that is independent of patient respiratory effort.
    D. All of the above.

25. A delivery system that allows for nitric oxide (NO) to have a long residence time in the ventilator circuit can lead to high concentrations of which of the following toxic metabolites?

    A. NO_2
    B. NO
    C. N_2O
    D. N_2O_2

26. Which of the following cardiac rhythm abnormalities is most likely to be seen on an ECG based on the CVP waveform provided below?

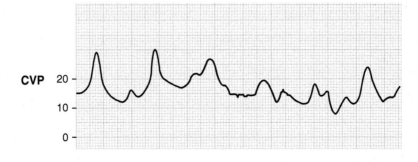

A. Normal sinus rhythm
B. Wenckebach heart block
C. Complete heart block
D. Atrial fibrillation

27. The following waveform is obtained after wedging a pulmonary artery catheter. Which point on the waveform correctly represents the wedge pressure?

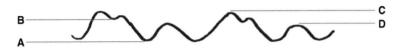

A. Point A
B. Point B
C. Point C
D. Point D

28. A typical CVP waveform is depicted below. What is the reason for the positive deflection pointed out by the arrow in the figure?

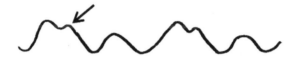

A. Right atrial contraction
B. Bulging of the tricuspid valve during right ventricular systole
C. Transmitted pressure wave from left atrial contraction
D. Interventricular conduction delay
E. Artifact due to movement of the central venous catheter

29. A 44-year-old patient is scheduled to undergo elective pericardiotomy for constrictive pericarditis. After insertion of a central venous catheter into the left internal jugular vein, which of the following CVP waveforms would most likely be seen?

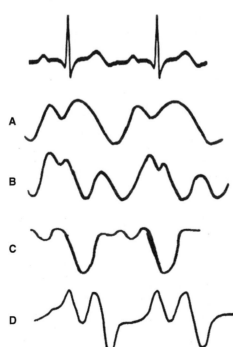

30. A 72-year-old woman is admitted to the intensive care unit (ICU) after sustaining an acute myocardial infarction 8 hours ago. She acutely develops increasing vasopressor requirements and worsening hypoxemia. A pulmonary artery catheter is inserted and wedged, revealing the waveform seen below. Which of the following is the most likely cause of her sudden decompensation?

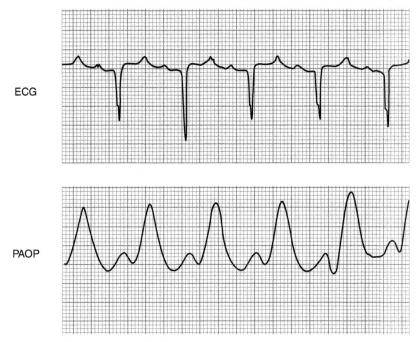

(Adapted from Daily EK. Hemodynamic waveform analysis. *J Cardiovasc Nurs.* 2001;15(2):6-22.)

    A. Ventricular septal defect
    B. Pulmonary embolism
    C. Mitral regurgitation
    D. Left ventricular failure
    E. Cardiac tamponade

31. Which of the following best describes the method for calculating of mean arterial pressure (MAP) using a noninvasive blood pressure monitor?

    A. Calculated from a proprietary algorithm based on systolic and diastolic blood pressure
    B. Inflation pressure at which maximum oscillometric pulse amplitude is detected
    C. Noninvasive blood pressure monitors do not give MAP
    D. Calculated using the equation, MAP = diastolic blood pressure + 1/3 (systolic-diastolic blood pressure)

32. A "square wave" test is performed to measure the dynamic response of a radial arterial line. Two oscillations are seen before the tracing returns to baseline. Which of the following best describes the state of the arterial pressure monitoring system?

    A. Underdamped
    B. Adequately damped
    C. Overdamped
    D. Cannot be determined

33. You are called to evaluate a patient in the ICU who has an indwelling pulmonary artery catheter. The nurse states that the waveform (below) appears markedly changed from 30 minutes ago. Which of the following best explains the portion of the waveform indicated by the arrow?

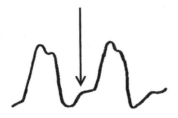

    A. Pulmonary regurgitation
    B. Right ventricular diastole
    C. Right ventricular systole
    D. Intermittent wedging of the pulmonary artery catheter

34. Which of the following conditions have the most insignificant effect on left ventricular end-diastolic pressure (LVEDP) estimation using a pulmonary artery catheter?

    A. Severe mitral regurgitation
    B. Tip of pulmonary artery catheter in West Zone I
    C. Severe tricuspid regurgitation
    D. Peak end-expiratory pressure at 15 cm H_2O.
    E. Left atrial myxoma

35. A patient with a permanent pacemaker undergoing general anesthesia for open cholecystectomy has the following ECG. The pacemaker function indicated by the arrow is best described as which of the following?

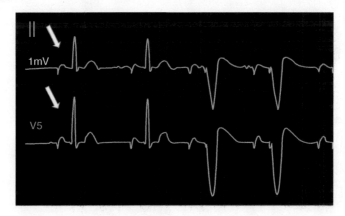

    A. A paced, V paced
    B. A sensed, V paced
    C. A paced, V sensed
    D. A sensed, V sensed

36. A 64-year-old woman is scheduled for laparoscopic cholecystectomy. Her medical history is significant for diabetes, hypertension, and mild chronic obstructive pulmonary disease (COPD). Before induction of anesthesia, the following rhythm is seen on the monitor. Her blood pressure is 120/72 mm Hg. What is the most appropriate next step in the treatment?

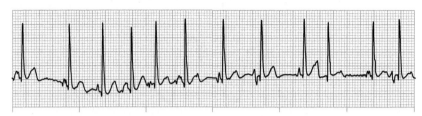

(From Badescu GC, Sherman B, Zaidan JR, Barash PG. Atlas of electrocardiography. In: Barash PG, Cullen BF, Stoelting RK, et al, eds. *Clinical Anesthesia*. 7th ed. Philadelphia: Lippincott Williams & Wilkins; 2013:1713, with permission.)

    A. β-Blockade
    B. Cardiology consultation before surgery
    C. DC cardioversion
    D. Dobutamine stress testing

37. A 68-year-old previously healthy woman becomes acutely hypotensive requiring high doses of phenylephrine while undergoing right hip arthroplasty under general anesthesia. A point-of-care cardiac ultrasonography is performed, which provides the following image. Which of the following is the most likely cause for the hypotension?

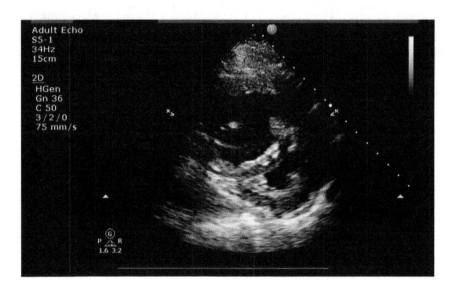

    A. Hemorrhage
    B. Pericardial tamponade
    C. Left ventricular failure
    D. Pulmonary embolism

38. After weaning from cardiopulmonary bypass, a patient undergoing coronary artery bypass grafting has an underlying heart rhythm of sinus bradycardia at 45 beats per minute. To augment her cardiac output, you decide to pace her in a VOO mode at 80 beats per minute, using epicardial pacing leads. Shortly after chest closure, she develops pulseless ventricular tachycardia, which is defibrillated with return of spontaneous circulation. Based on the rhythm strip provided below, which of the following interventions could most likely have prevented this event?

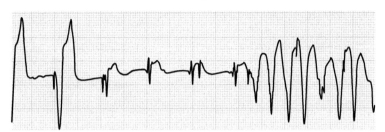

(Adapted from McLeod AA, Jokhi PP. Pacemaker induced ventricular fibrillation in coronary care units. *BMJ.* 2004;328(7450):1249-1250, with permission.)

A. Using a magnet after chest closure
B. Increasing the VOO rate to 100 beats per minute
C. Epinephrine infusion
D. Setting the pacemaker to DDD mode

39. Using the following measurements obtained from a patient with a pulmonary artery catheter that are listed below, what is the systemic vascular resistance (SVR) (in dynes/cm^5)?

Cardiac output	6.3 L/min
Mean arterial blood pressure	91 mm Hg
Mean pulmonary arterial pressure	24 mm Hg
Pulmonary capillary wedge pressure	12 mm Hg

A. 1003
B. 851
C. 673
D. Cannot be calculated with the given information

40. A 78-year-old woman with endocarditis develops hypotension after undergoing explantation of her permanent dual chamber pacemaker. Her medical history is significant for coronary artery disease and has had 3 drug-eluting stents placed 10 years ago. Focused echocardiography is performed to evaluate the cause of the patient's hypotension. Based on the image provided below, what is the most appropriate next step for management?

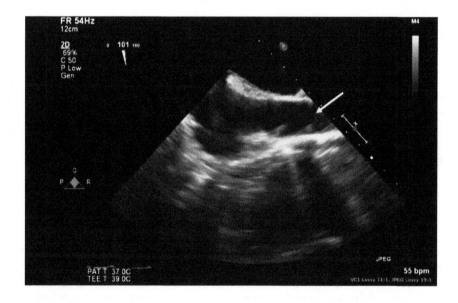

A. Pericardiocentesis
B. Cardiac catheterization
C. Transfusion for hemorrhage
D. Diuresis

41. **Transesophageal echocardiography is used for early detection of air embolism in a patient undergoing sitting craniotomy. Identify the structure pointed out by the arrow in the image.**

A. Inferior vena cava (IVC)
B. Superior vena cava
C. Right atrial appendage
D. Right ventricle
E. Patent foramen ovale

42. **A 23-year-old man was an unrestrained passenger in a motor vehicle crash. Primary and secondary survey revealed a left tibia and fibula fracture as well as a fracture of the posterior left fourth and fifth ribs. Although initially hemodynamically stable, he becomes hypotensive during transfer to the operating room. A bedside-focused ultrasonography is performed to determine the cause of the hypotension. Based on this image, which is the most likely cause of the patient's hypotension?**

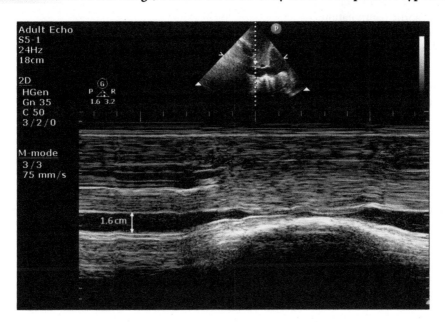

    A. Cardiac tamponade
    B. Tension pneumothorax
    C. Pulmonary embolism
    D. Hypovolemia

43. **A 42-year-old man with septic shock is undergoing exploratory laparotomy. You note that his norepinephrine requirement continues to increase and that his blood pressure continues to fall. The patient's arterial line tracing is seen below. What is the next best step to manage this patient's ongoing hypotension?**

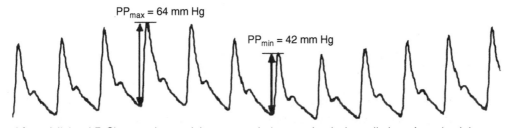

(Adapted from Michard F. Changes in arterial pressure during mechanical ventilation. *Anesthesiology*. 2005;103(2):419-428.)

    A. Give a fluid bolus
    B. Add epinephrine
    C. Add milrinone
    D. No further intervention

44. A patient is being monitored in the ICU using a noninvasive cardiac output monitoring device attached to radial arterial line. It uses arterial pressure contour for estimating stroke volume and cardiac output. In which of the following clinical scenarios would stroke volume estimated by this cardiac output monitor be most accurate?

    A. Rapid atrial fibrillation
    B. Acute aortic regurgitation
    C. During fluid resuscitation
    D. End-stage liver disease

45. Based on the Stewart-Hamilton equation, the relationship between thermodilution-based cardiac output and area under the temperature curve is best characterized by which of the following?

    A. Directly proportional
    B. Inversely proportional
    C. Varies based on body surface area
    D. Not related

46. Which of the following statements regarding the Bispectral index (BIS) for monitoring depth of anesthesia is most correct?

    A. BIS is superior to end-tidal anesthetic gas monitoring in preventing awareness.
    B. BIS correlates with probability of patient movement to noxious stimuli.
    C. BIS is an American Society of Anesthesiology standard monitor.
    D. BIS is unreliable during total intravenous anesthesia.

47. An EEG monitor is being used to measure the depth of anesthesia for a patient receiving total intravenous anesthesia with propofol. Which of the following best describes the characteristics of an EEG in an awake patient and in a patient under general anesthesia?

    A. Awake: high frequency and high amplitude; general anesthesia: low frequency and low amplitude
    B. Awake: low frequency and low amplitude; general anesthesia: high frequency and high amplitude
    C. Awake: high frequency and low amplitude; general anesthesia: low frequency and high amplitude
    D. Awake: low frequency and high amplitude; general anesthesia: high frequency and low amplitude

48. The velocity of blood through the middle cerebral artery, measured using transcranial Doppler (TCD), is likely to be elevated in all the following scenarios, EXCEPT which one?

    A. Increased cerebral perfusion pressure (CPP)
    B. Increased intracranial pressure
    C. Cerebral vasospasm
    D. Carotid artery stenosis

49. Which of the following BEST represents the degree of influence of anesthetic agents on somatosensory evoked potential (SSEP) monitoring? (Arranged from most deleterious to the least deleterious agents.)

    A. Etomidate > isoflurane > propofol > opioids
    B. Isoflurane > propofol > opioids > etomidate
    C. Isoflurane > opioids > etomidate > propofol
    D. Propofol > isoflurane > opioids > etomidate

50. Which of the following modalities for monitoring evoked potentials (EPs) is least affected by inhalational anesthetics?

    A. Visual EP
    B. Somatosensory EP
    C. Motor EP
    D. Brainstem auditory EP

Chapter 12 ▪ Answers

1. **Correct answer: B**

Although trauma patients often suffer from early coagulopathies, traditional tests of coagulation status such as partial thromboplastin time, international normalized ratio, platelet count, and fibrinogen may not reflect the true extent of the coagulopathy until life-threatening organ dysfunction has occurred. TEG is a hemostatic test that measures the shear elasticity and the dynamics of clot formation and the strength and stability of formed clot. Four values that represent clot formation are determined by this test: the R value, the K value, the α angle, and the MA. The reaction (R) time is the time interval between deposition of blood into the cuvette and a 1-mm amplitude on the thromboelastogram. It reflects clot *formation* kinetics, and prolongation is consistent with a lack of functioning clotting factors. Prolongation of R can be treated with fresh frozen plasma.

Other important parameters in the thromboelastogram can be seen in the figure. Although the R time is a reflection of clot formation and presence of adequate clotting factors, the kinetic (K) time and the α angle reflect the rate of clot cross-linking and presence of fibrinogen and platelets. The MA of the thromboelastogram is dependent on platelet number and function. The fibrinolysis (F) time is the interval from MA back to a 0-amplitude baseline.

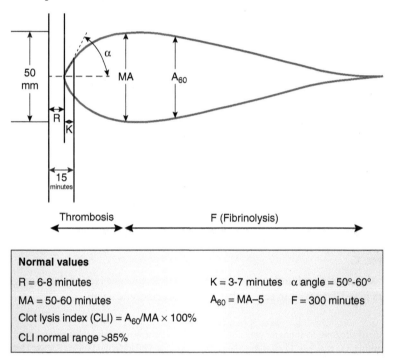

(From Figure 32-3, Tobin JM, Grabinsky A. Trauma and burn anesthesia. In: Barash PG, Cullen BF, Stoelting RK, et al, eds. *Clinical Anesthesia Fundamentals*. Philadelphia: Wolters Kluwer Health; 2015:607–627.)

Reference:
1. Tobin JM, Grabinsky A. Trauma and burn anesthesia. In: Barash PG, Cullen BF, Stoelting RK, et al, eds. *Clinical Anesthesia Fundamentals*. Philadelphia: Wolters Kluwer Health; 2015:607–627.

2. **Correct answer: D**

The figure shows several classic tracings of abnormal thromboelastograms. Thrombocytopenia or platelet blockers decrease the MA because clots cannot be normally stabilized by platelets. The R time, K time, and α angle can be affected by anticoagulants or lack of clotting factors (see explanation given for question 1). A decreased F time is found in fibrinolysis. Hypercoagulability can result in shortened R, K, and α angle, with an increased MA.

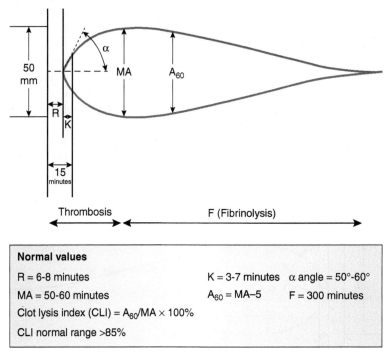

Thrombosis F (Fibrinolysis)

Normal values

R = 6-8 minutes K = 3-7 minutes α angle = 50°-60°

MA = 50-60 minutes A_{60} = MA–5 F = 300 minutes

Clot lysis index (CLI) = A_{60}/MA × 100%

CLI normal range >85%

(From Tobin JM, Grabinsky A. Trauma and burn anesthesia. In: Barash PG, Cullen BF, Stoelting RK, et al, eds. *Clinical Anesthesia Fundamentals*. Philadelphia: Wolters Kluwer Health; 2015:607–627, with permission.)

Reference:

1. Tobin JM, Grabinsky A. Trauma and burn anesthesia. In: Barash PG, Cullen BF, Stoelting RK, et al, eds. *Clinical Anesthesia Fundamentals*. Philadelphia: Wolters Kluwer Health; 2015:607–627.

3. **Correct answer: C**

The figure shows a decreased F time, reflecting increased fibrinolysis (see explanation given for question 1). Of the answers listed, tranexamic acid is the only antifibrinolytic agent.

References:

1. Krishnan S. Anesthetic considerations for patients with obesity, hepatic disease, and other gastrointestinal issues. In: Barash PG, Cullen BF, Stoelting RK, et al, eds. *Clinical Anesthesia Fundamentals*. Philadelphia: Wolters Kluwer Health; 2015:519–538.
2. Robertson AC, Pilla MA, Sandberg WS. Anesthesia for liver surgery and transplantation. In: Longnecker DE, Mackey SC, Newman MF, et al, eds. *Anesthesiology*. 3rd ed. New York: McGraw-Hill; 2018:971–999.

4. **Correct answer: E**

R is a reflection of clotting initiation and presence of adequate clotting factors. MA decrease is consistent with low platelets (see explanation given for question 1). This patient is likely in the late phase of disseminated intravascular coagulation, where many coagulation factors have already been consumed.

Reference:

1. Tsen LC. Anesthesia for obstetric care and gynecologic surgery. In: Longnecker DE, Mackey SC, Newman MF, et al, eds. *Anesthesiology*. 3rd ed. New York: McGraw-Hill; 2018:1063–1082.

5. **Correct answer: D**

The α angle is a reflection of clotting kinetics and can be decreased by insufficient fibrinogen (see explanation given for question 1). Cryoprecipitate will help replete the patient's fibrinogen.

Reference:
1. Tsen LC. Anesthesia for obstetric care and gynecologic surgery. In: Longnecker DE, Mackey SC, Newman MF, et al, eds. *Anesthesiology*. 3rd ed. New York: McGraw-Hill; 2018:1063–1082.

6. **Correct answer: D**

Risks of intra-arterial catheter placement include bleeding complications such as hemorrhage and hematoma, vascular complications such as ischemia, thrombosis, cerebral embolism, and fistula formation, and other complications such as nerve injury, skin necrosis, and infection. Although all of these complications are undesirable, a recent study found a relatively low incidence rate of ~3-18 per 10 000 patients of vascular and nerve complications secondary to arterial line placement, with the incidence rate varying depending on the catheter size.

References:
1. Fink RJ, Mark JB. Standard anesthesia monitoring techniques and instruments. In: Barash PG, Cullen BF, Stoelting RK, et al, eds. *Clinical Anesthesia Fundamentals*. Philadelphia: Wolters Kluwer Health; 2015:277–296.
2. Nuttall G, Burckhardt J, Hadley A, et al. Surgical and patient risk factors for severe arterial line complications in adults. *Anesthesiology*. 2016;124:590-597.

7. **Correct answer: A**

The median nerve is in close proximity to the brachial artery within the antecubital fossa and is at risk of nerve injury during brachial artery cannulation. Despite this risk, recent literature suggests that brachial artery catheterization may be a suitable alternative to radial artery catheterization in patients with complex medical comorbidities.

References:
1. Nuttall G, Burckhardt J, Hadley A, et al. Surgical and patient risk factors for severe arterial line complications in adults. *Anesthesiology*. 2016;124:590-597.
2. Handlogten KS, Wilson GA, Clifford L, et al. Brachial artery catheterization: an assessment of use patterns and associated complications. *Anesth Analg*. 2014;118:288-295.

8. **Correct answer: B**

Arterial pressure measurement systems consist of a column of fluid directly connecting the arterial system to a pressure transducer. The pressure waveform of the arterial pulse is transmitted via the column of fluid to a pressure transducer where it is converted into an electrical signal. This electrical signal is then processed, amplified, and converted into a visual display by a microprocessor.

To determine whether an arterial pressure monitoring system can adequately reproduce a patient's blood pressures, the dynamic response characteristics of the catheter system must be tested. Only when system accuracy, also termed fidelity, has been confirmed, can the analog waveform be accepted as an accurate reflection of a patient's status. The dynamic response of a hemodynamic monitoring system is defined by its natural frequency and the damping coefficient. The natural frequency indicates how fast the pressure monitoring system vibrates when excited by a signal such as the arterial pressure pulse or the pressure signal caused by a fast-flush test. The damping coefficient of a monitoring system is a measure of how quickly the oscillations of a shock-excited system dampen and eventually come to rest. An appropriately damped arterial line system will have one large and one small oscillation in response to a test flush.

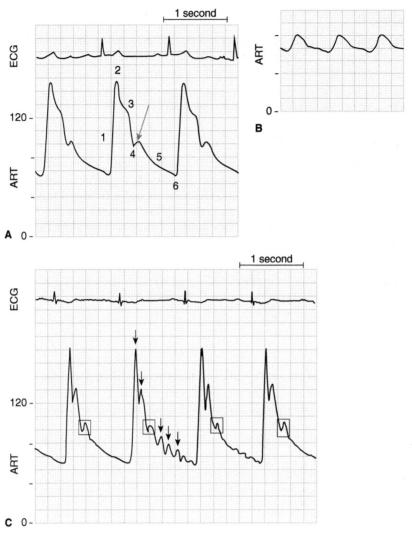

(From Fink RJ, Mark JB. Standard anesthesia monitoring techniques and instruments. In: Barash PG, Cullen BF, Stoelting RK, et al, eds. *Clinical Anesthesia*. Philadelphia: Wolters Kluwer Health; 2015:288, with permission.)

References:

1. Fink RJ, Mark JB. Standard anesthesia monitoring techniques and instruments. In: Barash PG, Cullen BF, Stoelting RK, et al, eds. *Clinical Anesthesia Fundamentals*. Philadelphia: Wolters Kluwer Health; 2015:277–296.
2. Bar-Yosef S, Schroeder RA, Mark JB. Hemodynamic monitoring. In: Longnecker DE, Mackey SC, Newman MF, et al, eds. *Anesthesiology*. 3rd ed. New York: McGraw-Hill; 2018:360–381.
3. Marino PL. Arterial pressure monitoring. In: *The ICU Book*. 4th ed. Philadelphia: Wolters Kluwer Health/Lippincott Williams & Wilkins; 2014:123–134.

9. **Correct answer: A**

Overdamped systems attenuate the true arterial pressure waveform, making the displayed systolic pressure and the pulse pressures appear erroneously low (see also explanation given for question 8). Obstruction of the arterial catheter with a thrombus or kink, as well as bubbles in the fluid tubing, can cause overdamping. An excessive length of tubing can result in underdampening, making the systolic blood pressure appear erroneously high.

References:

1. Fink RJ, Mark JB. Standard anesthesia monitoring techniques and instruments. In: Barash PG, Cullen BF, Stoelting RK, et al, eds. *Clinical Anesthesia Fundamentals*. Philadelphia: Wolters Kluwer Health; 2015:277–296.
2. Bar-Yosef S, Schroeder RA, Mark JB. Hemodynamic monitoring. In: Longnecker DE, Mackey SC, Newman MF, et al, eds. *Anesthesiology*. 3rd ed. New York: McGraw-Hill; 2018:360–381.
3. Marino PL. Arterial pressure monitoring. In: *The ICU Book*. 4th ed. Philadelphia: Wolters Kluwer Health/Lippincott Williams & Wilkins; 2014:123–134.

10. **Correct answer: C**

As the arterial pressure wave moves from its origin in the aorta, toward the periphery, the systolic portion becomes peaked and narrowed with increased amplitude. As a result, the systolic blood pressure in distal sites will be significantly higher (by as much as 20 mm Hg) than that recorded from a more central site. The diastolic portion of the waveform may display a secondary (reflectance) wave, as the monitoring site becomes more distal to the central aorta. The dicrotic notch becomes less defined, as the monitoring site is moved toward the periphery. These changes could also be intensified with significant doses of vasodilators or vasopressors. Because the systolic pressure wave narrows, the MAP remains the same between the aorta and distal arterial sites.

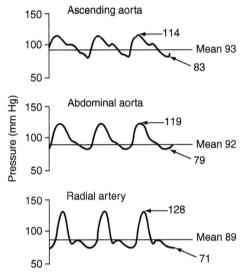

(From Frenzel JZ. Arterial wave form. In: Singh-Radcliff N, ed. *The 5-Minute Anesthesia Consult*. Philadelphia: Lippincott Williams & Wilkins; 2013:86, with permission.)

Reference:

1. Marino PL. Arterial pressure monitoring. In: *The ICU Book*. 4th ed. Philadelphia: Wolters Kluwer Health/Lippincott Williams & Wilkins; 2014:123–134.

11. **Correct answer: A**

The normal CVP waveform has 3 named peaks and descending segments. The a-wave is caused by atrial contraction at the end of diastole ("atrial kick"). The c-wave occurs during early systole and is a result of isovolumetric ventricular contraction against a closed tricuspid valve, resulting in back pressure through the atrium to the CVP catheter. The x-descent during midsystole is due to atrial relaxation and heart base descent, followed by the v-wave during late systole caused by filling of the right atrium against a closed tricuspid valve. This is followed by the y-descent, which occurs in early diastole, and is due to blood flow out of the right atrium into the right ventricle. In a junctional rhythm, contraction of the right atrium occurs when the tricuspid valve is still closed, resulting in an exaggerated a-wave, known as a "cannon a-wave."

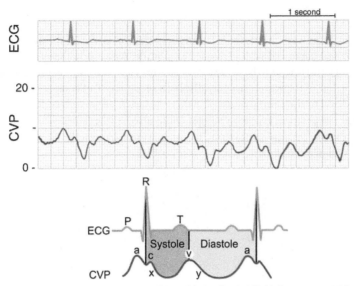

(From Mark JB. *Atlas of Cardiovascular Monitoring*. New York: Churchill Livingstone; 1998, with permission.)

Reference:
1. Fink RJ, Mark JB. Standard anesthesia monitoring techniques and instruments. In: Barash PG, Cullen BF, Stoelting RK, et al, eds. *Clinical Anesthesia Fundamentals*. Philadelphia: Wolters Kluwer Health; 2015:277–296.

12. Correct answer: B

See answer to previous question for explanation of the normal CVP waveform. In tricuspid regurgitation, the incompetent tricuspid valve causes abnormal systolic filling of the right atrium, resulting in an increase in the magnitudes of the c-wave (isovolumetric contraction of the right ventricle) and the v-wave (venous filling of the right atrium in late systole while the right ventricle is still contracting) and obliteration of the x-descent, causing a broad, tall systolic c-v wave. A cannon a-wave is associated with a junctional rhythm. An exaggerated x-descent is associated with pericardial tamponade. The y-descent represents a decrease in right atrial pressure after the tricuspid valve opens, and there is rapid filling of the right ventricle.

Reference:
1. Fink RJ, Mark JB. Standard anesthesia monitoring techniques and instruments. In: Barash PG, Cullen BF, Stoelting RK, et al, eds. *Clinical Anesthesia Fundamentals*. Philadelphia: Wolters Kluwer Health; 2015:277–296.

13. Correct answer: D

Anatomically, the internal jugular vein runs in a line from the suprasternal notch to the mastoid process under the sternocleidomastoid muscle. Although there can be anatomical variations, right internal jugular vein is most typically anterior and lateral to the carotid artery.

Reference:
1. Marino PL. Central venous access. In: *The ICU Book*. 4th ed. Philadelphia: Wolters Kluwer Health/Lippincott Williams & Wilkins; 2014:17–40.

14. Correct answer: D

The cephalic veins run on the lateral side of the arm, whereas the basilic veins run on the medial side of the arm. Of the 2 vessels, the basilic vein is typically larger in diameter and runs in a more linear course through the arm.

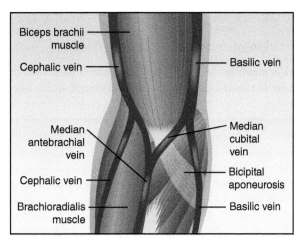

(From Marino PL. Central venous access. In: *Marino's The ICU Book*. 4th ed. Philadelphia: Wolters Kluwer Health/Lippincott Williams & Wilkins; 2014:31, with permission.)

Reference:
1. Marino PL. Central venous access. In: *The ICU Book*. 4th ed. Philadelphia: Wolters Kluwer Health/Lippincott Williams & Wilkins; 2014:17–40.

15. Correct answer: A

The proposed mechanisms responsible for catheter-induced PAR include lodging of the catheter tip into the vessel wall when the pulmonary artery catheter (PAC) is advanced with an uninflated balloon, retraction of a wedged balloon, and flushing of a wedged catheter. The initial presentation of PAR may be as obvious as a massive pulmonary hemorrhage or as subtle as a cough associated with minimal hemoptysis, or it may even be totally asymptomatic. Primary management of catheter-induced PAR focuses on the prevention of asphyxia. Hypoxia secondary to lung spillage or blood clots is the main factor leading to death. Preventing the contamination of the unaffected lung is therefore essential. Being a pulmonary, low-pressure bleeding, the blood loss is rarely massive enough to cause a great threat to the hemodynamic status, and slight hypotension may be treated with volume replacement. It is different from massive hemoptysis secondary to bronchial systemic high-pressure bleeding.

Reference:
1. Bussières JS. Iatrogenic pulmonary artery rupture. *Curr Opin Anaesthesiol.* 2007;20(1):48-52.

16. Correct answer: A, C, and F

Lung protective mechanical ventilation aims to keep transpulmonary pressures in the linear portion of the pressure-volume curve for the lung but avoid both alveolar derecruitment and overdistension. Several large studies have suggested that use of lung protective ventilation in the operating room reduces postoperative respiratory complications for surgical patients. Ventilatory parameters that have been associated with intraoperative lung protection include tidal volume of 6-8 mL/kg ideal body weight, PEEP of at least 5 cm H_2O, and a median plateau pressure of 16 cm H_2O or less.

Reference:
1. Ruscic KJ, Grabitz SD, Rudolph MI, Eikermann M, Prevention of respiratory complications of the surgical patient: actionable plan for continued process improvement. *Curr Opin Anesthesiol.* 2017;30:399-408.
2. Ladha K, Vidal Melo MF, McLean DJ, et al. Intraoperative protective mechanical ventilation and risk of postoperative respiratory complications: hospital based registry study. *BMJ.* 2015;351:h3646.

17. Correct answer: A

Compliance is a measure of distensibility, or how much volume a given entity can hold at a given pressure, which is mathematically expressed as $C = \Delta V/\Delta P$. For calculating lung compliance, the delivered tidal volume, V_T, is the volume in question, whereas the relevant pressure when considering static lung compliance is the difference between the plateau pressure, $P_{plateau}$, and the PEEP. This is expressed as follows:

$$C_{stat} = V_T/(P_{plateau} - PEEP)$$

$$= 400 \text{ mL}/(12 \text{ cm H}_2O - 2 \text{ cm H}_2O) = 40 \text{ mL/cm H}_2O$$

The plateau pressure is measured by an end-expiratory hold maneuver in volume control ventilation. The peak airway pressure is affected by upper airway resistance and is not linearly related to the static thoracic compliance.

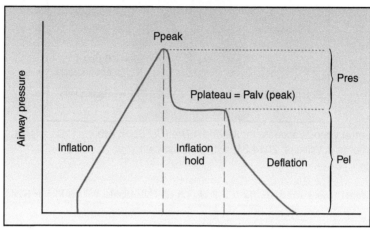

(From Marino PL. Positive pressure ventilation. In: *Marino's The ICU Book*. 4th ed. Philadelphia: Wolters Kluwer Health/Lippincott Williams & Wilkins; 2014:489, with permission.)

Reference:

1. Marino PL. Positive pressure ventilation. In: *The ICU Book*. 4th ed. Philadelphia: Wolters Kluwer Health/Lippincott Williams & Wilkins; 2014:487–504.

18. Correct answer: C

In *volume control* ventilation (A), pressure steadily increases during inspiration, as gas (typically at a constant flow rate) fills the lungs, and pressure drops quickly during expiration as the chest and diaphragm passively recoil. In *pressure control* ventilation (B), the ventilator quickly reaches the "control" pressure and maintains this throughout the breath. This requires an increased respiratory flow at the outset of the breath and a small delay for the ventilator to reach the target pressure. Expiratory flows are passive and follow the same waveform as in volume control. In *pressure support* ventilation (C), the patient initiates each pressure-controlled breath by generating negative pressure (note the downward deflections before the pressure support wave), and thus inspiratory timing is dependent on patient effort. In SIMV (synchronized intermittent mandatory ventilation) (D), a volume-controlled breath is delivered with each inspiratory effort. If the patient fails to initiate a breath after a set interval, the ventilator will deliver a volume-controlled breath regardless.

Reference:

1. Marino PL. Conventional modes of ventilation. In: *The ICU Book*. 4th ed. Philadelphia: Wolters Kluwer Health/Lippincott Williams & Wilkins; 2014:505–520.

19. Correct answer: B and F

The closing pressure is defined as the transpulmonary pressure at which the distal airspaces start to collapse. Although normal closing pressure is approximately 3 cm H$_2$O, it is decreased in disease processes, causing decreases in lung compliance (such as acute respiratory distress syndrome and pulmonary fibrosis), and is increased with age and with obstructive processes (such as COPD). When the airway pressure at the end of expiration falls below the closing pressure, the distal airways collapse (atelectasis), resulting in a reduction in the functional residual capacity. PEEP helps prevent the end-expiratory pressure from falling below the closing pressure and, when in the appropriate range, can help promote recruitment of collapsed alveoli. The recruitment of alveoli results in an increase in pulmonary compliance. Of note, high PEEP can overdistend alveoli in regions of lung that are not atelectatic, thereby decreasing lung compliance. See answer to question 17 for further explanation of compliance.

Reference:

1. Marino PL. Conventional modes of ventilation. In: *The ICU Book*. 4th ed. Philadelphia: Wolters Kluwer Health/Lippincott Williams & Wilkins; 2014:505–520.

20. Correct answer: A

PPV decreases preload via multiple mechanisms. The increased intrathoracic pressure caused by PPV reduces the pressure gradient that normally drives venous return into the thoracic cavity. Furthermore, the increased intrathoracic pressure decreases the distensibility of the heart, which decreases diastolic cardiac filling. Lastly, pulmonary vascular resistance is increased by compression of the pulmonary vasculature by the increased intrathoracic pressure, which can impede right ventricular emptying; this in turn decreases the volume available for left ventricular filling.

Although PPV impedes diastolic filling of the heart, the same compressive positive pressure facilitates systolic emptying of the heart. Peak systolic transmural wall pressure is a determinant of left ventricular afterload. Thus, because PPV causes peak systolic transmural wall pressure to be decreased, ventricular afterload is decreased. Because PPV decreases both preload and afterload, the net effect on cardiac output will depend on which effect predominates. If the intravascular volume is normal, the intrathoracic pressures are kept low (as in lung-protective ventilation), and the cardiac function is normal, the net effect is typically an overall increase in cardiac stroke output. If a patient is hypovolemic, the preload reduction can predominate, and the cardiac output can be decreased by PPV.

Reference:

1. Marino PL. Positive pressure ventilation. In: *The ICU Book*. 4th ed. Philadelphia: Wolters Kluwer Health/Lippincott Williams & Wilkins; 2014:487–504.

21. Correct answer: D

Low flow supplemental oxygen inhalation systems work on the principle that a constant flow of oxygen fills a reservoir, which then admixes with entrained room air to enrich the oxygen content of the air. For a simple face mask, the oxygen reservoir is the face mask itself, with a reservoir capacity of 150-250 mL. When nasal cannula is used, the patients' own nasopharynx and oropharynx serve as the oxygen reservoir and have a capacity of approximately 50 mL. Of note, this reservoir mechanism is the reason that nasal cannula still delivers an Fio_2 above that of room air even when the patient is a "mouth breather."

If a patient's minute ventilation exceeds the flow rate of the oxygen delivery device, the reservoir is drained of supplemental oxygen and the resulting Fio_2 delivered is decreased. For example, at a flow rate of 6 L/min, the Fio_2 for nasal cannula is 0.6 when the minute ventilation is 5 L/min, but decreases to 0.44 and 0.32 if the minute ventilation is increased to 10 L/min or 20 L/min, respectively. Thus, for patients with a high minute ventilation (for example, in respiratory distress, where minute ventilation can increase to 30-100 L/min), a substantively increased Fio_2 cannot be achieved with nasal cannula. Face masks increase the reservoir volume and allowing for increased enrichment of inspired air with supplemental oxygen (see table below).

Low-Flow Oxygen Inhalation Systems

DEVICE	RESERVOIR CAPACITY (mL)	OXYGEN FLOW (L/min)	APPROXIMATE (Fio_2)[a]
Nasal cannula	50	1	0.21-0.24
		2	0.24-0.28
		3	0.28-0.34
		4	0.34-0.38
		5	0.38-0.42
		6	0.42-0.46
Oxygen face mask	150-250	5-10	0.40-0.60
Mask reservoir bag:	750-1250		
Partial rebreather		5-7	0.35-0.75
Nonrebreather		5-10	0.40-1.0

[a]*Estimated value based on a tidal volume of 500 mL, a respiratory rate of 20 breaths per minute, and an inspiratory:expiratory time ratio of 1:2. From Vines DA, Shelledy DC, Peters J. Current respiratory care: oxygen therapy, oximetry, bronchial hygiene. J Crit Illness. 2000;15:507-515.*

Reference:
1. Marino PL. Oxygen therapy. In: *The ICU Book*. 4th ed. Philadelphia: Wolters Kluwer Health/Lippincott Williams & Wilkins; 2014:427–446.

22. Correct answer: A

Both partial rebreather and nonrebreather masks have a reservoir bag of 600-1000 mL attached to a standard face mask; this increases the face mask reservoir size from 150-250 to 750-1250 mL. When the reservoir bag is fully inflated, the patient's inspired tidal volume comes completely from the reservoir bag. A partial rebreather mask allows some exhaled gases to enter the reservoir bag (once expired flow decreases and the oxygen flow rate into the reservoir bag is greater than the patient's expired flow, the remaining expired gas is breathed out through the 1-way flaps on the face mask). As the portion of the expired gas going to the partial rebreather is from the start of exhalation, which contains upper airway gas (dead space), not much CO_2 is rebreathed. However, as the expired gas does not have an Fio_2 of 1.0, it is not possible to reach an Fio_2 of 1.0 with a partial rebreather mask (maximum is 70%-80%). A nonrebreather mask differs from a partial rebreather mask by a 1-way valve that does not allow expired gas to enter into the reservoir bag; thus all expired gas exits via 1-way flaps in the face mask. It is theoretically possible to achieve an Fio_2 of 1.0 with a nonrebreather mask (although an imperfect fit of the face mask portion may lead to some entrained room air). As both partial rebreather and nonrebreather masks require a tight-fitting seal on the face, patients cannot have aerosolized bronchodilator therapy or enteral or nasoenteral feeding in place, as the seal would be compromised.

Reference:
1. Marino PL. Oxygen therapy. In: *The ICU Book*. 4th ed. Philadelphia: Wolters Kluwer Health/Lippincott Williams & Wilkins; 2014:427–446.

23. Correct answer: B

Low-flow oxygen devices, such as nasal cannula and face mask, deliver a variable Fio_2, which is dependent on the minute ventilation of the patient and the oxygen flow rate (see explanation given for question 21). If a patient's minute ventilation increases, more air will be entrained and the delivered Fio_2 will decrease. In contrast, regulated air entrainment devices allow for control and delivery of a constant Fio_2 independent of changes in the patient's minute ventilation. While low-flow oxygen is delivered to the Venturi mask, the orifice port at the end of the oxygen inlet is narrowed, creating a high-velocity jet stream of gas at a flow rate exceeding 60 L/min. The size of the air entrainment port determines the proportion of room air pulled into the mask, thus determining the delivered Fio_2. An Fio_2 of 0.24 to 0.5 can be achieved depending on the entrainment port size. If the flow rate of oxygen delivered to the mask is increased, a proportionally greater volume of air is pulled into the mask, thus ensuring a constant delivered Fio_2.

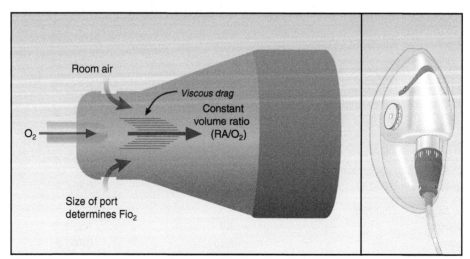

(From Marino PL. Oxygen therapy. In: *Marino's The ICU Book*. 4th ed. Philadelphia: Wolters Kluwer Health/Lippincott Williams & Wilkins; 2014:435, with permission.)

Reference:

1. Marino PL. Oxygen therapy. In: *The ICU Book*. 4th ed. Philadelphia: Wolters Kluwer Health/Lippincott Williams & Wilkins; 2014:427–446.

24. Correct answer: D

Traditional nasal prongs and face mask are not usually used beyond flow rates of ~10 L/min, as inhaling cold, dry oxygen leads to patient discomfort, drying of the upper airway, and potentially impaired mucociliary function. The inspired gas provided by HFNC is produced by a blending of air and oxygen to obtain the desired Fio_2. The resulting gas mixture then passes through a heated humidifier, which warms the gas to 37°C and saturates the gas with water. As its name suggests, HFNC is run at high flows, typically between 30 and 60 L/min. Because a patients' peak inspiratory flow and minute ventilation are unlikely to exceed this flow rate, even under respiratory distress, the Fio_2 provided by the HFNC will not vary with patient inspiratory effort (unlike traditional nasal cannulae and face mask oxygen; see explanation given for question 21). The high flow also creates PEEP in the airway. One study measured PEEP of 3 cm H_2O at a HFNC flow rate of 50 L/min with patients breathing with their mouths closed. Because the flow rate in the HFNC system is constant, a variable amount of pressure is generated in the airway, depending on the thoracic compliance and breathing effort. Interestingly, HFNC can also help with carbon dioxide clearance by washing out the gas in the airway dead space. The combined effects of improved thoracic compliance from PEEP and CO_2 flushing can result in decreased inspiratory effort and minute ventilation in patients with acute respiratory failure, making HFNC a potentially attractive alternative approach to traditional noninvasive ventilation.

References:

1. Hernandez G, Roca O, Colinas L. High-flow nasal cannula support therapy: new insights and improving performance. *Crit Care.* 2017;21:62.
2. Frat J, Coudroy R, Marjanovic N, Thille A. High-flow nasal oxygen therapy and noninvasive ventilation in the management of acute hypoxemic respiratory failure. *Ann Transl Med.* 2017;5(14):297.
3. Marino PL. Oxygen therapy. In: *The ICU Book*. 4th ed. Philadelphia: Wolters Kluwer Health/Lippincott Williams & Wilkins; 2014:427–446.

25. Correct answer: A

NO selectively dilates the pulmonary vasculature when administered by inhalation. Its action is rapid in onset, and effects are short-lived because of its short half-life (15-30 s). Inhaled NO is administered by mixing pressurized NO and oxygen and adjusting the amount of NO using bleeder valves. Because it is inhaled, it is selectively delivered only to ventilated regions of the pulmonary system. Thus, only ventilated regions are subject to the vasodilating effects of NO, and ventilation/perfusion mismatch is reduced.

NO is rapidly oxidized to the more stable metabolites nitrite dioxide (NO_2) and nitrite trioxide (NO_3). At high levels, NO_2 can have toxic effects on the lung resulting in pulmonary edema, alveolar hemorrhage, alterations in surfactant formation and function, and fibrin accumulation. NO binds to heme- and iron-containing intracellular proteins, resulting in oxidation of the heme iron with production of methemoglobin. The production of both NO_2 and methemoglobin are dependent on the dose and length of time of exposure to NO.

There are several different commercially available systems for delivery of NO to ICU ventilators and anesthesia workstation ventilators. Systems utilizing an inspiratory flow sensor to inject a proportional flow of NO into the ventilator circuit may help minimize NO_2 formation.

References:

1. Kirmse M, Hess D, Fujio Y, Kacmarek R, Hurford W. Delivery of inhaled nitric oxide using the Ohmeda INOvent Delivery System. *Chest.* 1998;113:1650-1657.
2. Steudel W, Hurford W, Zapol W. Inhaled nitric oxide. *Anesthesiology.* 1999;91:1090-1121.

26. Correct answer: C

This CVP wave demonstrates large, "cannon" a-waves. Cannon a-waves occur when the right atrium contracts against a closed tricuspid valve, thereby creating high pressure in the right atrium. This is commonly seen in complete heart block but may also occur with aberrant rhythms, where atrium depolarizes by retrograde conduction (eg, junctional rhythm and ventricular tachycardia), causing atrial contraction to occur during ventricular systole. Organized atrial contraction does not occur in atrial fibrillation, and thus no a-waves are generated.

Reference:

1. Connor CW. Commonly used monitoring techniques. In: Barash PG, Cullen BF, Stoelting RK, et al, eds. *Clinical Anesthesia*. 7th ed. Philadelphia: Lippincott Williams & Wilkins; 2013:699–722.

27. Correct answer: B

The wedge pressure (or pulmonary artery occlusion pressure) reflects changes in the left atrial pressure and is used as a means for estimating the LVEDP, a measure of left ventricular preload. During early diastole, the atrial pressure is higher than the ventricular pressure, which favors the flow of blood from atrium to ventricle. However, at the end of diastole (at the very end of ventricular filling), the atrial pressure equilibrates with the ventricular pressure. Measurement of the wedge pressure (left atrial pressure) at the end of diastole provides the best opportunity to capture ventricular filling pressure. The location on the left atrial pressure wave that best reflects end-diastolic pressure is the point just before the c-wave.

Reference:

1. Schroeder R, Barbeito A, Bar-Yosef S, et al. Cardiovascular monitoring. In: Miller RD, Eriksson LI, Fleisher LA, et al. *Miller's Anesthesia*. 8th ed. Philadelphia: W B Saunders Company; 2015:1345–1395.

28. Correct answer: B

The region of the CVP waveform depicted by the arrow is called c-wave. The c-wave reflects the period of isovolumetric contraction of the right ventricle. As the pressure builds in the right ventricle, the closed tricuspid valve begins to bulge into the atria, producing a small rise in the pressure represented as the c-wave on the CVP pressure tracing. The c-wave typically coincides with the QRS complex in the ECG. The physiological explanations for the typical positive and negative deflections that characterize the CVP waveform are summarized below:

a-wave	Atrial contraction
c-wave	Bulging of the atrioventricular valve from ventricular systole
v-wave	Filling of the atria during systole (atrioventricular valves closed)
x-descent	Atrial relaxation
y-descent	Early ventricular filling during ventricular diastole

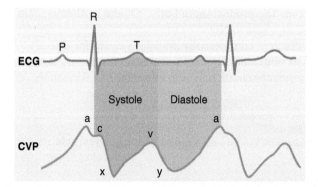

(Redrawn from Mark JB. Central venous pressure monitoring: clinical insights beyond the numbers. *J Cardiothorac Vasc Anesth*. 1991;5:163-173, with permission.)

References:

1. Connor CW. Commonly used monitoring techniques. In: Barash PG, Cullen BF, Stoelting RK, et al, eds. *Clinical Anesthesia.* 7th ed. Philadelphia: Lippincott Williams & Wilkins; 2013:699–722.
2. Schroeder R, Barbeito A, Bar-Yosef S, et al. Cardiovascular monitoring. In: Miller RD, Eriksson LI, Fleisher LA, et al. *Miller's Anesthesia.* 8th ed. Philadelphia: W B Saunders Company; 2015:1345–1395.

29. Correct answer: D

The atrial pressure contour seen in constrictive pericarditis is unique. The pericardium in constrictive pericarditis is nondistensible, thickened, and scarred, thereby impeding normal diastolic cardiac filling. This limits the maximum quantity of blood that the 4 chambers of the heart can collectively hold. Ejection of blood out of the heart during systole rapidly generates space within the pericardium, resulting in increased filling of atria during atrial relaxation and creating an exaggerated x-descent on the contour tracing. The y-descent in constrictive pericarditis results from the ventricle's ability to allow passive filling, with initial relief of atrial and venous pressures. Once filling begins, the ventricle is abruptly restrained by the rigid pericardium, resulting in a rapid filling wave followed by a plateau—referred to as "the square root sign"—which is typical of constrictive pericarditis.

Pericardial tamponade has a similar physiology but a different waveform, as represented in option C. In tamponade, the pericardial space is hydraulically distended under sufficient tension to raise filling pressures equally in all chambers and impair diastolic filling. As in constrictive pericarditis, ejection of blood from the ventricles momentarily relieves tamponade, allowing for a surge of blood into atria, causing an exaggerated x-descent. However, the venous input matches the ventricular output by the end of systole, and the intrapericardial space is once again full. When diastolic ventricular relaxation ensues, loss of blood from the atria does not relieve atrial pressure because the hydraulic action of the displaced pericardial fluid now impinges on the emptying atria. Hence, a high level of pressure is maintained in the atria during diastole, preventing the y-descent.

Reference:

1. Schroeder R, Barbeito A, Bar-Yosef S, et al. Cardiovascular monitoring. In: Miller RD, Eriksson LI, Fleisher LA, et al. *Miller's Anesthesia.* 8th ed. Philadelphia: W B Saunders Company; 2015:1345–1395.

30. Correct answer: C

The differential diagnosis for the acute development of hypotension after a recent myocardial infarction includes rupture of papillary muscle, leading to mitral regurgitation, ischemic perforation of interventricular septum causing a ventricular septal defect, ventricular free wall rupture, and cardiogenic shock. In this case, the presence of mitral regurgitation (likely from ruptured papillary muscles or chordae tendinae) results in entry of blood into the left atrium during ventricular systole, resulting in large v-waves. Other causes of large v-waves include hypervolemia, an atrial septal defect, and diastolic dysfunction (all of which are related to increased blood volume in the left atrium).

Reference:

1. Martin DE, Chambers CE. Monitoring the cardiac surgical patient. In: Hensley FA, Martin DE, Gravlee GP, eds. *A Practical Approach to Cardiac Anesthesia.* Philadelphia: Lippincott Williams & Wilkins; 2012:117–155.

31. Correct answer: B

Noninvasive blood pressure monitors use pulse wave oscillations generated by the arterial pulse at different inflation pressures to measure the blood pressure. During measurement of the noninvasive blood pressure, the cuff initially inflates to a predetermined high pressure. Then, the inflation pressure is decreased in a stepwise fashion, and the amplitude of pulse wave oscillations is recorded at each inflation pressure. MAP is the cuff pressure where the highest pulse amplitude is detected.

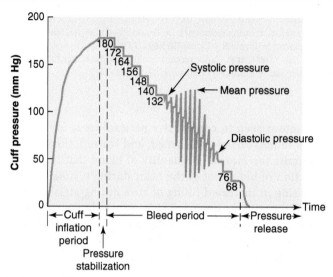

(Modified from Dorsch JA, Dorsch SE. *Understanding Anesthesia Equipment.* 4th ed. Baltimore: Williams & Wilkins; 1999, with permission.)

Reference:

1. Connor CW. Commonly used monitoring techniques. In: Barash PG, Cullen BF, Stoelting RK, et al, eds. *Clinical Anesthesia.* 7th ed. Philadelphia: Lippincott Williams & Wilkins; 2013:699–722.

32. Correct answer: B

The "square wave" or the dynamic response test is used to measure the damping of a pressure monitoring system. This is performed by squeezing the flush valve and exposing the transducer to 300 mm Hg pressure from the pressurized saline bag. This produces a waveform that rises sharply, plateaus, and drops off sharply when the flush valve is released again. An accurate, responsive, and adequately damped arterial line waveform will typically generate 1 or 2 oscillations that occur after the flush valve is released. In an overdamped tracing the arterial waveform is reached after a delay and without any oscillations and will result in an underestimation of the systolic blood pressure. In contrast an underdamped waveform will have multiple oscillations (typically 3 or more) before reaching baseline and will overestimate the systolic blood pressure.

References:

1. Martin DE, Chambers CE. Monitoring the cardiac surgical patient. In: Hensley FA, Martin DE, Gravlee GP, eds. *A Practical Approach to Cardiac Anesthesia.* Philadelphia: Lippincott Williams & Wilkins; 2012:117–155.
2. Connor CW. Commonly used monitoring techniques. In: Barash PG, Cullen BF, Stoelting RK, et al, eds. *Clinical Anesthesia.* 7th ed. Philadelphia: Lippincott Williams & Wilkins; 2013:699–722.

33. Correct answer: B

This waveform represents a right ventricular pressure waveform and not a pulmonary artery waveform. After insertion, a pulmonary artery catheter appears to have been pulled back into the right ventricle. Right ventricular pressure increases during diastole (as shown in the figure), whereas pulmonary artery pressure decreases during diastole, which can be used to distinguish between the 2 waveforms. The normal pulmonary artery waveform also has a dicrotic notch, whereas the right ventricular waveform does not. The arrow indicates the increase in right ventricular pressure, which occurs during diastole due to filling of the right ventricle (as pointed out by the arrow). Inflating the balloon may wedge the catheter, if it is in the pulmonary artery.

References:

1. Connor CW. Commonly used monitoring techniques. In: Barash PG, Cullen BF, Stoelting RK, et al, eds. *Clinical Anesthesia.* 7th ed. Philadelphia: Lippincott Williams & Wilkins; 2013:699–722.
2. Schroeder R, Barbeito A, Bar-Yosef S, et al. Cardiovascular monitoring. In: Miller RD, Eriksson LI, Fleisher LA, et al. *Miller's Anesthesia.* 8th ed. Philadelphia: W B Saunders Company; 2015:1345–1395.

34. Correct answer: C

LVEDP is estimated by measuring the pulmonary artery wedge pressure. The ability of the wedge pressure to accurately estimate LVEDP is dependent on the presence of an uninterrupted column of blood from the tip of the pulmonary artery catheter to the left ventricle. Factors that can influence the pressure along this column of blood (pulmonary capillaries, pulmonary vein, left atria, and mitral valve) may result in inaccurate estimation of LVEDP. Thus, abnormalities that alter left atrial pressure, such as mitral stenosis, or a large atrial septal defect will alter the estimation of LVEDP. Similarly, a left atrial myxoma can cause intermittent obstruction of the mitral inlet, resulting in an elevation of left atrial pressure. Severe mitral regurgitation can cause large v-waves in the wedge waveform, thereby impacting the pressure estimation. In contrast, tricuspid does not affect the pressure on the column of blood (from the tip of the catheter to the left ventricle) at end diastolic and thus will have no influence on the wedge pressure.

Based on variations in pulmonary blood flow resulting from pressure differences between pulmonary artery (Pa), alveolar (Palv), and pulmonary venous (Pv) pressures, lung regions have been categorized into 3 distinct zones—West Zone I (Palv > Pa > Pv), West Zone II (Pa > Palv > Pv), and West Zone III (Pa > Pv > Palv). Only Zone III permits an uninterrupted column of blood between the tip of the pulmonary artery catheter and the left ventricle. In Zone I or II, alveolar pressure changes will influence the wedge pressure because it is higher than the pulmonary venous pressure. Flow-directed placement of the pulmonary artery catheter usually favors the tip being positioned to the lung region with the highest blood flow (Zone III). However, increases in alveolar pressure (high PEEP), decreases in perfusion, or changes in the position of the patient can convert areas of Zone III into either Zone II or I, thus leading to a faulty estimation of LVEDP. Characteristics of a pulmonary artery catheter outside Zone III are wedge pressure greater than pulmonary artery diastolic pressure, nonphasic wedge waveform, and inability to aspirate blood from the distal port when the catheter is wedged.

Reference:
1. Connor CW. Commonly used monitoring techniques. In: Barash PG, Cullen BF, Stoelting RK, et al, eds. *Clinical Anesthesia*. 7th ed. Philadelphia: Lippincott Williams & Wilkins; 2013:699–722.

35. Correct answer: C

In the rhythm illustrated in the figure, atrial pacing is represented by a spike preceding the p-wave. This atrial pacing then results in the typical pattern of ventricular contraction via the atrioventricular node, resulting in a narrow QRS complex beat (and the absence of a ventricular pacemaker spike). Thus the ventricular activity is sensed by the pacemaker and not paced. The second half of the ECG shows an A paced rhythm followed by a V paced beat shown by the wide complex QRS and the pacing spike right before the QRS complex.

Reference:
1. Badescu GC, Sherman B, Zaidan JR, et al. Appendix 1: Atlas of electrocardiography. In: Barash PG, Cullen BF, Stoelting RK, et al, eds. *Clinical Anesthesia*. 7th ed. Philadelphia: Lippincott Williams & Wilkins; 2013:1701–1720.

36. Correct answer: A

The ECG strip demonstrates a multifocal atrial tachycardia (MAT). MAT is a form of supraventricular tachycardia where the atrial contraction occurs from the impulse generated by different clusters of cells outside the sinoatrial node. Thus, different morphologies of P waves are present in MAT. It is typically seen in older patients and is often associated with exacerbations of COPD or other lung diseases, and treatment of the underlying cause typically results in its resolution. There is no role for DC cardioversion in MAT. This rhythm is typically not representative of an ischemic etiology and further cardiac workup is not necessary. It is reasonable to proceed with surgery by achieving heart rate control with β-blockers.

Reference:
1. Badescu GC, Sherman B, Zaidan JR, et al. Appendix 1: Atlas of electrocardiography. In: Barash PG, Cullen BF, Stoelting RK, et al, eds. *Clinical Anesthesia*. 7th ed. Philadelphia: Lippincott Williams & Wilkins; 2013:1701–1720.

37. Correct answer: D

The figure below shows transthoracic short-axis views of the heart in the midpapillary level, showing cross sections of the right and left ventricles. This view is important for identifying the causes of undifferentiated shock, specifically cardiac tamponade, hemorrhage, pulmonary embolism, and left ventricular failure. In the short-axis view, the left ventricle is typically circular under normal conditions (Figure B). A hemodynamically significant pulmonary embolism results in acute dilation of the right ventricle. This causes bowing of the interventricular septum toward the left ventricle, resulting in a D-shaped left ventricle (Figure A). Smaller pulmonary embolisms may not result in right ventricular pressure overload; however, they are also less likely to cause hemodynamic compromise.

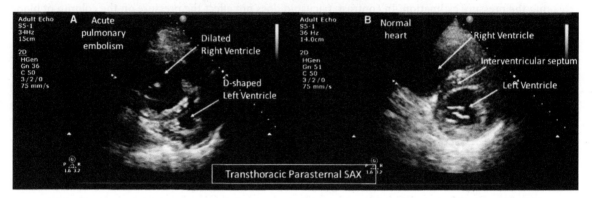

References:

1. Kaplan A. Echocardiographic diagnosis and monitoring of right ventricular function. In: Levitov AB, Mayo PH, Slonim AD, eds. *Critical Care Ultrasonography*. The McGraw-Hill Companies; 2014:125–134.

2. Desjardins G, Vezina DP, Johnson KB. Perioperative echocardiography. In: Miller RD, Eriksson LI, Fleisher LA, et al, eds. *Miller's Anesthesia*. 8th ed. Philadelphia: W B Saunders Company; 2015:1396–1428.

38. Correct answer: D

VOO mode or asynchronous ventricular pacing results in delivery of ventricular pacing impulses at a set rate, irrespective of the underlying rhythm. As shown in the figure, a paced beat is delivered on the preceding T wave, resulting in an R-on-T phenomenon and precipitating ventricular fibrillation. Changing the pacemaker mode from an asynchronous to a sensing mode (DDD, VVI, or AAI) would likely have prevented the event. Occasionally a pacemaker in a sensing mode fails to sense the intrinsic cardiac activity because of lead malfunction, called undersensing. Undersensing can also lead to R-on-T phenomenon when the presence of a ventricular contraction is not adequately sensed by the ventricular lead.

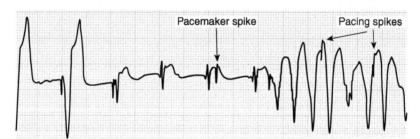

(Adapted from McLeod AA, Jokhi PP. Pacemaker induced ventricular fibrillation in coronary care units. *BMJ*. 2004;328(7450):1249-1250, with permission.)

Reference:

1. Badescu GC, Sherman B, Zaidan R, Barash PG. Appendix: Pacemaker and implantable cardiac defibrillator protocols. In: Barash PG, Cullen BF, Stoelting RK, et al, eds. *Clinical Anesthesia*. 7th ed. Philadelphia: Lippincott Williams & Wilkins; 2013:1721–1731.

39. **Correct answer: D**

SVR is a frequently used clinical index for estimating left ventricular afterload or the peripheral arterial tone. Calculation of SVR helps to differentiate between different types of shock. Hemorrhagic shock typically results in a high SVR because of vasoconstriction, whereas distributive shock will result in a low SVR. The SVR cannot be measured directly but rather is calculated using MAP, central venous pressure, and cardiac output:

$$SVR(dynes/cm^5)$$
$$= \frac{(\text{Mean arterial pressure in mm Hg} - \text{Central venous pressure in mm Hg}) \times 80}{\text{Cardiac output in L/min}}$$

where 80 is the conversion factor to the units dynes/cm^5. The normal range of SVR is 900-1200 dynes/cm^5.
    Because CVP is not provided in the question, SVR cannot be calculated.

Reference:
1. Hensley FA, Martin DE, Gravlee GP. Cardiovascular physiology. In: *A Practical Approach to Cardiac Anesthesia*. Philadelphia: Lippincott Williams & Wilkins; 2012:1-22.

40. **Correct answer: A**

Focused cardiac ultrasonography is a useful tool for identifying causes of undifferentiated shock. In a patient with new-onset hypotension, it can be used to diagnose cardiac tamponade, left ventricular failure, hemodynamically significant pulmonary embolism, and hypovolemia.

The ultrasound image is a transthoracic parasternal short-axis view of the heart at the midpapillary level, showing the left and right ventricles in cross section, labeled below.

The point-of-care echocardiographic image obtained for this patient shows a large pericardial effusion seen as echo-free (black) space outside the ventricle but within the pericardium. The echocardiographic features of cardiac tamponade include early-diastolic right ventricular collapse and late-diastolic right atrial collapse.

A small effusion that occurs after pacemaker lead explant can often be managed conservatively, whereas larger effusions may cause hemodynamic compromise and require pericardial drainage. Ongoing bleeding into pericardial cavity may even require repair of the right ventricular defect via sternotomy.

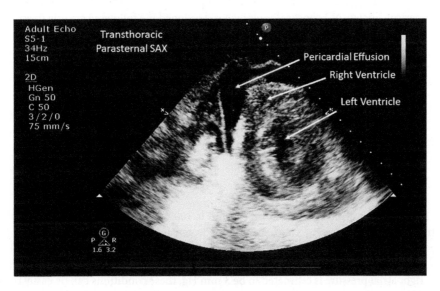

References:
1. Sweeny DA, McAreavy D. Echocardiographic diagnosis of cardiac tamponade. In: Levitov AB, Mayo PH, Slonim AD, eds. *Critical Care Ultrasonography*. The McGraw-Hill Companies; 2014:135–142.
2. Desjardins G, Vezina DP, Johnson KB. Perioperative echocardiography. In: Miller RD, Eriksson LI, Fleisher LA, et al. *Miller's Anesthesia*. 8th ed. Philadelphia: W B Saunders Company; 2015:1396–1428.

41. **Correct answer: B**

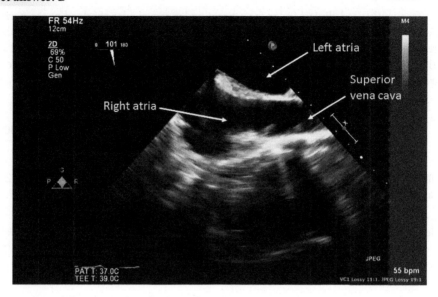

This image depicts a midesophageal bicaval view obtained using transesophageal echocardiography. This view is commonly used for venous air embolism monitoring and is obtained at a multiplane angle between 90° and 120°. The structures seen in a bicaval view are labeled in the figure. This view is also used for investigating the presence of atrial septal defect or patent foramen ovale.

Reference:

1. Perrino AC, Popescu WM, Skubas NJ. Echocardiography. In: Barash PG, Cullen BF, Stoelting RK, et al, eds. *Clinical Anesthesia.* 7th ed. Philadelphia: Lippincott Williams & Wilkins; 2013:723–762.

42. **Correct answer: D**

This ultrasound image is an M-mode image of the IVC subcostal view. This view is commonly used to assess volume status. M-mode is used to measure movement of structures in time. Here it allows measurement of the change in the IVC diameter with patient's respirations referred to as the collapsibility index. American Society of Echocardiography has developed the following criteria to estimate right atrial pressure (CVP) based on IVC diameter and collapsibility.

IVC DIAMETER (cm)	IVC COLLAPSIBILITY (%)	ESTIMATED RIGHT ATRIAL PRESSURE (mm Hg)
<2.1	>50	3
<2.1	<50	8
>2.1	>50	8
>2.1	<50	15

The IVC diameter of this patient is 1.6 cm and is 100% collapsible. Based on the table, the patient's right atrial pressure is 3 mm Hg. Cardiac tamponade, tension pneumothorax, and pulmonary embolism impede forward flow of blood through the heart and thereby cause obstructive shock. This typically results in markedly elevated right ventricular and consequently high right atrial pressures. Because the patient's right atrial pressure is estimated to be 3 mm Hg, these conditions can be easily ruled out. On the other hand, a low right atrial pressure is expected in a patient with hypovolemia.

References:

1. Desjardins G, Vezina DP, Johnson KB. Perioperative echocardiography. In: Miller RD, Eriksson LI, Fleisher LA, et al. *Miller's Anesthesia.* 8th ed. Philadelphia: W B Saunders Company; 2015:1396–1428.
2. Lang RM, Badano LP, Mor-Avi V, et al. Recommendations for cardiac chamber quantification by echocardiography in adults: an update from the American Society of Echocardiography and the European Association of Cardiovascular Imaging. *J Am Soc Echocardiogr.* 2015;28(1):1-39.

43. Correct answer: A

Dynamic parameters of fluid responsiveness are calculated based on measurement of variations in stroke volume resulting from respiratory (inspiration and expiration)-based changes in left ventricular preload. If stroke volume decreases significantly from the increase in intrathoracic pressure resulting from PPV, then administration of a fluid bolus will also likely increase stroke volume. Because stroke volume is difficult to measure, changes in pulse pressure obtained from an arterial line tracing are a commonly used surrogate.

Various studies have shown that variations in pulse pressure or stroke volume (called pulse pressure variation or stroke volume variation) of a magnitude greater than 15% are associated with positive response to fluid challenge (increased cardiac output). Conversely, when variations are less than 10%, no hemodynamic benefit to volume resuscitation is seen. However, most studies evaluating variations in pulse pressure (or stroke volume) and fluid responsiveness required the patient to be paralyzed and on PPV. A patient under general anesthesia with an endotracheal tube satisfies these conditions, thus making interpretation of pulse pressure variation useful.

Such dynamic indices of volume responsiveness have been found to be superior to static indices such as CVP in predicting the response to volume challenge. Predicting fluid responsiveness obviates the need for unnecessary volume challenge. Pulse pressure variation is calculated based on the equation:

$$\text{Pulse pressure variation}(\%) = \frac{\text{PP}_{max} - \text{PP}_{min}}{\left(\text{PP}_{max} + \text{PP}_{min}\right)/2} \times 100$$

This patient has a pulse pressure variation of 41%, based on the figure. This favors administration of more intravenous fluids to treat hypotension.

Reference:

1. Eisenkraft JB, Cohen E, Neustein SM. Anesthesia for thoracic surgery. In: Barash PG, Cullen BF, Stoelting RK, et al, eds. *Clinical Anesthesia*. 7th ed. Philadelphia: Lippincott Williams & Wilkins; 2013:1030–1076.

44. Correct answer: C

Although pulmonary artery catheter–based thermodilution remains the gold standard for determining cardiac output, it is invasive and is not without risks. On the other hand, arterial waveform–based cardiac output monitors are minimally invasive and can estimate cardiac output from an arterial pressure waveform. Three such devices are well established in the market: FloTrac (Edwards Lifesciences, Irvine, CA), PiCCO (PULSION Medical Systems AG, Munich, Germany), and LiDCO rapid (LiDCO Ltd, London, England).

Calculation of cardiac output by these monitors is based on certain basic assumptions. While calculating the cardiac output, a proprietary algorithm uses population-based assumptions for SVR and arterial compliance. Clinical scenarios where these values are vastly different from the expected population norms may lead to inaccurate estimation of cardiac output. This may occur in patients with sepsis or other high-output states such as cirrhosis. Reduction in vascular compliance from use of vasopressors may also cause similar inaccuracies.

All cardiac output monitors use arterial pressure contour data from over 20 preceding seconds to calculate cardiac output and assume that stroke volume remains relatively unchanged during this time. Presence of an irregular heart rhythm such as rapid atrial fibrillation violates this assumption because of the large beat-to-beat variability in stroke volume. Hence, noninvasive cardiac output measurements are not reliable in patients with atrial fibrillation. Arterial waveform analysis assumes no further flow in the arterial system at the end of systole. However, in aortic insufficiency part of ejected stroke volume flows back into the left ventricle, making stroke volume assessment inaccurate. However, arterial waveform–based cardiac output devices appear to be quite reliable at assessing changes in cardiac output caused by fluid resuscitation.

Reference:

1. Connor CW. Commonly used monitoring techniques. In: Barash PG, Cullen BF, Stoelting RK, et al, eds. *Clinical Anesthesia*. 7th ed. Philadelphia: Lippincott Williams & Wilkins; 2013:699–722.

45. **Correct answer: B**

Indicator dilution method is a method for cardiac output measurement where a known amount of tracer (dye) is injected into the blood stream (right atrium), and its concentration is measured over time at a downstream site (pulmonary artery). The change in concentration with time is related to the rate of flow. The flow in this case is the cardiac output (CO). The Stewart-Hamilton equation can be used to calculate the CO, which may be simplistically represented as follows:

$$CO \propto \frac{\text{Amount of injected indicator}}{\text{Area under the dilution curve}}$$

The thermodilution method is based on the indicator dilution principle. A known volume and temperature (usually, room temperature) of normal saline is injected into the right atrium. The temperature change produced by the colder injectate is measured by a thermistor at the tip of the pulmonary artery catheter. A lower CO results in slower equilibration of the injectate temperature to body temperature, whereas a higher CO will result in quicker equilibration and a smaller area under the curve.

Reference:

1. Schroeder R, Barbeito A, Bar-Yosef S, et al. Cardiovascular monitoring. In: Miller RD, Eriksson LI, Fleisher LA, et al. *Miller's Anesthesia*. 8th ed. Philadelphia: W B Saunders Company; 2015:1345–1395.

46. **Correct answer: B**

Processed EEG monitors were developed to quantitatively measure the depth of anesthesia. They use statistical signal processing techniques to calculate a weighted sum of several electroencephalographic subparameters, resulting in an easily interpretable number. This number, which is typically an integer between 0 and 100, correlates with the depth of anesthesia of the patient. The most commonly used processed EEG monitors are the BIS (Covidien) and SedLine (Masimo), and the operation of these devices is similar.

These monitors have been extensively studied for their ability to identify awareness under anesthesia. In patients receiving inhaled anesthetics for general anesthesia, BIS has not been demonstrated to be superior to end-tidal agent concentration monitoring in the prevention of awareness under anesthesia. However, it may be useful during total intravenous anesthesia where the real-time blood concentration of the agent is unknown. Here, it can provide real-time feedback on the pharmacodynamics effects of the administered agents when there is no end-tidal agent concentration to measure.

When hypnotic drugs such as propofol or halogenated anesthetics are used as the primary anesthetic agent, changes in BIS correlate with probability of movement to skin incision. However, when opioid analgesics are used at higher doses, the correlation becomes less significant. In its current stage of development, depth of anesthesia monitoring with processed EEG is not an essential component of monitoring during delivery of anesthesia and is not classified as a standard American Society of Anesthesiology monitor. However, the decision on using processed EEG for monitoring depth of anesthesia should be made on an individual patient basis.

Reference:

1. Connor CW. Commonly used monitoring techniques. In: Barash PG, Cullen BF, Stoelting RK, et al, eds. *Clinical Anesthesia*. 7th ed. Philadelphia: Lippincott Williams & Wilkins; 2013:699–722.

47. **Correct answer: C**

The EEG has a complex waveform that is typically far less organized and less regular than the electrocardiogram waveform. Most depth of anesthesia monitors process the EEG to generate an absolute number, thereby providing clinicians a simple and easily interpretable guide to depth of anesthesia. However, some monitors also provide unprocessed EEG waveforms, which are measured by the frontal electrodes. The numerical value generated by the processed EEG monitors can be influenced by factors other than the anesthetic depth such as the electrical activity of the muscles, whereas the unprocessed EEG waveforms may be more reliable. Its interpretation, however, is dependent on the anesthesiologist's ability to interpret unprocessed EEG.

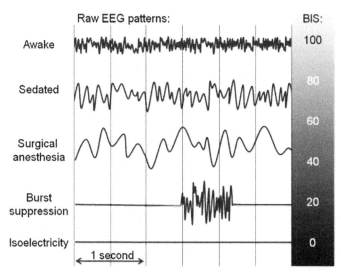

(Adapted from Kertai MD, Whitlock EL, Avidan MS. Brain monitoring with electroencephalography and the electroencephalogram-derived bispectral index during cardiac surgery. *Anesth Analg.* 2012;114(3):533-446, with permission.)

A typical EEG waveform is made up of several waves. The component waves contribute to the overall waveform seen, but different waves predominate during different states of wakefulness or sleep. The figure depicts the predominant type of waves seen with increasing depth of anesthesia. The high-frequency and low-amplitude waves (gamma [>30 Hz] and beta [12-30 Hz]) are more prominent during wakefulness. With sleep, sedation, and general anesthesia, slower frequency waves (alpha [8-12 Hz], theta [4-8 Hz], and delta [0-4 Hz]) become more prominent.

References:

1. Connor CW. Commonly used monitoring techniques. In: Barash PG, Cullen BF, Stoelting RK, et al, eds. *Clinical Anesthesia.* 7th ed. Philadelphia: Lippincott Williams & Wilkins; 2013:699–722.
2. Brown E, Solt K, Purdon PL, et al. Monitoring brain state during general anesthesia and sedation. In: Miller RD, Eriksson LI, Fleisher LA, et al, eds. *Miller's Anesthesia.* 8th ed. Philadelphia: W B Saunders Company; 2015:1524–1540.

48. Correct answer: B

TCD is a noninvasive monitor for evaluating relative changes in flow through the large basal arteries of the brain, which form the circle of Willis. TCD does not measure flow directly and therefore cannot provide information on the absolute cerebral blood flow. On the other hand, TCD measures flow velocity, which is directly proportional to flow as long as the diameter of the vessels remains constant. The flow velocity measured by TCD increases when either the flow increases or the diameter decreases.

An increase in CPP results in increased cerebral blood flow, thereby increasing TCD signals. On the other hand, increased intracranial pressure decreases CPP, thereby decreasing flow through the cranial blood vessels. TCD is commonly used to diagnose cerebral vasospasm, which may occur as a complication of subarachnoid hemorrhage. The reduced diameter of vessels in vasospasm results in a high flow velocity through the arteries. Although TCD measures velocity of blood flow in intracranial vessels, a stenotic lesion in the distal internal carotid artery can result in elevated flow velocity in the ipsilateral cerebral vessels.

Reference:

1. Dagal A, Lam AM. Anesthesia for neurosurgery. In: Barash PG, Cullen BF, Stoelting RK, et al, eds. *Clinical Anesthesia.* 7th ed. Philadelphia: Lippincott Williams & Wilkins; 2013:996–1029.

49. Correct answer: B

SSEP monitoring is used to monitor the intactness of the neural pathway from peripheral skin sensory receptors to cerebral sensory cortex. This is achieved by measuring EEG signals from sensory cortex, in response to cutaneous electrical stimulation. SSEP monitoring is used during surgical procedures, which may interrupt this pathway, allowing early identification and thereby permitting modification of the surgical technique. Decreases in SSEP amplitude by 50% and an increase in latency by 10% are considered clinically significant.

Anesthetic agents can have a significant influence on amplitude and latency of SSEP. Inhalation agents, including nitrous oxide, generally have more depressant effects on SSEP monitoring than intravenous agents. Opioids and benzodiazepines have negligible effects on recording of SSEP. Propofol and thiopental attenuate the amplitude of SSEPs but do not obliterate them. In contrast, ketamine and etomidate have been reported to enhance the quality of signals in patients with weak baseline SSEP signals; however, the clinical significance on interpretation of SSEPs is unclear.

Reference:

1. Dagal A, Lam AM. Anesthesia for neurosurgery. In: Barash PG, Cullen BF, Stoelting RK, et al, eds. *Clinical Anesthesia*. 7th ed. Philadelphia: Lippincott Williams & Wilkins; 2013:996–1029.

50. Correct answer: D

Although EEG is a cerebral function monitor that detects spontaneous activity, EP monitoring methods detect signals that occur as a result of a specific stimulus applied to the patient. Various EP modalities include somatosensory EP, brainstem auditory EP, visual EP, and motor EP. The proposed benefit is early identification of deterioration in neuronal function, thereby providing an opportunity to institute corrective measures or remove the offending factor before their effects become permanent.

Each modality tests a certain neural pathway. Somatosensory EP detects cortical EEG in response to cutaneous sensory (electrical) stimulus. In brainstem auditory EP, a clicking sound is applied to stimulate the eighth cranial nerve, which is useful in acoustic neuroma surgical procedures. Visual EP measures stimulation of the retina by light, made possible by wearing light-emitting goggles. In contrast to measurement of ascending sensory pathways by other EPs, motor EP evaluates the descending motor pathways. It measures the motor response (using electromyography) to a transcranial stimulus applied to the motor cortex.

Cortical EP with long latency involving multiple synapses is exquisitely sensitive to anesthetic agents, whereas the short-latency brainstem and spinal components are resistant. Thus, brainstem auditory EP can be recorded under any anesthetic technique, whereas visual and somatosensory EPs are extremely sensitive. Motor EP is markedly sensitive to the depressant effects of inhalation anesthetics, including nitrous oxide, and is best measured during total intravenous anesthesia.

Reference:

1. Dagal A, Lam AM. Anesthesia for neurosurgery. In: Barash PG, Cullen BF, Stoelting RK, et al, eds. *Clinical Anesthesia*. 7th ed. Philadelphia: Lippincott Williams & Wilkins; 2013:996–1029.

13

PAIN

Alexandra Raisa Adler

1. A 67-year-old man is scheduled for a Whipple procedure and is offered an epidural for postoperative pain control. Which of the following is an absolute contraindication to placement of an epidural?

   A. Aortic stenosis with a valve area of 1.2 cm²
   B. Recent upper respiratory tract infection
   C. Patient refusal
   D. Scoliosis

2. You are called to the postanesthesia care unit because a patient with an epidural placed at T12-L1 is complaining of pain at the site of his lower abdominal incision but cannot move his legs. He was initially very comfortable. His motor examination has not changed since arrival in the postanesthesia care unit. Which of the following local anesthetics is most likely to have been used?

   A. Etidocaine 1.5%
   B. Lidocaine 2%
   C. Bupivacaine 0.5%
   D. Chloroprocaine 3%

3. A 67-year-old woman is on the first postoperative day following a Whipple procedure. She has a thoracic epidural in place and is receiving a mix of bupivacaine and dilaudid. She reports good pain relief but states that she is incredibly itchy, especially in her face and on her nose. Which of the following is LEAST likely to relieve her itching?

   A. Naloxone
   B. Propofol
   C. Diphenhydramine
   D. Elimination of opioids from epidural mix

4. A 100-kg, 71-year-old man with a history of asthma, snoring, and emphysema undergoes thoracotomy and wedge resection for removal of a lung tumor. Which of the following treatments would be most effective to control his pain postoperatively while also maintaining adequate ventilation?

   A. Thoracic epidural with a continuous infusion of bupivacaine and hydromorphone
   B. As-needed doses of hydromorphone administered by the nurse
   C. Patient-controlled analgesia (PCA) with hydromorphone
   D. Lumbar epidural with a continuous infusion of bupivacaine and hydromorphone

5. A 67-year-old woman who is 9 hours status post gastrectomy is noted to have a respiratory rate of 6 and is also somewhat somnolent. Which of the following neuraxial medications or combinations of medications would be predicted to cause respiratory depression within 6-12 hours of exposure?

   A. Morphine
   B. Fentanyl
   C. Bupivacaine
   D. Bupivacaine plus sufentanil

6. Compared with a single epidural dose of morphine, a single epidural dose of fentanyl has a longer half-time in the epidural space secondary to which of the following properties?

   A. Lipid solubility
   B. Ionization state
   C. Molecular size
   D. Molecular weight

7. A 42-year-old woman undergoes total colectomy under general anesthesia with a thoracic epidural (T10-T11) in place. At the conclusion of the procedure, she receives an infusion of bupivacaine 0.1% and hydromorphone 20 µg/mL at 6 mL/h through her epidural catheter. You are called to see her 8 hours postoperatively and find that she is complaining of pain at the site of her incision. Her heart rate is 100 beats per minute and her blood pressure is 160/92 mm Hg. What is the most appropriate next step to manage this patient's pain?

   A. Administer a bolus of 5 cc of 1.5% lidocaine with epinephrine 1:200 000 through her epidural catheter.
   B. Add PCA with hydromorphone to her current regimen.
   C. Add Toradol to her current regimen.
   D. Check a serum bupivacaine level.

8. You are caring for a 77-year-old man with no significant medical history who underwent an L5-S1 fusion yesterday for spinal stenosis. He was taking oxycodone at home for his chronic back pain, and you decide to write him for a PCA. Which of the following medications should be avoided?

   A. Hydromorphone
   B. Morphine
   C. Meperidine
   D. Fentanyl

9. Which of the following settings is *not* recommended for a PCA pump using hydromorphone for an opioid-naive patient in the postoperative period?

   A. Continuous background infusion
   B. Initial lockout interval of 10 minutes
   C. Initial hourly dose limit of 1-2 mg
   D. Addition of opioid-sparing medications to the analgesic regimen

10. A 65-year-old woman with Parkinson disease and esophageal cancer is receiving an intravenous PCA with hydromorphone after undergoing Ivor Lewis esophagectomy. She reports excellent pain control but is experiencing nausea. Which of the following antiemetics is the most appropriate selection for this patient?

   A. Ondansetron
   B. Haldol
   C. Promethazine
   D. Droperidol

11. **Which of the following best describes the mechanism of acetaminophen?**

    A. Central inhibition of cyclooxygenase (COX) activation
    B. Inhibition of lipoxygenase activation
    C. Activation of lipoxygenase central a2 receptors
    D. Activation of GABA receptors

12. **You are consulted on a patient with a history of chronic back pain who is now on the first postoperative day from a L4-L5 fusion surgery. He tells you that he has a "high tolerance" to opioids and his pain is currently 8/10 when he moves, so you decide to start him on a multimodal regimen for pain control. His medical history is significant for chronic kidney disease and depression. He is currently taking ciprofloxacin per his surgical team. Which of the following medications should *not* be included as part of a multimodal regimen?**

    A. Ketamine
    B. Hydromorphone
    C. Tizanidine
    D. Tylenol

13. **Which of the following agents or drugs is most likely to have a similar mechanism of action to ketamine?**

    A. Sevoflurane
    B. Nitrous oxide
    C. Midazolam
    D. Clonidine

14. **A 60-year-old man with bilateral radicular pain in his legs presents 4 weeks after implantation of a spinal cord stimulator (SCS) with dual percutaneous leads. He had reported greater than 50% pain relief with his SCS trial and also reports feeling well after implantation of his SCS. He has therefore greatly increased his daily activity. He now complains of paresthesias in his lower abdominal region and worsening pain in his legs. His neurologic exam is unremarkable. There is no pain on palpation of his lower back. His incision site is clean, dry, and intact and he is afebrile. Which of the following most likely explains this presentation?**

    A. Epidural abscess
    B. Migration of leads
    C. Disc herniation
    D. Infection of the SCS leads

15. **Which of the following areas is targeted by SCSs?**

    A. Dorsal columns
    B. Lateral corticospinal tract
    C. Botzinger complex
    D. Peripheral nerves

16. **A patient with a history of unresectable pancreatic cancer presents to your office because his current pain control regimen, Tylenol and hydromorphone (2-4 mg every 4 h as needed), is no longer sufficient. He reports that when he began this regimen 6 months ago, his pain was under good control and he could remain active. However, now he reports worsening back pain that limits his ability to walk. He asks whether it would be reasonable to increase his dose of hydromorphone at this time. Which of the following phenomena best describes this situation?**

    A. Opioid-induced hyperalgesia (OIH)
    B. Pseudotolerance
    C. Drug-seeking behavior
    D. Addiction

17. A patient with a history of prostate cancer with metastases to his spine causing back pain presents to your office. You have been managing his opioid prescriptions for over a year, and during that time he has required increasing doses of hydromorphone to treat his back pain. He currently takes 8-10 mg of dilaudid every 3 hours. When questioned about his pain, he describes a diffuse pain that affects his arms and legs. His back pain is also present. Which of the following receptors or family of receptors is thought to be involved in this phenomenon?

   A. GABA-A
   B. NMDA
   C. GABA-B
   D. Dopamine-2

18. In the perioperative period, patients maintained on Suboxone will most likely experience which of the following?

   A. Increased postoperative opioid requirements
   B. Increased sensitivity to opioids
   C. Withdrawal symptoms within 24 hours of discontinuing Suboxone
   D. Increased risk of postoperative delirium

19. Which of the following effects would be likely to occur after parenteral injection of Suboxone in a patient actively taking heroin?

   A. Respiratory depression
   B. Withdrawal
   C. Euphoria
   D. Miosis

20. A 76-year-old man with pancreatic cancer and chronic abdominal pain admits to his pain specialist that he has been giving his son, who has chronic back pain, some of his oxycodone pills. Which of the following terms best characterizes this situation?

   A. Abuse
   B. Misuse
   C. Pseudoaddiction
   D. Addiction

21. A patient with metastatic prostate cancer complains of back pain. He is found to have metastases to his vertebral bodies. He has no neurologic deficits. Which of the following is the first-line definitive treatment for this pain?

   A. Physical therapy
   B. Glucocorticoids
   C. Radiation therapy
   D. Surgical decompression

22. Which of the following would you expect to see in a patient receiving continuous thoracic epidural analgesia as compared with one receiving PCA with morphine after undergoing open nephrectomy?

   A. Faster return of bowel function
   B. Comparable requirements for antiemetic medications
   C. Inferior pain control at the surgical site
   D. Similar patient satisfaction

23. An immunocompromised patient undergoing treatment for lymphoma presents to the emergency department with altered mental status. He has recently tested positive for coccidiomycosis, and there is a concern that he has a disseminated infection. He undergoes a lumbar puncture, which is negative. His mental status clears later that night, but 2 days later he returns to the emergency department with a positional headache, consistent with a postdural puncture headache (PDPH). Every time he sits up, he reports severe pain and nausea. He fails treatment with rest, intravenous fluids, and medications. Which of the following epidural injections is most appropriate?

    A. Normal saline
    B. Autologous blood
    C. Allogeneic blood
    D. Autologous blood with fibrin glue

24. A patient with unresectable pancreatic cancer presents for a celiac plexus block. Which of the following organs or structures does not receive innervation from the celiac plexus?

    A. Biliary tract
    B. Mesentery
    C. Descending colon
    D. Adrenal glands

25. A patient with unresectable pancreatic cancer presents for celiac plexus neurolysis via a posterior approach. He asks what the risks of the procedure are. Which of the following is the most common complications?

    A. Constipation
    B. Lower-extremity paralysis
    C. Anterior abdominal pain
    D. Orthostatic hypotension

26. When used for neurolytic blocks, compared with ethanol, which of the following is true about phenol?

    A. Painless on injection
    B. More effective
    C. Provides a longer duration of block
    D. More likely to cause hypotension

27. According to the World Health Organization (WHO) pain ladder, what is the next treatment step for a patient who has inadequate pain control for back pain secondary to metastatic prostate cancer after trying Tylenol, ibuprofen, aspirin as well as multiple nonnarcotic adjuvant pain medications such as gabapentin, tizanidine, and lidocaine patches?

    A. Paracetamol
    B. Fentanyl patch
    C. Tramadol
    D. Morphine

28. Which of the following statements is most consistent with the WHO pain ladder?

    A. The oral form of analgesics should be used over other forms whenever possible.
    B. Analgesics should be given only as needed.
    C. Standardized dosing of opioids should be used for adult patients.
    D. Treatment of cancer pain should begin with an opioid medication.

29. **All of the following are part of the diagnostic criteria for fibromyalgia EXCEPT which one?**

A. Allodynia to digital pressure at 11 or more of 18 anatomically defined tender points
B. A history of widespread pain for at least 3 months
C. A history of sleep disturbance
D. A history of radicular pain in both arms and legs

30. **Which of the following medications has been shown to be efficacious in the treatment of fibromyalgia?**

A. Duloxetine
B. Amitriptyline
C. Pregabalin
D. Hydrocodone

31. **Which of the following scenarios is suggestive of complex regional pain syndrome (CRPS) type II?**

A. A patient burns his right foot and develops pain, hyperalgesia, and allodynia in his right lower leg that continues more than 6 months after his burn. His right foot is noted to be shiny and without hair.
B. A patient's right forearm is crushed by a falling object. She reports pain, hyperalgesia, and allodynia of the forearm more than a year later. Her forearm is noted to be shiny and without hair.
C. A patient's left forearm is crushed by a falling object. She reports pain, hyperalgesia, and allodynia of the forearm more than a year later. Atrophy of the muscles of the forearm is noted.
D. After surgery, a patient develops numbness over his right lateral thigh. He reports pain, hyperalgesia, and allodynia of the lateral thigh more than a year later. The area is noted to be shiny and without hair.

32. **What is the greatest risk factor for the development of postherpetic neuralgia (PHN)?**

A. Increasing age
B. Male sex
C. Lack of a prodrome
D. Use of antiviral agents during acute herpes zoster infection

33. **All of the following are risk factors for the development of phantom limb pain EXCEPT which one?**

A. Preamputation pain
B. Depression
C. Distal amputation
D. Proximal amputation

34. **Which of the following is most characteristic with facetogenic back pain?**

A. Pain in the low back that radiates to the ipsilateral posterior thigh
B. Nonradiating pain in the low back
C. Pain in the ipsilateral buttocks
D. Numbness over the lower back

35. **A patient with a history of pain in the lower back that radiates to his ipsilateral thigh presents to a pain clinic for a facet joint injection. Which nerve fibers innervate the facet joints?**

A. Medial branch of the dorsal ramus of spinal nerve
B. Lateral branch of the dorsal ramus of spinal nerve
C. Lateral branch of the posterior cutaneous branch of the dorsal ramus
D. Medial branch of the posterior cutaneous branch of the dorsal ramus

36. **Which of the following would you expect to find in a patient who presents with pain originating from the sacroiliac joint?**

    A. Back pain that radiates to the ipsilateral buttocks
    B. Back pain accompanied by pain extending down the ipsilateral leg when the ipsilateral leg is passively raised straight in the air up to 60°
    C. Numbness of the anterolateral thigh
    D. Back pain accompanied by a leg length discrepancy

37. **A patient presents with pain in the left buttock. He reports that he frequently carries his wallet in the left pocket and that his wallet is quite large. Furthermore, he sits on the wallet throughout most of the day at a desk job. You suspect piriformis syndrome and plan to inject a combination of local anesthetic and steroid. Which anatomic relationship between the piriformis muscle and the sciatic nerve is most common?**

    A. The undivided sciatic nerve passes below the piriformis muscle.
    B. The divided sciatic nerve passes through and below the piriformis muscle.
    C. The divided sciatic nerve passes through and above the piriformis muscle.
    D. The undivided nerve passes through the piriformis muscle.

38. **A 56-year-old man with a history of hypertension, chronic obstructive pulmonary disease, and diabetes presents for a lumbar epidural steroid injection (ESI) for lower-back pain that radiates into his right leg. He receives an injection of methylprednisone and lidocaine. Which of the following is most likely to occur after he receives this injection?**

    A. Arachnoiditis
    B. Headache
    C. Infection
    D. Hyperglycemia

39. **Which of the following statements about new, acute onset low-back pain is most accurate?**

    A. Bed rest is recommended for up to 1 week.
    B. In the absence of "red flag" symptoms, imaging is not indicated in the acute setting.
    C. Opioids are the first-line therapy for this type of pain.
    D. A short course of oral steroids may be helpful in treating this pain.

40. **A patient presents to you with pain on the left side of her face. She states that the pain began a month ago and that chewing food is excruciating. She also notes the sensation of "shooting" pain on the left side of her face. Which of the following statements about this condition is most likely true?**

    A. Pain on the left side of the face is more common than the right side.
    B. Involvement of the V1 distribution is uncommon.
    C. Autonomic symptoms such as tearing or nasal discharge are common.
    D. The most common first-line drug is oxycodone.

41. **A 38-year-old man with a history of HIV well managed on antiretroviral agents presents with painful neuropathy in both feet. He describes the pain as burning and constant. It gets worse when he does his job as a postal carrier. Initially he responded to tramadol but no longer finds it helpful. Which of the following is the next most appropriate step to manage this patient's foot pain?**

    A. Further evaluate the patient's antiviral regimen.
    B. Initiate antiepileptic therapy.
    C. Perform an ESI.
    D. Initiate oxycontin.

42. **In a patient taking methadone, which of the following is most likely to contribute to development of torsades de pointes?**

   A. Methadone dose of 10 mg a day
   B. HIV
   C. Male sex
   D. Obesity

43. **A lumbar sympathetic block is appropriate for diagnosis and/or treatment of all the following conditions EXCEPT which one?**

   A. CRPS type I of the right calf
   B. Phantom limb pain of the left lower extremity
   C. PHN of the right thigh
   D. Coccydynia

44. **Which of the following is the most likely cause of a "failed" spinal?**

   A. Resistance to local anesthetics
   B. Displacement of the tip of a pencil-point needle
   C. Dural ectasia
   D. Use of lidocaine instead of bupivacaine

45. **An otherwise healthy 42-year-old patient who has received a spinal anesthetic for outpatient total knee arthroplasty reports severe pain in his legs and buttocks. The pain began a few hours after surgery and has persisted on the first postoperative day. Which medication was most likely used for the spinal anesthetic?**

   A. Bupivacaine
   B. Lidocaine
   C. Bupivacaine and fentanyl
   D. 2-Chloroprocaine

46. **Six months after undergoing a right inguinal hernia repair, a 27-year-old man presents to your office with continuing pain in the groin. He describes the pain as a constant burning sensation that is also occasionally sharp. He has seen his surgeon and does not have a recurrence of his hernia. Which of the following nerve blocks might be helpful in diagnosing this condition?**

   A. Genitofemoral nerve block
   B. Pudendal nerve block
   C. Transversus abdominus plane (TAP) block
   D. Lateral femoral cutaneous nerve (LFCN) block

47. **The pudendal nerve can become entrapped at all the following locations EXCEPT which one?**

   A. Inside the Alcock canal
   B. Between the sacrospinous and sacrotuberous ligaments
   C. Across the inner margin of the falciform process of the sacrotuberous ligament
   D. Inside the deep inguinal ring

48. **Which of the following nerve blocks is associated with a nearly 100% chance of ipsilateral diaphragmatic palsy?**

   A. Superficial cervical plexus block
   B. Infraclavicular block
   C. Greater auricular nerve block
   D. Axillary nerve block

49. **Which one of the following is the benefit of transcutaneous electrical stimulation (TENS)?**

    A. It can be applied by the patient at home.
    B. It has shown to be effective for chronic pain management.
    C. It is cost-effective.
    D. It improves the level of disability due to back pain.

50. **A 56-year-old type 1 diabetic man comes to your office to complaining of bilateral "stocking distribution" neuropathy. When questioned about his glucose control, the patient states that he normally maintains tight glucose control and he follows a strict low-carbohydrate diet. Which of the following is not a risk factor for development of peripheral neuropathy?**

    A. Poorly controlled blood glucose
    B. Duration of diabetes
    C. Gender
    D. Patient age

Chapter 13 ▪ Answers

1. Correct answer: C

There are few absolute contraindications to placement of an epidural. However, one of the most important is patient refusal. Although it may be appropriate to further explore the reasons for refusal and/or to educate the patient, it is ultimately the patient's choice. Other absolute contraindications include coagulopathy and bacteremia or infection near/at needle insertion site. The presence of spine pathology such as scoliosis is only a relative contraindication—placement may be more technically complicated or the treatment may fail if the anatomy is distorted and there is not even distribution of medication in the epidural space. A recent upper respiratory tract infection would not represent a contraindication, although a current infection in a febrile patient would give the clinician pause when considering an epidural. Finally, patients with aortic stenosis require afterload to continue to perfuse their heart. An epidural can be inserted but must be dosed carefully and slowly with careful hemodynamic monitoring.

References:
1. Vincent RD, Chestnut DH. Epidural analgesia during labor. *Am Fam Physician*. 1998;58(8):1785-1792.
2. Slevin KA, Ballantyne JC. Management of acute postoperative pain. In: Longnecker DE, Brown DL, Newman MF, Zapol WM, eds. *Anesthesiology*. 2nd ed. New York: McGraw Hill; 2012:1297-1314.

2. Correct answer: A

This question essentially asks which of the given local anesthetics would be expected to cause a prolonged motor blockade despite regression of a sensory blockade. Of the local anesthetics listed, etidocaine produces the most intense motor blockade, which may considerably outlast its sensory blockade. In a study, the duration between injection and total regression of motor blockade was just more than 600 minutes for etidocaine, whereas it was just more than 360 minutes for bupivacaine.

Of the local anesthetics considered in this question, the length of sensory block is shortest for chloroprocaine (100-160 min), moderate for lidocaine (160-200 min), and similar for bupivacaine and etidocaine (300-460 min). Balancing sensory blockade (which is helpful for postoperative pain control) and motor blockade (which is distressing to the patient and prevents movement postoperatively) is a goal when considering a choice of epidural local anesthetic.

Although the profound motor blockade may assist the surgeon intraoperatively by causing muscle relaxation, many anesthesiologists no longer use etidocaine because of the prolonged motor block in the absence of a sensory block. A prolonged motor block provides no benefit to the patient, especially in the absence of good pain control. Bupivacaine, on the other hand, at low concentrations (0.5%-0.75%) produces a sensory blockade that is relatively more intense than the motor blockade.

Although this question asks for specifics regarding the relative length and extent of motor versus sensory blockade for epidural local anesthetics, it is always important to consider a wide differential diagnosis when a patient develops a neurologic deficit after neuraxial anesthesia. For example, severe pain (most likely in the back, not at the site of a surgical incision) and paralysis raise the concern for epidural hematoma, which requires emergent management.

References:
1. Bernards CM, Hostetter LS. Epidural and spinal anesthesia. In: Barash PG, Cullen BF, Stoelting RK, et al, eds. *Clinical Anesthesia*. 7th ed. Philadelphia: Lippincott; 2013:905-936.
2. Axelsson K, Nydahl PA, Philipson L, et al. Motor and sensory blockade after epidural injection of mepivacaine, bupivacaine, and etidocaine—a double-blind study. *Anesth Analg*. 1989;69:739.

3. Correct answer: C

A well-known side effect of opioids, regardless of route of administration, is pruritus or itching. Pruritus that occurs following neuraxial opioid administration frequently affects the upper face and nose, although the whole body can be affected. This distribution may occur because the spinal nucleus of the trigeminal nerve is rich in opioid receptors. Pruritus associated with neuraxial opioids is not uncommon—the incidence has been stated to be 69% in patients (both women and men). There are several methods to address pruritus associated with neuraxial opioids. One option is to simply discontinue the opioid and use only a local anesthetic for pain control. Given that the mu (μ) receptor is responsible for some opioid-induced side effects, such as pruritus and nausea, it is not surprising that a μ receptor antagonist, such as naloxone, could help prevent or reduce pruritus.

The literature suggests that a continuous, low-dose infusion of naloxone can be used to prevent opioid-induced pruritus in adults. The recommendation is to use doses under 2 μg/kg/h to avoid potential reversal of analgesia. Propofol, given as small boluses, has been used for the treatment and prevention of pruritus. It is believed to work by inhibition of posterior horn transmission in the spinal cord. H1 blockers such as diphenhydramine or hydroxyzine do not have an effect on centrally induced pruritus. They may cause sedation, which could help provide a patient with pruritus a chance to rest, but they will not affect the severity of the pruritus itself.

References:
1. Kumar K, Singh SI. Neuraxial opioid-induced pruritus: an update. *J Anaesthesiol Clin Pharmacol*. 2013;29(3):303-307.
2. Macres SM, Moore PG, Fishman SM. Acute pain management. In: Barash PG, Cullen BF, Stoelting RK, et al, eds. *Clinical Anesthesia*. 7th ed. Philadelphia: Lippincott; 2013:1611-1644.

4. Correct answer: A

A patient with underlying lung disease who has undergone thoracotomy is at high risk of postoperative pulmonary complications. Therefore, maximizing pain control (which will improve ventilation) while avoiding suppression of respiratory drive is paramount. Patients with obesity, sleep apnea (which this patient might have given his history of snoring), and neuromuscular disorders and elderly patients are at higher risk for opioid-related respiratory depression. Patients who have pain that impacts their breathing (ie, a chest incision) are also at further risk for hypoventilation. Although episodes of hypoxemia may be recognized using continuous pulse oximetry, hypoventilation is harder to monitor unless the patient has an arterial line and is undergoing frequent arterial blood gas checks.

Opioids, however, need not be totally avoided in patients similar to the one mentioned in this question. The goal is to minimize their use while maximizing pain relief. Of the options listed, the best way to do this is using neuraxial opioids plus a local anesthetic. A continuous infusion in an epidural will provide superior pain relief compared with as-needed doses given by a nurse (which may only be given every 3-4 h). Although PCA does give patients more control, they can fall behind on pain control when they are asleep. The dose of opioid received via the epidural will almost always be smaller than what would be given intravenously. For example, with a PCA device, a patient might receive a maximum of 0.5 mg of hydromorphone an hour. With a standard epidural mix of bupivacaine and 10-20 μg/mL of hydromorphone run at a rate of 6 mL/h, they will only receive 0.06-0.12 mg of hydromorphone per hour. A lumbar epidural with the same infusion might be appropriate for a lower abdominal surgery but will not cover a thoracotomy incision and therefore would not be helpful to this patient.

References:
1. Macres SM, Moore PG, Fishman SM. Acute pain management. In: Barash PG, Cullen BF, Stoelting RK, et al, eds. *Clinical Anesthesia*. 7th ed. Philadelphia: Lippincott; 2013:1611-1644.
2. Practice Guidelines for the Prevention, Detection, and Management of Respiratory Depression Associated with Neuraxial Opioid Administration: An Updated Report by the American Society of Anesthesiologists Task Force on Neuraxial Opioids and the American Society of Regional Anesthesia and Pain Medicine. *Anesthesiology*. 2016;124(3):535-552.

5. Correct answer: A

Opioids via any route place a patient at risk for respiratory depression. However, the most important factor to consider with neuraxial opioids and respiratory depression is the lipid solubility of the drug. Of the opioids listed, fentanyl and sufentanil are both lipophilic. When these lipid-solid opioids are administered, they enter the cerebrospinal fluid (CSF) and would be expected to cause respiratory depression in around 2 hours. By the same token, once they enter the CSF, they are quickly absorbed by lipophilic body tissues and thus eliminated. Thus, not only will respiratory depression occur quickly, but the time it will last is also short. Morphine is hydrophilic compared with these opioids. The onset of respiratory depression may not occur until 6-12 hours after injection. Once morphine does enter the CSF, it tends to stay and affect the respiratory centers for hours.

References:
1. Wong CA. Epidural and spinal analgesia/anesthesia for labor and vaginal delivery. In: Chestnut DH, Polley LS, Tsen LC, et al, eds. *Chestnut's Obstetric Anesthesia Principles and Practice*. 4th ed. Philadelphia: Elsevier; 2009:429-492.
2. Chaney MA. Side effects of intrathecal and epidural opioids. *Can J Anaesth*. 1995;42:891-903.

6. Correct answer: A

The behavior of fentanyl and that of morphine in the epidural space differ in some aspects because of the relative lipid solubilities of these drugs. Morphine is hydrophilic, whereas fentanyl is fairly lipophilic. There is a linear relationship between the lipophilicity of an opioid and its terminal elimination half-time in the epidural space. Compared with hydrophilic opioids such as morphine, more lipophilic opioids (ie, fentanyl) will spend more time in the epidural space. There will also be less net transfer to the intrathecal space for lipophilic opioids. The degree of ionization and the molecular size/weight do not appear to have as profound an effect.

References:
1. Bernards CM, Hostetter LS. Epidural and spinal anesthesia. In: Barash PG, Cullen BF, Stoelting RK, et al, eds. *Clinical Anesthesia.* 7th ed. Philadelphia: Lippincott; 2013:905-936.
2. Bernards CM, Shen DD, Sterling ES, et al. Epidural, cerebrospinal fluid, and plasma pharmacokinetics of epidural opioids (part 1): differences among opioids. *Anesthesiology.* 2003;99:455.

7. Correct answer: A

When you are called to see a patient who is experiencing pain and has an epidural in place, the first consideration is whether or not the epidural is working. Administering lidocaine and then checking for a level 10-15 minutes later is a good way to assess this. Keep in mind that the patient should be monitored during and after this bolus and a pressor, such as phenylephrine, should be available in case of hypotension. Although Toradol could be helpful, a working epidural will provide her with the best pain control, so the most appropriate first step would be to determine whether or not the epidural is working. A hydromorphone PCA might improve pain control, but it is generally better not to administer both neuraxial and peripheral opioids, given the risks of sedation and respiratory depression.

There is little role for checking a bupivacaine level in this case. The bupivacaine level does not necessarily correlate to accurate pain relief. Even if the epidural had become dislodged and was in the subcutaneous tissue, it is possible to have a nonzero serum bupivacaine level.

References:
1. Macres SM, Moore PG, Fishman SM. Acute pain management. In: Barash PG, Cullen BF, Stoelting RK, et al, eds. *Clinical Anesthesia.* 7th ed. Philadelphia: Lippincott; 2013:1611-1644.
2. Macintyre PE. Safety and efficacy of patient-controlled analgesia. *Br J Anaesth.* 2001;87(1):36-46.

8. Correct answer: C

Although all these choices might be appropriate for a single bolus, meperidine is generally avoided for PCA, given its potentially toxic metabolic (normeperidine). Normeperidine can decrease the seizure threshold. Given that meperidine is metabolized by both the liver and kidney, patients with dysfunction of these organs would be at risk for toxicity. And, not surprisingly, given that acute kidney injury is not uncommon in the perioperative period, there have been reports of toxicity (central nervous system excitation and seizures) from meperidine PCAs in the postoperative period.

In a patient with normal renal function, the other 3 choices would be safe. In a patient with renal dysfunction, however, morphine should be avoided. Morphine has 3 main metabolites: normorphine, morphine-3-glucuronide, and morphine-6-glucuronide. All 3 are excreted by the kidneys. Morphine-6-glucuronide can build up and lead to respiratory depression and hypotension. Although M6G can cause excessive sedation, normeperidine actually has a unique toxicity separate from its parent compound. Importantly, although respiratory depression associated with M6G may be improved by naloxone, there is no antagonist for normeperidine and some studies have reported that its effects are actually exacerbated by naloxone.

Hydromorphone does have a metabolic product (hydromorphone-3-glucuronide) that is thought to be neuroexcitatory. However, hydromorphone can be used in patients with renal dysfunction with appropriate monitoring. Fentanyl has no active metabolites and is safe for use in patients with renal dysfunction. However, given its short half-life, it may not be the most appropriate medication for PCA use.

References:
1. Macintyre PE. Safety and efficacy of patient-controlled analgesia. *Br J Anaesth.* 2001;87(1):36-46.
2. Geller RJ. Meperidine in patient-controlled analgesia: a near-fatal mishap. *Anesth Analg.* 1993;76(3):655-657.

9. **Correct answer: A**

In adults, continuous background infusions are generally not recommended, especially in opioid-naive patients. It was initially thought that by using an infusion in addition to bolus doses of medication on demand, a patient would receive better analgesia and could also sleep through the night without waking up in pain and needing to press the PCA button. However, most studies that have compared PCA with and without a background infusion have not shown improved pain relief with a continuous background infusion. These studies have shown an increase in the incidence of side effects, such as respiratory depression, however. Therefore, a continuous background infusion should generally not be used in adult patients, especially those who are opioid-naive.

As an aside, in children, the use of a background infusion is thought to improve sleep, but it also fails to improve pain relief and may increase the risk of hypoxemia. For a hydromorphone PCA in an opioid-naive adult, a reasonable starting regimen includes a demand dose of 0.1-0.2 mg, an hourly lockout of 1-2 mg, and a lockout interval of 10 minutes. For example, if a patient is placed on a PCA that has a demand dose of 0.2 mg and a lockout interval of 10 minutes, they can receive up to 1.2 mg/h. These settings should be adjusted based on the patient's age and comorbidities.

References:

1. Macres SM, Moore PG, Fishman SM. Acute pain management. In: Barash PG, Cullen BF, Stoelting RK, et al, eds. *Clinical Anesthesia*. 7th ed. Philadelphia: Lippincott; 2013:1611-1644.
2. Macintyre PE. Safety and efficacy of patient-controlled analgesia. *Br J Anaesth*. 2001;87(1):36-46.

10. **Correct answer: A**

The most appropriate choice for this patient is a 5-HT$_3$ blocker such as ondansetron.

Dopamine antagonists (phenothiazines such as promethazine and prochlorperazine, droperidol, haldol, and metoclopramide) should be avoided because these medications can exacerbate the symptoms of Parkinson disease.

References:

1. Dierdorf SE, Walton JS, Stasic AF. Rare coexisting diseases. In: Barash PG, Cullen BF, Stoelting RK, et al, eds. *Clinical Anesthesia*. 7th ed. Philadelphia: Lippincott; 2013:612-640.
2. Katus L, Shtilbans A. Perioperative management of patients with Parkinson's disease. *Am J Med*. 2014;127(4):275-280.

11. **Correct answer: A**

Acetaminophen is both an analgesic and antipyretic. It is thought to act centrally by inhibiting activation of COX. It does not actually bind the COX enzyme but instead prevents the activation of COX by reducing heme at its peroxidase site. Acetaminophen also may modulate descending inhibitory serotonergic pathways. Acetaminophen is opioid-sparing and frequently comprises part of a multimodal analgesic regimen.

Lipoxygenase is part of the pathway of arachidonic acid metabolism to leukotrienes. It is not involved in analgesia. Central a2 receptors are activated by clonidine and tizanidine. Both of these drugs have sedative, anxiolytic, and analgesic properties, but tizanidine has a shorter duration of action than clonidine and is also thought to have less effect on heart rate and blood pressure. This leads to decreased release of norepinephrine at both central and peripheral sites, which in part explains the roles these drugs play in a multimodal regimen. Both of these medications can cause hypotension. GABA receptors are activated by many anesthetic agents, such as benzodiazepines, but not acetaminophen.

References:

1. Giovannitti Jr JA, Thoms SM, Crawford JJ. Alpha-2 adrenergic receptor agonists: a review of current clinical applications. *Anesth Prog*. 2015;62(1):31-39.
2. Hinz B, Brune K. Paracetamol and cyclooxygenase inhibition: is there a cause for concern? *Ann Rheum Dis*. 2012;71(1):20-25.
3. Macres SM, Moore PG, Fishman SM. Acute pain management. In: Barash PG, Cullen BF, Stoelting RK, et al, eds. *Clinical Anesthesia*. 7th ed. Philadelphia: Lippincott; 2013:1611-1644.

12. **Correct answer: C**

All of these drug choices could be part of a multimodal analgesic regimen. However, in a patient on ciprofloxacin, care must be taken when prescribing tizanidine. Ciprofloxacin has been shown to increase both the concentration and the hypotensive effect of tizanidine. Although one of the goals of using multimodal analgesia is to reduce opioid consumption, a patient who is in the immediate postoperative period may require some opioids. A multimodal regimen does not necessitate avoiding opioids altogether. Hydromorphone is a safe choice in a patient with chronic kidney disease.

Tylenol is an excellent adjunctive pain medication and could be used safely in this patient. A low-dose ketamine infusion could also be considered (ie, 5-10 µg/kg/min). Multiple trials have demonstrated that a low-dose ketamine infusion in the postoperative period can reduce opioid requirements. Ketamine has known side effects, including nausea, vomiting, increased secretions, and vivid dreams or hallucinations. However, in a meta-analysis of the use of postoperative ketamine, the likelihood of these adverse events was not significantly higher in the groups that received ketamine.

References:

1. Granfors MT, Backman JT, Neuvonen M, Neuvonen PJ. Ciprofloxacin greatly increases concentrations and hypotensive effect of tizanidine by inhibiting its cytochrome P450 1A2-mediated presystemic metabolism. *Clin Pharmacol Ther*. 2004;76(6):598-606.
2. Jouguelet-Lacoste J, La Colla L, Schilling D, Chelly JE. The use of intravenous infusion or single dose of low-dose ketamine for postoperative analgesia: a review of the current literature. *Pain Med*. 2015;16(2):383-403.
3. Helander EM, Menard BL, Harmon CM, et al. Multimodal analgesia, current concepts, and acute pain considerations. *Curr Pain Headache Rep*. 2017:1-10.

13. **Correct answer: B**

Ketamine acts as a noncompetitive *N*-methyl-D-aspartate (NMDA) receptor antagonist. It binds to the phencyclidine site on the NMDA receptor protein. This medication comes as a racemic mixture of S(+) and R(−) enantiomers, with the former having 4 times the affinity for the NMDA receptor than the latter. Nonhalogenated inhaled anesthetics, in particular xenon and nitrous oxide, also act as NMDA antagonists. Nitrous oxide noncompetitively inhibits the NMDA receptor. Compared with ketamine, it is a less specific and less potent NMDA antagonist. The halogenated inhaled anesthetics (ie, sevoflurane) do not act as NMDA antagonists.

Midazolam is a benzodiazepine that enhances the effect of GABA on GABA-A receptors. Clonidine is an a2 antagonist.

References:

1. Hillier SC, Mazurek MS, Havidich JE. Monitored anesthesia care. In: Barash PG, Cullen BF, Stoelting RK, et al, eds. *Clinical Anesthesia*. 7th ed. Philadelphia: Lippincott; 2013:824-843.
2. Helander EM, Menard BL, Harmon CM, et al. Multimodal analgesia, current concepts, and acute pain considerations. *Curr Pain Headache Rep*. 2017:1-10.

14. **Correct answer: B**

Traditional SCSs aim to create a paresthesia in the area in which the patient experiences pain, thereby masking the pain. Although the exact mechanism is unclear, SCS creates a depolarizing electric field that stimulates the dorsal column of the spinal cord via surgically implanted paddles or percutaneous leads. Energy is delivered at approximately 40-60 Hz, which causes depolarization of the Aβ fibers of the dorsal column. This depolarization may essentially "distract" from signals from the small Aδ and C pain fibers in the spinal cord.

When patients experience good pain relief after implantation of an SCS, they may increase their activity. One of the largest adverse events reported in trials of SCSs is lead migration. Lead migration literally means that the percutaneous leads have moved and thereby cause paresthesia in a different anatomical area. Therefore, a patient who presents with paresthesias in a different area should be assessed for lead migration (in this case, the leads have likely migrated caudally). This problem can be treated but sometimes requires reoperation. The first step after examining the patient is to have radiographs taken and compare them with the radiographs taken when the device was implanted.

Given that the patient does not have any significant findings on neurologic examination, new back pain, fever, or evidence of surgical site infection, infection and epidural abscess are unlikely. New disc herniation is certainly possible with increased activity but again would be unlikely to cause a shift in the distribution of paresthesias.

References:

1. Baranidharan G, Titterington J. Recent advances in spinal cord stimulation for pain treatment. *Pain Manag*. 2016;6(6):581-589.
2. Kumar K, Taylor RS, Jacques L, et al. The effects of spinal cord stimulation in neuropathic pain are sustained: a 24-month follow-up of the prospective randomized controlled multicenter trial of the effectiveness of spinal cord stimulation. *Neurosurgery*. 2008;63(4):762-770.

15. **Correct answer: A**

SCS leads are generally placed at the midline of the epidural space to stimulate the dorsal column tracts. The dorsal column tracts contain the axons of second-order spinal cord projection neurons in addition to the ascending axons of primary afferent neurons that relay touch, pressure, and vibratory sensation. It is by stimulation of the dorsal column tract that an SCS creates a paresthesia.

The lateral corticospinal tract is a descending motor pathway. It begins in the cerebral cortex and ends in the contralateral side of the spinal cord. The Botzinger complex is a group of neurons located in the rostral ventrolateral medulla and ventral respiratory column. This group of neurons is important in the control of breathing. Peripheral nerve field stimulation is an approach to address, among other complaints, chronic low-back pain in certain clinical contexts. Unlike SCSs, in peripheral nerve field stimulation, the device is placed directly over the nerve at the targeted pain area and not near the spinal cord, where the nerve actually originates.

References:

1. Benzon HT, Hurley RW, Deer T, Buvanendran A. Chronic pain management. In: Barash PG, Cullen BF, Stoelting RK, et al, eds. *Clinical Anesthesia*. 7th ed. Philadelphia: Lippincott; 2013:1645-1671.
2. Baranidharan G, Titterington J. Recent advances in spinal cord stimulation for pain treatment. *Pain Manag.* 2016;6(6):581-589.
3. Song JJ, Popescu A, Bell RL. Present and potential use of spinal cord stimulation to control chronic pain. *Pain Physician.* 2014;17(3):235-246.

16. **Correct answer: B**

In patients with unresectable cancer, it is inevitable that the cancer will progress. As this occurs, there is frequently an increase in the level of nociception, which may be due to destruction of nerves in the area of the tumor. This can result in worsening of pain and can lead to neuropathic pain. Unfortunately, the latter may be poorly responsive to escalating doses of opioids. This phenomenon is known as pseudotolerance.

OIH is a phenomenon in which there is a paradoxical increase in pain sensitivity in a patient being treated with opioids. This can occur during long-term and/or high-dose treatments, rapid escalation of doses, or administration of quickly metabolized opioids (ie, remifentanil). The treatment for this involves weaning the patient from opioids and possibly opioid rotation to a different opioid. Although a patient with chronic pain from cancer is certainly at risk for OIH, the situation described above does not suggest OIH as the most likely explanation.

It is also possible that the patient is displaying drug-seeking behavior. However, the natural history of unresectable pancreatic cancer would support the development of pseudotolerance, as the disease progresses and the tumor enlarges. Addiction is a very general term. It is characterized by a compulsion to repeatedly expose oneself to a stimulus that is reinforcing and rewarding. It should not be confused with tolerance to medications, by which there is a progressive lack of effect of a drug, leading to dose escalation. Tolerance is part of the natural history of long-term opioid use and can also be seen with other classes of medications.

References:

1. Dahan A, Niesters M, Olofsen E, Smith T, Overdyk F. Opioids. In: Barash PG, Cullen BF, Stoelting RK, et al, eds. *Clinical Anesthesia*. 7th ed. Philadelphia: Lippincott; 2013:501-522.
2. Lee M, Silverman SM, Hansen H, Patel VB, Manchikanti L. A comprehensive review of opioid-induced hyperalgesia. *Pain Physician.* 2011;14(2):145-161.

17. **Correct answer: B**

There are several important features to consider when a patient with chronic cancer-related pain presents with an increase in pain. They include disease progression, change in functional status (ie, increased physical activity), misuse of opioids, and both time course and dose of opioids. In this case, the patient has chronic pain and is on a fairly high dose of hydromorphone. He presents with diffuse pain, which is new, in addition to his chronic back pain.

OIH is difficult to differentiate from other causes of pain, such as progression of a cancer, increased activity, new injury, and tolerance. It can also present similarly to pain associated with opioid withdrawal, although with withdrawal, one would expect other symptoms such as nausea, diarrhea, restless legs, agitation, and yawning. It tends to produce more diffuse pain that affects other distributions than the patient's baseline pain. Unlike these other problems, increasing the dose of opioids should worsen the pain instead of making it better.

There is currently no standard treatment for OIH. If OIH is suspected, a practitioner could try and wean the patient from opioids while adding nonopioid adjunct medications. Studies have examined whether low-dose ketamine could be helpful, but this remains an area of active investigation.

OIH is a complex phenomenon that we are only beginning to understand. It is thought to involve pathologic activation of NMDA receptors, leading to the development of central sensitization. However, other mechanisms may well be involved. There is currently no evidence to suggest a role for GABA receptors (activated by benzodiazepines) or dopamine-2 receptors (activated by multiple antipsychotics such as haloperidol).

References:
1. Dahan A, Niesters M, Olofsen E, Smith T, Overdyk F. Opioids. In: Barash PG, Cullen BF, Stoelting RK, et al, eds. *Clinical Anesthesia.* 7th ed. Philadelphia: Lippincott; 2013:501-522.
2. Lee M, Silverman SM, Hansen H, Patel VB, Manchikanti L. A comprehensive review of opioid-induced hyperalgesia. *Pain Physician.* 2011;14(2):145-161.

18. Correct answer: A

Suboxone is a combination of buprenorphine and naloxone. Buprenorphine is derived from an opium alkaloid (thebaine) and acts as a partial agonist-antagonist at the μ-opioid receptor. It has a much higher affinity for this receptor than other opioids (such as morphine, oxycodone, and fentanyl) and also dissociates slowly, with a half-life of 20-40 hours. The naloxone is added to prevent diversion of the medication. It is not absorbed when Suboxone is taken as intended (sublingually) but will be absorbed if the drug is administered intravenously (ie, not as intended).

Perioperative management of Suboxone varies. Some providers recommend stopping it several days preoperatively and giving a short course of oral opioids, whereas others continue it. If Suboxone is continued, patients are likely to have increased opioid requirements postoperatively. It is difficult to determine how much more they will require. Therefore, they can be treated by titrating a short-acting opioid to meet their pain requirements while continuing Suboxone.

Given Suboxone's long half-life, withdrawal would not be expected to occur within 24 hours. There is no clear link between Suboxone and postoperative delirium. However, there is a link between inadequate pain control and postoperative delirium.

References:
1. Benzon HT, Hurley RW, Deer T, Buvanendran A. Chronic pain management. In: Barash PG, Cullen BF, Stoelting RK, et al, eds. *Clinical Anesthesia.* 7th ed. Philadelphia: Lippincott; 2013:1645-1671.
2. Bryson EO, Lipson S, Gevirtz C. Anesthesia for patients on buprenorphine. *Anesthesiol Clin.* 2010;28(4):611-617.

19. Correct answer: B

Buprenorphine is a semisynthetic opioid that acts as a partial agonist/antagonist at the μ opioid receptor. It is also an antagonist at the κ opioid receptor. It binds very strongly to the μ opioid receptor and dissociates slowly, with a half-life of 20-40 hours. When it is combined with naloxone, it can be administered as a sublingual preparation as a part of an opioid. This combination can be used for pain treatment or as a treatment for opioid addiction. When Suboxone is administered sublingually, the naloxone is not absorbed in clinically relevant amounts, and thus the patient receives only the effects of the buprenorphine. However, if it is injected, the naloxone will be active and can precipitate withdrawal. Symptoms of withdrawal include nausea, restless legs, agitation, diarrhea, mydriasis, piloerection, and yawning. Respiratory depression would not be expected.

References:
1. Benzon HT, Hurley RW, Deer T, Buvanendran A. Chronic pain management. In: Barash PG, Cullen BF, Stoelting RK, et al, eds. *Clinical Anesthesia.* 7th ed. Philadelphia: Lippincott; 2013:1645-1671.
2. Bryson EO, Lipson S, Gevirtz C. Anesthesia for patients on buprenorphine. *Anesthesiol Clin.* 2010;28(4):611-617.

20. Correct answer: B

The patient described above is misusing his medication. Misuse is defined as use of a medication for nonmedical use or for reasons other than the one it is prescribed. Misuse includes altering the dosing of a medication (such as taking it 6 times a day instead of 4 times) or sharing the medication. Abuse, on the other hand, is similar to misuse but is the correct term when harmful consequences occur. It is also use of a substance with an intention of altering one's mood or state of mind in a manner that is either harmful to oneself or others or illegal.

Addiction is a disease and is characterized by 1 or more behaviors. These include lack of control over use of the drug or substance, compulsive use, use despite harm, and cravings. Pseudoaddiction is a syndrome characterized by addictionlike behaviors, such as doctor shopping or trying to fill prescriptions early, to relieve pain, not to achieve pleasure or altered state of mind. Patients characterized as having pseudoaddiction may require a different pain regimen to adequately control their pain.

References:
1. Chang Y-P, Compton P. Management of chronic pain with chronic opioid therapy in patients with substance use disorders. *Addic Sci Clin Pract.* 2013;8(1):21.
2. Katz NP, Adams EH, Chilcoat H, et al. Challenges in the development of prescription opioid abuse-deterrent formulations. *Clin J Pain.* 2007;23(8):648-660.
3. Savage SR, Joranson DE, Covington EC, Schnoll SH, Heit HA, Gilson AM. Definitions related to the medical use of opioids: evolution towards universal agreement. *J Pain Symptom Manage.* 2003;26(1):655-667.

21. Correct answer: C

Bone metastases are the most prevalent cause of chronic pain in cancer patients. Skeletal metastases are a common manifestation of distant disease spread from many types of solid cancers, especially those arising in the lung, breast, and prostate.

For most patients with bony metastases, radiation therapy is the first-line treatment. Glucocorticoids may be used temporarily to relieve pain while the patient is awaiting radiation therapy. If the tumor is radio-resistant and high grade or if neurologic status deteriorates despite radiation, surgical decompression may be required. Physical therapy may be helpful in mobilizing patients with chronic cancer pain but is not a definitive first-line treatment.

References:
1. Huisman M, van den Bosch MAAJ, Wijlemans JW, van Vulpen M, van der Linden YM, Verkooijen HM. Effectiveness of reirradiation for painful bone metastases: a systematic review and meta-analysis. *Radiat Oncol Biol.* 2012;84(1):8-14.
2. Nielsen OS. Palliative radiotherapy of bone metastases: there is now evidence for the use of single fractions. *Radiother Oncol.* 1999;52(2):95-96.

22. Correct answer: A

There is abundant evidence to support the use of continuous epidural anesthesia for analgesia after open abdominal surgical procedures. There are several benefits to this type of analgesia, including improved pain control, faster return of bowel function, and reduced rates of nausea.

A recent prospective randomized study demonstrated that thoracic epidural anesthesia provided improved postoperative analgesia, reduced postoperative morphine and antiemetic requirements, shorter ICU stay, and faster recovery of bowel function compared with a control group who received PCA with morphine. A meta-analysis also found that when compared with PCA, continuous epidural anesthesia provided superior postoperative analgesia up to 3 days after surgery.

References:
1. Capdevila X, Moulard S, Plasse C, et al. Effectiveness of epidural analgesia, continuous surgical site analgesia, and patient-controlled analgesic morphine for postoperative pain management and hyperalgesia, rehabilitation, and health-related quality of life after open nephrectomy. *Anesth Analg.* 2017;124(1):336-345.
2. Wu CL, Cohen SR, Richman JM, et al. Efficacy of postoperative patient-controlled and continuous infusion epidural analgesia versus intravenous patient-controlled analgesia with opioids: a meta-analysis. *Anesthesiology.* 2005;103(5):1079-1088-quiz 1109-1110.
3. Bernards CM, Hostetter LS. Epidural and spinal anesthesia. In: Barash PG, Cullen BF, Stoelting RK, et al, eds. *Clinical Anesthesia.* 7th ed. Philadelphia: Lippincott; 2013:905-936.

23. Correct answer: C

Although in many cases, PDPH will resolve spontaneously, it can present enough of a functional impairment that it requires treatment. An epidural blood patch (EBP) is considered to be the definitive treatment for PDPH that fails conservative therapy. In most cases, an EBP is performed with autologous blood (ie, the patient's own blood). However, in a patient with cancer or a disseminated severe infection (especially a patient who is immunocompromised), it may be unsafe to use autologous blood. In this patient, for example, there would be the risk of causing coccidioidomycosis meningitis, which could be fatal. In rare cases such as this, it would be appropriate to give the patient allogeneic (donor) blood that is drawn from a volunteer in a sterile fashion. This is, of course, not without risk.

Normal saline has not been shown to be as effective as blood for an EBP. The addition of fibrin glue has been used in some refractory cases of PDPH but would not be used for the initial EBP.

References:
1. Trentman TL, Hoxworth JM, Kusne S, Torloni AS, Patel NP, Rosenfeld DM. Allogeneic epidural blood patch in the setting of persistent spinal headache and disseminated coccidioidomycosis. *Pain Physician.* 2009;12(3):639-643.
2. Elwood JJ, Dewan M, Smith JM, Mokri B, Mauck WD, Eldrige JS. Efficacy of epidural blood patch with fibrin glue additive in refractory headache due to intracranial hypotension: preliminary report. *Springer Plus.* 2016:1-5.
3. Bernards CM, Hostetter LS. Epidural and spinal anesthesia. In: Barash PG, Cullen BF, Stoelting RK, et al, eds. *Clinical Anesthesia.* 7th ed. Philadelphia: Lippincott; 2013:905-936.

24. Correct answer: C

The celiac plexus is located over the anterolateral surface of the aorta near the origins of the celiac and superior mesenteric arteries. It is predominantly made up of preganglionic sympathetic efferent nerve fibers derived from the greater splanchnic (T5 through T9), lesser splanchnic (T10 through T11), and least splanchnic (T12) nerves. There are also contributions from the preganglionic parasympathetic efferent fibers from the posterior trunk of the vagus nerve and the visceral afferent fibers carrying nociceptive stimuli from the upper abdominal viscera. The celiac plexus supplies the following organs: pancreas, liver, biliary tract, gallbladder, spleen, adrenal glands, kidneys, mesentery, stomach, small bowel, and large bowel (ascending and transverse colon only). Nerve block of this plexus is used as a pain treatment in several conditions including pancreatic cancer, chronic pancreatitis, and cancers of the upper gastrointestinal tract/biliary system (gastric, esophageal, liver, and gallbladder). The descending colon receives innervation from the inferior mesenteric plexus.

References:
1. Kambadakone A, Thabet A, Gervais DA, Mueller PR, Arellano RS. CT-guided celiac plexus neurolysis: a review of anatomy, indications, technique, and tips for successful treatment. *Radiographics.* 2011;31(6):1599-1621.
2. Benzon HT, Hurley RW, Deer T, Buvanendran A. Chronic pain management. In: Barash PG, Cullen BF, Stoelting RK, et al, eds. *Clinical Anesthesia.* 7th ed. Philadelphia: Lippincott; 2013:1645-1671.

25. Correct answer: D

Celiac plexus block and/or neurolysis is indicated for several abdominal pain conditions, including pain from malignancy (ie, pancreatic cancer). It has been also reported as a treatment for chronic abdominal pain or pain secondary to chronic pancreatitis. The celiac plexus is located anterolateral to the aorta and around the origin of the celiac trunk, usually at T12-L1. It is a relay center for nociceptive stimuli that originate from the upper abdominal viscera (stomach to proximal transverse colon). Thus, pain from such structures may be treated via this approach.

A common complication of celiac plexus block or neurolysis is orthostatic hypotension, which affects 10%-52% of patients. It results from sympathetic blockade, which causes vasodilatation. This risk may be minimized by maintaining the patient's volume status and undergoing bed rest for approximately 12 hours postprocedure.

Another common complication is diarrhea. The reason for this is not exactly understood but likely relates to sympathetic blockade, leading to unblocked parasympathetic tone, increased peristalsis, quicker transport, and thus diarrhea. The diarrhea is usually self-limited.

When a posterior approach is taken to celiac plexus neurolysis, the most common but transient complication is back pain. Abdominal pain (anteriorly) is not common and should raise the question of possible peritoneal irritation.

Lower-extremity paralysis is exceedingly uncommon, occurring in about 0.15% of people.

References:
1. Kambadakone A, Thabet A, Gervais DA, Mueller PR, Arellano RS. CT-guided celiac plexus neurolysis: a review of anatomy, indications, technique, and tips for successful treatment. *Radiographics.* 2011;31(6):1599-1621.
2. Rana MV, Candido KD, Raja O, Knezevic NN. Celiac plexus block in the management of chronic abdominal pain. *Curr Pain Headache Rep.* 2014;18(2):220-227.
3. Benzon HT, Hurley RW, Deer T, Buvanendran A. Chronic pain management. In: Barash PG, Cullen BF, Stoelting RK, et al, eds. *Clinical Anesthesia.* 7th ed. Philadelphia: Lippincott; 2013:1645-1671.

26. Correct answer: A

Both ethanol and phenol can be used to perform neurolytic block of, for example, the celiac plexus. Very few differences have been found between the 2 agents—they provide equal efficacy and the same duration of block. However, phenol is painless on injection, whereas ethanol is painful. To address this issue, bupivacaine is sometimes injected before the ethanol or the ethanol is diluted.

A common complication of celiac plexus neurolytic block is orthostatic hypotension, which is usually not permanent. There is no difference between ethanol and phenol in the incidence of hypotension.

References:
1. Kambadakone A, Thabet A, Gervais DA, Mueller PR, Arellano RS. CT-guided celiac plexus neurolysis: a review of anatomy, indications, technique, and tips for successful treatment. *Radiographics*. 2011;31(6):1599-1621.
2. Benzon HT, Hurley RW, Deer T, Buvanendran A. Chronic pain management. In: Barash PG, Cullen BF, Stoelting RK, et al, eds. *Clinical Anesthesia*. 7th ed. Philadelphia: Lippincott; 2013:1645-1671.
3. Koyyalagunta D, Engle MP, Yu J, Feng L, Novy DM. The effectiveness of alcohol versus phenol based splanchnic nerve neurolysis for the treatment of intra-abdominal cancer pain. *Pain Physician*. 2016;19(4):281-292.

27. Correct answer: C

The WHO pain ladder was developed in 1986 as an approach to cancer pain management. This ladder is frequently used for noncancer pain treatment as well, although some physicians have more recently expressed concern that it may emphasize overuse of opioids for the treatment of chronic pain. It outlines an approach to pain control that is based on the severity of pain. Pharmacologic treatment begins with step 1 with Tylenol (paracetamol) and nonsteroidal anti-inflammatory drugs (NSAIDs) plus or minus adjuvant medications. For moderate pain not controlled by these, step 2 is used. This includes weak opioids, including codeine, oxycodone, tramadol, and hydrocodone. Finally, for more severe pain, stronger opioids, such as morphine or fentanyl, are added as a part of step 3. A fentanyl patch is unlikely to be appropriate for an opioid-naive patient.

STEP	SYMPTOMS	TREATMENT
1	Pain	Nonopioid analgesic ± adjuvant
2	Persistent or increasing pain	Weak opioid ± nonopioid ± adjuvant
3	Persistent or increasing pain	Strong opioid ± nonopioid ± adjuvant

References:
1. Vargas-Schaffer G. Is the WHO analgesic ladder still valid? Twenty-four years of experience. *Canadian Family Physician Medecin De Famille Canadien*. 2010;56(6):514-517-e202-e205.
2. Cancer pain relief and palliative care. Report of a WHO Expert Committee. *World Health Organ Tech Rep Ser*. 1990;804:1-75.

28. Correct answer: A

Concepts central to the WHO pain ladder are that oral administration is preferred whenever possible, analgesics should be given at regular intervals, and pain regimens should be adapted to the patient's individual needs instead of using a standard dosing regimen. Even for cancer pain, treatment begins with nonopioid medications.

References:
1. Vargas-Schaffer G. Is the WHO analgesic ladder still valid? Twenty-four years of experience. *Canadian Family Physician Medecin De Famille Canadien*. 2010;56(6):514-517-e202-e205.
2. Cancer pain relief and palliative care. Report of a WHO Expert Committee. *World Health Organ Tech Rep Ser*. 1990;804:1-75.

29. Correct answer: D

The American College of Rheumatology (ACR) initially established criteria to classify fibromyalgia in 1990 and at that point stated that the diagnosis requires 2 components: a history of widespread pain for at least 3 months and allodynia to pressure applied by a finger at 11 or more of 18 anatomically defined points. These points include the following:
- Occiput
- Intertransverse spaces between C5 and C7

- Trapezii (bilateral)
- Supraspinatus (bilateral)
- Second rib (bilateral)
- Lateral to the costochondral junctions (bilateral)
- Lateral epicondyles (bilateral)
- Glutei (bilateral)
- Greater trochanters (bilateral)
- Knees (bilateral)

In an update published in 2010, the ACR acknowledged that many fibromyalgia diagnoses were made in primary care and many primary care physicians did not know how to examine tender points or chose not to. Thus, fibromyalgia diagnosis was frequently based on symptoms. Therefore, the ACR created a system that takes into account symptoms and their severity. These include somatic symptoms, waking unrefreshed, cognitive symptoms, fatigue, sleep problems, mood problems, and pain. Radicular pain, however, is not part of the diagnostic criteria for fibromyalgia.

References:

1. Benzon HT, Hurley RW, Deer T, Buvanendran A. Chronic pain management. In: Barash PG, Cullen BF, Stoelting RK, et al, eds. *Clinical Anesthesia*. 7th ed. Philadelphia: Lippincott; 2013:1645-1671.
2. Wolfe F, Clauw DJ, Fitzcharles M-A, et al. The American College of Rheumatology preliminary diagnostic criteria for fibromyalgia and measurement of symptom severity. *Arthritis Care Res*. 2010;62(5):600-610.
3. Wolfe F, Smythe HA, Yunus MB, et al. The American College of Rheumatology 1990 Criteria for the Classification of Fibromyalgia. Report of the Multicenter Criteria Committee. *Arthritis Rheum*. 1990;33(2):160-172.

30. Correct answer: A

Treatment of fibromyalgia requires a multidisciplinary approach that includes medication combined with nonpharmacologic therapies such as low-intensity, low-impact exercise; physical therapy; cognitive behavioral therapy; and patient education. Medications thought to be efficacious for the treatment of fibromyalgia include serotonin and norepinephrine uptake inhibitors, specifically duloxetine and milnacipran, pregabalin, amitriptyline, gabapentin, and γ-hydroxybutyrate.

Hydrocodone and other opioids are not a treatment of choice for fibromyalgia. A 2015 systematic review noted that there is more evidence available on the harms of opioid therapy in chronic nonmalignant pain than on the benefits. They also reported that there was insufficient evidence to support long-term use of opioid therapy in patients with chronic nonmalignant pain.

References:

1. Gilron I, Chaparro LE, Tu D, et al. Combination of pregabalin with duloxetine for fibromyalgia: a randomized controlled trial. *Pain*. 2016;157(7):1532-1540.
2. Chou R, Turner JA, Devine EB, et al. The effectiveness and risks of long-term opioid therapy for chronic pain: a systematic review for a National Institutes of Health Pathways to Prevention Workshop. *Ann Intern Med*. 2015;162(4):276-286.
3. Benzon HT, Hurley RW, Deer T, Buvanendran A. Chronic pain management. In: Barash PG, Cullen BF, Stoelting RK, et al, eds. *Clinical Anesthesia*. 7th ed. Philadelphia: Lippincott; 2013:1645-1671.

31. Correct answer: D

CRPS is a disorder in which a patient develops ongoing pain and other sensory changes that are unusual, given the expected time course of their initial injury or trauma. Criteria proposed by the International Association for the Study of Pain suggest that patients should have at least 1 symptom in each of the following general areas: sensory (ie, increased sensitivity to sensory stimulation), vasomotor (temperature abnormalities or skin color changes), trophic (changes in hair or nail growth), sudomotor (sweating abnormalities or edema), or motor (decreased range of movement or weakness).

The differentiation between types I and II CRPS is difficult. The symptoms of both are the same. However, there is a clear preceding nerve injury in CRPS type II. A patient who undergoes a positioning injury during surgery (in this case, possibly injury to the LFCN) is at risk for development of CRPS type II. In the other examples, a mechanism of injury can be clearly defined, but the injury and the distribution of pain do not suggest a clear peripheral nerve injury.

References:
1. Benzon HT, Hurley RW, Deer T, Buvanendran A. Chronic pain management. In: Barash PG, Cullen BF, Stoelting RK, et al, eds. *Clinical Anesthesia*. 7th ed. Philadelphia: Lippincott; 2013:1645-1671.
2. Littlejohn G, Dutton K. Terminology, criteria, and definitions in complex regional pain syndrome: challenges and solutions. *J Pain Res*. 2015:871-877.

32. Correct answer: A

PHN is a somewhat arbitrarily defined pain condition that occurs after acute herpes zoster infection. The most common definition is the continuation of pain 3 or more months after the original infection. The greatest risk factor for developing PHN is age—it is uncommon in people below the age of 50 years, but in those above 60 years of age, the risk of developing it is at least 20% and increases with age. There is some evidence that treating the initial herpes zoster infection with oral antiviral agents (such as acyclovir, famciclovir, and valacyclovir) may reduce the duration of PHN if it does develop.

Other risk factors for developing PHN include greater rash severity, presence of a prodrome, and severe pain in the area of the initial herpes zoster infection. Male sex does not appear to be a risk factor.

References:
1. Watson PN. Postherpetic neuralgia. *BMJ Clin Evid*. 2010;2010.
2. Fashner J, Bell AL. Herpes zoster and post herpetic neuralgia: prevention and management. *Am Fam Physician*. 2011;83(12): 1432-1437.
3. Benzon HT, Hurley RW, Deer T, Buvanendran A. Chronic pain management. In: Barash PG, Cullen BF, Stoelting RK, et al, eds. *Clinical Anesthesia*. 7th ed. Philadelphia: Lippincott; 2013:1645-1671.

33. Correct answer: C

Phantom limb pain is a phenomenon whereby a patient experiences pain in a part of the body that has been removed. It is most commonly thought in terms of traumatic or surgical loss of a limb but can also occur after mastectomy or amputation of other parts of the body. Its prevalence varies greatly between studies from 30% to 90%.

Risk factors that have been described for the development of phantom limb pain include the presence of pain before the amputation (especially in patients who have vascular damage), the loss of the dominant upper limb, bilateral amputation, lower limb amputation, proximal amputation, the presence of stump pain, and psychologic disorders such as depression.

Distal amputation carries a lower risk for the development of phantom limb pain than proximal amputation.

References:
1. Dijkstra PU, Geertzen JHB, Stewart R, van der Schans CP. Phantom pain and risk factors: a multivariate analysis. *J Pain Symptom Manage*. 2002;24(6):578-585.
2. Flor H. Phantom-limb pain: characteristics, causes, and treatment. *Lancet Neurol*. 2002;1(3):182-189.

34. Correct answer: A

Low-back pain has multiple causes. Common causes include musculoskeletal disease, herniated discs, spinal stenosis, and arthritis/degeneration of joints such as the facet and sacroiliac joints. Pain from herniated discs, spinal stenosis, and facet joint disease tends to be radicular (radiating), whereas pain from the sacroiliac joints typically presents as buttock pain although it can present as low-back pain. Musculoskeletal pain tends to be localized to the affected area but can also radiate. The facet joints are bilateral and are located between the articular processes of 2 adjacent vertebrae. Patients with low-back pain due to degeneration of the facet joints often have pain that radiates into the ipsilateral posterior thigh, ending at the knee. There is typically paraspinal tenderness, and extension plus rotation of the back on the ipsilateral side may reproduce the pain. Numbness over the lower back would be unlikely to occur with any of the common conditions causing back pain.

References:
1. Benzon HT, Hurley RW, Deer T, Buvanendran A. Chronic pain management. In: Barash PG, Cullen BF, Stoelting RK, et al, eds. *Clinical Anesthesia*. 7th ed. Philadelphia: Lippincott; 2013:1645-1671.
2. Filippiadis DK, Kelekis A. A review of percutaneous techniques for low back pain and neuralgia: current trends in epidural infiltrations, intervertebral disk and facet joint therapies. *Br J Radiol*. 2016;89(1057):20150357.

35. **Correct answer: A**

The facet joints are innervated by nerve fibers from the medial branch of the dorsal ramus of the spinal nerves. Each facet joint has a dual nerve supply—it is innervated by the nerves at its level and also from the level above. The medial branch of the dorsal ramus arises from the spinal nerves soon after they exit the intervertebral foramina and divide into ventral and dorsal rami (branches). The ventral rami travel laterally and anteriorly to supply musculature, subcutaneous tissue, and skin of the neck, trunk, and the upper and lower extremities. The dorsal rami travel posteriorly to supply the paravertebral muscles, subcutaneous tissues, and skin of the back close to the midline. Both the lateral and medial branches innervate musculature and skin of the back. However, only the medial branch innervates the facet joints. The posterior cutaneous branches of the dorsal ramus arise from the medial branch and provide innervation to the skin of the midline of the back.

Blockade of the facet joint or of the medial branch of the dorsal ramus can serve to diagnose and also treat facetogenic pain. A facet joint block involves injecting a mixture of local plus or minus corticosteroid intra-articularly, whereas a medial branch block involves injecting the mixture right next to the medial branch, usually where the superior articular process connects to the base of the transverse process. A facet joint injection can be performed under fluoroscopy as shown below.

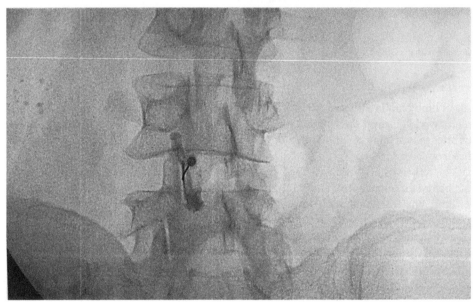

(From Benzon HT, Hurley RW, Deer T, Buvanendran A. Chronic pain management. In: Barash PG, Cullen BF, Stoelting RK, et al, eds. *Clinical Anesthesia*. Philadelphia: Wolters Kluwer Health; 2015:1654, with permission.)

References:
1. Benzon HT, Hurley RW, Deer T, Buvanendran A. Chronic pain management. In: Barash PG, Cullen BF, Stoelting RK, et al, eds. *Clinical Anesthesia*. 7th ed. Philadelphia: Lippincott; 2013:1645-1671.
2. Filippiadis DK, Kelekis A. A review of percutaneous techniques for low back pain and neuralgia: current trends in epidural infiltrations, intervertebral disk and facet joint therapies. *Br J Radiol*. 2016;89(1057):20150357.

36. **Correct answer: A**

Low-back pain has many causes. The origin of a particular patient's low-back pain can be ascertained from a combination of patient history, physical examination, and imaging. In a patient with a normal hip examination (no pain with passive hip joint motion), pain that radiates into the ipsilateral buttocks that can be provoked by the FABER test (Patrick test) is consistent with pain originating from the sacroiliac joint. To perform this test, the examiner flexes, abducts, externally rotates, and extends the affected leg so that the ankle of that leg is on top of the contralateral knee. Then, the examiner applies pressure to slowly lower the affected leg toward the table. This test is positive if the affected leg remains above the contralateral leg.

Numbness of the anterolateral thigh is most suggestive of meralgia paresthetica or entrapment of the LFCN. The usual site of entrapment is where the nerve passes under the inguinal ligament. Obesity is a risk factor for the development of meralgia paresthetica. This condition usually resolves spontaneously.

Back pain accompanied by a positive straight leg raise test suggests nerve root irritation, which can be caused by disc herniation. Usually, the L5 or S1 nerve root is irritated. This test is sensitive, but not specific, for nerve root irritation. A positive straight leg raise test should not be confused with hamstring tightness, with which patients will have pain in the hamstring during passive raising of their leg.

Back pain accompanied by a leg length discrepancy can be caused by scoliosis or severe muscle spasm of the ipsilateral paraspinal muscles.

References:
1. Benzon HT, Hurley RW, Deer T, Buvanendran A. Chronic pain management. In: Barash PG, Cullen BF, Stoelting RK, et al, eds. *Clinical Anesthesia*. 7th ed. Philadelphia: Lippincott; 2013:1645-1671.
2. Casazza BA. Diagnosis and treatment of acute low back pain. *Am Fam Physician*. 2012;85(4):343-350.
3. Maslowski E, Sullivan W, Harwood JF, et al. The diagnostic validity of hip provocation maneuvers to detect intra-articular hip pathology. *PM R*. 2010;2(3):174-181.

37. Correct answer: A

There are thought to be 6 possible anatomic relationships between the piriformis muscle and the sciatic nerve. They are as follows:
1. Whole sciatic nerve passes below the piriformis muscle.
2. Divided sciatic nerve passes through and below the piriformis muscle.
3. Divided sciatic nerve passes through and above the piriformis muscle.
4. Divided sciatic nerve passes above and below the piriformis muscle.
5. Whole sciatic nerve passes through the piriformis muscle.
6. Whole sciatic nerve passes above the piriformis muscle.

The most common arrangement by far is that the whole sciatic nerve passes below the piriformis muscle. In various cadaver studies, the rate of this relationship has been reported to be between 78% and 98.5%. Understanding these relationships is important because blocks can be used both for diagnosis and treatment. Block failure may not only occur because the patient does not have piriformis syndrome, but it may also occur because of inadequate coverage of the nerve, given anatomical variants.

References:
1. Benzon HT, Hurley RW, Deer T, Buvanendran A. Chronic pain management. In: Barash PG, Cullen BF, Stoelting RK, et al, eds. *Clinical Anesthesia*. 7th ed. Philadelphia: Lippincott; 2013:1645-1671.
2. Benzon HT, Katz JA, Benzon HA, Iqbal MS. Piriformis syndrome: anatomic considerations, a new injection technique, and a review of the literature. *Anesthesiology*. 2003;98(6):1442-1448.

38. Correct answer: D

ESIs are a common treatment modality for patients with low-back pain or radiculitis secondary to disc degeneration, leading to stenosis or disc herniation. In patients with diabetes, several studies have documented a rise in blood glucose levels that can persist for up to 7 days after the injection of a steroid. This phenomenon depends on the dose and type of steroid. It appears that preinjection glucose control does not affect this phenomenon, so it is important to counsel diabetic patients before performing an ESI and also to consider reducing the dose of steroids. The reasons corticosteroids cause a transient hyperglycemia are multiple: they affect the hypothalamic-pituitary axis and also act as insulin antagonists, inhibit peripheral glucose uptake, and promote hepatic gluconeogenesis.

Headache is a possible reaction after ESI. In the case of accidental dural puncture, a PDPH (positional headache) is possible. If the steroid is injected intrathecally, arachnoiditis can occur as well. However, these outcomes are not as likely as transient hyperglycemia in a diabetic patient.

Infections occur after about 1%-2% of ESIs. Severe infections, such as meningitis, occur less than 1% of the time.

References:
1. Goodman BS, Posecion LWF, Mallempati S, Bayazitoglu M. Complications and pitfalls of lumbar interlaminar and transforaminal epidural injections. *Curr Rev Musculoskelet Med*. 2008;1(3-4):212-222.
2. Even JL, Crosby CG, Song Y, McGirt MJ, Devin CJ. Effects of epidural steroid injections on blood glucose levels in patients with diabetes mellitus. *Spine*. 2012;37(1):E46-E50.
3. Kim WH, Sim WS, Shin BS, et al. Effects of two different doses of epidural steroid on blood glucose levels and pain control in patients with diabetes mellitus. *Pain Physician*. 2013;16(6):557-568.

39. Correct answer: B

Low-back pain is one of the most common reasons that people present to their primary care doctor and then, subsequently, pain specialists. It is likely that by the age of 40 years, many people will have experienced an episode of acute low-back pain. And in many people, the pain improves (if not resolves) in 4-6 weeks.

When discussing low-back pain, it is common to look for "red flag" symptoms or symptoms of potentially severe pathology. These include significant trauma, a marked or progressive motor or sensory deficit, new-onset bowel or bladder incontinence or urinary retention, loss of anal sphincter tone, saddle anesthesia, a history of cancer (and especially a history of cancer metastatic to the bones), and fevers or other signs of infection that could point to spinal infection. Although most people presenting with new, acute onset low-back pain do not require imaging, people with red flag symptoms should at least be considered for imaging. Unfortunately, red flags are not perfect predictors of severe pathology, but the presence of more than one may raise the suspicion for severe pathology.

An appropriate first-line therapy is treatment with NSAIDs. Opioids are both commonly sought after and prescribed for patients with severe, acute low-back pain. However, there is little in support of this therapy. Studies have shown no difference in pain relief or time to return to work between oral opioids and NSAIDs or acetaminophen. There are, however, serious risks with opioids. There is also no evidence that a short course of oral corticosteroids provides much benefit.

References:
1. Henschke N, Maher CG, Refshauge KM, et al. Prevalence of and screening for serious spinal pathology in patients presenting to primary care settings with acute low back pain. *Arthritis Rheum.* 2009;60(10):3072-3080.
2. Casazza BA. Diagnosis and treatment of acute low back pain. *Am Fam Physician.* 2012;85(4):343-350.

40. Correct answer: B

Trigeminal neuralgia is a painful condition in which a patient experiences recurrent episodes of lancinating pain in the distribution of the trigeminal nerves. The pain may be triggered by many stimuli to the face, such as chewing, tooth brushing, or even light touch. The pain tends to be unilateral (more common in the right side than the left side) and most commonly involves the V2 and V3 distributions. The V1 distribution is only involved about 5% of the time. Therefore forehead involvement is uncommon. In addition, autonomic symptoms such as nasal discharge and tearing are also uncommon and should raise the question of cluster headaches or other phenomena.

There is grade A evidence that the initial treatment for trigeminal neuralgia should be carbamazepine. It has been found to be successful in many cases. According to a Cochrane review, the number needed to treat for carbamazepine for patients with trigeminal neuralgia is 2.5 and the number needed to harm (minor adverse events) is 3.6. However, although most patients respond at least initially to carbamazepine, for some it will lose effect. Other medications used include phenytoin, lamotrigine, topiramate, gabapentin, clonazepam, and valproic acid.

References:
1. Wiffen PJ, Derry S, Moore RA, Kalso EA. Carbamazepine for chronic neuropathic pain and fibromyalgia in adults. *Cochrane Database Syst Rev.* 2014;(4):CD005451.
2. Krafft RM. Trigeminal neuralgia. *Am Fam Physician.* 2008;77(9):1291-1296.
3. Tsui BCH, Rosenquist RW. Peripheral nerve blockade. In: Barash PG, Cullen BF, Stoelting RK, et al, eds. *Clinical Anesthesia.* 7th ed. Philadelphia: Lippincott; 2013:937-995.

41. Correct answer: A

The most common neurologic complication that occurs in individuals infected with HIV is peripheral neuropathy. The most common type of peripheral neuropathy is a distal symmetrical sensory neuropathy. The neuropathy can not only be due to HIV infection, but it can also be caused by some antiretroviral therapies (ARTs). Risk factors for sensory neuropathy in HIV-infected individuals include advanced age, lower CD4 nadir, current use of antiretroviral drugs, and past use of specific ARTs (dideoxynucleosides) such as didanosine, zalcitabine, and stavudine. Some protease inhibitors have also been implicated in the pathogenesis of distal symmetric peripheral neuropathy (indinavir, saquinavir, and ritonavir). Therefore the first step in treating this patient would be to evaluate his/her ART regimen.

The treatment of HIV-associated peripheral neuropathy is complicated. Once an idiopathic cause is eliminated (ie, peripheral neuropathy secondary to ARTs), treatment can proceed as for other sensory peripheral neuropathies. Patients are treated with antiepileptics and antidepressant drugs. Unfortunately, the literature for antiepileptic drugs suggests mixed results, with a large trial finding pregabalin to be ineffective. It would be reasonable to consider initiation of antiepileptic therapy in this patient. As for other chronic nonmalignant pain, the data for opioids do not support a role for long-term usage. An ESI is unlikely to be helpful, given that this is a distal peripheral neuropathy, not a nerve root irritation.

References:
1. Gabbai AA, Castelo A, Oliveira ASB. HIV peripheral neuropathy. *Handb Clin Neurol.* 2013;115:515-529.
2. Simpson D M, Schifitto G, Clifford DB, et al. Pregabalin for painful HIV neuropathy: a randomized, double-blind, placebo-controlled trial. *Neurology.* 2010;74(5):413-420.

42. Correct answer: B

Methadone is an opioid used both to treat pain and also as a part of a treatment in people who abuse heroin or other opioids. It has multiple mechanisms including μ receptor agonism, antagonism at the NMDA receptor antagonism, and also reuptake inhibition of serotonin and norepinephrine. Patients on methadone require monitoring for multiple reasons, including that it prolongs the QTc interval and can put patients at increased risk of developing torsades de pointes. There are multiple factors that increase a patient's likelihood of developing torsades de pointes while on methadone. These include the following:

PRE-EXISTING QTc >450 ms
Female sex
Bradycardia
Atrial fibrillation
Dose >60 mg/d and especially >100-120 mg/d
Use of other QT-prolonging drugs
Liver dysfunction
HIV
Hypokalemia or hypomagnesemia
Anorexia nervosa
Heart disease
hERG mutation
Metabolic (CYP) drug interactions
Cocaine use

Before prescribing methadone, a provider must carefully consider the other medications a patient takes. Methadone is primarily metabolized by CYP3A4, CYP2B6, and CYP2C19. Although this is by no means a complete list, some drugs that inhibit these enzymes include antibiotics (eg, clarithromycin, sulfamethoxazole/trimethoprim, ciprofloxacin), antifungals (eg, itraconazole, voriconazole), sertraline, fluoxetine, and ritonavir. A baseline ECG is also needed.

References:
1. Vieweg WVR, Hasnain M, Howland RH, et al. Methadone, QTc interval prolongation and torsade de pointes: case reports offer the best understanding of this problem. *Ther Adv Psychopharmacol.* 2013;3(4):219-232.
2. Stringer J, Welsh C, Tommasello A. Methadone-associated Q-T interval prolongation and torsades de pointes. *Am J Health Syst Pharm.* 2009;66(9):825-833.

43. Correct Answer: D

The sympathetic nervous system plays a role in many types of visceral, vascular, and neuropathic pain. A block of the lumbar sympathetic plexus can be used both as a diagnostic modality for pain syndromes of the lower extremities and as a treatment modality. For example, in vascular diseases such as Buerger disease, diabetic neuropathy, and diabetic ulcers, a sympathetic block can improve circulation to local nerves and potentially improve or relieve pain. Pain from coccydynia (tailbone pain) may benefit from sympathetic blockade, but the blockade would need to be done at the ganglion of impar (which receives input from sacral, not lumbar, nerves), not the lumbar sympathetic plexus.

References:
1. Benzon HT, Hurley RW, Deer T, Buvanendran A. Chronic pain management. In: Barash PG, Cullen BF, Stoelting RK, et al, eds. *Clinical Anesthesia*. 7th ed. Philadelphia: Lippincott; 2013:1645-1671.
2. Menon R, Swanepoel A. Sympathetic blocks. Continuing education in anaesthesia. *Crit Care Pain*. 2010;10(3):88-92.

44. Correct answer: B

Spinal anesthesia is usually a straightforward way to provide analgesia and muscle relaxation for surgical procedures of the lower extremities and also for C-sections. However, spinal anesthesia can fail, meaning that the block is inadequate for the surgical procedure to be performed. The rate of spinal failure by experienced practitioners may be as low as 1% but may be as high as 17% at academic centers.

Displacement of the tip of the spinal needle is a particular issue with pencil-point needles, which are more commonly used these days to reduce the incidence of PDPH. Because the opening of these needles is proximal to the tip, if the needle moves backward during the injection process, it will straddle the dura and it is possible that only some of the solution will enter the CSF, whereas the rest may enter the epidural space.

The idea of local anesthetic resistance exists in the literature, but there has never been a sodium channel mutation defined that would actually confer resistance. Failure is more likely to be due to technique or anatomical variation.

Using lidocaine would result in a shorter duration of the spinal block than bupivacaine but it would not necessarily provide an inadequate block for the surgery. Lidocaine is avoided for spinals by some practitioners because of the association with transient neurologic syndrome (TNS). The risk of developing TNS, which is characterized by mild to severe buttock and leg pain that usually lasts up to 5 days, is higher with lidocaine than with other local anesthetics.

References:
1. Zaric D, Pace NL. Transient neurologic symptoms (TNS) following spinal anaesthesia with lidocaine versus other local anaesthetics. *Cochrane Database Syst Rev*. 2009;(2):CD003006.
2. Fettes PDW, Jansson J-R, Wildsmith JAW. Failed spinal anaesthesia: mechanisms, management, and prevention. *Br J Anaesth*. 2009;102(6):739-748.
3. Bernards CM, Hostetter LS. Epidural and spinal anesthesia. In: Barash PG, Cullen BF, Stoelting RK, et al, eds. *Clinical Anesthesia*. 7th ed. Philadelphia: Lippincott; 2013:905-936.

45. Correct answer: B

Lidocaine is avoided for spinals by some practitioners because of the association with TNS. The risk of developing TNS, which is characterized by mild to severe buttock and leg pain that develops within a few hours (or up to 24 h) after anesthesia and usually lasts up to 5 days (although some sources say 10 d), is higher with lidocaine than with other local anesthetics. There is no weakness associated with TNS. Compared with other local anesthetics such as bupivacaine, 2-chloroprocaine, ropivacaine, prilocaine, procaine, and levobupivacaine, the relative risk for developing TNS with lidocaine is 4.16-12.86. However, patients can develop TNS with any local anesthetic. The value of lidocaine is that it is shorter acting than many of the other local anesthetics, making it ideal for outpatient surgery.

References:
1. Zaric D, Pace NL. Transient neurologic symptoms (TNS) following spinal anaesthesia with lidocaine versus other local anaesthetics. *Cochrane Database Syst Rev*. 2009;(2):CD003006.
2. Fettes PDW, Jansson J-R, Wildsmith JAW. Failed spinal anaesthesia: mechanisms, management, and prevention. *Br J Anaesth*. 2009;102(6):739-748.
3. Bernards CM, Hostetter LS. Epidural and spinal anesthesia. In: Barash PG, Cullen BF, Stoelting RK, et al, eds. *Clinical Anesthesia*. 7th ed. Philadelphia: Lippincott; 2013:905-936.

46. Correct answer: A

After inguinal hernia repair, patients can develop chronic groin pain. The cause of the pain is not clear, but it is believed to occur from entrapment of the ilioinguinal, iliohypogastric, or genital branch of the genitofemoral nerve in the sutures, mesh, or scar tissue. Preservation of the latter of these nerves has been suggested to be a way to prevent pain. A nerve block of the genitofemoral nerve (arises from L1 and L2) can be used to both diagnose and treat this problem. (Frequently a combination of local anesthetic and steroid is used.)

The LFCN also runs under the inguinal ligament but gives sensation to the anterolateral thigh. Compression or injury to this nerve can cause meralgia paresthetica, or paresthesia, numbness, or pain in the anterolateral thigh. Risks for development of this condition include obesity, diabetes, and wearing tight garments around the waist.

A TAP block is done both for postoperative pain control and also for some chronic pain conditions, such as anterior cutaneous nerve entrapment syndrome, which is the most common cause of chronic abdominal wall pain. This block is effective in the T7-T12 dermatomes. To do this block, an ultrasound probe is placed lateral to the rectus sheath so that all 3 layers of the abdominal muscles can be visualized (viz., external oblique, internal oblique, and transversus abdominus). Local anesthetic or a combination of steroid plus local anesthetic is then injected between the fascial layer of the internal oblique and transversus abdominis. A TAP block would not cover this patient's area of pain.

A pudendal nerve block can be done for pudendal neuralgia or pain in the area of the external genitals, anus and perineum. This condition is thought to result from pudendal nerve entrapment. The pudendal nerve arises from S2, S3, and S4. This nerve passes between the piriformis and coccygeus muscle, crosses over the lateral aspect of the sacrospinous ligament, and then reenters the pelvis through the lesser sciatic foramen. It would be unlikely to be injured during an inguinal hernia repair.

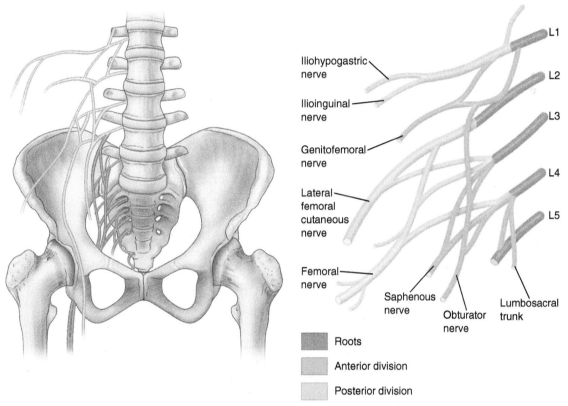

(From Anderson MK, Parr GP. *Foundations of Athletic Training: Prevention, Assessment, and Management.* 5th ed. Philadelphia: Lippincott Williams & Wilkins; 2013, with permission.)

References:
1. Aroori S, Spence RAJ. Chronic pain after hernia surgery–an informed consent issue. *Ulster Med J.* 2007;76(3):136-140.
2. Sahoo RK, Nair AS. Ultrasound guided transversus abdominis plane block for anterior cutaneous nerve entrapment syndrome. *Korean J Pain.* 2015;28(4):284-286.

47. **Correct answer: D**

The pudendal nerve arises from the S2-S4 nerve roots. It supplies sensation to external genitalia and also motor fibers to the external anal and urethral sphincters. It can be injured during vaginal delivery or by blunt trauma such as from a bicycle seat. Once the pudendal nerve is formed from S2-S4, it first travels through the greater sciatic foramen, below the piriformis muscles, and then exits the gluteal region via the lesser sciatic foramen (between the sacrotuberous and sacrospinous ligaments). It then enters the pudendal canal, which lies on the obturator fascia.

Compression or entrapment of the pudendal nerve or its branches is typically between the sacrospinous and sacrotuberous ligaments, inside the Alcock canal or across the inner margin of the falciform process (part of the sacrotuberous ligament). A nerve block of this nerve can be diagnostic and potentially therapeutic for pudendal neuralgia.

The nerve that travels through the deep inguinal ring is the genitofemoral nerve. It can be compressed at this location and cause pain over the groin that may extend into the genital region.

References:

1. Aroori S, Spence RAJ. Chronic pain after hernia surgery–an informed consent issue. *Ulster Med J.* 2007;76(3):136-140.
2. Filippiadis DK, Velonakis G, Mazioti A. CT-guided percutaneous infiltration for the treatment of Alcock's neuralgia. *Pain.* 2011;14(2):211-215.
3. Bendtsen TF, Parras T, Moriggl B, et al. Ultrasound-guided pudendal nerve block at the entrance of the pudendal (Alcock) canal. *Reg Anesth Pain Med.* 2016;41(2):140-145.

48. **Correct answer: A**

The superficial cervical plexus contains nerves that arise from C1 to C4. These nerves travel deep to the superficial cervical fascia (which surrounds the sternocleidomastoid muscle) and can be blocked at this location at approximately the midpoint of the sternocleidomastoid. A risk of this block is an almost 100% chance of ipsilateral diaphragmatic palsy. For most patients this will not pose a problem. However, for patients with hemidiaphragmatic elevation on the contralateral side or severe underlying lung disease, this block should not be performed.

A greater auricular nerve block is purely a sensory block that is performed anteriorly to the tragus. There is no known risk of phrenic nerve palsy with this block. Infraclavicular blocks are used for surgery of the arm (but not the shoulder). The risk of phrenic nerve block is much lower than with blocks performed higher in the neck such as an interscalene block. Finally, an axillary nerve block is performed at the level of the nerves near the axilla. The phrenic nerve does not travel here.

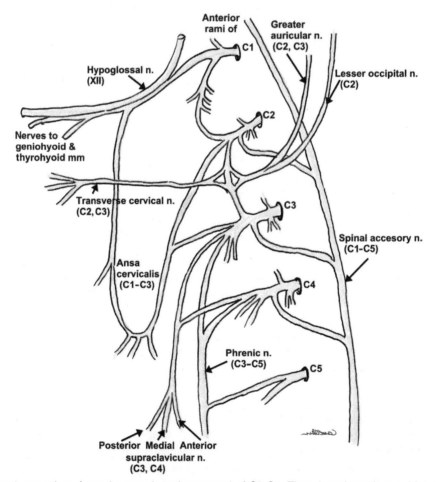

Note how the plexus arises from the anterior primary rami of C2-C4. The motor branches, which include the phrenic nerve, usually travel anteriorly around the anterior scalene muscle. (From Tsui BCH, Rosenquist RW. Peripheral nerve blockade. In: Barash PG, Cullen BF, Stoelting RK, et al, eds. *Clinical Anesthesia.* Philadelphia: Wolters Kluwer Health; 2015:952, with permission.)

References:

1. Pandit JJ, Satya-Krishna R, Gration P. Superficial or deep cervical plexus block for carotid endarterectomy: a systematic review of complications. *Br J Anaesth*. 2007;99(2):159-169.
2. Tsui BCH, Rosenquist RW. Peripheral nerve blockade. In: Barash PG, Cullen BF, Stoelting RK, et al, eds. *Clinical Anesthesia*. 7th ed. Philadelphia: Lippincott; 2013:937-995.

49. Correct answer: A

TENS is a relatively safe therapy for pain that can be used easily by patients at home. Pads are applied over the painful area and provide stimulation in different patterns and at different frequencies. Unfortunately, no large trials have shown major benefits of TENS therapy. It has not been shown to improve the level of disability because of back pain, and more research is needed to see whether it is effective or cost-effective. However, given that it is safe and seems to help some patients, it is worth considering in patients with chronic pain.

References:

1. Nnoaham KE, Kumbang J. Transcutaneous electrical nerve stimulation (TENS) for chronic pain. *Cochrane Database Syst Rev*. 2008;(3):CD003222.
2. Khadilkar A, Odebiyi DO, Brosseau L, Wells GA. Transcutaneous electrical nerve stimulation (TENS) versus placebo for chronic low-back pain. *Cochrane Database Syst Rev*. 2008;(4):CD003008.

50. Correct Answer: C

Peripheral neuropathies are common in type 1 diabetics occurring in approximately 65% of this patient population. Distal symmetric polyneuropathies are the most common neuropathy, afflicting diabetics followed by median nerve neuropathy and visceral autonomic neuropathy. Several factors are associated with the occurrence of diabetic painful neuropathy. These include duration of diabetes, age, and degree of hyperglycemia. In general, neuropathies occur after several years of persistent hyperglycemia because the pathophysiology of this disease involves glycosylation end products and microvascular changes, which eventually lead to nerve ischemia.

Treatment includes tight glucose control in conjunction with pharmacologic interventions. Both gabapentin and pregabalin are effective in the treatment of diabetic painful neuropathy as are tricyclic antidepressants. Selective serotonin reuptake inhibitors have not been found to be effective, whereas newer norepinephrine-serotonin reuptake inhibitors have been found to be a good treatment modality and in fact are considered by some to be a first-line treatment option.

Reference:

1. Benzon HT, Hurley RW, Deer T, Buvanendran A. Chronic pain management. In: Barash PG, Cullen BF, Stoelting RK, et al, eds. *Clinical Anesthesia*. 7th ed. Philadelphia: Lippincott; 2013:1645-1671.

14

PEDIATRIC ANESTHESIA

Mara Kenger

1. A 42-day-old infant is brought to the operating room (OR) for repair of hypertrophic pyloric stenosis. After appropriate rapid sequence induction and intubation of the trachea, the surgeons begin the procedure. One hour into the procedure you notice that the infant's body temperature has dropped from 37°C to 35.5°C. Which of the following is the LEAST effective method of maintaining thermal homeostasis in an infant?

   A. Raising the room temperature from 24°C to 29°C
   B. Running maintenance IV fluids through a fluid warmer
   C. Wrapping the infant's head in plastic
   D. Applying a forced-air warming device to exposed body areas
   E. Using a circulating warm-water mattress

2. When considering premedication with midazolam in the pediatric patient, all of the following are true EXCEPT which one?

   A. Midazolam's fast onset of action is due to its water insolubility.
   B. Midazolam can be administered via the oral, nasal, intramuscular (IM), buccal, intravenous (IV), and rectal routes.
   C. As age decreases, required midazolam dose in mg/kg for effective anxiolysis increases.
   D. Oral midazolam has a bioavailability of 30% compared with IV administration.
   E. Time to peak plasma concentration of rectally administered midazolam is 15-20 minutes.

3. Of the various types of Mapleson circuits, which one has the fresh gas inflow furthest from the patient/T-piece?

   A. Mapleson A
   B. Mapleson B
   C. Mapleson C
   D. Mapleson D
   E. Mapleson E

4. Of the various types of Mapleson circuits, which has a spring-loaded pop-off valve located at the distal end of the circuit (furthest from the patient/T-piece?)

   A. Mapleson A
   B. Mapleson B
   C. Mapleson C
   D. Mapleson D
   E. Mapleson E

5. The Bain modification is a coaxial circuit where fresh gas flows through an inner tube through the corrugated reservoir tubing of which Mapleson circuit?

   A. Mapleson A
   B. Mapleson B
   C. Mapleson C
   D. Mapleson D
   E. Mapleson E

6. All of the following are acceptable agents for induction of anesthesia in children EXCEPT which one?

   A. Sevoflurane
   B. Ketamine
   C. Halothane
   D. Desflurane
   E. Methohexital

7. When evaluating a 4-month-old for elective circumcision revision in the preoperative area, the patient's mother tells you that she fed the child expressed breastmilk fortified with formula powder 3.5 hours ago. According to the ASA NPO status guidelines, how many hours must pass between this feeding and the induction of general anesthesia?

   A. 2 hours
   B. 4 hours
   C. 6 hours
   D. 8 hours
   E. 12 hours

The following vignette applies to questions 8, 9, and 10.

A 2-year-old, 12.5-kg girl with history of a ventriculoperitoneal shunt that was placed in infancy for congenital aqueductal stenosis presents to your OR for emergent shunt revision in the setting of lethargy, vomiting, and irritability. Her parents tell you she "ate some crackers" 2 hours ago. The patient is otherwise healthy with no known drug allergies.

8. The MOST appropriate medication and dosage for neuromuscular blockade for rapid sequence intubation in this patient is which of the following?

   A. Rocuronium 10 mg IV
   B. Rocuronium 25 mg IV
   C. Succinylcholine 12.5 mg IV
   D. Succinylcholine 25 mg IV
   E. Succinylcholine 25 mg IM

9. The MOST appropriate blade and endotracheal tube for this patient would be which of the following?

   A. Miller 1 blade, size 4.0 uncuffed endotracheal tube
   B. Miller 1 blade, size 4.0 cuffed endotracheal tube
   C. Miller 1 blade, size 4.5 cuffed endotracheal tube
   D. Wis-Hipple 1.5 blade, size 4.0 cuffed endotracheal tube
   E. Wis-Hipple 1.5 blade, size 5.0 uncuffed endotracheal tube

10. After successful intubation and initiation of general anesthesia, you decide you would like to attempt to decrease the patient's chance of emergence excitation. With that in mind, which of the following would be the least appropriate choice for maintenance anesthesia?

   A. Desflurane at 0.5 minimum alveolar concentration (MAC), dexmedetomidine infusion at 0.5 μg/kg/h
   B. Propofol and fentanyl total IV anesthesia
   C. Sevoflurane at 1.0 MAC, oxygen, and air
   D. Isoflurane at 1.0 MAC, oxygen, and air
   E. Ketamine infusion, 50% nitrous oxide/50% oxygen

11. **At what age is MAC of isoflurane the highest?**

    A. Newborn
    B. 6 months of age
    C. 12 months of age
    D. 2 years of age
    E. 5 years of age

12. **One MAC of isoflurane in a neonate equates to what percentage of end-tidal isoflurane concentration?**

    A. 0.9
    B. 1.1
    C. 1.3
    D. 1.6
    E. 2.2

13. **When considering the relative ED95 in µg/kg of nondepolarizing neuromuscular blocking drugs (NMBDs), the impact of age on relative pharmacodynamics is which of the following?**

    A. Neonates require less than children who require less than adults.
    B. Neonates require more than children who require more than adults.
    C. Neonates require more than children, but children require less than adults.
    D. Neonates require less than children, but children require more than adults.

14. **The estimated circulating blood volume of a 4-kg, full-term neonate is which of the following?**

    A. 200 mL
    B. 240 mL
    C. 340 mL
    D. 420 mL
    E. 480 mL

15. **The benefits of leukoreduction of donor blood products include all of the following EXCEPT which one?**

    A. Prevention of cytomegalovirus transmission
    B. Prevention of nonhemolytic febrile transfusion reactions
    C. Prevention of graft-versus-host disease
    D. Prevention of human leukocyte antigen alloimmunization

16. **A 2500-g infant is born at approximately 35 weeks' gestation to a woman who had received minimal prenatal care. Shortly after birth, the infant is noted to be tachypneic with respiratory rates in the 60s, an Spo$_2$ of 85%, and a heart rate of 180 beats per minute. A concave abdomen is noted, and breath sounds are minimal in the left thorax but present on the right. A chest X-ray demonstrates a mediastinal shift to the right and loops of bowel in the thorax. Which of the following is the best initial management of this infant's airway?**

    A. Application of continuous positive airway pressure (CPAP), with ventilation goals titrated to an ETco$_2$ of 35-40 mm Hg
    B. Application of CPAP, with ventilation goals titrated to an ETco$_2$ of 40-45 mm Hg
    C. Intubation and pressure control ventilation, with ventilation goals titrated to ETco$_2$ of 40-45 mm Hg
    D. Intubation and pressure support ventilation with permissive hypercapnia and peak inspiratory pressures <25 cm H$_2$0
    E. Spontaneous ventilation with high-flow oxygen therapy via nasal cannula

The following vignette applies to questions 17, 18, and 19.

A 37-week infant is born uneventfully to a 39-year-old G3P2002 mother via normal spontaneous vaginal delivery. He is noted to have small palpebral fissures and mild hypotonia. 24 hours after birth, the infant has repeated vomiting of bilious emesis.

17. **Which of the following is the most likely cause of the emesis?**

    A. Pyloric stenosis
    B. Duodenal atresia
    C. Choanal atresia
    D. Necrotizing enterocolitis
    E. Intussusception

18. **Which of the following is the most common radiologic finding that would be seen in this infant during workup for bilious emesis?**

    A. Gastric bubble above the diaphragm
    B. Multiple dilated loops of bowel
    C. Pneumatosis
    D. "Double-bubble" sign on X-ray
    E. Target sign on abdominal ultrasonography

19. **The patient undergoes successful surgical repair in the neonatal period. At 6 months of age he returns for an esophagogastroduodenoscopy. He has appropriately fasted, and an inhalational induction is planned. While your resident is managing the airway, you attempt to place an IV. The patient slightly withdraws to the needle, so your resident increases the inhaled sevoflurane concentration from 4% to 8% to aid with depth of anesthesia. The most likely hemodynamic response to this would be which of the following?**

    A. Hypotension
    B. Tachycardia
    C. Bradycardia
    D. Decreased respiratory rate
    E. Increased tidal volume

20. **Compared with adults, infants desaturate more quickly during induction of anesthesia because of which of the following?**

    A. Increased respiratory rate
    B. Increased cardiac output in mL/kg/min
    C. Decreased O_2 consumption in mL/kg/min compared with adults
    D. Decreased closing capacity
    E. Decreased functional residual capacity (FRC) in mL/kg

21. **A 14-week-old infant, who was born at 36 weeks' gestational age, presents for elective repair of a right-sided inguinal hernia. He is otherwise healthy and does not have any known allergies, and his parents have not noted any symptoms that would indicate a recent upper respiratory tract infection. The infant did not spend any time in the NICU and has never had an apneic or bradycardic spell. The surgeon asks you about the patient's disposition after surgery. Which of the following is true?**

    A. Preterm infants who are less than 60 weeks' postconceptual age (PCA) need to undergo extended apnea monitoring after general anesthesia but not after light sedation with a natural airway.
    B. This patient does not have a history of apnea or bradycardia and therefore does not meet criteria for postanesthetic admission for apnea monitoring.
    C. This patient will need to be admitted for apnea monitoring after general anesthesia with the requirement that 24 hours of apnea-free time elapse before discharge.
    D. Spinal and regional anesthesia without supplemental sedation does not abolish the need for postoperative apnea monitoring in former preterm infants less than 60 weeks' PCA.
    E. Prophylactic administration of caffeine is recommended for this patient after general anesthesia to prevent apnea.

22. Of the following pediatric surgical patients, which one would have the lowest risk of postoperative nausea and vomiting (PONV)?

   A. A 3-year-old undergoing open reduction of a radial fracture
   B. A 16-year-old undergoing hernia repair
   C. A 5-year-old undergoing strabismus repair
   D. An 8-year-old undergoing tonsillectomy
   E. A 12-year-old undergoing orchiopexy

23. All of the following are efficacious in preventing and managing PONV in children EXCEPT which one?

   A. Intraoperative fluid restriction
   B. Ondansetron
   C. Dexamethasone
   D. Total IV anesthesia with propofol
   E. Postoperative oral fluid restriction

24. Considerations in anesthetizing a neonate with meningomyelocele include which of the following?

   A. It is necessary to avoid succinylcholine because these patients are at higher risk for hyperkalemia.
   B. There is high likelihood of a difficult airway.
   C. Evaporative heat and fluid loss through the defect results in hypothermia and hypovolemia.
   D. Defect should be repaired within 12 hours of birth to avoid infection and worsening neurologic damage.
   E. Cardiac anomalies are commonly present.

25. A 12-day-old, 875-g infant born at 25 weeks' gestational age is brought to the OR for exploratory laparotomy for concern for necrotizing enterocolitis. The patient's vital signs on entry to the OR are notable for HR 160, RR 40, SPo$_2$ of 98%, and BP 70/40. The patient has appropriate IV access, and the decision is made to do an awake intubation after administration of 1 μg/kg of fentanyl. The laryngoscopy is more difficult than anticipated, but successful tracheal intubation occurs within 60 seconds. Despite this, the infant desaturates during laryngoscopy from 98% to 65%. The Spo$_2$ recovers with gentle positive pressure ventilation. With regard to the respiratory mechanics and anatomy of the newborn as compared with adults, which of the following is false?

   A. Tidal volumes in mL/kg are decreased compared with adults.
   B. FRC is equal in neonates and adults.
   C. Neonates have a higher rate of O$_2$ consumption in mL/kg/min.
   D. Neonates have a higher closing capacity than adults.
   E. Neonates have a decreased total lung capacity (TLC) in mL/kg compared with adults.

The following vignette pertains to questions 26 and 27.

   A 3-year-old, 16-kg unvaccinated child presents to the emergency department with fever, dysphagia, and drooling. His parents attempted herbal remedies for his fever and sought medical evaluation once he started drooling out of fear that he had been accidentally poisoned by the herbs. Vital signs include HR 120, BP 90/50, RR 40, Spo$_2$ 98%, and T 39.8°C. On examination the patient is in visible respiratory distress, drooling, and sitting leaning forward on one arm.

26. Which of the following is the most likely diagnosis?

   A. Fifth disease
   B. Pneumonia
   C. Foreign body ingestion
   D. Epiglottitis
   E. Coxsackie virus

27. The emergency department physicians decide that the child needs a secure airway, given that he is rapidly decompensating from a respiratory standpoint. The best strategy for airway management in this patient would be which of the following?

    A. Immediate placement of an IV in the emergency department followed by rapid sequence intubation with pediatric anesthesia on standby
    B. IM ketamine and glycopyrrolate, followed by IV placement and intubation in the emergency department with pediatric anesthesiology on standby
    C. Expedited transfer to the OR with pediatric anesthesiologists followed by rapid sequence intubation with succinylcholine, propofol, and fentanyl
    D. Expedited transfer to the OR, inhalational induction, and direct laryngoscopy with rigid bronchoscope and surgical personnel present on standby

28. A 7-day-old, 3.5-kg neonate with severe coarctation of the aorta has failed percutaneously repair in the catheterization laboratory and comes to the OR for an open repair. In addition to placing noninvasive blood pressure cuffs on both upper and lower extremities to monitor precoarctation and postcoarctation blood pressures, where should the pulse oximeter probe be placed in this patient?

    A. Right upper extremity
    B. Right lower extremity
    C. Left upper extremity
    D. Left lower extremity

29. An 18-month-old, 12-kg child with hypoplastic left heart syndrome is following a Norwood procedure at day 4 of life and a bidirectional Glenn (BDG) shunt at the age of 6 months. She is returning now for a Fontan procedure. During induction, her O_2 saturation falls from baseline of 90% to 75% where it remains after successful placement of an endotracheal tube. Which of the following interventions would be least helpful in improving oxygen delivery in this patient?

    A. 10 mL/kg crystalloid bolus
    B. Hypoventilation, 100% oxygen
    C. Transfusion of whole blood to achieve hematocrit of 39% from 33%
    D. Hyperventilation with 100% oxygen

30. A 3-year-old, 16-kg boy with unrepaired tetralogy of Fallot is presenting to the OR for repair. Preinduction vitals are BP 88/52, HR 100, and SpO_2 90%. He receives sevoflurane and nitrous oxide for induction of anesthesia, followed by IV placement and rocuronium. Airway placement is unexpectedly difficult, and the patient's vitals after successful intubation are BP 69/40, HR 135, and SpO_2 60% and falling, despite confirmation of $ETCO_2$ and bilateral breath sounds. Which of the following would be an appropriate pharmacologic intervention?

    A. Phenylephrine
    B. Ephedrine
    C. Lasix
    D. Epinephrine

31. Which of the following conditions seen in pediatric patients confers the lowest risk for development of hyperkalemia after succinylcholine administration?

    A. Central core disease
    B. Duchenne muscular dystrophy
    C. Spastic paraplegia
    D. 10% total-body surface area burns
    E. Werdnig-Hoffman syndrome (spinal muscular atrophy type 1)

32. A 5-year-old, 20-kg boy comes to the OR for laparoscopic appendectomy in the setting of acute appendicitis. He is otherwise healthy with no known allergies, and he takes no medications. Surgery is uneventful, and before emergence you administer 10 mg of ketorolac and 2 mg of morphine IV for analgesia. Compared with an adult, the clearance of morphine in this patient is which of the following?

    A. Less
    B. Equal
    C. Greater
    D. Cannot be determined

33. A 6-month-old male infant, who was born healthy at full term, is presenting for bilateral herniorrhaphy. His parents have read recent warnings about exposure to general anesthesia in infants and inquire about other anesthetic techniques available for this procedure. You decide to administer a spinal anesthetic. In infants, the spinal cord terminates at which of the following?

    A. T12
    B. L1
    C. L3
    D. L4

34. You are administering anesthesia to a healthy 14-month-old girl for an inguinal herniorrhaphy. You decide to perform a caudal epidural block for postoperative analgesia. The proper level of needle entry for a caudal block is which of the following?

    A. At the center of a line drawn connecting the posterior-superior iliac spines
    B. At the cornua of the sacral hiatus
    C. Between the sacrum and coccyx, piercing the sacrococcygeal ligament
    D. 1 cm above the crease of the buttocks

35. According to ASA practice guidelines, all of the following are required before discharge to home from the postanesthesia care unit (PACU) EXCEPT which one?

    A. Return to baseline level of consciousness
    B. Nausea/vomiting adequately controlled
    C. Pain adequately controlled with oral analgesics
    D. Patient's ability to void
    E. Stable blood pressure and heart rate

36. You are caring for an ex-25-week, 1-kg premature infant at 6 days of life who has necrotizing enterocolitis. You are concerned about the risk for retinopathy of prematurity in this very premature infant. To reduce his risk of developing this complication, your goals for management of his vital signs include which of the following?

    A. $Spo_2 > 94\%$ with no greater than 50% Fio_2
    B. Spo_2 90%-94% with the minimum Fio_2 necessary to achieve stable Spo_2
    C. Permissive hypercapnia with $ETco_2$ goals of 42-47 mm Hg
    D. Normotension, mean arterial pressure > 60 mm Hg
    E. Normotension, mean arterial pressure > 50 mm Hg

37. An infant is born at 38 weeks with omphalocele and macroglossia. Birth weight is 4500 g. Which of the following is the most likely diagnosis?

    A. Beckwith-Wiedemann syndrome
    B. Angelman syndrome
    C. Treacher-Collins syndrome
    D. Hurler syndrome
    E. Trisomy 21

38. **A 1-year-old child has mandibular hypoplasia, macrostomia, and cleft palate. His airway is expected to become more difficult with age. Which of the following is the most likely diagnosis?**

   A. Beckwith-Wiedemann syndrome
   B. Angelman syndrome
   C. Treacher-Collins syndrome
   D. Hurler syndrome
   E. Trisomy 21

39. **Of the following syndromes, which one typically causes cognitive impairment, skeletal abnormalities, short stature, cardiac disease, and restrictive lung disease and is considered to present one of the greatest airway challenges in pediatric anesthesia because of the progressive craniofacial anomalies that can make both intubation and mask ventilation extremely challenging?**

   A. Beckwith-Wiedemann syndrome
   B. Angelman syndrome
   C. Treacher-Collins syndrome
   D. Hurler syndrome
   E. Trisomy 21

40. **Which of the following is the most common type of tracheoesophageal fistula (TEF) seen in neonates?**

   A. Esophageal atresia with a blind esophageal pouch and a distal TEF
   B. TEF in the absence of esophageal atresia
   C. Proximal TEF with proximal esophageal pouch ending distal to the fistula
   D. Esophageal atresia with 2 TEFs, one each between the proximal and distal esophagus and the trachea

41. **Which of the following scenarios would be least appropriate for a parent-present induction of anesthesia?**

   A. An anxious 4-year-old girl here for tonsillectomy with her mother, who is tearful but cooperative
   B. A crying 7-year-old for unilateral orchiopexy here with his father, who states he prefers to be with his son when he goes to sleep
   C. A 5-month-old girl for diagnostic MRI under general anesthesia here with her mother, who is an anesthesiologist
   D. A 17-year-old boy with Down syndrome for general anesthesia in the cardiac catheterization suite here with his mother, who attends all of his medical appointments

42. **A woman who has received little prenatal care presents in labor with a frank breech fetus. Fetal age is estimated by ultrasonography to be 33 weeks. Her labor proves unstoppable and she undergoes an emergency cesarean delivery. A live-born, 2-kg female infant is delivered. Shortly after the birth, the infant is noted to have grunting, nasal flaring, and retractions. Cardiac examination is within normal limits. There are no structural abnormalities noted, and oral secretions are of the usual amount. Which of the following radiologic findings is/are most likely on chest X-ray of this infant?**

   A. Lung hyperinflation with diaphragmatic flattening and layering of fluid in horizontal lung fissures
   B. Diffuse ground-glass opacities and reduced lung volumes
   C. Loops of bowel in the left thorax with mediastinal shift to the right
   D. Right-sided pneumothorax
   E. Pulmonary edema

43. An 8-year-old, 45-kg girl with severe obstructive sleep apnea (OSA) presents for tonsillectomy and adenoidectomy. She has an uneventful inhalational induction and is intubated after IV placement and administration of propofol, rocuronium, and 50 μg of fentanyl. Intraoperatively, she receives 500 mg of IV Tylenol and 2 mg of IV morphine. At the end of her procedure she is extubated uneventfully and brought to the recovery room. Approximately 2 hours later, she begins to complain of pain. Which of the following is the most appropriate analgesic choice for her?

   A. 500 mg of PO Tylenol elixir
   B. 30 mg of IV ketorolac
   C. 25 μg of IV fentanyl
   D. 5 mg of IV morphine
   E. 1 mg of IV hydromorphone

44. The P50 of fetal hemoglobin is which of the following?

   A. 15
   B. 20
   C. 27
   D. 32

45. With regard to the fetal circulatory system, which of the following sites will possess the most oxygenated blood?

   A. The inferior vena cava (IVC)
   B. The superior vena cava (SVC)
   C. The right atrium
   D. The left atrium
   E. The aorta

46. A 6-year-old girl who has been diagnosed with a Wilms tumor presents to the OR for resection. You obtain consent from the parents for epidural placement to aid with postoperative analgesia. The safest technique for placement of a thoracic epidural in this age group is which of the following?

   A. Awake with minimal sedation, in the seated position, using the paramedian approach
   B. Under general anesthesia, in the right lateral decubitus position, using the paramedian approach
   C. Awake with moderate sedation, in the seated position, using the midline approach
   D. Under general anesthesia, in the right lateral decubitus position, using the midline approach

47. A 10-year-old, 40-kg boy is involved in a motor vehicle accident along with his parents. He is transported by ambulance to the emergency department after intubation in the field for decreased level of consciousness and hypotension. He is found in the emergency department to have a rigid abdomen concerning for intra-abdominal hemorrhage and is brought emergently to the OR for exploratory laparotomy. His father, who was injured minorly in the crash, accompanies him to the preoperative area and says to you as you take the patient into the OR, "We are Jehovah's Witnesses. He is not to receive blood transfusions." During the case, the patient is hypotensive with BP 60/30, HR 130, and Spo$_2$ 94%. Upon entry to the abdomen, 500 mL of frank blood is appreciated. An arterial blood gas is obtained, which shows a hematocrit of 20% with ongoing blood loss. The most appropriate course of action in this case is which of the following?

   A. Begin fluid resuscitation with nonblood products, including crystalloid and nonhuman colloid.
   B. Call the hospital lawyer to obtain an emergency court order to transfuse blood.
   C. Consult the hospital Ethics Committee.
   D. Transfuse blood.
   E. Ask a colleague to go discuss with the parents that without permitting blood transfusion, their child will die.

48. **Differences in required dosing of propofol between children and adults can be attributed to which of the following?**

    A. Increased clearance of propofol in children
    B. Larger volume of distribution in children
    C. More rapid redistribution of propofol from vessel-rich organs in children
    D. A and B
    E. B and C

49. **Dexmedetomidine can be safely used in children for all of the following situations EXCEPT which one?**

    A. Prevention of emergence delirium
    B. Treatment of opioid withdrawal
    C. As an analgesic adjunct
    D. Induction of general anesthesia with a loading dose of 2-4 µg/kg over 10 minutes
    E. Procedural sedation

50. **When administering sedation outside the OR, which of the following corresponds to a plane of moderate sedation?**

    A. Normal response to verbal stimuli; patent-unassisted airway
    B. Responsive to touch or verbal stimuli; may require assistance to maintain patency of airway
    C. Responsive to touch or verbal stimuli; patent-unassisted airway
    D. Purposeful response to painful stimuli but not verbal stimuli; patent-unassisted airway
    E. No response to painful stimuli; requires assistance to maintain patency of airway

Chapter 14 ▪ Answers

1. Correct answer: B

The impact of warming maintenance IV fluids in a neonate on thermal homeostasis is minimal. The volume of fluid warmed is small, and heat is lost during circulation of the small volume of fluid through the length of IV tubing, thereby rendering the effect ineffective. Raising the room temperature (A) is an effective means of preventing radiant heat loss, which accounts for most of the heat loss seen under anesthesia in infants (40%). Both forced-air warming blankets (D) and wrapping the child (C) are effective at preventing both radiant and convective heat loss, with forced-air warming blankets being the best strategy for maintaining thermal regulation in infants. Warm-water circulating mattresses are effective for small infants and children, preventing conductive heat loss. However, as conduction only accounts for a small amount of heat loss (5%) under anesthesia, this is less effective than other methods and is generally only effective in children <10 kg.

Reference:

1. Gazal EA, Mason LJ, Cote CJ. Preoperative evaluation, premedication and induction of anesthesia. In: Cote CJ, Lerman J, Anderson BJ, eds. A Practice of Anesthesia for Infants and Children. 5th ed. Philadelphia: Elsevier Saunders; 2013:31–63.

2. Correct answer: A

Midazolam is a water-soluble drug that exists as water-soluble salts at pH <4 but exists as a highly lipophilic closed ring at pH >4 (including physiologic pH 7.4). Its rapid onset of action is due to its ability to convert to the lipophilic form at higher pH.

Midazolam can be administered by multiple effective routes (B) with variable bioavailbilities and time to onset.

Similar to MAC, as age decreases, the effective dose of midazolam in mg/kg increases, with younger children requiring higher doses for adequate anxiolysis and sedation. This is due in part to the increased volume of distribution in younger children and increased clearance.

The bioavailability of oral midazolam (D) is 30%; rectal ~40%-50%; intranasal 60%; IM 90%.

Time to peak plasma concentrations (E) after rectal administration is ~15 minutes. After intranasal administration, it is ~10 minutes and after oral administration, it is ~50 minutes, although sedation and anxiolysis begin to occur within about 15-20 minutes.

References:

1. Gazal EA, Mason LJ, Cote CJ. Preoperative evaluation, premedication and induction of anesthesia. In: Cote CJ, Lerman J, Anderson BJ, eds. A Practice of Anesthesia for Infants and Children. 5th ed. Philadelphia: Elsevier Saunders; 2013:31–63.
2. Kanto JH. Midazolam: the first water-soluble benzodiazepine. Pharmacology, pharmacokinetics and efficacy in insomnia and anesthesia. *Pharmacotherapy*. 1985;5(3):138-155.

3. Correct answer: A

The Mapleson A circuit has the fresh gas inflow at the end of the reservoir tubing, distal from the T-piece that connects to the patient's mask, or endotracheal tube. The Mapleson B, C, D, and E circuits all have fresh gas inflow more proximal to the T-piece.

References:

1. Riutort KT, Eisenkraft JB. The anesthesia work station and delivery systems for inhaled anesthetics. In: Barash PG, Cullen BF, Stoelting RK, Calahan MK, Stock C, Ortega R, eds. Clinical Anesthesia. 7th ed. Philadelphia: Lippincott; 2013:641–698.
2. Dorsch JA, Dorsch SE. Mapleson breathing systems. In: *Understanding Anesthesia Equipment*. 5th ed. Baltimore: Lippincott Williams & Wilkins; 2007:209–222.

4. Correct answer: D

The Mapleson D circuit, from distal to proximal to the patient, consists of a reservoir bag, pop-off valve, length of reservoir/corrugated tubing, fresh gas inflow, and T-piece. The distal pop-off valve allows for excess expired gas to be released during expiration. The Mapleson D circuit is good for both controlled and spontaneous ventilation, preventing rebreathing of CO_2 at a fresh gas flow (FGF) approximately 2× minute ventilation. It is more efficient during controlled ventilation than the Mapleson A circuit, which allows for a large proportion of FGF to leak out of the adjustable pressure-limiting valve during positive pressure ventilation. However, the Mapleson A circuit is the most efficient for spontaneous ventilation, preventing rebreathing of CO_2 at a FGF of only 1× the minute ventilation.

For efficiency during spontaneous ventilation, the Mapleson circuit order is A > BC > DEF. During controlled ventilation, it is the opposite: DEF > BC > A. The Mapleson A circuit requires extremely high FGF during controlled ventilation to prevent rebreathing of gas, approximately 20× the minute ventilation.

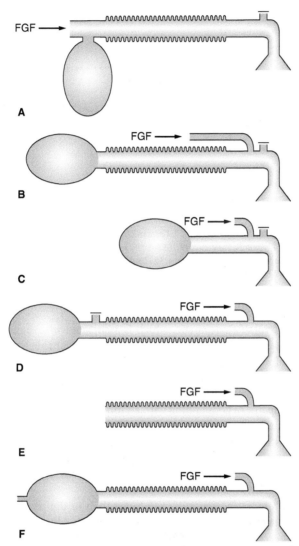

(From Riutort KT, Eisenkraft JB. The anesthesia workstation and delivery systems for inhaled anesthetics. In: Barash PG, Cullen BF, Stoelting RK, et al, eds. *Clinical Anesthesia*. Philadelphia: Wolters Kluwer Health; 2015:672, with permission.)

References:
1. Riutort KT, Eisenkraft JB. The anesthesia work station and delivery systems for inhaled anesthetics. In: Barash PG, Cullen BF, Stoelting RK, Calahan MK, Stock C, Ortega R, eds. Clinical Anesthesia. 7th ed. Philadelphia: Lippincott; 2013:641–698.
2. Dorsch JA, Dorsch SE. Mapleson breathing systems. In: *Understanding Anesthesia Equipment*. 5th ed. Baltimore: Lippincott Williams & Wilkins; 2007:209–222.

5. **Correct answer: D**

The Bain modification is a modified Mapleson D circuit where FGF is delivered via a smaller inner tube running coaxially inside the reservoir tubing. The main advantage of the Bain circuit is that the expired gases inside the reservoir tubing, without mixing with FGF until right before the patient, maintain more heat and humidity within the circuit. For this reason, it is one of the most common semiopen circuits used in neonatal anesthesia. The FGF requirements for preventing nonrebreathing of CO_2 are similar to other systems.

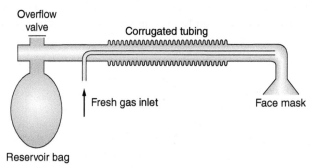

(From Riutort KT, Eisenkraft JB. The anesthesia workstation and delivery systems for inhaled anesthetics. In: Barash PG, Cullen BF, Stoelting RK, et al, eds. *Clinical Anesthesia*. Philadelphia: Wolters Kluwer Health; 2015:673, with permission.)

References:
1. Riutort KT, Eisenkraft JB. The anesthesia work station and delivery systems for inhaled anesthetics. In: Barash PG, Cullen BF, Stoelting RK, Calahan MK, Stock C, Ortega R, eds. Clinical Anesthesia. 7th ed. Philadelphia: Lippincott; 2013:641–698.
2. Blum RH, Cote CJ. Pediatric equipment. In: Cote CJ, Lerman J, Anderson BJ, eds. A Practice of Anesthesia for Infants and Children. 5th ed. Philadelphia: Elsevier Saunders; 2013:1053–1080.
3. Dorsch JA, Dorsch SE. Mapleson breathing systems. In: *Understanding Anesthesia Equipment*. 5th ed. Baltimore: Lippincott Williams & Wilkins; 2007:209–222.

---

6. **Correct answer: D**

Desflurane is a pungent volatile anesthetic, which is associated with significant airway irritability. As such, it increases the likelihood of laryngospasm, making it unsuitable for mask induction in children. Sevoflurane (A) and halothane (C) have both been used successfully for mask induction, with sevoflurane being the most common modern agent used for inhaled induction in children. Sevoflurane, especially when used in conjunction with nitrous oxide, produces a smooth, relatively rapid induction of anesthesia in children capable of cooperating with an inhaled technique.

Ketamine (B) can be administered as an IM injection at 2-4 mg/kg to induce deep sedation/general anesthesia in uncooperative or larger patients who will not tolerate a mask induction or an IV. Onset of sedation is 3-5 minutes when given intramuscularly. The addition of midazolam to the IM injection is commonly used to promote anxiolysis and sedation and prevent nightmares, which can be associated with ketamine administration.

Methohexital (E), while less commonly used today than in the past, can be used intravenously or rectally as an induction agent. Rectally, a dose of 15-25 mg/kg is administered. This method of induction has fallen out of favor because of variability in absorption and bioavailability, as well as the availability of a wider range of medications and induction agents.

References:
1. Lerman J. Pediatric anesthesia. In: Barash PG, Cullen BF, Stoelting RK, Calahan MK, Stock C, Ortega R, eds. Clinical Anesthesia. 7th ed. Philadelphia: Lippincott; 2013:1216–1256.
2. Gazal EA, Mason LJ, Cote CJ. Preoperative evaluation, premedication and induction of anesthesia. In: Cote CJ, Lerman J, Anderson BJ, eds. A Practice of Anesthesia for Infants and Children. 5th ed. Philadelphia: Elsevier Saunders; 2013:31–63.

---

7. **Correct answer: C**

Although breastmilk is considered easier to digest than cow's milk-based formulas and therefore has a recommended NPO interval of just 4 hours, formula ingestion mandates an NPO interval of 6 hours between ingestion and induction of anesthesia to be properly fasted. This scenario is unusual because although most of the feeding was breastmilk, the addition of formula powder to fortify the breastmilk makes this feeding more akin to a formula feeding in terms of digestibility and gastric transit time. Thus, the appropriate NPO interval is 6 hours.

Clear liquids can be ingested up to 2 hours before induction of anesthesia. A light meal (toast with no fat) can be ingested up to 6 hours before anesthesia. Solids or fatty food mandates an 8-hour NPO time.

References:

1. Gazal EA, Mason LJ, Cote CJ. Preoperative evaluation, premedication and induction of anesthesia. In: Cote CJ, Lerman J, Anderson BJ, eds. A Practice of Anesthesia for Infants and Children. 5th ed. Philadelphia: Elsevier Saunders; 2013:31–63.
2. Practice guidelines for preoperative fasting and the use of pharmacologic agents to reduce the risk of pulmonary aspiration: application to healthy patients undergoing elective procedures. *Anesthesiology.* 2011;114:495-511.

8. Correct answer: D

The rapid sequence intubation dose of succinylcholine, which is the most appropriate choice for intubation in a patient with full stomach for emergent surgery, is dosed at 2 mg/kg intravenously for young children. The adult dose of 1 mg/kg intravenously (C) is incorrect because children have a larger volume of distribution and therefore require higher doses. Although there are concerns in the pediatric population about unknown muscular dystrophy diagnoses causing exaggerated hyperkalemia and rhabdomyolysis with succinylcholine administration, one should remember that muscular dystrophies are more common in males (this patient is female), and in most cases of a full stomach, the benefit of a rapid onset of muscle relaxation is greater than the risk. When there is no IV access or IV access is lost during induction, succinylcholine can be administered intramuscularly at 4 mg/kg for young children (5 mg/kg in infants). At large doses of succinylcholine, or with a second dose, preemptive atropine or glycopyrrolate can mitigate the bradycardia often seen.

In cases of known contraindication to succinylcholine, such as spinal cord injury with immobility or severe burns, rocuronium (1.2 mg/kg) can provide similar intubating conditions as succinylcholine, in about 30 seconds. For this patient, 10 mg (A) would be too small a dose for effective rapid sequence intubation and 25 mg (B) would be too large.

Reference:

1. Gazal EA, Mason LJ, Cote CJ. Preoperative evaluation, premedication and induction of anesthesia. In: Cote CJ, Lerman J, Anderson BJ, eds. A Practice of Anesthesia for Infants and Children. 5th ed. Philadelphia: Elsevier Saunders; 2013:31–63.

9. Correct answer: D

Although blade selection is somewhat operator-dependent, some general guidelines for intubating the pediatric patient are as follows:
- Premature neonate: Miller 0 (or Miller 00)
- Neonate/infant under age 1 year: Miller 1
- Toddler age 1-3 years: Wis-Hipple 1.5
- Preschooler age 3-5 years: Mac 2

Tube size selection can be performed using Cole formula: (Age + 16)/4 or (Age/4) + 4. This calculates the recommended uncuffed endotracheal tube size. Most pediatric anesthesiologists will size down 0.5 mm for cuffed endotracheal tubes. Thus, for this patient: (2/4) + 4 = 4.5 uncuffed, 4.0 cuffed. Of course, this formula is merely a guideline, and larger or smaller children will require appropriate adjustments in both blade selection and tube size.

Reference:

1. Everett LL. Anesthesia for children. In: Longnecker D, Brown DL, Newman MF, Zapol W, eds. Anesthesiology. 2nd ed. New York: McGraw-Hill Education; 2012:1185–1193.

10. Correct answer: C

Volatile agents with quick onset and offset of anesthesia, such as sevoflurane and desflurane, are associated with emergence agitation/delirium in children. The mechanism of this is poorly understood. Some hypothesize that it is due to the more rapid emergence from general anesthesia than seen with other agents with longer washout (ie, isoflurane.) The incidence of emergence delirium can be reduced with the use of hypnotic or analgesic agents either intraoperatively or nearing the time of emergence. Agents such as dexmedetomidine, propofol, and fentanyl have been shown to reduce the incidence of emergence delirium. Thus, although A includes desflurane as maintenance anesthesia, the addition of dexmedetomidine to the anesthetic makes it a better choice for preventing emergence excitation than choice C. Choices B, D, and E are all acceptable choices for reducing the risk of emergence delirium.

Reference:

1. Everett LL. Anesthesia for children. In: Longnecker D, Brown DL, Newman MF, Zapol W, eds. Anesthesiology. 2nd ed. New York: McGraw-Hill Education; 2012:1185–1193.

11. Correct answer: B

MAC, defined as the end-tidal inhalational concentration that renders 50% of the population immobile to a noxious stimulus, is highest for isoflurane between ages 1 and 6 months, peaking during this period and then steadily falling thereafter. This differs from the behavior of sevoflurane, which is highest in the neonatal period for full-term neonates (3.3%), falling to 2.5% after 6 months and remaining there through 10 years. The differences in pharmacodynamics of the various inhaled agents are not well understood.

MAC is affected by other variables including temperature; for each 1°C decrease in body temperature, MAC decreases by approximately 5%. Other factors including acid-base balance, electrolyte balance, and cardiac output also affect MAC to varying degrees.

References:

1. Anderson BJ, Lerman J, Cote CJ. Pharmacokinetics and pharmacology of drugs used in children. In: Cote CJ, Lerman J, Anderson BJ, eds. A Practice of Anesthesia for Infants and Children. 5th ed. Philadelphia: Elsevier Saunders; 2013:77–149.
2. Eger EI. Age, minimum alveolar anesthetic concentration, and minimum alveolar anesthetic concentration-awake. *Anesth Analg.* 2001;93:947-953.
3. Lerman J, Sikich N, Kleinman S, Yentis S. The pharmacology of sevoflurane in infants and children. *Anesthesiology.* 1994;80(4):814-824.
4. Nickalls RW, Mapleson WW. Age-related iso-MAC charts for isoflurane, sevoflurane and desflurane in man. *Br J Anaesth.* 2003;91:170-174.

12. Correct answer: D

As discussed in question 11, MAC in neonates and infants is higher than adults. In neonates, 1 MAC of isoflurane equates to approximately 1.6% end-tidal isoflurane compared with ~1.2% in adults. For sevoflurane, it is 3.3% end-tidal sevoflurane, compared with ~3.2% in older infants, 2.5% in children, and 2.1% in adults.

Reference:

1. Anderson BJ, Lerman J, Cote CJ. Pharmacokinetics and pharmacology of drugs used in children. In: Cote CJ, Lerman J, Anderson BJ, eds. A Practice of Anesthesia for Infants and Children. 5th ed. Philadelphia: Elsevier Saunders; 2013:77–149.

13. Correct answer: D

Neonates are more sensitive to NMBDs than older children, requiring lower doses in μg/kg to achieve ED95 in population norms. However, the relationship between dose requirement and age is not linear because children require higher doses than adults in μg/kg. Hypotheses for why neonates are more sensitive to NMBDs than children include immaturity of neuromuscular transmission in the neonatal period and a more rapid depletion of acetylcholine vesicles after stimulation. The time to onset is shorter and time to recovery is longer in neonates as well. It is hypothesized that children require higher doses than adults for blockade because of increased relative muscle bulk compared with adults.

References:

1. Anderson BJ, Lerman J, Cote CJ. Pharmacokinetics and pharmacology of drugs used in children. In: Cote CJ, Lerman J, Anderson BJ, eds. A Practice of Anesthesia for Infants and Children. 5th ed. Philadelphia: Elsevier Saunders; 2013:77–149.
2. Goudsouzian NG. Maturation of neuromuscular transmission in the infant. *Br J Anaesth.* 1980;52:205-214.
3. Goudsouzian NG, Standaert FG. The infant and the myoneural junction. *Anesth Analg.* 1986;65:1208-1217.
4. Meretoja OA, Wirtavuori K, Neuvonen PJ. Age-dependence of the dose-response curve of vecuronium in pediatric patients during balanced anesthesia. *Anesth Analg.* 1988;67:21-26.

14. Correct answer: C

A full-term neonate has an estimated blood volume (EBV) of 80-90 mL/kg. A preterm neonate has an EBV of 90-100 mL/kg. Infants 3 months to 1 year have an EBV of 70-80 mL/kg, and children above 1 year, 70 mL/kg. Estimating the child's EBV is critical when calculating the estimated maximum allowable blood loss. As the absolute circulating blood volume of children is so much less than that of adults, small volumes of estimated blood loss during surgery can cause wide fluctuations in the child's hematocrit, making it important for the anesthesiologist caring for children to pay close attention to blood loss in the field, the starting hematocrit, and the maximum allowable blood loss.

Reference:
1. Cote CJ, Grabowski EF, Stowell CP. Strategies for blood product management and reducing transfusions. In: Cote CJ, Lerman J, Anderson BJ, eds. A Practice of Anesthesia for Infants and Children. 5th ed. Philadelphia: Elsevier Saunders; 2013:198–220.

15. Correct answer: C

Graft-versus-host disease in relation to blood transfusion is mediated by donor lymphocytes, and these lymphocytes are disabled by exposure to γ radiation, not leukoreduction. Leukoreduction is useful in preventing the transmission of cytomegalovirus, human leukocyte antigen alloimmunization, and non-hemolytic febrile transfusion reactions.

Reference:
1. Cote CJ, Grabowski EF, Stowell CP. Strategies for blood product management and reducing transfusions. In: Cote CJ, Lerman J, Anderson BJ, eds. A Practice of Anesthesia for Infants and Children. 5th ed. Philadelphia: Elsevier Saunders; 2013:198–220.

16. Correct answer: D

The infant in this question has a congenital diaphragmatic hernia (CDH), with herniation of the abdominal viscera into the thorax through a congenital defect in the diaphragm. Infants with CDH have poorly developed lung parenchyma in the side of the thorax with the herniation (typically left) but also have high pulmonary vascular resistance in the other lung. Ventilation strategies in the past focused on aggressive ventilation to decrease $PaCO_2$ and promote pulmonary vasodilatation, but aggressive positive pressure ventilation has been associated with worse outcomes, likely due to barotrauma of the already underdeveloped lung. Currently, the most common ventilation strategy is to secure the airway and allow spontaneous ventilation (with pressure support as needed), with permissive hypercapnia and low peak inspiratory pressures (<25 cm H_2O).

Application of CPAP (A and B) via mask airway is not recommended because of the risk of increasing distension of gastric viscera and further compressing the pulmonary structures. Positive pressure ventilation through an endotracheal tube (answer C) with targeted normocapnia may result in aggressive ventilation that can injure remaining lung tissue. Spontaneous ventilation through high-flow nasal cannula leaves the airway unprotected, and the addition of high-flow oxygen may further gastric distension and pulmonary compromise (answer choice E).

References:
1. Boloker J, Bateman D, Wung J, Stolar C. Congenital diaphragmatic hernia in 120 infants treated consecutively with permissive hypercapnea/spontaneous respiration/elective repair. *J Pediatr Surg*. 2002;37(3);357-366.
2. Bachiller PR, Chou JH, Romanelli TM, et al. Neonatal emergencies. In: Cote CJ, Lerman J, Anderson BJ, eds. A Practice of Anesthesia for Infants and Children. 5th ed. Philadelphia: Elsevier Saunders; 2013:746–765.

17. Correct answer: B

The infant in the vignette likely has a diagnosis of trisomy 21, Down syndrome. 30%-40% of infants with Down syndrome will have duodenal atresia, which presents as bilious emesis in the first 24-48 hours of life. Pyloric stenosis (A) presents between 4 and 10 weeks of life, most commonly with nonbilious, projectile vomiting after feeds, but otherwise normal development. It is more common in males. Choanal atresia (C) is malformation of the nasopharynx during fetal development, resulting in blocked nasal passages and inability to breathe through the nose. It can be associated with CHARGE syndrome, a constellation of congenital anomalies including coloboma, heart defects (tetralogy of Fallot and atrial/ventricular septal disorders) atresia of choanae, retardation of growth, genital anomalies, and ear anomalies. Necrotizing enterocolitis (answer D) is associated with preterm-birth and low-birth-weight neonates. Infants affected have a distended, tender abdomen and signs of severe illness, including acidosis and temperature instability. The associated mortality rate is high, between 10% and 30%. Intussusception (E) general presents in older infants. Symptoms include pain, with babies classically pulling their knees to their chest and crying during an episode. Nausea, vomiting, and passage of "currant jelly" stools are classically associated findings.

Reference:
1. Gertler R, Miller-Hance WC. Essentials of cardiology. In: Cote CJ, Lerman J, Anderson BJ, eds. A Practice of Anesthesia for Infants and Children. 5th ed. Philadelphia: Elsevier Saunders; 2013:291–326.

18. Correct answer: D

The "double-bubble" sign is classic for duodenal atresia, reflecting distension of the stomach and the proximal duodenum. It can be seen in other forms of duodenal obstruction, including webs and strictures, but is most commonly associated with atresia. A gastric bubble above the diaphragm (A) is associated with CDH. Dilated loops of bowel and pneumatosis (B and C) are associated with multiple intra-abdominal pathologies, resulting in bowel obstruction or necrosis, the most notable in the neonatal period being necrotizing enterocolitis. A target sign on ultrasonography is associated with intussusception, in which the bowel "telescopes" in on itself, causing pain, nausea, and intermittent bowel obstruction.

Reference:
1. Traubici J. The double bubble sign. *Radiology*. 2001;220:463-464.

19. Correct answer: C

Children with trisomy 21 are prone to bradycardia during inhalational inductions with high concentrations of sevoflurane. The mechanism of this conduction disturbance is poorly understood and occurs in children with and without associated congenital heart disease. For this reason, pretreatment with atropine may be wise; if the child is not pretreated, it is essential to have atropine or glycopyrrolate available, along with succinylcholine (in case of laryngospasm before IV access is obtained) for immediate IM administration during inhalational inductions. Whereas hypotension (A) and tachycardia (B) are possible responses to inhalational anesthesia, in Down syndrome the more common hemodynamically significant response is bradycardia. Increased respiratory rate and decreased tidal volume are common reactions to inhalational anesthesia, with the increased respiratory rate thought to be a compensatory mechanism for shallower tidal volumes that occur, as the anesthetic is deepened. In children with Down syndrome in particular, obstruction from a large tongue can lead to decreased tidal volumes, necessitating an oral airway. Because many children with Down syndrome may have atlantoaxial instability, repositioning of the airway during mask induction should be done cautiously.

Reference:
1. Gertler R, Miller-Hance WC. Essentials of cardiology. In: Cote CJ, Lerman J, Anderson BJ, eds. A Practice of Anesthesia for Infants and Children. 5th ed. Philadelphia: Elsevier Saunders; 2013:291–326.

20. Correct answer: E

Infants have a decreased FRC for their body weight compared with adults. This is due to a more compliant chest wall with less compliant lungs, such that lung recoil more forcefully empties the lungs at the end of passive expiration. Given their lower FRC, periods of apnea are less well tolerated, and desaturation can occur quite rapidly.

Reference:
1. Firth PG, Kinane TB. Essentials of pulmonology. In: Cote CJ, Lerman J, Anderson BJ, eds. A Practice of Anesthesia for Infants and Children. 5th ed. Philadelphia: Elsevier Saunders; 2013:221–236.

21. Correct answer: D

Although spinal and regional anesthesia are associated with respiratory and cardiovascular benefits over general anesthesia, they do not obviate the need for postoperative apnea monitoring because there is insufficient evidence to establish official guidelines. Generally, preterm infants less than 60 weeks' PCA will require either extended PACU stays or admission to the hospital for apnea monitoring after any anesthetic (A). History of apneic events increases risk of postoperative apnea, but lack of history of apneic events does not obviate the need for postoperative monitoring (B). Generally, healthy former preterm infants above 46 weeks' PCA should be monitored for anywhere from 6 to 12 apnea-free hours (C) before discharge (although longer periods are often employed and the length of stay is institution-dependent). Although caffeine can be administered to patients at high risk for apnea (40-44 wk' PCA, history of apnea and bradycardia, familial history of sudden infant death syndrome, anemia), doing so is not recommended as a prophylactic move in this patient, who is an otherwise healthy former late preterm infant now at 50 weeks' PCA with no history of apnea.

References:
1. Taenzer AH, Havidich JE. The postanesthesia care unit and beyond. In: Cote CJ, Lerman J, Anderson BJ, eds. A Practice of Anesthesia for Infants and Children. 5th ed. Philadelphia: Elsevier Saunders; 2013:980–992.
2. Walther-Larsen S, Rasmussen LS. The former preterm infant and risk of postoperative apnea: recommendations for management. *Acta Anaesthesiol Scand.* 2006;50:888-893.

22. Correct answer: A

The incidence of PONV is related to age; the youngest pediatric patients are at the least risk, with risk increasing at school age and peaking in adolescence. Thus, a teenager (B) undergoing hernia repair is at higher risk than a preschooler (A). High-risk surgical procedures include strabismus repair, tonsillectomy, orchiopexy, hernia repair, and intracranial procedures (C, D, and E).

Reference:
1. Taenzer AH, Havidich JE. The postanesthesia care unit and beyond. In: Cote CJ, Lerman J, Anderson BJ, eds. A Practice of Anesthesia for Infants and Children. 5th ed. Philadelphia: Elsevier Saunders; 2013:980–992.

23. Correct answer: A

One strategy for prevention of PONV is adequate intraoperative fluid administration. There are data that hydration, not fluid restriction, is effective at diminishing the likelihood of PONV. Postoperatively, administration of PO fluids can precipitate vomiting, especially if narcotic analgesics have been used (E). Ondansetron (B) and dexamethasone (C) are effective pharmacologic prophylactic agents for PONV, and in children, dual therapy is even more effective and should be used in high-risk patients (adolescents, children undergoing tonsillectomy or strabismus surgery, etc) Propofol is an effective antiemetic agent, and total intravenous anesthesia is one strategy to reduce PONV, as inhalational anesthetics can be emetogenic.

Reference:
1. Taenzer AH, Havidich JE. The postanesthesia care unit and beyond. In: Cote CJ, Lerman J, Anderson BJ, eds. A Practice of Anesthesia for Infants and Children. 5th ed. Philadelphia: Elsevier Saunders; 2013:980–992.

24. Correct answer: C

Especially with large defects, evaporative heat loss and fluid loss can be significant for a neonate. Appropriate warming devices should be used intraoperatively, with careful monitoring of the infant's volume status. Neural tube defects are not associated with exaggerated succinylcholine-induced hyperkalemia (A). Whereas large defects that hinder positioning may make tracheal intubation more difficult, neural tube defects by themselves are not associated with an anatomically difficult airway (B). Although these defects used to be repaired immediately after birth for fear of infection or worsened permanent neurologic damage, the data have shown that outcomes are no worse when there is delayed repair, and some neurosurgeons may prefer to wait until up to 72 hours postbirth to allow for thorough interdisciplinary planning and planning of surgical approach (D). There is no association with cardiac anomalies (E).

Reference:
1. McClain CD, Soriano SG, Rockoff MA. Pediatric neurosurgical anesthesia. In: Cote CJ, Lerman J, Anderson BJ, eds. A Practice of Anesthesia for Infants and Children. 5th ed. Philadelphia: Elsevier Saunders; 2013:510–532.

25. Correct answer: A

In terms of respiratory mechanics, tidal volumes for full-term neonates, infants, and adults are 6-7 cc/kg. FRC is very similar on a cc/kg basis; however, the ability of the neonate to mobilize this intrapulmonary oxygen is compromised when compared with adults. Additionally, the increased metabolic rate of neonates can contribute to rapid hypoxemia that can be seen in the anesthetized infant. For full-term neonates the oxygen consumption is roughly twice that of adults (4-6 cc/kg/min vs 2-3 cc/kg/min), and the work of breathing in infants is mostly due to small-airway resistance, whereas in adults it is mostly due to nasal passages. Closing capacity is very closely related to age in that it declines throughout childhood and then increases. For neonates, closing capacity is above FRC, whereas for adults, it is well below; thus some airways remain closed throughout tidal breathing in neonates. TLC is decreased in neonates compared with that in adults even when examined on an mL/kg basis (63 vs 82 cc/kg), which reflects that TLC depends on the ability of the inspiratory muscles to function properly and efficiently.

References:

1. Firth PG, Kinane TB. Essentials of pulmonology. In: Cote CJ, Lerman J, Anderson BJ, eds. A Practice of Anesthesia for Infants and Children. 5th ed. Philadelphia: Elsevier Saunders; 2013:221–236.
2. Litman RS, Fiadjoe JE, Striker PA, et al. The pediatric airway. In: Cote CJ, Lerman J, Anderson BJ, eds. A Practice of Anesthesia for Infants and Children. 5th ed. Philadelphia: Elsevier Saunders; 2013:237–276.
3. Marciniak B. Growth and development. In: Cote CJ, Lerman J, Anderson BJ, eds. A Practice of Anesthesia for Infants and Children. 5th ed. Philadelphia: Elsevier Saunders; 2013:7–20.

26. Correct answer: D

Drooling, dysphagia, and tripoding (sitting leaning forward on one arm, resembling a tripod) with elevated temperature are indicative of epiglottitis, especially in an unvaccinated child. Vaccination for *Haemophilus influenza* type B has decreased rates of epiglottitis. More recently, with an increase in parents electing against vaccinations, epiglottitis must be high on the differential with presentations of respiratory distress, particularly with drooling. Epiglottitis can also be caused by *Streptococcus*. Although foreign body ingestion (answer C) can present with respiratory distress and, in some cases, drooling or leaning forward to relieve airway obstruction, it is less likely to present first with fever. Fifth disease (A) is a viral syndrome causing rash and fever. Pneumonia may present with respiratory distress and fever, but tripoding and drooling make epiglottitis more likely. Coxsackie virus, or hand-foot-mouth disease, can present with lesions in the oropharynx, causing discomfort, refusal to swallow because of pain, or even drooling, but it is less likely to present with true respiratory distress, tripoding, or high fever.

Reference:

1. Hannallah RS, Brown KA, Verghese ST. Otorhinolaryngologic procedures. In: Cote CJ, Lerman J, Anderson BJ, eds. A Practice of Anesthesia for Infants and Children. 5th ed. Philadelphia: Elsevier Saunders; 2013:653–682.

27. Correct answer: D

A child with epiglottitis should not be made upset, as complete airway obstruction can occur with aggravation or discomfort. Thus, attempts to place an IV may be inappropriate, and the patient should be taken to the OR for intubation with anesthesia and surgery personnel present. The child should remain sitting up because supine positioning can worsen airway obstruction. A seated gentle mask induction of anesthesia with parents present if necessary, followed by IV placement once anesthetic depth is adequate, and gentle direct laryngoscopy is preferred. A rigid bronchoscope should be ready in the event that direct laryngoscopy is unsuccessful. If rigid bronchoscopy fails, emergency tracheotomy should be performed.

Reference:

1. Hannallah RS, Brown KA, Verghese ST. Otorhinolaryngologic procedures. In: Cote CJ, Lerman J, Anderson BJ, eds. A Practice of Anesthesia for Infants and Children. 5th ed. Philadelphia: Elsevier Saunders; 2013:653–682.

28. Correct answer: A

The pulse oximeter probe should be placed on the only limb that should not be affected during coarctation repair, which is the right upper extremity. The left upper extremity will likely be compromised during the repair as the left subclavian artery is often transected and used in patch angioplasty repair, and this left upper extremity Spo_2 will give inaccurate readings. The lower extremities are postcoarctation and should not be used for Spo_2 monitoring because they will be compromised during the repair.

Reference:

1. McEwan A. Anesthesia for children undergoing heart surgery. In: Cote CJ, Lerman J, Anderson BJ, eds. A Practice of Anesthesia for Infants and Children. 5th ed. Philadelphia: Elsevier Saunders; 2013:327–353.

29. Correct answer: D

Patients with a BDG shunt have a cavopulmonary connection where all blood flow through the lungs is dependent on passive movement from the cerebral circulation to the SVC. In hyperventilation, the resultant hypocarbia restricts cerebral blood flow and decreases the amount of blood coming to the pulmonary circulation via the SVC, thus lowering the amount of blood (and subsequently, oxygen) available to the systemic circulation. Hypoventilation, even with a small rise in pulmonary vascular resistance from hypercarbia, has been shown to increase systemic oxygenation in patients with BDG shunts. Volume status is important in these patients, so a fluid bolus is reasonable if one suspects dehydration.

Reference:

1. Bradley SM, Simsic JM, Mulvihill DM. Hypoventilation improves oxygenation after bidirectional superior cavopulmonary connection. *J Thorac Cardiovasc Surg.* 2003;126(4):1033-1039.

30. Correct answer: A

The patient had a decrease in systemic vascular resistance (SVR) with induction of anesthesia, causing increased right to left shunting across the ventricular septal defect. Thus, despite adequate ventilation, oxygenation will continue to suffer so long as the SVR is low. Phenylephrine will increase SVR and decrease the right to left shunting, thereby lessening the amount of mixing of deoxygenated and oxygenated blood leaving the left ventricle. Ephedrine (B) and epinephrine (D) will also increase SVR but will further increase heart rate. Because the cause of the hypoxia is shunting rather than volume overload, Lasix is not the best choice.

Reference:

1. Schnure AY, DiNardo JA. Cardiac physiology and pharmacology. In: Cote CJ, Lerman J, Anderson BJ, eds. A Practice of Anesthesia for Infants and Children. 5th ed. Philadelphia: Elsevier Saunders; 2013:354–385.

31. Correct answer: A

Central core disease is a syndrome involving hypotonia with muscle weakness, hip dislocation, contractures, and scoliosis. It is associated with an increased risk of malignant hyperthermia after exposure to triggering agents but is not generally associated with an increased risk of hyperkalemia. Duchenne muscle dystrophy, paraplegia, burns >8% of total body surface area, and spinal muscular atrophy type 1 (Werdnig-Hoffman syndrome) are all associated with hyperkalemia after succinylcholine administration, and succinylcholine should be avoided in patients known to have these conditions.

Reference:

1. Crean P, Peake D. Essentials of neurology and neuromuscular disorders. In: Cote CJ, Lerman J, Anderson BJ, eds. A Practice of Anesthesia for Infants and Children. 5th ed. Philadelphia: Elsevier Saunders; 2013:475–491.

32. Correct answer: B

Clearance of morphine in L/h is significantly lower in neonates than in adults but raises to adult levels between ages 6 and 12 months. Because of the reduced clearance of morphine in neonates, caution dosing is important to prevent respiratory depression. The typical morphine dosing for a pediatric patient is 0.05-0.2 mg/kg.

Reference:

1. Anderson BJ, Lerman J, Cote CJ. Pharmacokinetics and pharmacology of drugs used in children. In: Cote CJ, Lerman J, Anderson BJ, eds. A Practice of Anesthesia for Infants and Children. 5th ed. Philadelphia: Elsevier Saunders; 2013:77–149.

33. Correct answer: C

The spinal cord terminates at the conus medullaris, which lies at L3 in neonates, as opposed to L1 in adults. For this reason, in infants, targeted level for a spinal tap or administration of spinal anesthesia should be at L4-L5 or L5-S1 to ensure safely being below the conus medullaris.

Reference:

1. Suresh S, Polaner DM, Cote CJ. Regional anesthesia. In: Cote CJ, Lerman J, Anderson BJ, eds. A Practice of Anesthesia for Infants and Children. 5th ed. Philadelphia: Elsevier Saunders; 2013:835–879.

34. Correct answer: B

The proper landmarks for a caudal block include palpation of the cornua of the sacral hiatus, which can be found often directly where the crease of the buttocks begins (rather than above, D) appreciated as 2 bony ridges a narrow width apart, above where the sacrum meets the coccyx (C) but well below the posterior-superior iliac spine (A).

Reference:

1. Suresh S, Polaner DM, Cote CJ. Regional anesthesia. In: Cote CJ, Lerman J, Anderson BJ, eds. A Practice of Anesthesia for Infants and Children. 5th ed. Philadelphia: Elsevier Saunders; 2013:835–879.

35. Correct answer: D

The ability to void is not part of the ASA guidelines for criteria for discharge from PACU. All of the other answers (baseline level of consciousness, adequate control of nausea/vomiting and pain, and stable hemodynamics) are necessary before discharge from the PACU after ambulatory surgery.

Reference:

1. Apfelbaum J, Silverstein JH, Chung FF, et al. Practice guidelines for postanesthetic care: an updated report by the American Society of Anesthesiologists Task Force on Postanesthetic Care. *Anesthesiology*. 2013;118(2):291-307.

36. Correct answer: B

Retinopathy of prematurity has been associated with hyperoxia (as well as hypoxia), and avoidance of delivery of high inspired oxygen concentrations is recommended to allay this risk. A stable low-normal Spo_2 at the minimum necessary Fio_2 is the goal rather than aiming for higher Spo_2. Although permissive hypercapnia has a role in management of lung injury and normotension is always an appropriate goal when managing a sick neonate, these are not associated with retinopathy of prematurity.

References:

1. Mariani G, Cifuentes J, Carlo W. Randomized trial of permissive hypercapnia in preterm infants. *Pediatrics*. 1999;104:1082-1088.
2. Spaeth JP, Kurth CD. The extremely premature infant (Micropremie). In: Cote CJ, Lerman J, Anderson BJ, eds. A Practice of Anesthesia for Infants and Children. 5th ed. Philadelphia: Elsevier Saunders; 2013:733–745.

37. Correct answer: A

Beckwith-Wiedemann syndrome is characterized by macrosomia, perinatal hypoglycemia, macroglossia, cardiac abnormalities, as well as omphalocele. Omphalocele is a midline defect in which the bowels protrude through the abdominal wall, covered by a membrane. It differs from gastroschisis in that gastroschisis is periumbilical, has no membrane covering, and is less likely to have associated defects.

References:

1. Litman RS, Fiadjoe JE, Striker PA, et al. The pediatric airway. In: Cote CJ, Lerman J, Anderson BJ, eds. A Practice of Anesthesia for Infants and Children. 5th ed. Philadelphia: Elsevier Saunders; 2013:237–276.
2. Bachiller PR, Chou JH, Romanelli TM, et al. Neonatal emergencies. In: Cote CJ, Lerman J, Anderson BJ, eds. A Practice of Anesthesia for Infants and Children. 5th ed. Philadelphia: Elsevier Saunders; 2013:746–765.

38. Correct answer: C

Children affected by Treacher-Collins syndrome are often noted to have mandibular hypoplasia, macrostomia (wide mouth), and cleft palate. These patients also can have hypoplastic zygomatic arches, sloping palpebral fissures, notched lower eyelids, cardiovascular defects, and renal abnormalities. Unlike the other syndromes/genetic abnormalities listed, those affected by Treacher-Collins syndrome have known difficult airways, which worsen with age.

Reference:

1. Engelhardt T, Crawford MW, Subramanyam R, et al. Plastic and reconstructive surgery. In: Cote CJ, Lerman J, Anderson BJ, eds. A Practice of Anesthesia for Infants and Children. 5th ed. Philadelphia: Elsevier Saunders; 2013:697–711.

39. Correct answer: D

These are features of Hurler syndrome, a lysosomal storage disease involving deficient metabolism of mucopolysaccharidoses, which presents one of the greatest airway challenges in all of anesthesia because of crowded facial anatomy and craniofacial abnormalities, including narrowed nasal passages, hypertrophy of adenoids and tonsils, large tongue, and tracheomalacia. Fiberoptic intubation is often necessary, and case reports with impossible intubation and mask ventilation have been published (in one case, a laryngeal mask airway was used for successful ventilation).

References:
1. Litman RS, Fiadjoe JE, Striker PA, et al. The pediatric airway. In: Cote CJ, Lerman J, Anderson BJ, eds. A Practice of Anesthesia for Infants and Children. 5th ed. Philadelphia: Elsevier Saunders; 2013:237–276.
2. Walker R, Belani KG, Braunlin EA, et al. Anaesthesia and airway management in mucopolysaccharidosis. *J Inherit Metab Dis.* 2013;36(2):211-219.

40. Correct answer: A

The most common form of TEF is answer choice A, the "C-type". This consists of esophageal atresia with a dilated proximal esophageal pouch and a connection between the distal esophagus and the trachea. Infants with this form of TEF present with excessive secretions, regurgitation of feeds, and respiratory distress during feeds. Repair is often staged, and alternate routes of feeding need to be established until definitive repair can be performed. TEF commonly, but not always, co-occurs with one or more associated anomalies of the VACTERL association (**v**ertebral anomalies, imperforate **a**nus, **c**ardiac anomalies, **TE** fistula, **r**enal abnormalities, and **l**imb deformities.)

Reference:
1. Bachiller PR, Chou JH, Romanelli TM, et al. Neonatal emergencies. In: Cote CJ, Lerman J, Anderson BJ, eds. A Practice of Anesthesia for Infants and Children. 5th ed. Philadelphia: Elsevier Saunders; 2013:746–765.

41. Correct answer: C

A 5-month-old is not developmentally expected to have separation anxiety yet and therefore has no need for a parent present at induction. The mother's occupation is of little consequence. Ultimately, the decision to have a parent present at induction rests with the anesthesiologist and requires an assessment of the child's needs, the parental ability to be present without interference in the induction or medical treatment of their child, and the comfort level of the anesthesiologist. Although parents may be tearful or anxious before their child's anesthetic, if they are able to remain calm enough to provide reassurance to the child, their presence at induction can be permitted. Data supporting parent-present inductions are mixed, and some suggest that parental presence, particularly in the case of an anxious parent, is not always beneficial. However, the trend in many children's hospitals is to offer parent present induction when appropriate, with necessary preinduction preparation of the parent regarding what they may observe as their child goes under anesthesia (including jerking movements during stage 2, eye rolling, and flaccidity). Whereas a 17-year-old teenager without delays would not normally require a parent-present induction, in the case of a child with developmental delays, the presence of a parent can be quite helpful and should be considered if the parent and child would benefit.

References:
1. Kain ZM, Fortier MA, Mayes LC. Perioperative behavioral stress in children. In: Cote CJ, Lerman J, Anderson BJ, eds. A Practice of Anesthesia for Infants and Children. 5th ed. Philadelphia: Elsevier Saunders; 2013:21–30.
2. Gazal EA, Mason LJ, Cote CJ. Preoperative evaluation, premedication and induction of anesthesia. In: Cote CJ, Lerman J, Anderson BJ, eds. A Practice of Anesthesia for Infants and Children. 5th ed. Philadelphia: Elsevier Saunders; 2013:31–63.

42. Correct answer: B

This infant most likely is suffering from acute respiratory distress syndrome (RDS) of the newborn, common in preterm infants and caused by insufficient surfactant production and immature lung development. Treatment is supportive, with positive pressure ventilation and exogenous surfactant administration as mainstays of treatment. In women who are at risk for preterm delivery, administration of glucocorticoids has been found to reduce the incidence of RDS of the newborn. RDS is different from transient tachypnea of the newborn, which is the most common form of neonatal respiratory distress and is caused by inadequate clearance of amniotic fluid from the lungs during delivery (often found in infants who are born via cesarean delivery without labor). Transient tachypnea of the newborn generally resolves soon after delivery. Loops of bowel in the left thorax would be pathognomonic for CDH, which would be expected to be associated with a scaphoid abdomen on examination. There is no reason to suspect a pneumothorax or pulmonary edema in this newborn where RDS is much more likely and consistent with the clinical picture.

References:
1. Bachiller PR, Chou JH, Romanelli TM, et al. Neonatal emergencies. In: Cote CJ, Lerman J, Anderson BJ, eds. A Practice of Anesthesia for Infants and Children. 5th ed. Philadelphia: Elsevier Saunders; 2013:746–765.
2. Saccone G, Berghella V. Antenatal corticosteroids for maturity of term or near term fetuses: systematic review and meta-analysis of randomized controlled trials. *BMJ.* 2016.

43. **Correct answer: C**

Small doses of fentanyl titrated postoperatively are appropriate in this patient, but caution must be exercised, given her history of severe sleep apnea. It is too early for a repeat dose of Tylenol (A). 30 mg of IV ketorolac is too high a dose for her (0.5 mg/kg IV in children is appropriate), and many ENT surgeons do not favor ketorolac in tonsillectomies, given the risk of posttonsillectomy bleeding. IV morphine or hydromorphone could be administered at low doses, but again, caution must be used, given her OSA, which would not be instantly cured by surgery (and may even be worse on the first postoperative night after surgery). The doses listed for morphine and hydromorphone here are too high to start with in the PACU. Although morphine dosed at 0.1 mg/kg and hydromorphone dosed at 20 μg/kg may be appropriate for major surgical procedures in patients not at risk for OSA, the listed doses here are slightly higher than that and are inappropriate for this relatively minor surgery in a patient at risk for apnea.

Reference:

1. Hannallah RS, Brown KA, Verghese ST. Otorhinolaryngologic procedures. In: Cote CJ, Lerman J, Anderson BJ, eds. A Practice of Anesthesia for Infants and Children. 5th ed. Philadelphia: Elsevier Saunders; 2013:653–682.

44. **Correct answer: B**

Fetal hemoglobin has a higher affinity for oxygen than does adult hemoglobin (P50 of 27). This facilitates oxygen delivery to fetal tissues preferentially. Additionally, the concentration of fetal hemoglobin is higher, allowing for greater oxygen carrying capacity. Shortly after birth, the predominant hemoglobin produced switches from fetal (2 α and 2 γ subunits) to adult (2 α and 2 β subunits). The presence of fetal hemoglobin at birth is protective in children who have sickle cell disease, and current investigation into genetic therapy aimed at reawakening the production of fetal hemoglobin as a treatment for hemoglobinopathies is ongoing.

References:

1. Brusseau R. Fetal intervention and the EXIT procedures. In: Cote CJ, Lerman J, Anderson BJ, eds. A Practice of Anesthesia for Infants and Children. 5th ed. Philadelphia: Elsevier Saunders; 2013:766–788.
2. Lettre G, Bauer D. Fetal haemoglobin in sickle-cell disease: from genetic epidemiology to new therapeutic strategies. *Lancet.* 2016;387:2554-2564.

45. **Correct answer: A**

Oxygenated blood from placenta travels through the umbilical vein to the IVC. Approximately one-third to one-half of this blood is shunted across the ductus venosus to the IVC; the remainder travels through the hepatic circulation. Both meet up in the IVC, which empties into the right atrium (RA). The blood in the fetal IVC has the highest percentage oxygenation of all of the answer choices. The SVC carries deoxygenated blood back from the brain and upper half of the body to the RA where it mixes with oxygenated blood from the IVC. From the RA, some blood is shunted to the left atrium, through the foramen ovale, and the rest goes through the right ventricle → the pulmonary artery. A small fraction travels through the pulmonary artery to supply oxygen to the nonfunctional lungs, and the rest travels through the ductus arteriosus to the aorta. All of the blood traveling through the fetal circulation is mixed except the relatively highly oxygenated blood from the placenta, which empties through the umbilical vein directly into the IVC, thus making the IVC the location of the highest oxygenated blood in the fetus.

Reference:

1. Brusseau R. Fetal intervention and the EXIT procedures. In: Cote CJ, Lerman J, Anderson BJ, eds. A Practice of Anesthesia for Infants and Children. 5th ed. Philadelphia: Elsevier Saunders; 2013:766–788.

46. **Correct answer: D**

Although neuraxial blockade in adults is frequently performed awake with minimal to moderate sedation, there is no evidence that performing epidurals in awake children confers any safety benefit. In fact, with an experienced anesthesiologist performing the block, the data show that inadvertent dural puncture or nerve injury is quite rare in the anesthetized pediatric patient. There are anatomic differences between children and adults, which necessitate familiarity with placing pediatric epidurals to allow for this success. First, the ligamentum flavum is thinner and less rigid in children, making the tactile differences when passing through tissue planes more subtle. A cautious approach is required to not move the needle past the epidural space. Second, the bony structures in children are less well ossified than in adults, making a paramedian approach more difficult, as the needle can drill into the lamina rather than crisply "walking off" as it would in an adult. Thus, a midline approach is generally used.

Reference:

1. Suresh S, Polaner DM, Cote CJ. Regional anesthesia. In: Cote CJ, Lerman J, Anderson BJ, eds. A Practice of Anesthesia for Infants and Children. 5th ed. Philadelphia: Elsevier Saunders; 2013:835–879.

47. Correct answer: D

In emergent situations, the anesthesiologist should act in the best interests of the child legally and medically. In this case, with ongoing blood loss and a hematocrit of 20% with hemodynamic instability, the child will require a blood transfusion to save his life. It is essential to transfuse blood promptly and obtain a court order after the fact. Discussion with the hospital counsel and Ethics Committee are appropriate steps but should be undertaken after the child is stabilized, not before.

Reference:

1. Waisel DB. Ethical issues in pediatric anesthesiology. In: Cote CJ, Lerman J, Anderson BJ, eds. A Practice of Anesthesia for Infants and Children. 5th ed. Philadelphia: Elsevier Saunders; 2013:64–76.

48. Correct answer: E

Children have a larger volume of distribution and faster redistribution of propofol from vessel-rich organs to vessel-poor compartments, terminating propofol's effectiveness more quickly than in adults. However, actual clearance of propofol in children is similar to clearance rates in adults.

Reference:

1. Anderson BJ, Lerman J, Cote CJ. Pharmacokinetics and pharmacology of drugs used in children. In: Cote CJ, Lerman J, Anderson BJ, eds. A Practice of Anesthesia for Infants and Children. 5th ed. Philadelphia: Elsevier Saunders; 2013:77–149.

49. Correct answer: D

Dexmedetomidine is used in pediatric anesthesia for all of the answer choices except induction of general anesthesia. Although large bolus doses can confer moderate to deep sedation, the amount required to produce anesthetic-level unconsciousness is unknown, and it is not used for induction of GA. When children are administered these large bolus doses, care must be taken, as in adults, to prevent bradycardia, which children may tolerate less well than adults owing to the fact that their heart rates are higher at baseline.

Reference:

1. Anderson BJ, Lerman J, Cote CJ. Pharmacokinetics and pharmacology of drugs used in children. In: Cote CJ, Lerman J, Anderson BJ, eds. A Practice of Anesthesia for Infants and Children. 5th ed. Philadelphia: Elsevier Saunders; 2013:77–149.

50. Correct answer: C

Under moderate sedation, children should respond to touch or verbal stimuli and should not require assistance to maintain airway patency. If the airway becomes compromised, this signals a transition from moderate to deep sedation, which can occur quickly in children, and appropriate airway assistance should be provided by trained providers. A normal response to verbal stimuli is consistent with light sedation. Response to verbal stimuli or light touch is consistent with moderate sedation. Response to painful, but not verbal, stimuli is consistent with deep sedation. Unresponsiveness to painful stimuli is consistent with general anesthesia.

Reference:

1. Cote CJ, Wilson S. Guidelines for monitoring and management of pediatric patients before, during, and after sedation for diagnostic and therapeutic procedures: update 2016. *Pediatrics*. July 2016;138(1).

15

OBSTETRIC ANESTHESIA

Emily Naoum

1. **Which of the following cardiovascular parameters increases with pregnancy?**

   A. Left ventricular end-systolic volume
   B. Left ventricular end-diastolic volume
   C. Central venous pressure
   D. Pulmonary artery diastolic pressure
   E. Pulmonary vascular resistance

2. **Which of the following is NOT consistent with supine hypotensive syndrome of pregnancy?**

   A. Bradycardia
   B. Decreased right atrial filling pressure
   C. Normal blood flow in the upper extremities
   D. Increased femoral vein velocity

3. **Which of the following characteristics of local anesthetic administration for spinal anesthesia is more common in a parturient than in a nonpregnant patient?**

   A. Increased dose requirement for the same level and duration of block
   B. Slower onset of neuraxial blockade
   C. Longer duration of neuraxial blockade
   D. Decreased neural sensitivity to local anesthetics
   E. Increased risk of local anesthetic systemic toxicity

4. **Which of the following pharmacokinetic physiologic changes in drug metabolism do you anticipate in a pregnant woman at term?**

   A. Decreased requirement of isoflurane for maintenance of general anesthesia
   B. Slower increase in alveolar concentration of inhaled anesthetics due to increased cardiac output
   C. Increased susceptibility to propofol induction
   D. Prolonged paralysis after succinylcholine administration
   E. Increased dose requirements for aminosteroidal neuromuscular blockers (such as vecuronium and rocuronium)

5. **During which time period of a normal pregnancy does the Paco$_2$ decrease to reach a level of 30 mm Hg?**

    A. 8 weeks
    B. 12 weeks
    C. 20 weeks
    D. 28 weeks

6. **Which of the following changes in lung volume occurs in a pregnant patient at term compared with prepregnancy?**

    A. Increased functional residual capacity (FRC)
    B. Increased vital capacity
    C. Decreased inspiratory capacity
    D. Decreased expiratory reserve volume
    E. Decreased inspiratory reserve volume

7. **Which of the following renal physiologic adaptations is NOT commonly seen in pregnancy?**

    A. Increased creatinine clearance
    B. Increased glomerular filtration rate
    C. Increased protein excretion
    D. Decreased serum bicarbonate
    E. Decreased glucose excretion

8. **Which of the following statements is correct regarding biliary disease during pregnancy?**

    A. Hormonal changes in pregnancy account for altered bile acid content.
    B. Alkaline phosphatase (AP) levels increase during pregnancy because of biliary stasis.
    C. Intrahepatic cholestasis of pregnancy is a normal phenomenon that is not associated with increased risk to the fetus.
    D. Computerized tomography is the gold standard for diagnosis of gallstones in pregnancy.
    E. Laparoscopic surgery is significantly safer during pregnancy in reducing fetal loss as compared with open cholecystectomy.

9. **Which of the following statements regarding gastrointestinal (GI) changes during pregnancy is true?**

    A. Gastroesophageal reflux disease is common, and lower esophageal sphincter pressures are significantly reduced during the first trimester.
    B. Gastric emptying becomes progressively more delayed during the later trimesters of pregnancy.
    C. Preoperative fasting guidelines for scheduled cesarean section required increased fasting periods compared with other surgical procedures.
    D. Intestinal transit and peristalsis are slowed during pregnancy, resulting in constipation.
    E. The use of nonparticulate antacids to increase gastric pH has demonstrated a significant decrease in clinical aspiration events.

10. **Which of the following statements regarding hematologic changes during pregnancy is false?**

    A. Plasma volume increases more in pregnancy than red blood cell (RBC) volume, resulting in a physiologic anemia of pregnancy.
    B. There is increased fibrinolytic activity during pregnancy, resulting in elevated fibrin degradation products.
    C. Procoagulant proteins including factors I, VII, VIII, IX, and X are increased during pregnancy, resulting in a prothrombotic state.
    D. White blood cell function is impaired during pregnancy.
    E. Platelet consumption during pregnancy is unchanged compared with that during prepregnancy.

11. **Which of the following drugs when administered to the mother is *least* likely to have clinical effects on the neonate?**

    A. Vecuronium
    B. Propofol
    C. Morphine
    D. Diazepam
    E. Ketamine

12. **Which of the following drugs administered for postpartum hemorrhage (PPH) is *incorrectly* paired with a commonly associated side effect?**

    A. Carbetocin—hypotension
    B. Oxytocin—hypernatremia
    C. Misoprostol—fever
    D. Methylprostaglandin—bronchoconstriction
    E. Methylergonovine—arteriolar constriction

13. **Which of the following drugs administered to reduce preterm labor is *least likely* to reduce preterm birth?**

    A. β-Adrenergic agonists
    B. Magnesium sulfate
    C. Progesterone
    D. Calcium channel blockers
    E. Indomethacin

14. **A 22-year-old G2P1 is seen preoperatively for an anesthesia consultation at 32 weeks. She has a history of complex partial seizures since the age of 8 years and has been maintained on carbamazepine for the last several years with good control, and her last seizure was 19 months ago. Which of the following is NOT a common perinatal consequence of maternal antiepileptic drug use?**

    A. Small for gestational age
    B. Decreased Apgar scores
    C. Thromboembolic events
    D. Admission to NICU
    E. Preterm delivery

15. **You are called to assist with an emergent general anesthesia for a 34-year-old G1P0 for nonreassuring fetal heart tones and persistent fetal bradycardia. During induction, you give propofol, succinylcholine, and fentanyl intravenously. Which of the following pharmacologic drug characteristics is most likely to be associated with an increased transfer of drugs across the placental membrane?**

    A. Lipophilic substances
    B. Charged molecules
    C. Molecular weight >1000 Da
    D. Low free drug fraction
    E. α-1-Acid glycoprotein binding

16. **Which of the following statements comparing chorionic villus sampling (CVS) with amniocentesis is most accurate?**

    A. Amniocentesis is associated with a risk of Rh isoimmunization; however, CVS is not.
    B. CVS is safer than amniocentesis before 15 weeks of gestation.
    C. Pregnancy loss following CVS and amniocentesis is directly related to provider experience.
    D. Both techniques evaluate amniotic fluid and desquamated fetal cells (amniocytes) to perform genetic analysis.
    E. Amniocentesis is contraindicated in patients with a history of pregnancy loss.

17. **Which of the following statements regarding oligohydramnios is most accurate?**

   A. The amniotic fluid volume can be influenced by acute fetal hypoxia or acute fetal CNS dysfunction.
   B. Oligohydramnios secondary to amniocentesis carries a worse prognosis than other causes and rarely reverts to normal volumes of amniotic fluid.
   C. The most common cause of oligohydramnios is fetal anomalies.
   D. Uteroplacental insufficiency is not associated with oligohydramnios.
   E. Hydrops fetalis is classically associated with oligohydramnios.

18. **Which of the following statements regarding the etiology of hydrops fetalis is *most correct*?**

   A. Since the introduction of Rho(D) immune globulin, the most common causes of hydrops fetalis are nonimmune.
   B. Maternal viral infections are not associated with hydrops fetalis.
   C. Although the etiology of this condition must be addressed after delivery, the overall perinatal mortality associated with hydrops fetalis is <10%.
   D. Non-ABO RBC antigens such as Kell, Rh(E), Rh(c), and Duffy are not associated with severe immune hydrops.
   E. Isolated blunt abdominal trauma to a pregnant woman is not an indication for Rho(D) immune globulin.

19. **Which of the following variables is NOT included in a biophysical profile (BPP)?**

   A. Fetal limb movements
   B. Fetal breathing movements
   C. Fetal response to stimulation
   D. Qualitative amniotic fluid volume
   E. Fetal body movements

20. **A 23-year-old G2P0 undergoes ultrasound at 38 weeks, which demonstrates an estimated fetal weight (EFW) of 4850 g. Which of the following statements is the correct statement regarding fetal macrosomia?**

   A. An EFW greater than 4500 g in a nondiabetic woman or greater than 5000 g in a diabetic woman may warrant an elective cesarean delivery.
   B. Fetal macrosomia is associated with an increased risk of cesarean and instrumental vaginal delivery.
   C. Fetal macrosomia is more accurately predicted by ultrasound than by Leopold maneuvers.
   D. Induction of labor at 38 weeks for suspected fetal macrosomia is associated with improved maternal and fetal outcomes.
   E. The risk of PPH is unchanged by the presence of fetal macrosomia.

21. **For which of the following urgent obstetric conditions would it be considered most appropriate to perform neuraxial anesthesia?**

   A. Placenta previa
   B. Preterm footling breech
   C. Uterine rupture with hemodynamic compromise
   D. Severe obstetric hemorrhage
   E. Profound fetal bradycardia

22. **Which of the following symptoms is not consistent with a postdural puncture headache (PDPH)?**

   A. Improves with lying flat, worsened by sitting or standing
   B. Neck stiffness
   C. Tinnitus
   D. Bifrontal distribution
   E. Scalp tenderness

23. **What is the anticipated change in oxygen consumption during a normal second stage of labor?**

    A. Unchanged
    B. Increased by 20%
    C. Increased by 50%
    D. Increased by 70%
    E. Increased by 100%

24. **You are participating in the care of a complex obstetric patient who has a history of severe pulmonary arterial hypertension and is undergoing induction of labor. She is a G3P2 at 37 weeks with 2 prior vaginal deliveries and has had progressive dyspnea over the last month, and a multidisciplinary discussion with her cardiologist, maternal fetal medicine specialist, and anesthesia team took place before her admission. She has an epidural in place and is now fully dilated and beginning to push. During which phase of labor and delivery is the cardiac output the greatest?**

    A. At the beginning of the first stage of labor (onset of contractions, cervical dilation <5 cm)
    B. At the end of the first stage of labor (full cervical dilation)
    C. At the end of the second stage of labor (immediate postpartum period)
    D. At the end of 24 hours after delivery
    E. At the end of 72 hours after delivery

25. **A 23-year-old G1P0 woman with an uncomplicated pregnancy is now beginning the second stage of labor. Which of the following changes in respiratory physiology would be expected for this patient compared with prepregnancy?**

    A. Decreased tidal volume and increased respiratory rate
    B. Increased tidal volume and increased minute ventilation
    C. Decreased tidal volume and increased minute ventilation
    D. Increased tidal volume and decreased respiratory rate
    E. Increased tidal volume and decreased minute ventilation

26. **Which of the following statements regarding the effect of combined spinal epidural (CSE) anesthesia on progress of labor is most correct?**

    A. CSE anesthesia techniques accelerate the progress of the second stage of labor.
    B. CSE anesthesia techniques increase the rate of instrumental vaginal delivery.
    C. Early placement CSE anesthesia increases the risk of cesarean delivery when compared with later placement.
    D. CSE anesthesia has no greater effect on the progress of labor than epidural anesthesia.
    E. CSE has been shown to increase the risk of requiring a cesarean delivery compared with epidural anesthesia alone.

27. **A 31-year-old G2P0 woman with an epidural in place for labor analgesia has been actively pushing for the last 2 hours and 15 minutes. Her partner inquires whether this is a concerning duration of time. What would be considered a prolonged second stage of labor in this patient?**

    A. Second stage lasting more than 1 hour with neuraxial anesthesia
    B. Second stage lasting more than 1 hour without neuraxial anesthesia
    C. Second stage lasting more than 2 hours with neuraxial anesthesia
    D. Second stage lasting more than 3 hours with neuraxial anesthesia
    E. Second stage lasting more than 4 hours with neuraxial anesthesia

28. **Which of the following is not a strong indication for cesarean delivery?**

    A. Previous Pfannenstiel incision cesarean delivery
    B. Placenta previa
    C. Breech presentation
    D. Prolapsed umbilical cord
    E. Prior myomectomy

29. **For which of the following conditions would general anesthesia be considered the preferred technique for a cesarean delivery?**

    A. High body mass index (BMI)/obesity
    B. History of malignant hyperthermia
    C. Severe psychiatric disorder
    D. History of pulmonary disease
    E. History of difficult intubation

30. **Which of the following pregnancy-related changes is least likely to contribute to airway complications during intubation?**

    A. Presence of a Mallampati class III or IV airway
    B. Friable oral mucosa
    C. Increased metabolic need and oxygen consumption
    D. Decreased lower esophageal sphincter tone
    E. Decreased duration of paralysis following succinylcholine administration

31. **You are asked to provide an anesthesia consultation for a 33-year-old G1P0 with a medical history significant for relapsing and remitting multiple sclerosis that was diagnosed 4 years before this pregnancy. She is currently not taking any medications, and her last relapse was 15 months ago. Her physical examination is significant only for right foot drop. Which of the following is the most appropriate management for her obstetric anesthesia?**

    A. Spinal and epidural analgesia are contraindicated for labor.
    B. Spinal techniques are significantly safer than epidural techniques and are preferred for analgesia or anesthesia.
    C. Epidural techniques are significantly safer than spinal techniques and are preferred for analgesia or anesthesia.
    D. Spinal and epidural techniques are both considered to be safe and can be pursued for analgesia or anesthesia.
    E. General anesthesia has been implicated in relapses of multiple sclerosis and should be avoided.

32. **A 24-year-old G2P0 woman, 7 weeks pregnant based on the last menstrual period, presents to the ED with right lower quadrant pain, tachycardia, and vaginal bleeding concerning for threatened abortion. Which of the following statements is correct?**

    A. If on physical examination she has cervical dilation without fetal or placental expulsion, this would be considered a threatened abortion.
    B. Spontaneous abortions are most commonly related to maternal immunologic phenomena.
    C. Methotrexate may be used to treat this patient with suspected ectopic pregnancy.
    D. The rate of serum β-hCG concentration rise is not reliable for the diagnosis of ectopic pregnancies.
    E. Transvaginal ultrasound is the best modality to image if an ectopic pregnancy is suspected.

33. **Which of the following statements is not true regarding systemic lupus erythematosus (SLE) in pregnancy?**

    A. Patients with SLE have an increased risk of preterm delivery.
    B. The presence of atypical blood antibodies may make it challenging to obtain a blood type and crossmatch.
    C. The presence of lupus anticoagulant increases the patient's risk of bleeding complications from neuraxial anesthesia.
    D. Patients with SLE are at risk of pericarditis and cardiac tamponade.
    E. Infants born to mothers with SLE may be born with congenital heart block.

34. **Which of the following hematologic disorders is not associated with an increased risk of thrombotic events in pregnancy?**

    A. Protein C deficiency
    B. Antithrombin III deficiency
    C. Disseminated intravascular coagulation
    D. Von Willebrand disease
    E. Antiphospholipid syndrome

35. **Which of the following statements regarding management of a parturient with mitral stenosis is most correct?**

    A. Percutaneous mitral balloon valvuloplasty may be considered during pregnancy in patients with severe disease who are refractory to medical management.
    B. The physiologic changes of pregnancy are well tolerated with the peak period of symptoms in the first trimester that typically improves throughout gestation.
    C. Peripartum β-blockers may be used but have been associated with worse maternal outcomes.
    D. Percutaneous valvuloplasty should be performed postconception in patients with moderate or severe mitral stenosis, as the clinical course during pregnancy is widely variable.
    E. Epidural labor analgesia is not recommended given the risk of cardiovascular collapse.

36. **Which of the following associations between findings from fetal heart rate (FHR) monitoring and their causes is most accurately paired?**

    A. Early decelerations—umbilical cord compression
    B. Variable decelerations—fetal head compression
    C. Late decelerations—umbilical cord compression
    D. Sinusoidal pattern—fetal anemia
    E. Accelerations—fetal distress

37. **A 36-year-old G1P0 at 37 weeks' gestation presents to triage complaining of a severe headache and blurry vision. Her vital signs include T 37.8, HR 84, RR 28, and BP 190/114. Her laboratory evaluation is significant for proteinuria and shows a platelet count of 86 000/ mm³ with normal coagulation studies. Which of the following steps of management is inappropriate?**

    A. Treatment of hypertension to a goal of 15%-25% reduction in mean arterial pressure with intravenous (IV) hydralazine
    B. Initiating seizure prophylaxis with magnesium sulfate
    C. Performing an epidural for labor analgesia
    D. Placement of a radial arterial blood pressure catheter
    E. Platelet transfusion to achieve a platelet count of >100 000 mm³ before performing neuraxial anesthesia

38. **A 42-year-old G1P0 woman complains of shortness of breath 3 hours after undergoing cesarean delivery of a term infant. She was initially admitted for preeclampsia and had a prolonged induction during which time she received 5 L of crystalloid infusions. Which of the following is the most likely etiology of her hypoxemia?**

    A. Pulmonary embolism
    B. Pulmonary edema
    C. Spontaneous pneumothorax
    D. Atelectasis
    E. Pneumonia

39. **Which of the following statements is *most correct* regarding umbilical cord prolapse during labor?**

   A. Vaginal delivery may be attempted if the diagnosis is made during the first stage of labor; however, if diagnosed in the second stage, then cesarean delivery should be performed.
   B. Manual elevation of the presenting limb is contraindicated.
   C. Neuraxial anesthesia should be attempted before the use of general anesthesia.
   D. Macrosomia is associated with an increased risk of umbilical cord prolapse.
   E. The risk of complications is decreased with a shorter interval from diagnosis to delivery.

40. **Which of the following interventions is not recommended for aspiration prophylaxis in pregnant patients?**

   A. Ondansetron
   B. Metoclopramide
   C. H_2-receptor antagonists
   D. Nonparticulate antacids
   E. Avoidance of solid foods during labor

41. **A 23-year-old G1P0 woman who just had a successful vaginal delivery with epidural analgesia now has persistent bleeding suspected to be related to retained placenta. Which of the following actions is the least appropriate to pursue for this patient's anesthetic management?**

   A. Use of oxytocin for increased uterine tone after manual removal of the placenta
   B. Neuraxial anesthesia to achieve a block height of T6
   C. Intermittent boluses of ketamine to facilitate extraction
   D. Administering nitroglycerin spray to the mother
   E. Transport to OR and induction of general anesthesia with 1.5-2 MAC (minimum alveolar concentration) of volatile anesthetic

42. **You are called to the bedside to evaluate a 31-year-old G2P1 at term who is attempting a trial of labor after cesarean (TOLAC) and is complaining of abrupt onset of abdominal pain despite previously adequate epidural analgesia. She has a history of a prior cesarean delivery for arrest of descent at 39 weeks. Which of the following statements regarding TOLAC and vaginal birth after cesarean (VBAC) is false?**

   A. Contraindications to VBAC include a previous classic incision uterine surgery.
   B. Risk of uterine rupture is significantly increased in patients attempting a TOLAC.
   C. The risk of maternal mortality is less in a TOLAC than that in an elective cesarean section.
   D. Gestation beyond 40 weeks carries a higher risk of uterine rupture in an attempted TOLAC.
   E. Increased BMI (>30) significantly decreases the likelihood of a successful VBAC.

43. **A 24-year-old G1P0 patient at 33 weeks' gestation with twins presents to triage with uterine contractions and a concern for preterm premature rupture of membranes. Which of the following complications of pregnancy is not consistently associated with multiple gestations?**

   A. Preterm labor
   B. Acute fatty liver of pregnancy
   C. Placental abruption
   D. Postpartum hemorrhage
   E. Gestational diabetes

44. **Which of the statements below regarding preterm labor is most correct?**

   A. Preterm labor complicates roughly 5% of all pregnancies in the United States.
   B. Birth weight of preterm neonates does not correlate with morbidity and mortality.
   C. Urinary tract infections may predispose patients to preterm labor.
   D. Neonatal benefits of maternal administration of corticosteroids in preterm labor are limited to pulmonary maturation.
   E. Magnesium sulfate is preferred as a first-line agent for tocolysis in preterm labor.

45. **Which of the following statements is false regarding breech presentation and delivery?**

   A. External cephalic version is more likely to be successful if performed with general anesthesia.
   B. Perinatal morbidity and mortality are greater in planned cesarean delivery than those in planned vaginal delivery.
   C. Maternal morbidity is lower in planned cesarean delivery than that in planned vaginal delivery.
   D. Institutional protocols for vaginal breech delivery to select appropriate candidates and labor management may be appropriate.
   E. Fetal head entrapment during delivery may require administration of nitroglycerin to the mother.

46. **A neonate, born with a heart rate of 109 beats per minute, is taking gasping irregular breaths, appears cyanotic, grimaces to stimulation, and flexes the extremities. Which of the following is the infant's Apgar score?**

   A. 2
   B. 4
   C. 5
   D. 7
   E. 8

47. **A neonate is delivered at 38 weeks via cesarean section after a failed induction for intrauterine growth restriction. Which of the following is most likely to be associated with increased neonatal morbidity?**

   A. Two separate episodes of FHR late decelerations each lasting 90 seconds
   B. An Apgar score of 6 at 1 minute after delivery
   C. Umbilical artery pH of 7.18 and base deficit of 10 mmol/L
   D. Umbilical artery pH less than 7.0 and base deficit of 14 mmol/L
   E. Stage I hypoxic-ischemic encephalopathy

48. **A neonate is delivered at 35 weeks via an emergent cesarean section and is noted to have rapid shallow gasping, appears cyanotic, and has a heart rate of 110 beats per minute. Which of the following is the most appropriate next step in fetal resuscitation?**

   A. Continue to observe.
   B. Provide positive pressure ventilation.
   C. Provide blow-by supplementary oxygen.
   D. Administer epinephrine.
   E. Begin chest compressions.

49. **You are caring for a 29-year-old G2P1 at 28 weeks' gestation with the pregnancy complicated by a fetal sacrococcygeal teratoma, who is presenting for an intrauterine surgical intervention. Which of the following statements is NOT true regarding intrauterine surgery?**

   A. Volatile anesthetic agents are used at 2-3 MAC for maintenance of anesthesia.
   B. Magnesium and nitroglycerin may be used to provide tocolysis.
   C. Maternal administration of paralytic agents is needed to ensure maternal and fetal immobility.
   D. Vasopressor use to maintain placental perfusion is frequently required.
   E. Subsequent pregnancies should be delivered via cesarean section rather than allowing labor.

50. **A healthy 24-year-old G2P1 at term with an epidural in place for analgesia who is currently at 7 cm cervical dilatation develops a late deceleration in the FHR tracing. Her current heart rate is 108 beats per minute, blood pressure is 80/47 mm Hg, and oxygen saturation is 97% on room air. Which of the following interventions is least likely to be beneficial for correction of fetal distress?**

   A. IV fluid bolus
   B. IV bolus of phenylephrine
   C. Terbutaline
   D. Maternal repositioning
   E. Maternal oxygen supplementation

Chapter 15 ■ Answers

1. Correct answer: B

Cardiovascular changes during pregnancy begin early during the first trimester. Cardiac output increases by 40% during the first trimester and continues to increase to 50% greater than prepregnancy values by the end of the third trimester. The increased cardiac output results from increases in heart rate and stroke volume; the stroke volume in the third trimester is 30% greater than prepregnancy values. While the left ventricular end-diastolic volume increases, the left ventricular end-systolic pressure remains unchanged, which results in an increased ejection fraction. Left ventricular mass and myocardial contractility also increase. Central venous pressure, pulmonary artery diastolic pressure, and pulmonary capillary wedge pressure remain unchanged.

Changes in Cardiovascular Parameters During Pregnancy

INCREASE	REMAIN UNCHANGED	DECREASE
• Cardiac output • Heart rate • Stroke volume • LV end-diastolic volume • Ejection fraction • Myocardial contractility	• LV end-systolic volume • LV stroke work index • Pulmonary capillary wedge pressure • PA diastolic pressure • Central venous pressure	• Systemic vascular resistance • Pulmonary vascular resistance

References:
1. Clark SL, Cotton DB, Lee W, et al. Central hemodynamic assessment of normal term pregnancy. *Am J Obstet Gynecol.* 1989;161(6 Pt 1):1439-1242.
2. Gaiser R. Physiologic changes of pregnancy. In: Chestnut DH, Polley LS, Tsen LC, Wong CA, eds. *Chestnut's Obstetric Anesthesia Principles and Practice.* 4th ed. Philadelphia: Elsevier; 2009:15–36.
3. Robson SC, Hunter S, Boys RJ, Dunlop W. Serial study of factors influencing changes in cardiac output during human pregnancy. *Am J Physiol.* 1989;256(4 Pt 2):H1060-H1065.

2. Correct answer: D

Supine hypotensive syndrome occurs in up to 15% of parturients and is the result of compression of the inferior vena cava (IVC), which reduces venous return of blood from the lower extremities to the heart. The femoral artery pressure is significantly lower than brachial artery pressure in patients in this setting, as the upper extremities continue to have normal blood flow. Uterine blood flow can fall by up to 20%, and lower extremity blood flow, by up to 50%. In patients with supine hypotensive syndrome, the femoral veins have decreased blood flow velocity secondary to impeded obstruction. The hemodynamic response to decreased venous return includes hypotension, decreased cardiac output, and tachycardia that may transition to bradycardia in some cases.

Despite this well-described hemodynamic phenomenon of pregnancy and the advocacy for traditional positioning to reduce the incidence, the benefit of left lateral uterine displacement has been questioned. Some studies suggest that manual displacement is better than with a wedge and that left displacement may be better than right; however, the evidence for any single intervention is limited and does not clearly demonstrate superiority of any specific positioning. MRI studies have shown that the aorta is not compressed in term parturients in the supine position; however, the IVC is significantly more compressed than that in nonpregnant patients. The recommended 15° left lateral tilt position may not effectively reduce IVC compression, and a full 30° tilt may be needed to improve IVC compression.

References:
1. Chestnut DH, Polley LS, Tsen LC, Wong CA. Physiologic changes of pregnancy. In: Conklin KA, Chang BA. *Chestnut's Obstetric Anesthesia Principles and Practice.* 4th ed. Philadelphia: Elsevier; 2009:25–36.
2. Cluver C, Novikova N, Hofmeyr GJ, Hall DR. Maternal position during caesarean section for preventing maternal and neonatal complications. *Cochrane Database Syst Rev.* 2013;(3):CD007623.
3. Higuchi H, Takagi S, Zhang K, et al. Effect of lateral tilt angle on the volume of the abdominal aorta and inferior vena cava in pregnant and nonpregnant women determined by magnetic resonance imaging. *Anesthesiology.* 2015;122(2):286-293.

4. Kinda P, Velraj J, Amirthalingam U, et al. Effect of positioning from supine and left lateral positions to left lateral tilt on maternal blood flow velocities and waveforms in full-term parturients. *Anaesthesia.* 2012;67(8):889-893.
5. Kinsella SM, Lohmann G. Supine hypotensive syndrome. *Obstet Gynecol.* 1994;83(5 Pt 1):774-788.

3. Correct answer: C

Pregnant women have an increased neural sensitivity to local anesthetics and demonstrate a faster onset and prolonged duration of neuraxial block than nonpregnant patients. The dose requirement of hyperbaric local anesthetic in term pregnant women is 25%-35% lower than that in nonpregnant women. This phenomenon results from multiple factors including decreased CSF volume, distended epidural venous plexus, enhanced neural susceptibility to local anesthetics, and increased rostral spread due to widening of the pelvis. These pregnancy-induced changes are short-lived, as the spinal dose requirements rapidly return to those of nonpregnant women within 2 days of postpartum as CSF volume expands and vena caval compression is relieved. Pregnancy does not enhance the susceptibility to neurotoxicity of lidocaine or bupivacaine in animal studies.

References:
1. Abouleish EI. Postpartum tubal ligation requires more bupivacaine for spinal anesthesia than dose cesarean section. *Anesth Analg.* 1986;65:897-900.
2. Gaiser R. Physiologic changes of pregnancy. In: Chestnut DH, Polley LS, Tsen LC, Wong CA, eds. *Chestnut's Obstetric Anesthesia Principles and Practice.* 4th ed. Philadelphia: Elsevier; 2009:15–36.
3. Hirabayashi Y, Shimizu R, Saitoh K, Fukuda H. Spread of subarachnoid hyperbaric amethocaine in pregnant women. *Br J Anaesth.* 1995;74(4):384-386.
4. Zhan Q, Huang S, Geng G, Xie Y. Comparison of relative potency of intrathecal bupivacaine for motor block in pregnant versus non-pregnant women. *Int J Obstet Anesth.* 2011;20(3):219-223.

4. Correct answer: A

The MAC for volatile anesthetics is decreased in term pregnancy by up to 40%. The rate of rise of alveolar anesthetic concentration with inhalational anesthetic administration is faster in pregnant women than that in a nonpregnant woman because of the increased minute ventilation and decreased FRC in pregnant women despite the increased cardiac output, which typically slows inhalational induction. Despite the traditional teaching that MAC is decreased, there is an increased risk of awareness with general anesthesia in pregnant women with rates reported up to 1/670. This may be related to the increased risk of emergency surgery, difficult airway, and lack of adjunctive agents due to concern for fetal depression.

IV anesthetic effects are variable, as pregnant women require decreased thiopental dosing by about 35%, whereas propofol, etomidate, and ketamine dosing is unchanged. Early pregnancy studies fail to demonstrate changes in propofol requirements compared with nonpregnant women. It is recommended that for cesarean delivery, given the increased volume of distribution and lack of premedication, propofol, etomidate, and ketamine dosing for general anesthesia remain unchanged from nonpregnant women. Other drug requirements during pregnancy are variable, as pregnant women have a larger volume of distribution and altered protein binding. At term, plasma levels of α-1-acid glycoprotein and albumin are both reduced. Pseudocholinesterase activity is decreased by up to 30% at term; however, this is rarely clinically relevant in regard to return of neuromuscular activity after a single dose of succinylcholine. Pregnant women demonstrate an increased sensitivity to the aminosteroid muscle relaxants vecuronium and rocuronium.

References:
1. Gaiser R. Physiologic changes of pregnancy. In: Chestnut DH, Polley LS, Tsen LC, Wong CA, eds. *Chestnut's Obstetric Anesthesia Principles and Practice.* 4th ed. Philadelphia: Elsevier; 2009:15–36.
2. Higuchi H, Adachi Y, Arimura S, Kanno M, Satoh T. Early pregnancy does not reduce the C(50) of propofol for loss of consciousness. *Anesth Analg.* 2001;93(6):1565-1569.
3. Pandit JJ, Andrade J, Bogod DG, et al. 5th National Audit Project (NAP5) on accidental awareness during general anesthesia: summary of main findings and risk factors. *Br J Anaesth.* 2014;113:549.
4. Palahniuk RJ, Shnider SM, Eger EI. Pregnancy decreases the requirement for inhaled anesthetic agents. *Anesthesiology.* 1974;41:82-83.

5. Correct answer: B

Resting alveolar minute ventilation rises during pregnancy largely because of an increase in tidal volume up to 45% higher than prepregnancy values. These changes are mediated by hormones (principally progesterone), increased carbon dioxide production, and increased chemosensitivity. They occur early in the pregnancy, resulting in a decreased $Paco_2$ to approximately 30 mm Hg by 12 weeks' gestation, where it plateaus throughout the remainder of the pregnancy. Metabolic compensation for the respiratory alkalosis of pregnancy is incomplete but results in a serum bicarbonate concentration of about 20 mEq/L. Controlled ventilation during general anesthesia should be adjusted to maintain the $Paco_2$ of 30 mm Hg, as allowing it to rise to that of a nonpregnant woman will result in respiratory acidosis.

The increased minute ventilation often produces dyspnea in women by the third trimester, and this sensation is worsened by the increased pulmonary blood volume, anemia, and upper airway congestion.

References:
1. Gaiser R. Physiologic changes of pregnancy. In: Chestnut DH, Polley LS, Tsen LC, Wong CA, eds. *Chestnut's Obstetric Anesthesia Principles and Practice*. 4th ed. Philadelphia: Elsevier; 2009:15–36.
2. Conklin KA. Maternal physiologic adaptations during gestation, labor, and the puerperium. *Semin Anesth*. 1991;10:221-234.
3. Rampton AJ, Mallaiah S, Garrett CP. Increased ventilation requirements during obstetric general anaesthesia. *Br J Anaesth*. 1988;61:730-737.
4. Zwillich CW, Natalino MR, Sutton FD, Weil JV. Effects of progesterone on chemosensitivity in men. *J Lab Clin Med*. 1978;92(2):262-269.

6. Correct answer: D

FRC decreases by about 20% at term because of elevation of the diaphragm from uterine enlargement. Vital capacity is relatively unchanged at term, whereas inspiratory capacity increases by 15%, and expiratory reserve volume decreases by 25%. The anesthetic implications of these changes include rapid oxygen desaturation in the setting of apnea with Pao_2 decreasing at twice the rate of that in nonpregnant women. This rapid oxygen desaturation is due to increased oxygen consumption and reduced FRC. In addition, the closing capacity is higher than FRC in up to 50% of supine parturients, resulting in airway closure during tidal breathing.

Changes in Respiratory Parameters During Pregnancy

INCREASE (% RELATIVE TO NONPREGNANT STATE)	REMAIN UNCHANGED	DECREASE (% RELATIVE TO NONPREGNANT STATE)
• Inspiratory reserve volume (+5%) • Tidal volume (+45%) • Inspiratory capacity (+15%) • Dead space (+45%) • Minute ventilation (+45%)	• Vital capacity • Respiratory rate • Forced expiratory volume (FEV1)	• Expiratory reserve volume (−25%) • Residual volume (−15%) • Functional residual capacity (−20%) • Total lung capacity (−5%)

References:
1. Archer GW, Marx GF. Arterial oxygen tension during apnea in parturient women. *Br J Anaesth*. 1974;46:358-360.
2. Gaiser R. Physiologic changes of pregnancy. In: Chestnut DH, Polley LS, Tsen LC, Wong CA, eds. *Chestnut's Obstetric Anesthesia Principles and Practice*. 4th ed. Philadelphia: Elsevier; 2009:15–36.
3. Conklin KA. Maternal physiologic adaptations during gestation, labor, and the puerperium. *Semin Anesth*. 1991;10:221-234.
4. Milne JA, Mills RJ, Howie AD, Pack AI. Large airways function during normal pregnancy. *Br J Obstet Gynaecol*. 1977;84(6):448-451.
5. Russell IF, Chambers WA. Closing volume in normal pregnancy. *Br J Anaesth*. 1981;53(10):1043-1047.

7. Correct answer: E

Renal volume increases during pregnancy by up to 30% with dilation of the renal calyces, pelvis, and ureters. Hydronephrosis can be observed with imaging and is seen during pregnancy in up to 65% of women, thus increasing the potential for pyelonephritis during pregnancy. Glomerular filtration rate and renal plasma flow increase by up to 50% and 75%, respectively, compared with prepregnancy values. Creatinine clearance increases by up to 40%, resulting in decreased blood concentrations of nitrogenous metabolites as well as serum creatinine. Total protein and urinary albumin excretion are also increased compared with nonpregnant values. Owing to the increase in alveolar ventilation and the resultant respiratory alkalosis that occur in normal pregnancy, the kidney compensates by increasing bicarbonate excretion from the kidneys to decrease serum bicarbonate levels. Glucose excretion is increased during pregnancy because of changes in the capacity to resorb glucose in the proximal tubules that persists for about a week after delivery.

References:

1. Gaiser R. Physiologic changes of pregnancy. In: Chestnut DH, Polley LS, Tsen LC, Wong CA, eds. *Chestnut's Obstetric Anesthesia Principles and Practice*. 4th ed. Philadelphia: Elsevier; 2009:15–36.
2. Cheung KL, Lafayette RA. Renal physiology of pregnancy. *Adv Chronic Kidney Dis*. 2013;20(3):209-214.
3. Davison JM, Hytten FE. The effect of pregnancy on the renal handling of glucose. *Br J Obstet Gynaecol*. 1975;82:374-381.

8. Correct answer: A

Pregnancy is associated with biliary stasis and changes in bile composition, which increase the risk of biliary sludge and gallbladder disease. Estrogen increases cholesterol production, and progesterone inhibits the contractility of the GI smooth muscle, inhibiting gallbladder emptying. Progesterone also alters the composition of bile to favor insoluble acids, thereby encouraging stone formation. AP levels increase during pregnancy by up to 4 times of prepregnancy values because of placental production of AP, not biliary stasis.

Intrahepatic cholestasis of pregnancy is a disease specific to pregnancy that typically develops in the third trimester and is associated with pruritus and elevated serum bile acids in the mother. It is associated with increased rates of adverse pregnancy outcomes including preterm labor, fetal distress, and intrauterine fetal demise. Treatment is typically with ursodeoxycholic acid, which improves maternal symptoms and may be protective for the fetus.

Ultrasonography is the most sensitive imaging test for detecting gallstones and has the additional benefit that it does not expose the mother or fetus to radiation. Multiple studies have been unable to draw formal conclusions regarding the superiority of open versus laparoscopic approaches for cholecystectomy during pregnancy in regard to maternal or fetal outcomes, and the decision is made based on surgeon and center experience as well as the individual case.

References:

1. Gaiser R. Physiologic changes of pregnancy. In: Chestnut DH, Polley LS, Tsen LC, Wong CA, eds. *Chestnut's Obstetric Anesthesia Principles and Practice*. 4th ed. Philadelphia: Elsevier; 2009:15–36.
2. Dixon PH, Williamson C. The pathophysiology of intrahepatic cholestasis of pregnancy. *Clin Res Hepatol Gastroenterol*. 2016;40(2):141-153.
3. Gilo NB, Amini D, Landy HJ. Appendicitis and cholecystitis in pregnancy. *Clin Obstet Gynecol*. 2009;52(4)586-596.
4. Nasioudis D, Tsilimigras D, Economopoulos KP. Laparoscopic cholecystectomy during pregnancy: a systematic review of 590 patients. *Int J Surg*. 2016;27:165-175.

9. Correct answer: D

Hormonal changes of pregnancy result in reduced lower esophageal sphincter tone and contribute to an increased risk of gastroesophageal reflux during pregnancy. Reflux symptoms are further exacerbated by the enlarging uterus, which displaces the stomach and intra-abdominal esophageal segment upward into the thorax. The lower esophageal sphincter pressure typically remains normal until the second trimester when it is reduced to about 50% of prepregnancy levels. Multiple imaging studies have demonstrated that the gastric emptying of both liquid and solid meals is not altered during pregnancy. Preoperative fasting guidelines for cesarean section are unchanged compared with those of other surgical procedures (2 h for clear liquids, 6 h for solids, and 8 h for fatty meals). In general, solid foods should be avoided in laboring patients. Esophageal peristalsis and intestinal transit are delayed during pregnancy, which is attributed to the effect of progesterone on GI motility as well as decreased concentrations of serum motilin.

It is considered standard of care to administer at least one medication for aspiration prophylaxis in laboring patients. Nonparticulate antacids and H_2 antagonists are commonly administered to increase gastric pH in this setting.

References:

1. Gaiser R. Physiologic changes of pregnancy. In: Chestnut DH, Polley LS, Tsen LC, Wong CA, eds. *Chestnut's Obstetric Anesthesia Principles and Practice*. 4th ed. Philadelphia: Elsevier; 2009:15–36.
2. Chiloiro M, Darconza G, Piccioli E, et al. Gastric emptying and orocecal transit time during pregnancy. *J Gastroenterol*. 2001;36:538-543.
3. Goldszmidt E. Principles and practices of obstetric airway management. *Anesthesiol Clin*. 2008;26(1):109-125.
4. Paranjothy S, Griffiths JD, Broughton HK, et al. Interventions at caesarean section for reducing the risk of aspiration pneumonitis. *Cochrane Database Syst Rev*. 2014;5(2):CD004943.
5. Practice guidelines for obstetric anesthesia: an updated report by the American Society of Anesthesiologist Task Force on Obstetric Anesthesia and the Society for Obstetric Anesthesia and Perinatology. *Anesthesiology*. 2016;124(2):270-300.

10. Correct answer: E

Plasma volume increases by 50% and RBC mass, by about 40% compared with prepregnancy values, resulting in physiologic anemia. Iron deficiency is also more common during pregnancy because of fetal iron requirements for development. Fibrinolytic activity is increased during pregnancy, and plasminogen concentration also rises. Several coagulation factors (I, VII, VIII, IX, X, and XII) are increased during pregnancy by up to 100% of prepregnancy values and contribute to the hypercoagulable state present during pregnancy and the peripartum period. Polymorphonuclear lymphocyte chemotaxis and adherence is reduced during pregnancy and may account for the increased incidence of infection during pregnancy. Platelet consumption is greater during pregnancy; however, studies suggest that increased platelet production compensates for this greater activation, consumption, and clearance. Thrombocytopenia occurs in 8%-10% of pregnancies, and most cases are mild. Severely decreased platelets counts merit investigation and management.

References:
1. Gaiser R. Physiologic changes of pregnancy. In: Chestnut DH, Polley LS, Tsen LC, Wong CA, eds. *Chestnut's Obstetric Anesthesia Principles and Practice*. 4th ed. Philadelphia: Elsevier; 2009:15–36.
2. Conklin KA. Maternal physiologic adaptations during gestation, labor, and the puerperium. *Semin Anesth*. 1991;10:221-234.
3. Krause PJ, Ingardia CJ, Pontius LT, et al. Host defense during pregnancy: neutrophil chemotaxis and adherence. *Am J Obstet Gynecol*. 1987;157:274-280.
4. Townsley DM. Hematologic complications of pregnancy. *Semin Hematol*. 2013;50(3):222-231.

11. Correct answer: A

Many of the induction agents used for general anesthesia are lipophilic and therefore readily cross the placenta into the fetal circulation. Propofol, ketamine, morphine, and diazepam all cross the placenta and are more likely to have a clinical effect on the neonate than a drug that does not have high placental transfer. High lipid solubility allows drugs to penetrate the lipid bilayer and cross the placenta. Drugs with lower protein binding also cross the placenta more readily. Morphine has been shown to reduce fetal breathing movements and decrease FHR variability. Hydrophilic, charged drugs with high molecular weight (>1000 Da) are less likely to transfer across the placenta. Vecuronium and other ionized, quaternary ammonium salt nondepolarizing muscle relaxants do not readily cross the placenta, have low fetal/maternal drug ratios, and have no significant clinical effect on neonates born to mothers who received them while under general anesthesia.

References:
1. Zakowski MI, Herman NL. The placenta: anatomy, physiology, and transfer of drugs. In: Chestnut DH, Polley LS, Tsen LC, Wong CA, eds. *Chestnut's Obstetric Anesthesia Principles and Practice*. 4th ed. Philadelphia: Elsevier; 2009:55–72.
2. Dailey PA, Fisher DM, Shnider SM, et al. Pharmacokinetics, placental transfer, and neonatal effects of vecuronium and pancuronium administered during cesarean section. *Anesthesiology*. 1984;60(6):569-574.

12. Correct answer: B

PPH is one of the most common and potentially devastating complications of pregnancy occurring in approximately 5% of deliveries. Primary PPH is defined as a blood loss greater than 500 mL within 24 hours after birth, and severe PPH occurs when blood loss exceeds 1000 mL after delivery. The most common cause of PPH is uterine atony, and other risk factors include prolonged labor, chorioamnionitis, multiple gestations, macrosomia, polyhydramnios, high parity, and medications including tocolytic agents and volatile anesthetic agents. First-line treatment includes bimanual compression, uterine massage, and oxytocin infusion. Other commonly used agents for PPH include the ergot alkaloids (methylergonovine), prostaglandin analogues (methylprostaglandin $F_2\alpha$), and other oxytocin agonists (carbetocin). Off-label use of prostaglandin E1 (misoprostol) is also often used when bleeding is uncontrolled with other agents or there are contraindications to any of the other uterotonics.

Each of the uterotonic drugs has unique side effects. Oxytocin is associated with systemic vasodilation, hypotension, flushing, headache, nausea/vomiting, and rarely hyponatremia (not hypernatremia), elevated pulmonary artery pressures, and pulmonary edema. Carbetocin is a long-acting oxytocin agonist with a significantly longer half-life than oxytocin; it shares a similar hemodynamic side effect profile to oxytocin including hypotension. Misoprostol is commonly associated with pyrexia, shivering, and nausea. Methylprostaglandin is associated with nausea, headache, shivering, pyrexia, and life-threatening bronchospasm, therefore relatively contraindicated in patients with reactive airway disease such as asthma. Methylergonovine is associated with hypertension and vasospasm and occasionally results in coronary or cerebral ischemia; consequently methylergonovine is relatively contraindicated in patients with preeclampsia or hypertension.

References:
1. Mayer DC, Smith KA. Antepartum and postpartum hemorrhage. In: Chestnut DH, Polley LS, Tsen LC, Wong CA, eds. *Chestnut's Obstetric Anesthesia Principles and Practice.* 4th ed. Philadelphia: Elsevier; 2009:811–836.
2. Bohlmann MK, Rath W. Medical prevention and treatment of postpartum hemorrhage: a comparison of different guidelines. *Arch Gynecol Obstet.* 2014;289(3):555-567.

13. Correct answer: B

Preterm labor is defined as labor before 37 weeks' gestation and can be associated with significant neonatal morbidity and mortality. Risk factors for preterm labor and delivery include premature activation of physiologic contractions, uterine overdistension (due to multiple gestation, polyhydramnios, etc), placental ischemia, decidual hemorrhage, premature rupture of membranes, abnormal uterine or cervical anatomy, cervical insufficiency, history of preterm delivery, and maternal systemic or vaginal infection. The goal of tocolytic therapy is to delay delivery to allow for further fetal maturation. Tocolytic agents are administered when the gestation is between 20 and 34 weeks, fetal status is reassuring, and there is no evidence of infection.

β-Adrenergic agonists are effective at preventing preterm delivery; however, they are associated with significant cardiovascular side effects including dysrhythmias, hypotension, tachycardia, palpitations, and occasionally severe complications including pulmonary edema. Progesterone reduces intracellular calcium and prostaglandin synthesis and has been shown to reduce preterm births in patients at risk of preterm delivery. Calcium channel blockers cause uterine relaxation by decreasing intracellular calcium and have relatively benign side effects including headache, flushing, and mild hypotension. Indomethacin is a cyclooxygenase inhibitor that decreases the prostaglandin synthesis that is associated with uterine contractions and has been demonstrated to have tocolytic effects in preterm labor. It is however associated with premature closure of the ductus arteriosus, and its use is typically limited to the second trimester. Magnesium sulfate is a calcium antagonist, which was historically used for preterm labor; however, the current evidence suggests that it does not have a beneficial role in preventing or delayed preterm labor. Despite a lack of benefit for preventing preterm delivery, it is frequently administered during preterm labor, as it has been associated with neonatal neuroprotective effects.

References:
1. Muir HA, Wong CA. Preterm labor and delivery. In: Chestnut DH, Polley LS, Tsen LC, Wong CA, eds. *Chestnut's Obstetric Anesthesia Principles and Practice.* 4th ed. Philadelphia: Elsevier; 2009:749–778.
2. Hubinont C, Debieve F. Prevention of preterm labour: 2011 update on tocolysis. *J Pregnancy.* 2011:941057.

14. Correct answer: C

Women with a history of epilepsy may be on long-term anticonvulsant agents before pregnancy that require continuation for the duration of pregnancy. Changes in drug absorption, metabolism, clearance, volume of distribution, and hormonal levels during pregnancy cause varying levels of drug concentrations and require monitoring to maintain therapeutic drug levels and prevent seizures. Maternal seizures during pregnancy can have dramatic and severe consequences to both the mother and fetus, so it is important to monitor these women closely during pregnancy with the guidance of a neurologist.

Several studies have found associations with epilepsy and antiepileptic drugs with adverse perinatal outcomes including preterm delivery, low birth weight, small-for-gestational age, low Apgar scores, respiratory complications, NICU admissions, microcephaly, and neurodevelopmental deficits. Epilepsy and antiepileptic drugs may also be associated with increased risk of pregnancy complications such as preeclampsia and gestational hypertension.

In patients taking long-term antiepileptic agents that induce hepatic enzymes, such as carbamepazine, phenobarbital, and phenytoin, infants are at an increased risk of vitamin K–dependent coagulation factor deficiencies. As a result, affected infants are at an increased risk of neonatal hemorrhage (not thrombosis) and it is recommended to give intramuscular vitamin K after delivery to prevent hemorrhagic complications of the newborn. Although vitamin K is often given prenatally in mothers taking these medications, there is not enough evidence to support the use of maternal antenatal vitamin K supplementation to avoid newborn bleeding complications.

References:
1. Bader AM. Neurologic and neuromuscular disease. In: Chestnut DH, Polley LS, Tsen LC, Wong CA, eds. *Chestnut's Obstetric Anesthesia Principles and Practice.* 4th ed. Philadelphia: Elsevier; 2009:1053–1078.
2. Patel SI, Pennell PB. Management of epilepsy during pregnancy: an update. *Ther Adv Neurol Disord.* 2016;9(2):118-129.
3. Zhao Y, Hebert MF, Venkataramanan R. Basic obstetric pharmacology. *Semin Perinatol.* 2014;38(8):475-486.

15. Correct answer: A

Studies have been done to evaluate fetal-maternal ratios of drug concentration, and these data have been used to extrapolate pharmacokinetics of anesthetics and other drugs across the human placenta.

Factors that contribute to **increased** transfer across the placenta include the following:
- Molecules <1000 Da
- Uncharged molecules
- Lipophilic substances
- Lower proportion of ionized drug in maternal plasma
- Absence of a placental efflux transporter protein
- Albumin protein binding (lower binding affinity)
- High free (unbound) drug fraction

Factors that contribute to **decreased** transfer across the placenta include the following:
- Molecules >1000 Da
- Charged molecules
- Hydrophilic substances
- Higher proportion of ionized drug in maternal plasma
- Presence of a placental efflux transporter protein
- α-1-Acid glycoprotein binding (higher binding affinity)
- Low free (unbound) drug fraction

References:
1. Zakowski MI, Herman NL. The placenta: anatomy, physiology, and transfer of drugs. In: Chestnut DH, Polley LS, Tsen LC, Wong CA, eds. *Chestnut's Obstetric Anesthesia Principles and Practice.* 4th ed. Philadelphia: Elsevier; 2009:55–72.
2. Pacifici GM, Nottoli R. Placental transfer of drugs administered to the mother. *Clin Pharmacokinet.* 1995;28(3):235-269.

16. Correct answer: B

CVS and amniocentesis are procedures performed to evaluate fetal karyotype together with a number of other antenatal markers. Chorionic villus samples include placental cells and trophoblasts, rather than amniocytes. The major risks associated with both procedures are pregnancy loss (see below) and infection (0.3% for CVS, <0.1% for amniocentesis), and minor risks include vaginal spotting and amniotic fluid leakage. Early amniocentesis is associated with club foot in the fetus, while CVS performed before 9 weeks is associated with limb reduction defects.

CVS is typically performed between 9 and 14 weeks of gestation, whereas amniocentesis is typically performed in the second trimester after 18 weeks. Overall, second trimester amniocentesis is safer and associated with a decreased rate of pregnancy loss than CVS; however, CVS is safer than early (performed between 9 and 14 wk) amniocentesis. The risk of pregnancy loss is 0.25%-1% for late amniocentesis, 1%-1.5% for CVS, and 2.2%-4.8% for early amniocentesis. Neither technique is contraindicated in patients with a history of pregnancy loss; however, the risk of procedure-related pregnancy loss should be discussed with the patient when obtaining informed consent.

Both procedures carry a risk of isoimmunization, and Rh-negative women should receive Rh(D) immune globulin before the procedure. Provider experience may influence the rate of pregnancy loss in CVS; however, it has not been shown to alter outcomes with amniocentesis.

References:
1. American College of Obstetricians and Gynecologists (ACOG), Committee on Practice Bulletins. *Prevention of RhD Alloimmunization. Practice Bulletin No. 4.* Washington, DC: American College of Obstetricians and Gynecologists; 1999, reaffirmed in 2016.
2. Alfirevic Z, Sundberg K, Brigham S. Amniocentesis and chorionic villus sampling for prenatal diagnosis. *Cochrane Database Syst Rev.* 2003;(3):CD003252.
3. Campbell K, Park JS, Norwitz ER. Antepartum fetal assessment and therapy. In: Chestnut DH, Polley LS, Tsen LC, Wong CA, eds. *Chestnut's Obstetric Anesthesia Principles and Practice.* 4th ed. Philadelphia: Elsevier; 2009:89–122.

17. **Correct answer: C**

Amniotic fluid is composed almost entirely of fetal urine in the second and third trimesters. **Oligohydramnios** is a condition in pregnancy characterized by a deficiency of amniotic fluid. Adverse pregnancy outcomes are more common when oligohydramnios is present and include an increased risk of cesarean delivery for fetal distress and decreased Apgar scores.

The most common cause of oligohydramnios is fetal anomalies, occurring in roughly 50% of second and third trimester cases of oligohydramnios. Uteroplacental insufficiency is associated with oligohydramnios and can predispose the umbilical cord to compression, leading to intermittent fetal hypoxemia and meconium passage at the time of delivery. The volume of amniotic fluid is not affected by acute fetal hypoxia or CNS dysfunction.

Pregnancies complicated by preterm premature rupture of membranes after amniocentesis are associated with better perinatal outcomes compared with those pregnancies complicated by spontaneous preterm premature rupture of membranes at a similar gestational age, and amniotic fluid reaccumulates to normal volume in most cases. Hydrops fetalis is most commonly seen with polyhydramnios in up to 75% of cases, not oligohydramnios.

Causes of oligohydramnios include the following:
- Uteroplacental insufficiency due to maternal causes: preeclampsia, chronic hypertension, collagen vascular disease, nephropathy, and thrombophilia
- Maternal medications (ACE inhibitors)
- Placental abruption
- Twin-twin transfusion
- Placental thrombosis infarction
- Chromosomal abnormalities
- Congenital fetal anomalies (especially those associated with impaired urine production)
- Growth restriction
- Fetal demise
- Postterm pregnancy
- Ruptured fetal membranes
- Postamniocentesis
- Idiopathic

References:

1. Borgida AF, Mills AA, Feldman DM, et al. Outcome of pregnancies complicated by ruptured membranes after genetic amniocentesis. *Am J Obstet Gynecol.* 2000;183(4):937-939.
2. Chauhan SP, Sanderson M, Hendrix NW, et al. Perinatal outcome and amniotic fluid index in the antepartum and intrapartum periods: a meta-analysis. *Am J Obstet Gynecol.* 1999;181(6):1473.
3. Campbell K, Park JS, Norwitz ER. Antepartum fetal assessment and therapy. In: Chestnut DH, Polley LS, Tsen LC, Wong CA, eds. *Chestnut's Obstetric Anesthesia Principles and Practice.* 4th ed. Philadelphia: Elsevier; 2009:89–122.
4. Shipp TD, Bromley B, Pauker S, et al. Outcome of singleton pregnancies with severe oligohydramnios in the second and third trimesters. *Ultrasound Obstet Gynecol.* 1996;7(2):108-113.

18. **Correct answer: A**

Hydrops fetalis (fetal hydrops) is a serious fetal condition defined as abnormal accumulation of fluid in 2 or more fetal compartments, including ascites, pleural effusion, pericardial effusion, and skin edema. Immune hydrops fetalis is the result of maternal immune sensitization and antibodies directed toward fetal RBC proteins that are viewed as "foreign." IgG immunoglobulin antibodies can cross the placenta and destroy fetal RBCs, resulting in severe fetal anemia and high-output cardiac failure. The most antigenic protein on the surface of fetal RBCs is the D antigen of the Rhesus protein complex Rh(D); however, there are other non-ABO antigens that can also result in severe immune hydrops. These include non-ABO RBC antigens such as Kell, Rh(E), Rh(c), and Duffy. Antigens that are associated with less severe immune hydrops include ABO, Rh(e), Rh(C), Ce, k, and s. Rho(D) immune globulin is used to prevent immunization to fetal Rh(D)-positive RBCs and is given to Rh(D)-negative mothers whose fetus is a possible Rh(D)-positive when a risk of fetomaternal hemorrhage exists.

Causes of fetomaternal hemorrhage that can result in alloimmunization and are indications for Rho(D) immune globulin administration include delivery, manual placental removal, placental abruption, placenta previa, spontaneous or induced abortion, invasive prenatal diagnostic or therapeutic procedure, blunt abdominal trauma, external cephalic version, ectopic pregnancy, threatened abortion, fetal death in the second or third trimester, and antepartum hemorrhage in the second or third trimester.

Rho(D) immune globulin prophylaxis should be given after Rh(D)-negative women have delivered a known Rh(D)-positive newborn. Since the advent of Rho(D) immune globulin, the proportion of hydrops fetalis cases with immune etiology has decreased to 10%-15%.

Maternal infections are responsible for 5%-10% of nonimmune fetal hydrops fetalis and are mostly commonly due to parvovirus B19, CMV, toxoplasmosis, syphilis, rubella, or varicella. Other nonimmune etiologies include fetal cardiovascular, chromosomal, hematologic, and structural abnormalities, complications of monochorionic twinning, and placental abnormalities. The prognosis of hydrops fetalis depends on the etiology; however, the overall neonatal survival is often <50%.

References:
1. American College of Obstetricians and Gynecologists. ACOG Practice Bulletin No. 75: management of alloimmunization during pregnancy. *Obstet Gynecol.* 2006;108(2):457-464.
2. Campbell K, Park JS, Norwitz ER. Antepartum fetal assessment and therapy. In: Chestnut DH, Polley LS, Tsen LC, Wong CA, eds. *Chestnut's Obstetric Anesthesia Principles and Practice.* 4th ed. Philadelphia: Elsevier; 2009:89–122.
3. Society for Maternal-Fetal Medicine (SMFM), Norton ME, Chauhan SP, Dashe JS. Society for maternal-fetal medicine (SMFM) clinical guideline #7: nonimmune hydrops fetalis. *Am J Obstet Gynecol.* 2015;212(2):127-139.
4. Sohan K, Carroll SG, De La Fuente S, et al. Analysis of outcome in hydrops fetalis in relation to gestational age at diagnosis, cause and treatment. *Acta Obstet Gynecol Scand.* 2001;80(8):726-730.

19. Correct answer: C

Fetal nonstress testing (NST) evaluates changes in the FHR pattern during a 30- to 60-minute interval and reflects the maturity of the fetal autonomic nervous system (for this reason it is less useful in premature fetuses <28 wk). An NST can be classified as normal, atypical, or abnormal. A normal NST will show a baseline FHR between 110 and 160 beats per minute with moderate variability (5-25 interbeat variability) and 2 qualifying accelerations in 20 minutes with no decelerations. A "reactive" NST is reassuring for fetal well-being; however, interpretation of a "nonreactive" NST requires consideration of gestational age, underlying clinical circumstances, and previous FHR tracings before making management considerations because of concern for poor perinatal outcome.

A BPP is a sonographic scoring system ranging from 0 to 10 performed for more than 30 to 40 minutes to assess fetal well-being that has been validated in both preterm and term fetuses. The 5 components of the BPP are gross fetal body movements, fetal tone (flexion/extension of limbs), amniotic fluid volume, fetal breathing movements, and the NST. The BPP can also be interpreted without the NST. Each component of the BPP is graded either 0 or 2 points and then added up to yield a number between 0 and 10. A BPP of 8 or 10 is generally considered reassuring.

Vibroacoustic stimulation (VAS) is the response of the FHR to a vibroacoustic stimulus (82-95 dB for 3 s) applied to the maternal abdomen in the region of the fetal head. Accelerations in FHR are suggestive of fetal well-being and are considered a positive response. Absent FHR acceleration in response to VAS at term is associated with an increased risk of nonreassuring FHR in labor and increased risk of cesarean delivery.

Although VAS provides information regarding fetal responsiveness, it is not included in the scoring system of the BPP.

References:
1. Campbell K, Park JS, Norwitz ER. Antepartum fetal assessment and therapy. In: Chestnut DH, Polley LS, Tsen LC, Wong CA, eds. *Chestnut's Obstetric Anesthesia Principles and Practice.* 4th ed. Philadelphia: Elsevier; 2009:89–122.
2. Lalor JG, Fawole B, Alfirevic Z, Devane D. Biophysical profile for fetal assessment in high risk pregnancies. *Cochrane Database Syst Rev.* 2008;(1):CD000038.
3. Sarno AP, Ahn MO, Phelan JP, Paul RH. Fetal acoustic stimulation in the early intrapartum period as a predictor of subsequent fetal condition. *Am J Obstet Gynecol.* 1990;162(3):762-767.
4. Tan KH, Smyth RM, Wei X. Fetal vibroacoustic stimulation for facilitation of tests of fetal wellbeing. *Cochrane Database Syst Rev.* 2013;(12):CD002963.

20. Correct answer: B

Planned cesarean delivery for suspected fetal macrosomia remains controversial, as diagnosis is imprecise and it does not eliminate the risk of birth trauma and brachial plexus injury associated with fetal macrosomia. There also have not been any trials to establish a specific EFW at which an elective cesarean delivery should be recommended. The most current recommendations of ACOG suggest that prophylactic cesarean delivery may be considered with a suspected birth weight in excess of 4500 g in a diabetic woman or 5000 g in a nondiabetic woman, which is a reasonable threshold.

Counseling should be individualized for pregnant women with suspected fetal macrosomia regarding the risks and benefits of vaginal and cesarean delivery based on the degree of macrosomia and maternal comorbidities.

The primary risk associated with fetal macrosomia is increased risk of cesarean delivery, and there is also an increased risk of PPH and vaginal lacerations. Fetal injuries can include shoulder dystocia, clavicular fracture, and brachial plexus injury. Macrosomic infants also have an elevated risk of lower Apgar scores and increased risk of admission to the NICU.

Studies comparing ultrasound measurements for detection of macrosomia versus physical examination with Leopold maneuvers have been inconsistent and do not demonstrate any statistically significant difference in diagnostic accuracy.

Induction of labor at 38 weeks for suspected fetal macrosomia is not an indication for induction of labor in itself, as it has not consistently demonstrated to improve maternal or fetal outcomes. Although a meta-analysis did show that induction of labor reduced the risk of shoulder dystocia and fracture, there was no difference in brachial plexus injury or cesarean or instrumental delivery. The American Academy of Pediatrics recommends against delivery before 39 weeks unless it is medically indicated, and based on the current evidence, there is no benefit to intervention over expectant management for large-for-gestational-age infants.

References:

1. American College of Obstetricians and Gynecologists' Committee on Practice Bulletins—Obstetrics. Practice Bulletin No. 173: fetal macrosomia. *Obstet Gynecol.* 2016;128(5):e195-e209.
2. Boulvain M, Irion O, Dowswell T, Thornton JG. Induction of labour at or near term for suspected fetal macrosomia. *Cochrane Database Syst Rev.* 2016;22(5):CD000938.
3. Chauhan SP, Hendrix NW, Magann EF, Morrison JC, Kenney SP, Devoe LD. Limitations of clinical and sonographic estimates of birth weight: experience with 1034 parturients. *Obstet Gynecol.* 1998;91:72-77.
4. Campbell K, Park JS, Norwitz ER. Antepartum fetal assessment and therapy. In: Chestnut DH, Polley LS, Tsen LC, Wong CA, eds. *Chestnut's Obstetric Anesthesia Principles and Practice.* 4th ed. Philadelphia: Elsevier; 2009:89–122.
5. Kayem G, Grange G, Breart G, Goffinet F. Comparison of fundal height measurement and sonographically measured fetal abdominal circumference in the prediction of high and low birth weight at term. *Ultrasound Obstet Gynecol.* 2009;34:566-571.

21. Correct answer: A

Historically general anesthesia has been reserved for emergent cesarean deliveries for which there is insufficient time to pursue neuraxial anesthetic techniques. Some of the most commonly cited indications for emergent delivery that would most likely necessitate general anesthesia include preterm footling breech, uterine rupture, severe obstetric hemorrhage, severe placental abruption, umbilical cord prolapse, and profound fetal bradycardia. Severe, uncorrected hypovolemia is a contraindication to a neuraxial technique; however, if there is no evidence of fetal compromise, it is reasonable to resuscitate the mother with fluids and/or blood products as needed to consider neuraxial blockade. Placental previa and preeclampsia are not strict indications for general anesthesia, and both can potentially be managed and stabilized to provide adequate time to place a spinal or epidural catheter for surgical anesthesia.

References:

1. Tsen LC. Anesthesia for cesarean delivery. In: Chestnut DH, Polley LS, Tsen LC, Wong CA, eds. *Chestnut's Obstetric Anesthesia Principles and Practice.* 4th ed. Philadelphia: Elsevier; 2009:521–574.
2. Practice guidelines for obstetric anesthesia: an updated report by the American Society of Anesthesiologist Task Force on Obstetric Anesthesia and the Society for Obstetric Anesthesia and Perinatology. *Anesthesiology.* 2016;124(2):270-300.
3. Suwal A, Shrivastava VR, Giri A. Maternal and fetal outcome in elective versus cesarean section. *J Nepal Med Assoc.* 2013;52(192):563-566.

22. Correct answer: E

Headaches after labor and delivery are common ranging from benign to life-threatening causes, including tension headache, migraines, musculoskeletal pain, preeclampsia, cortical vein thrombosis, subarachnoid hemorrhage, subdural hematoma, posterior reversible leukoencephalopathy syndrome, brain tumors, cerebral infarction/ischemia, meningitis, caffeine withdrawal, lactation headache, and PDPH. Most postpartum headaches are due to primary headache disorders; however, of secondary causes, the most common is PDPH with an incidence of around 1.5%.

The classic symptoms of a PDPH include bilateral frontal or occipital headache, which may radiate to the neck, neck stiffness, photophobia, and nausea. With PDPH these symptoms improve with lying flat and worsen with the upright position. Symptoms including tinnitus, hearing loss, and diplopia can also result from traction on cranial nerves. The PDPH typically occurs on the first or second day following dural puncture. The vast majority of PDPHs resolve within a week of presentation; however, the symptoms can be very severe and interfere with normal daily activities. Risk factors for PDPH in parturients include age <40 years, multiple dural punctures, use of a cutting needle (compared with a pencil-point needle), and larger needle size. Treatment for PDPHs includes fluid hydration, caffeine, gabapentin, theophylline, hydrocortisone, and epidural blood patch.

Scalp tenderness and circumferential, constricting pain are more commonly associated with tension headaches. Unilateral, pulsating headaches associated with nausea, vomiting, photophobia, and/or phonophobia are more likely to be a migraine. Focal neurologic symptoms, seizures, or somnolence are not commonly associated with PDPHs and merit further investigation.

References:
1. Macarthur A. Postpartum headache. In: Chestnut DH, Polley LS, Tsen LC, Wong CA, eds. *Chestnut's Obstetric Anesthesia Principles and Practice*. 4th ed. Philadelphia: Elsevier; 2009:677–700.
2. Basurto OS, Osorio D, Bonfill CX. Drug therapy for treating post-dural puncture headache. *Cochrane Database Syst Rev*. 2015;15(7):CD007887.
3. Klein AM, Loder E. Postpartum headache. *Int J Obstet Anesth*. 2010;19(4):422-430.

23. Correct answer: D

Oxygen consumption increases above prelabor values by 40% in the first stage and by 70% in the second stage of labor. Increased oxygen consumption is secondary to increased metabolic demands of hyperventilation, uterine activity, and maternal expulsive efforts during pushing. Oxygen consumption exceeds demand during labor and is evidenced by a progressive increase in blood lactate levels.

Neuraxial anesthesia decreases these metabolic changes during both the first and second stages of labor. Patients with epidural analgesia have 20%-30% decreased oxygen consumption and significantly decreased lactate and acidosis compared with those with no analgesia or sedation during contractions with pushing.

References:
1. Gaiser R. Physiologic changes of pregnancy. In: Chestnut DH, Polley LS, Tsen LC, Wong CA, eds. *Chestnut's Obstetric Anesthesia Principles and Practice*. 4th ed. Philadelphia: Elsevier; 2009:15–36.
2. Hägerdal M, Morgan CW, Sumner AE, Gutsche BB. Minute ventilation and oxygen consumption during labor with epidural analgesia. *Anesthesiology*. 1983;59(5):425-427.
3. Pearson JF, Davies P. The effect of epidural analgesia on the acid-base status of maternal arterial blood during the first stage of labour. *J Obstet Gynaecol Br Commonw*. 1973;80:218-224.

24. Correct answer: C

Cardiac output during labor increases from prelabor measurements by 10% in early first stage, 25% in late first stage, and 50% in the second stage. In the immediate postpartum period, cardiac output may be up to 80% greater than predelivery measurements because of increases in venous return and stroke volume, as well as changes in sympathetic nervous system activity. There are also relief of vena caval compression, decreased lower extremity venous pressure, rapid mobilization of extracellular fluid, and a reduction of maternal vascular capacitance. Cardiac output falls just below prelabor measurements by 24 hours postpartum and returns to prepregnancy levels between 3 and 6 months postpartum.

References:
1. Gaiser R. Physiologic changes of pregnancy. In: Chestnut DH, Polley LS, Tsen LC, Wong CA, eds. *Chestnut's Obstetric Anesthesia Principles and Practice*. 4th ed. Philadelphia: Elsevier; 2009:15–36.
2. Ouzounian JG, Elkayam U. Physiologic changes during normal pregnancy and delivery. *Cardiol Clin*. 2012;30(3):317-329.

25. Correct answer: B

In patients without IV pain medication or neuraxial anesthesia, minute ventilation increases by 70%-140% in the first stage of labor and 120%-200% in the second stage of labor compared with prepregnancy level. The increased minute ventilation during pregnancy is primary due to increased tidal volume, whereas respiratory rate is unchanged or only slightly increased. These changes result from hormonal changes and increased carbon dioxide production. Tidal volume and minute ventilation remain elevated until at least 6-8 weeks after delivery.

References:

1. Gaiser R. Physiologic changes of pregnancy. In: Chestnut DH, Polley LS, Tsen LC, Wong CA, eds. *Chestnut's Obstetric Anesthesia Principles and Practice*. 4th ed. Philadelphia: Elsevier; 2009:15–36.
2. Elkus R, Popovich J. Respiratory physiology in pregnancy. *Clin Chest Med*. 1992;13(4):555-565.
3. Zwillich CW, Natalino MR, Sutton FD, Weil JV. Effects of progesterone on chemosensitivity in men. *J Lab Clin Med*. 1978;92(2):262-269.

26. Correct answer: D

The effect of neuraxial labor analgesia on the duration of the first stage of labor has been studied with variable findings. Neuraxial anesthesia may shorten labor in some women and lengthen it in others. Prolongation of the first stage of labor has not been shown to have adverse maternal or neonatal effects and is not clinically relevant.

There has been more conclusive evidence of the prolonging effect of neuraxial labor analgesia on the duration of the second stage of labor. The mean duration of the second stage is about 15 minutes longer in women who receive neuraxial analgesia compared with those who receive systemic opioid analgesia. Many studies suggest that this delay in the second stage is not harmful provided that the fetal heart tracing is reassuring, the mother is hydrated with adequate analgesia, and there is ongoing progress of fetal head descent.

Labor progress and outcome are similar among women receiving either combined spinal-epidural or epidural analgesia, and CSE is not associated with an increased frequency of anesthetic complications. Both techniques are demonstrated to provide adequate analgesia for mothers in labor.

Multiple randomized controlled studies comparing epidural analgesia with systemic opioid analgesia have concluded that conventional epidural analgesia is associated with a higher risk for instrumental vaginal delivery than systemic analgesia.

The effect of neuraxial analgesia on the mode of vaginal delivery has been assessed as a secondary but not primary outcome in multiple trials, and interpretation of these results is challenging. This may be due to many factors including the epidural dose and significance of motor blockade. In addition, practitioners may be more likely to perform an elective instrumental delivery in patients with adequate anesthesia than in a patient without analgesia.

There have been many studies over the years evaluating the impact of neuraxial analgesia on the incidence of cesarean delivery. The studies comparing neuraxial with systemic opioid analgesia have been reviewed in several meta-analyses and demonstrate that there is no difference in women assigned to neuraxial compared with those who receive opioid analgesia.

A meta-analysis of several randomized controlled trials and cohort studies comparing early versus late epidural placement concluded that early initiation of neuraxial analgesia does not increase the risk of cesarean delivery either.

References:

1. Wong CA. Epidural and spinal analgesia/anesthesia for labor. In: Chestnut DH, Polley LS, Tsen LC, Wong CA, eds. *Chestnut's Obstetric Anesthesia Principles and Practice*. 4th ed. Philadelphia: Elsevier; 2009:429–492.
2. Collis RE, Davies DW, Aveling W. Randomised comparison of combined spinal-epidural and standard epidural analgesia in labour. *Lancet*. 1995;345:1413-1416.
3. Katz M, Lunenfeld E, Meizner I, et al. The effect of the duration of the second stage of labour on the acid-base state of the fetus. *Br J Obstet Gynaecol*. 1987;94:425-430.
4. Marucci M, Cinnella G, Perchiazzi G, et al. Patient-requested neuraxial analgesia for labor: impact on rates of cesarean and instrumental vaginal delivery. *Anesthesiology*. 2007;106:1035-1045.
5. Norris MC, Fogel ST, Conway-Long C. Combined spinal-epidural versus epidural labor analgesia. *Anesthesiology*. 2001;95(4):913-920.
6. Sharma SK, McIntire DD, Wiley J, Leveno KJ. Labor analgesia and cesarean delivery: an individual patient meta-analysis of nulliparous women. *Anesthesiology*. 2004;100:142-148.
7. Wang TT, Sun S, Huang SQ. Effects of epidural labor analgesia with low concentrations of local anesthetics on obstetric outcomes: a systematic review and meta-analysis of randomized controlled trials. *Anesth Analg*. 2017;124(5):1571-1580.

27. Correct answer: D

The ACOG has defined a prolonged second stage in nulliparous women as more than 2 hours without neuraxial anesthesia and more than 3 hours with neuraxial anesthesia. In multiparous women, it is more than 1 hour without neuraxial anesthesia and more than 2 hours with neuraxial anesthesia. For most patients, little benefit is gained from allowing the second stage of labor to exceed 3 hours; however, ACOG has also stated that if progress is being made, the duration of the second stage alone does not mandate any intervention. The decision to perform surgical or instrumental delivery should be made based on the clinical assessment of the individual woman, the fetus, and the experience of the obstetrician.

References:
1. American College of Obstetricians and Gynecologists. Dystocia and augmentation of labor. ACOG Practice Bulletin No. 49, Washington, DC, December 2003. *Obstet Gynecol.* 2003;102:1445-1454.
2. Wong CA. Epidural and spinal analgesia/anesthesia for labor. In: Chestnut DH, Polley LS, Tsen LC, Wong CA, eds. *Chestnut's Obstetric Anesthesia Principles and Practice.* 4th ed. Philadelphia: Elsevier; 2009:429–492.
3. Kadar N, Cruddas M, Campbell S. Estimating the probability of spontaneous delivery conditional on time spent in the second stage. *Br J Obstet Gynaecol.* 1986;93:568-576.

28. Correct answer: A

A previous cesarean delivery with a Pfannenstiel incision does not require subsequent cesarean delivery, and a TOLAC can be attempted in most cases. There is however an increased risk of uterine rupture (0.47% vs 0.03% for scheduled cesarean) with TOLAC, and some patients and providers prefer to opt for a scheduled cesarean delivery rather than attempt a vaginal delivery. A prior classic incision cesarean delivery or uterine incision for myomectomy is considered to be associated with an unacceptably high risk of uterine rupture (up to 2%) to attempt a trial of labor, and it is recommended to perform a scheduled cesarean delivery in these cases. Other indications for cesarean delivery include the following:

Elective indications: maternal, fetal, obstetric issues
- Previous cesarean delivery, previous classic uterine incision
- Previous myomectomy
- Placental implantation anomalies
- Maternal request
- Concern for maternal to fetal transmission of infections including HIV, HCV, and HSV with active lesions
- Malpresentation including breech
- Fetal macrosomia
- High-order multiple gestation
- Twin gestation in which twin A is breech

Urgent indications: maternal, fetal issues
- Deteriorating maternal condition
- Arrest of labor
- Chorioamnionitis
- Fetal intolerance of labor
- Nonreassuring fetal heart tones
- Placental abruption

Emergent indications: maternal, fetal issues
- Uterine rupture
- Antepartum or intrapartum hemorrhage
- Prolapsed umbilical cord

References:
1. American College of Obstetricians and Gynecologists (College), Society for Maternal-Fetal Medicine, Caughey AB, Cahill AG, Guise JM, Rouse DJ. Safe prevention of the primary cesarean delivery. *Am J Obstet Gynecol.* 2014;210(3):179-193.
2. Betran AP, Merialdi M, Lauer JA, et al. Rates of caesarean section: analysis of global, regional and national estimates. *Paediatr Perinat Epidemiol.* 2007;21(2):98-113.
3. Tsen LC. Anesthesia for cesarean delivery. In: Chestnut DH, Polley LS, Tsen LC, Wong CA, eds. *Chestnut's Obstetric Anesthesia Principles and Practice.* 4th ed. Philadelphia: Elsevier; 2009:521–574.
4. Sabol B, Denman MA, Guise JM. Vaginal birth after cesarean: an effective method to reduce cesarean. *Clin Obstet Gynecol.* 2015;58(2):309-319.

29. Correct answer: C

In current obstetric anesthesia practice, neuraxial anesthesia is preferred over general anesthesia.
  Common reasons to prefer neuraxial anesthesia include the following:
- Potential difficult airway
- History of difficult intubation

- High BMI or obesity
- History of pulmonary disease
- History of complications with general anesthesia including malignant hyperthermia
- Plan for neuraxial analgesia after surgery
- Reduced exposure of fetus to general anesthesia
- Reduced blood loss
- Maternal desire to be alert and awake for delivery
- Ability to have presence of support person during delivery

Potential reasons to prefer general anesthesia include the following:
- Strong maternal preference and refusal of neuraxial blockade
- Severe psychiatric disorder, emotional immaturity, or developmental delay
- Coagulopathy
- Local infection at the site of neuraxial blockade
- Sepsis
- Severe uncorrected hypovolemia
- Intracranial mass with increased intracranial pressure
- Known allergy to local anesthetic
- Multiple failed attempts at neuraxial anesthesia
- Need for immediate induction of anesthesia and insufficient time to attempt neuraxial placement
- Known allergy to all local anesthetic agents

References:
1. Alfolabi BB, Lesi FE. Regional versus general anesthesia for caesarean section. *Cochrane Database Syst Rev.* 2012; 10:CD004350.
2. Hawkins JL, Koonin LM, Palmer SK, Gibbs CP. Anesthesia-related deaths during obstetric delivery in the United States, 1979-90. *Anesthesiology.* 1997;86(2):277-284.
3. Tsen LC. Anesthesia for cesarean delivery. In: Chestnut DH, Polley LS, Tsen LC, Wong CA, eds. *Chestnut's Obstetric Anesthesia Principles and Practice.* 4th ed. Philadelphia: Elsevier; 2009:521–574.

30. Correct answer: E

Studies evaluating the Mallampati classification of pregnant patients have demonstrated a correlation between class III or IV airways and difficulty with intubation. Obstetric patients often have airway edema related to labor, coexisting conditions such as preeclampsia, iatrogenic fluid administration, capillary engorgement, and/or weight gain that can result in friable tissue that may bleed more easily and complicate laryngoscopy. Oxygen consumption is increased significantly during pregnancy and labor and FRC is decreased, both of which can predispose pregnant patients to rapid desaturations and hypoxemia with airway management even with adequate preoxygenation. Lower esophageal sphincter tone is decreased and the gravid uterus displaces the stomach cephalad, and these changes predispose pregnant patients to aspiration of gastric contents, resulting in potentially severe pneumonitis. Given the GI changes associated with pregnancy, a rapid sequence induction is recommended with succinylcholine being the most common medication used given the speed of onset and duration of action. Pregnant patients do not require an increased dose of succinylcholine compared with nonpregnant patients, and the duration of action is unchanged from the nonpregnant population.

References:
1. Thomas JA, Hagberg CA. The difficult airway: risks, prophylaxis, and management. In: Chestnut DH, Polley LS, Tsen LC, Wong CA, eds. Chestnut's Obstetric Anesthesia Principles and Practice. 4th ed. Philadelphia: Elsevier; 2009:651–676.
2. Goldszmidt E. Principles and practices of obstetric airway management. *Anesthesiol Clin.* 2008;26(1):109-125.
3. Mhyre JM, Healy D. The unanticipated difficult intubation in obstetrics. *Anesth Analg.* 2011;112(3):648-652.

31. Correct answer: D

Multiple sclerosis is an autoimmune condition characterized by inflammation and demyelination in the CNS, resulting in multifocal neurologic symptoms. The clinical course is variable among patients and can be relapsing and remitting in nature or chronic and progressive. There is an increased rate of relapse following pregnancy thought to be due to immunologic changes during pregnancy and delivery.

Older studies suggested that neuraxial anesthesia and epidural analgesia in particular could provoke disease relapse; however, newer data challenge that notion. More recent studies suggest that the use of current neuraxial techniques (both spinal and epidural) in women with multiple sclerosis is not associated with disease progression and both techniques have similar safety profiles. There are data to suggest that the use of higher concentrations of epidural local anesthetics may be associated with more neurotoxicity in this population, so the use of a dilute solution with an opioid to reduce the total dose of anesthetic required is recommended. Despite newer evidence to support the safety of neuraxial anesthesia in these patients, providers may not be comfortable providing it and may be less likely to provide epidural anesthesia to women with shorter disease duration although this practice is not supported by the current evidence.

References:

1. Bader AM. Neurologic and neuromuscular disease. In: Chestnut DH, Polley LS, Tsen LC, Wong CA, eds. *Chestnut's Obstetric Anesthesia Principles and Practice.* 4th ed. Philadelphia: Elsevier; 2009:1053–1078.
2. Lu E, Zhao Y, Dahlgren L, et al. Obstetrical epidural and spinal anesthesia in multiple sclerosis. *J Neurol.* 2013;260(10):2620-2628.
3. Whitaker JN. Effects of pregnancy and delivery on disease activity in multiple sclerosis. *N Engl J Med.* 1998;339(5):339-340.
4. Makris A, Piperopoulos A, Karmaniolou I. Multiple sclerosis: basic knowledge and new insights into perioperative management. *J Anesth.* 2014;28(2):267-278.

32. Correct answer: E

Threatened abortions are uterine bleeding without cervical dilation at less than 20 weeks of gestation. Inevitable abortions occur with cervical dilation or rupture of membranes without expulsion of the fetus or placenta. An incomplete abortion is partial expulsion of the uterine contents, whereas a complete abortion is total, spontaneous expulsion of the fetus and placenta. A missed abortion may go unrecognized for days to weeks and consists of fetal demise without passage of fetus or placenta and can have severe consequences including infection or disseminated intravascular coagulopathy. The most common cause of spontaneous abortion is chromosomal abnormalities in the fetus and is responsible for up to 80% of cases.

Ectopic pregnancies are estimated to occur in about 0.16% of pregnancies and can occur in the fallopian tubes, cervix, ovary, abdomen, and cesarean scar. Risk factors include pelvic inflammatory disease, prior ectopic pregnancy, prior pelvic, abdominal, or tubal surgery, IUD contraceptive devices, and assisted reproductive technologies. Classic presenting symptoms include abdominal or pelvic pain, irregular menses, and vaginal bleeding. Severe complications can occur and include major hemorrhage, infection, and embolism. The best imaging technique for ectopic pregnancy is transvaginal ultrasound that can detect a pregnancy within 21 days of conception, whereas transabdominal ultrasound will not reliably detect a gestational sac until later.

Serial β-hCG testing is useful in monitoring the rate of rise in concentration, as the vast majority of nonviable pregnancies have concentrations that have subnormal rise, plateau, or a decrease over time. Management of ectopic pregnancy depends on the presentation, and in stable patients, expectant management or medical management may be appropriate. Methotrexate is a folate antagonist that inhibits the growth of the placental trophoblasts and has fairly high success in resolving ectopic pregnancies. In unstable patients, however, surgical intervention is indicated.

References:

1. Chantigian RC, Chantigian PDM. Problems of early pregnancy. In: Chestnut DH, Polley LS, Tsen LC, Wong CA, eds. *Chestnut's Obstetric Anesthesia Principles and Practice.* 4th ed. Philadelphia: Elsevier; 2009:319–335.
2. Cecchino GN, Araujo JE, Elito JJ. Methotrexate for ectopic pregnancy: when and how. *Arch Gynecol Obstet.* 2014;290(3):417-423.
3. Orazulike NC, Konie JC. Diagnosis and management of ectopic pregnancy. *Womens Health (Lond).* 2013;9(4):373-385.

33. Correct answer: C

SLE is an autoimmune inflammatory disease associated with autoantibodies against nuclear, cytoplasmic, and cell membrane antigens and is more common in women than in men (9:1) and affects many women of child-bearing age. Complications associated with SLE include pericarditis (usually asymptomatic; however, cardiac tamponade has been reported), cardiac valvular abnormalities, pulmonary hypertension, central and peripheral neuropathies, migraines, anemia, and thrombocytopenia. Patients with SLE are at increased risk of spontaneous abortion and preterm delivery compared with women without SLE.

Some patients may have atypical blood antibodies that make it challenging to obtain crossmatched blood. It is important to be aware of to communicate with the blood bank and allow adequate time to obtain appropriate blood products in the case of maternal hemorrhage. Lupus anticoagulant is present in up to 30% of patients with SLE, and its presence interferes with phospholipid-dependent coagulation testing, resulting in a prolonged partial thromboplastin time that gets corrected when normal plasma is added. Lupus anticoagulation is an in vitro laboratory artifact that does not cause clinical coagulopathy.

Neonatal lupus erythematosus may occur when maternal antibodies cross the placenta and bind to fetal tissue; however, it occurs in only a fraction of patients and is reversible when maternal antibodies clear from the newborn's circulation within the first year of life. Infants born to mothers affected by SLE with anti-Ro or anti-La antibodies may develop cardiac conduction abnormalities including congenital heart block requiring treatment with medications or pacing.

References:
1. Reid RW. Autoimmune disorders. In: Chestnut DH, Polley LS, Tsen LC, Wong CA, eds. *Chestnut's Obstetric Anesthesia Principles and Practice*. Philadelphia: Elsevier; 2009:869–880.
2. Davies SR. Systemic lupus erythematosus and the obstetrical patient – implications for the anaesthetist. *Can J Anaesth*. 1991;38(6):790-795.
3. Wetzl RG. Anasthesiological aspects of pregnancy in patients with rheumatic disease. *Lupus*. 2004;13(9):699-702.

34. **Correct answer: D**

The hematologic system changes throughout pregnancy, resulting in a hypercoagulable state at term with increased levels of factors VII, VIII, X, fibrinogen and von Willebrand factor activity. These changes may be associated with increased risk of complications in patients with inherited or acquired thrombophilias and can result in venous thrombosis, intrauterine fetal growth restriction, late and recurrent early miscarriage, preeclampsia, and placental abruption.

Protein C is a vitamin K–dependent protein synthesized in the liver that inhibits activated factors V and VIII. Normally, levels of protein C increase during pregnancy; however, in patients with protein C deficiency, this is less pronounced and can result in thrombosis without anticoagulation treatment. Antithrombin III is also produced in the liver and endothelial cells and inactivates thrombin as well as factors IXa, Xa, Xia, and XIIa. Quantitative and qualitative deficiencies increase the risk of thrombosis and should be treated with anticoagulation or antithrombin III replacement. Disseminated intravascular coagulation can occur in a number of different clinical scenarios and results from abnormal activation of the coagulation system, resulting in thrombin formation, depletion of coagulation factors, fibrinolysis, and hemorrhage. Patients demonstrate simultaneous coagulopathy and thrombophilia, and treatment is aimed to reverse the cause, support coagulation factors, and decrease ongoing fibrinolytic activity.

von Willebrand disease is a hemostatic disorder of the von Willebrand factor that normally aids in platelet binding. There are multiple forms of von Willebrand disease, but all are characterized by hemophilia with prolonged bleeding time. Treatment may include administration of DDAVP, fresh frozen plasma, cryoprecipitate, or factor VIII depending on the disease type.

Antiphospholipid syndrome (APLS) is a prothrombotic disorder characterized by the presence of lupus anticoagulation and anticardiolipin antibody. APLS is seen in some patients with SLE; however, it is also seen as a distinct and separate entity. APLS is associated with both arterial and venous thrombotic events, and it is recommended that pregnant patients with this syndrome be treated with aspirin and anticoagulation.

References:
1. Reid RW. Autoimmune disorders. In: Chestnut DH, Polley LS, Tsen LC, Wong CA, eds. *Chestnut's Obstetric Anesthesia Principles and Practice*. Philadelphia: Elsevier; 2009:869–880.
2. Sharma SK. Hematologic and coagulation disorders. In: Chestnut DH, Polley LS, Tsen LC, Wong CA, eds. *Chestnut's Obstetric Anesthesia Principles and Practice*. 4th ed. Philadelphia: Elsevier; 2009:943–960.
3. Rheaume M, Weber F, Durand M, Mabone M. Pregnancy-related venous thromboembolism risk in asymptomatic women with antithrombin deficiency: a systematic review. *Obstet Gynecol*. 2016;127(4):649-656.
4. Simcox LE, Ormesher L, Tower C, Greer IA. Thrombophilia and pregnancy complications. *Int J Mol Sci*. 2015;16(12):28418-28428.

35. Correct answer: A

Mitral stenosis is the most common valvular disease in pregnancy and is almost always associated with a history of rheumatic fever. Complications of mitral stenosis occur over time due to increased left atrial pressures, decreased stroke volume, decreased cardiac output, left atrial dilatation, and increased pulmonary arterial pressure. The classification of severity is based on the mean gradient and valve area. The hypervolemia and tachycardia associated with normal pregnancy physiology are not well tolerated by patients with severe mitral stenosis and may result in clinical deterioration and heart failure with pulmonary edema. The peak period of complications is during the second and third trimesters but can occur in peripartum or postpartum periods.

β-Blockers are a mainstay of treatment and are associated with a decreased incidence of pulmonary edema. In some patients, medical management is not sufficient to control maternal symptoms and if severe, a mitral valvotomy or valvuloplasty may be indicated to allow the mother to complete the pregnancy. Patients with symptomatic (NYHA functional class II or greater), moderate, or severe mitral stenosis (mitral valve area ≤1.5 cm² or mean gradient ≥5 mm Hg) should ideally be evaluated for percutaneous valvuloplasty preconception given the increased risk of pulmonary edema, arrhythmias, and potential maternal and fetal complications during pregnancy.

Epidural analgesia is recommended for parturients with mitral stenosis, as pain can contribute to tachycardia and worsen symptoms. Fluid hydration to maintain preload, appropriate vasopressor use, and maintenance of normal sinus rhythm are imperative to avoid cardiovascular complications related to hypotension or arrhythmias. General anesthetic management is aimed at maintaining a normal sinus rhythm, administering judicious amounts of fluids, preventing aortocaval compression, preserving systemic vascular resistance, and avoiding factors that may increase pulmonary pressures (pain, hypercarbia, hypoxia, and acidosis). It is beneficial to avoid abrupt increases in intrathoracic pressure that may occur with pushing during the second stage by providing adequate analgesia and assisted second stage delivery by the obstetrician.

References:

1. al Kasab SM, Sabag T, al Zaibag M, et al. Beta-adrenergic receptor blockade in the management of pregnant women with mitral stenosis. *Am J Obstet Gynecol.* 1990;163(1 Pt 1):37-40.
2. Harnett M, Tsen LC. Cardiovascular disease. In: Chestnut DH, Polley LS, Tsen LC, Wong CA, eds. *Chestnut's Obstetric Anesthesia Principles and Practice.* 4th ed. Philadelphia: Elsevier; 2009:881–912.
3. Pessel C, Bonanno C. Valve disease in pregnancy. *Semin Perinatol.* 2014;38(5):273-284.
4. Tsiaras S, Poppas A. Mitral valve disease in pregnancy: outcomes and management. *Obstet Med.* 2009;2(1):6-10.

36. Correct answer: D

Continuous FHR tracing is the most widespread form of intrapartum fetal assessment used today. External monitoring uses cardiac ultrasound to obtain FHR signals by securing transducers to the mother's abdomen with adjustable straps. FHR monitoring is commonly paired with uterine tocodynamometry to pair the FHR response with uterine activity. Normal baseline FHRs are 110-160 beats per minute, and interpretation of FHR tracing takes into account the baseline rate, variability, and presence of accelerations and decelerations.

Accelerations are increases over baseline and are generally considered to be reassuring and associated with fetal movement. Early decelerations occur as a symmetrical gradual decrease in heart rate with the nadir at the peak of uterine contraction. Early decelerations are related to fetal head compression and are thought to occur because of increased vagal tone. Variable decelerations are abrupt, variable in shape, and result from umbilical cord compression that activates the carotid baroreceptor reflex. Late decelerations are gradual, symmetric, and occur after the onset of uterine contraction with the nadir well after the peak of the uterine contraction. Late decelerations result from uteroplacental insufficiency and are a response to hypoxemia and may be associated with fetal acidosis. Sinusoidal tracings are regular, smooth, and wavelike heart rates that may signify fetal compromise and are associated with fetal anemia.

FHR tracings are classified using a 3-tiered system with Category 1 tracings being normal and reassuring, Category 2 tracings being neutral and not normal or abnormal, and Category 3 tracings being abnormal and warranting concern. Although FHR monitoring is widely used, there are very limited data to support improved fetal outcomes as a result of its use. The ACOG endorses the use of monitoring during labor, but the optimal interval for auscultation is unclear and likely different between low- and high-risk patients.

Three-Tier Fetal Heart Rate Interpretation System

Category I

Category I fetal heart rate (FHR) tracings include all of the following:

- Baseline rate: 110-160 beats per minute (bpm)
- Baseline FHR variability: moderate
- Late or variable decelerations: absent
- Early decelerations: present or absent
- Accelerations: present or absent

Category II

Category II FHR tracings include all FHR tracings not categorized as Category I or Category III. Category II tracings may represent an appreciable fraction of those encountered in clinical care. Examples of Category II FHR tracings include any of the following:

Baseline rate

- Bradycardia not accompanied by absent baseline variability
- Tachycardia

Baseline FHR variability

- Minimal baseline variability
- Absent baseline variability not accompanied by recurrent decelerations
- Marked baseline variability

Accelerations

- Absence of induced accelerations after fetal stimulation

Periodic or episodic decelerations

- Recurrent variable decelerations accompanied by minimal or moderate baseline variability
- Prolonged deceleration ≥2 minutes but <10 minutes
- Recurrent late decelerations with moderate baseline variability
- Variable decelerations with other characteristics, such as slow return to baseline, "overshoots," or "shoulders"

Category III

Category III FHR tracings include either:

- Absent baseline FHR variability and any of the following:
  - Recurrent late decelerations
  - Recurrent variable decelerations
  - Bradycardia
- Sinusoidal pattern

(From The 2008 National Institute of Child Health and Human Development workshop on electronic fetal monitoring: updates on definitions, interpretation, and reseach guidelines. *Obstet Gynecol.* 2008;112:661, with permission.)

References:

1. Braveman FR, Scavone BM, Blessing ME, Wong CA. Obstetric anesthesia. In: Barash PG, Cullen BF, Stoelting RK, et al, eds. *Clinical Anesthesia.* 7th ed. Philadelphia: Lippincott William & Wilkins; 2013:1144–1177.
2. Livingston EG. Intrapartum fetal assessment and therapy. In: Chestnut DH, Polley LS, Tsen LC, Wong CA, eds. *Chestnut's Obstetric Anesthesia Principles and Practice.* 4th ed. Philadelphia: Elsevier; 2009:141–154.
3. Smith JF, Onstad JH. Assessment of the fetus: intermittent auscultation, electronic fetal heart rate tracing, and fetal pulse oximetry. *Obstet Gynecol Clin North Am.* 2005;32(2):245-254.

37. **Correct answer: E**

Preeclampsia occurs in 4%-5% of all pregnancies, and it is a syndrome of new onset hypertension and proteinuria after 20 weeks' gestation and occurs as a syndrome of systemic abnormalities.

Management of severe, symptomatic hypertension is imperative, and the goal of therapy is to reduce the mean arterial pressure by 15%-25% with a target diastolic pressure of 100-105 mm Hg. Significant changes in maternal perfusion pressure may result in uteroplacental insufficiency and fetal distress, so antihypertensive medications should be carefully titrated so as not to decrease pressures abruptly. Commonly used antihypertensive agents for severe preeclampsia include hydralazine, labetalol, and sodium nitroprusside. Placement of an intra-arterial catheter for close monitoring of hemodynamics may be appropriate in cases of severe hypertension, and selection of patients for whom continuous arterial blood pressure monitoring is required is at the discretion of the anesthesia provider. Magnesium sulfate therapy is recommended for women with severe preeclampsia for prophylaxis for eclampsia.

Given the hematologic abnormalities that can be present with severe preeclampsia, performing neuraxial anesthesia may have a higher risk for epidural hematoma. There is no set guideline for a safe platelet count to perform neuraxial anesthesia, and the decision must be made based on the individual patient and clinical picture. In the absence of coagulopathy, most obstetric anesthesia providers would perform neuraxial anesthesia with a platelet count greater than 80 000/mm^3, while also considering the trend and evolving clinical picture. Platelet transfusion to achieve a count of 100 000/mm^3 is not recommended and unlikely to increase the margin of safety and carries the risk of transfusion reaction. Whenever a neuraxial technique has been used in the setting of thrombocytopenia or coagulopathy, close monitoring of neurologic examination is required and imaging should be obtained immediately if there is any concern of epidural hematoma, as prompt surgical intervention may be required to avoid permanent neurologic deficits.

References:

1. Braveman FR, Scavone BM, Blessing ME, Wong CA. Obstetric anesthesia. In: Barash PG, Cullen BF, Stoelting RK, et al, eds. *Clinical Anesthesia.* 7th ed. Philadelphia: Lippincott William & Wilkins; 2013:1144–1177.
2. Polley LS. Hypertensive disorders. In: Chestnut DH, Polley LS, Tsen LC, Wong CA, eds. *Chestnut's Obstetric Anesthesia Principles and Practice.* 4th ed. Philadelphia: Elsevier; 2009:975–1008.
3. Dennis AT. Management of pre-eclampsia: issues for anaesthetists. *Anaesthesia.* 2012;67(9):1009-1020.

38. Correct answer: B

Patients with preeclampsia have multisystem disease involvement including pulmonary complications with about 3% of affected women who develop pulmonary edema. Patients who receive large volumes of crystalloid infusions and magnesium therapy for seizure prophylaxis and/or those who undergo cesarean delivery are at increased risk of pulmonary edema; also, this should be high in the differential for hypoxemia after delivery. Management may include diuretic medications, fluid restriction, oxygen supplementation, and respiratory support via continuous positive pressure and potentially mechanical ventilation in severe cases.

References:

1. Polley LS. Hypertensive disorders. In: Chestnut DH, Polley LS, Tsen LC, Wong CA, eds. *Chestnut's Obstetric Anesthesia Principles and Practice.* 4th ed. Philadelphia: Elsevier; 2009:975–1008.
2. Dennis AT. Management of pre-eclampsia: issues for anaesthetists. *Anaesthesia.* 2012;67(9):1009-1020.

39. Correct answer: E

The incidence of umbilical cord prolapse is 0.1%-0.6%, and the prolapsed cord can be overt and visibly extruding from the vagina or occult where it presents alongside the presenting fetal. Risk factors including low birth weight (<1500 g), breech presentation, second born twin, and male sex. Cesarean delivery has decreased the rate of morbidity and mortality in cases of umbilical cord prolapse; however, vaginal delivery may be attempted when prolapse occurs in the second stage of labor (not the first). If the head is not engaged and the cervix is not fully dilated, a vaginal delivery should not be attempted and the recommendation is to perform a cesarean delivery expeditiously. Manual elevation of the presenting fetal part to decompress the cord is widely practiced to avoid the complications of prolonged cord occlusion. Instillation of fluid into the bladder has also been performed to elevate the presenting part.

Once the diagnosis is made, it is imperative to promptly deliver the fetus to reduce the risk of morbidity and mortality. Although neuraxial anesthesia is preferred in pregnant patients, if the FHR tracing remains nonreassuring, it would be inadvisable to pursue neuraxial blockade and rapid induction of general anesthesia is recommended. Although prompt delivery does not completely mitigate the risk of perinatal morbidity and mortality, it does reduce the risk of complications and should be pursued as soon as safely possible.

References:
1. Tsen LC. Anesthesia for cesarean delivery. In: Chestnut DH, Polley LS, Tsen LC, Wong CA, eds. *Chestnut's Obstetric Anesthesia Principles and Practice.* 4th ed. Philadelphia: Elsevier; 2009:521–574.
2. Holbook BD, Phelan ST. Umbilical cord prolapse. *Obstet Gynecol Clin North Am.* 2013;40(1):1-14.
3. Lin MG. Umbilical cord prolapse. *Obstet Gynecol Surv.* 2006;61(4):269-277.

40. Correct answer: A

Aspiration pneumonitis can range in severity from patients who are stable and only require supportive therapy to those requiring intubation and mechanical ventilation in the most severe cases. Supportive therapy includes bronchoscopy, appropriate antibiotics, and management of hypoxemia. Aspiration of acidic contents causes epithelial damage to the alveoli and results in alveolar damage, edema, reduced lung compliance, increased pulmonary vascular resistance, and an inflammatory response that can result in acute lung injury or acute respiratory distress syndrome.

The risk of aspiration in pregnant patients is increased because of the physiologic changes including lower esophageal relaxation and increased intra-abdominal pressure. Pregnant women undergoing cesarean delivery should receive pharmacologic prophylaxis for aspiration including nonparticulate antacids, H_2-receptor blockers, proton pump inhibitors, and/or metoclopramide. Treatment is aimed at increasing gastric pH and reducing gastric volume. Ondansetron is an effective antiemetic; however, it is not considered a prophylactic agent for aspiration pneumonitis. Oral administration of modest volumes of clear liquids up to 2 hours before surgery is considered to be safe in pregnant patients; however, solid foods should be avoided during labor and at least 8 hours before elective surgery.

References:
1. O'Sullivan G, Hari MS. Aspiration: risk, prophylaxis, and treatment. In: Chestnut DH, Polley LS, Tsen LC, Wong CA, eds. *Chestnut's Obstetric Anesthesia Principles and Practice.* 4th ed. Philadelphia: Elsevier; 2009:633–650.
2. Practice guidelines for obstetric anesthesia: an updated report by the American Society of Obstetric Anesthesiologists Task Force on Obstetric Anesthesia and the Society for Obstetric Anesthesia and Perinatology. *Anesthesiology.* 2016;124(2):270-300.

41. Correct answer: E

Retained placenta can occur in up to 3% of deliveries and contribute to significant morbidity because of the risk of both early and late PPH. The risk of hemorrhage increases when the time interval between delivery of the infant and the placenta is greater than 30 minutes. Oxytocin is frequently given following removal to enhance uterine tone.

Manual removal of the placenta can be very painful, and therefore, neuraxial anesthesia achieved by spinal or epidural routes to a block height of T6 may be pursued to facilitate the procedure. One should balance the benefits of neuraxial anesthesia while considering patient-specific factors including hemodynamic stability and the nature of the bleeding. In some cases, small boluses of ketamine or fentanyl can be sufficient to allow a skilled obstetrician to manually remove the placenta; however, it is critical to maintain maternal airway reflexes and be prepared for the potential need to provide general anesthesia.

Nitroglycerin spray or tablets may be given to provide uterine smooth muscle relaxation via nitric oxide release. Despite this common intervention, it has mixed data to support the efficacy in cases of retained placenta. There are limited data for any pharmacologic intervention being efficacious for treatment of retained placenta including oxytocin, nitroglycerin, and prostaglandins; however, the use of small doses of nitroglycerin has little hemodynamic consequence and may provide benefit. Uterine relaxation can be quickly accomplished with volatile anesthetic agents at high (1.5-2) MAC values to facilitate placental extraction; however, this is not an appropriate first step in management in an otherwise hemodynamically stable patient.

References:
1. Adams L, Menon R, Dresner M. Anaesthetic protocol for manual removal of placenta. *Anaesthesia.* 2013;68(1):104-105.
2. Mayer DC, Smith KA. Antepartum and postpartum hemorrhage. In: Chestnut DH, Polley LS, Tsen LC, Wong CA, eds. *Chestnut's Obstetric Anesthesia Principles and Practice.* 4th ed. Philadelphia: Elsevier; 2009:811–836.
3. Duffy JM, Mylan S, Showell M, Wilson MJ, Khan KS. Pharmacologic intervention for retained placenta: a systematic review and meta-analysis. *Obstet Gynecol.* 2015;125(3):711-718.

42. Correct answer: D

The risks associated with attempting a TOLAC include uterine rupture, hysterectomy, hemorrhage, transfusion of blood products, and death. In women with any uterine scar, the risk of uterine rupture is 0.3%

and the risks are significantly increased for women attempting TOLAC compared with elective repeat cesarean (0.47% vs 0.03%). Other risk factors for uterine rupture include fetal macrosomia, twin gestations, use of prostaglandins, and short interpregnancy interval (<24 mo). Gestation beyond 40 weeks does not increase the risk of uterine rupture in women attempting TOLAC.

The ACOG has published guidelines stating selective criteria for candidates for VBAC that include 1 prior low transverse cesarean delivery, clinically adequate pelvic anatomy, no other uterine scars or history of uterine rupture, physicians trained to monitor labor and perform emergency delivery immediately available throughout active labor, and availability of an anesthesia provider and/or other personnel for emergency cesarean delivery.

The ACOG has listed contraindications to VBAC that include previous uterine rupture, previous class or T-shaped incision or extensive transfundal uterine surgery, 2 prior uterine scares and no vaginal deliveries, medical or obstetric complications that preclude vaginal delivery, or an inability to perform emergency cesarean delivery due to unavailable medical personnel or facility access.

Factors that are associated with an increased likelihood of successful VBAC include history of prior VBAC, original cesarean for nonrecurring fetal issues (ie, breech), and spontaneous rupture of membranes or favorable cervix at time of presentation. Factors that are associated with a decreased likelihood of successful VBAC include BMI >30, fetal macrosomia >4000 g, gestation >40 weeks, advanced maternal age, maternal comorbid conditions, and African American or nonwhite Hispanic women.

References:
1. Chestnut DH. Vaginal birth after cesarean delivery. In: Chestnut DH, Polley LS, Tsen LC, Wong CA, eds. *Chestnut's Obstetric Anesthesia Principles and Practice.* 4th ed. Philadelphia: Elsevier; 2009:375–386.
2. Sabol B, Denman MA, Guise JM. Vaginal birth after cesarean: an effective method to reduce cesarean. *Clin Obstet Gynecol.* 2015;58(2):309-319.

43. Correct answer: E

Multiple gestations increase the incidence of maternal complications, morbidity, and mortality, and this increases in proportion to the number of fetuses. There are a number of complications associated with multiple gestations including

- Preterm labor
- Preterm premature rupture of membranes
- Prolonged labor
- Pregnancy-induced hypertension
- Peripartum cardiomyopathy
- Preeclampsia/eclampsia
- Acute fatty liver of pregnancy
- Placental abruption
- Need for operative delivery
- Obstetric trauma
- Uterine atony
- Postpartum hemorrhage

The evidence for increased incidence of gestational diabetes in multiple gestations is limited, and there are conflicting data. Although some studies have found a significant difference in rates of diabetes during pregnancy, there are several that have not been able to demonstrate an increased risk.

References:
1. Braveman FR, Scavone BM, Blessing ME, Wong CA. Obstetric anesthesia. In: Barash PG, Cullen BF, Stoelting RK, et al, eds. *Clinical Anesthesia.* 7th ed. Philadelphia: Lippincott William & Wilkins; 2013:1144–1177.
2. Buhling KJ, Henrich W, Starr E, et al. Risk for gestational diabetes and hypertension for women with twin pregnancy compared to singleton pregnancy. *Arch Gynecol Obstet.* 2003;269(1):33.
3. Koffel B. Abnormal presentation and multiple gestation. In: Chestnut DH, Polley LS, Tsen LC, Wong CA, eds. *Chestnut's Obstetric Anesthesia Principles and Practice.* 4th ed. Philadelphia: Elsevier; 2009:779–794.
4. Elkayam U, Akhter MW, Singh H, et al. Pregnancy-associated cardiomyopathy: clinical characteristics and a comparison between early and late presentation. *Circulation.* 2005;111(16)2050.
5. Henderson CE, Scarpelli S, LaRosa D, Divon MY. Assessing the risk of gestational diabetes in twin gestation. *J Natl Med Assoc.* 1995;87(10):757.
6. Schwartz DB, Daoud Y, Zazula P, et al. Gestational diabetes mellitus: metabolic and blood glucose parameters in singleton versus twin pregnancies. *Am J Obstet Gynecol.* 1999;181(4):912.

44. **Correct answer: C**

Preterm labor and delivery is estimated to occur in 10%-13% of pregnancies in the United States and can result in significant neonatal morbidity and mortality. Neonatal complications in preterm infants can be severe including intracranial hemorrhage, respiratory distress syndrome, hyperbilirubinemia, hypoglycemia, and developmental delay. Neonates with lower birth weights (<750 g) have significantly higher complication rates than those who weigh more, and the survival rate of preterm infants increases as birth weight and/or gestational age increases.

Risk factors for preterm labor include infections, multiple gestations, cervical incompetency, a history of preterm labor, nonwhite race, abnormal uterine or cervical anatomy, abdominal surgery during pregnancy, trauma, tobacco use, substance abuse, and fetal abnormalities. Proposed mechanisms of preterm labor include pathologic uterine distension, infection/inflammation, environmental toxins, behavioral/environmental influences, stress, autoimmune/allergy, and uterine factors that affect the decidua resulting in inflammation and prostaglandin synthesis. Systemic, genital tract, and periodontal infection can also contribute to preterm labor, and symptomatic urinary tract infections should be promptly treated if present during pregnancy.

Administration of corticosteroids in a pregnant woman with preterm labor reduces the incidence of respiratory distress syndrome and has demonstrated a decreased risk of intraventricular hemorrhage and neonatal death. Tocolysis in preterm labor may be achieved by use of calcium channel blockers, prostaglandin inhibitors, β-receptor adrenergic agonists, and magnesium sulfate. None of these agents have been proven to be superior to any others. There have not been studies to directly demonstrate tocolysis improving neonatal outcomes; however, they are effective at prolonging pregnancy, and this is presumed to be beneficial for preterm infants.

References:

1. ACOG. Committee Opinion No 652: magnesium sulfate use on obstetrics. *Obstet Gynecol.* 2016;127(1):e52-e53.
2. Braveman FR, Scavone BM, Blessing ME, Wong CA. Obstetric anesthesia. In: Barash PG, Cullen BF, Stoelting RK, et al, eds. *Clinical Anesthesia.* 7th ed. Philadelphia: Lippincott William & Wilkins; 2013:1144–1177.
3. Muir HA, Wong CA. Preterm labor and delivery. In: Chestnut DH, Polley LS, Tsen LC, Wong CA, eds. *Chestnut's Obstetric Anesthesia Principles and Practice.* 4th ed. Philadelphia: Elsevier; 2009:749–778.
4. Rundell K, Panchal B. Preterm labor: prevention and management. *Am Fam Physician.* 2017;95(6):366-372.

45. **Correct answer: C**

Breech presentation is defined as a fetus in a longitudinal lie with the buttocks or feet closest to the cervix. This occurs in 3%-4% of all deliveries. External cephalic version is the transabdominal manual rotation of the fetus from the breech into a cephalic presentation. External cephalic version is typically performed between 34 and 39 weeks and has been reported to have variable success rates anywhere from 35% to 85%. Uterine relaxation and tocolytics are frequently used to increase the likelihood of success. Several studies suggest that neuraxial anesthesia improves the likelihood of a successful version.

There is evidence that neonatal morbidity and mortality is significantly lower in planned cesarean delivery versus planned vaginal delivery (1.6% compared with 5%) with breech presentation.

Despite the concerns for increased risk to the neonate, some literature suggests that in hospitals with specific protocols to select candidates, it may be reasonable to pursue a vaginal delivery. ACOG highlights the importance of disclosing the risks to patients and the need for physicians to have adequate experience and comfort with performing a vaginal breech delivery if this is to be pursued. Criteria that should be considered for a trial of labor and vaginal delivery with a breech presentation include adequate pelvis dimensions, EFW between 2000 and 3500 g, flexion of the fetal head, continuous FHR monitoring, adequate progression of labor, and adequate skill of the obstetrician, assistant, anesthesiologist, and neonatal responder.

During vaginal delivery, one of the greatest concerns is fetal head entrapment. Anesthesia providers must be prepared to manage this complication by providing maternal muscle relaxation. Nitroglycerin is frequently used as a first-line agent for uterine relaxation to allow a brief period of uterine relaxation for delivery of the head. Induction of general anesthesia with use of muscle relaxants such as succinylcholine, nondepolarizing paralytic agents, and/or high doses of volatile anesthetics (2-3 MAC) may be required in some situations. Epidural analgesia is also thought be beneficial for relaxation of muscle in the perineum and pelvic floor, thereby reducing the risk of fetal head entrapment.

References:

1. ACOG Committee on Obstetric Practice. ACOG Committee Opinion No. 340. Mode of term singleton breech delivery. *Obstet Gynecol.* 2006;108(1):235-237.
2. Chalifoux LA, Sullivan JT. Anesthetic management of external cephalic version. *Clin Perinatol.* 2013;40(3):399-412.
3. Koffel B. Abnormal presentation and multiple gestation. In: Chestnut DH, Polley LS, Tsen LC, Wong CA, eds. *Chestnut's Obstetric Anesthesia Principles and Practice.* 4th ed. Philadelphia: Elsevier; 2009:779-794.

46. Correct answer: C

The Apgar score is a numeric system to clinically evaluate the neonate's well-being at the time of delivery. It is composed of 5 variables each with a score of graded from 0 to 2 for a minimum total score of 0 and maximum score of 10. The neonate in question has an Apgar score of 5 based on the description: heart rate >100 (2 points), irregular breathing (1 point), cyanosis (0 points), grimaces (1 point), and flexes extremities (1 point).

The Apgar score is used to determine need for resuscitation and evaluate the effectiveness of the resuscitation. Studies have shown an association between low Apgar scores and increased risks of neonatal and infant death as well as neonatal disability including developmental delay, cerebral palsy, and epilepsy. There is a dose-response pattern of mortality and disability outcomes with longer duration of lower scores. Preterm infants are more likely than term infants to have a lower Apgar score, as gestational age affects respiratory effort, muscle tone, and reflex irritability.

References:

1. Aucott SW, Zuckerman RL. Neonatal assessment and resuscitation. In: Chestnut DH, Polley LS, Tsen LC, Wong CA, eds. *Chestnut's Obstetric Anesthesia Principles and Practice.* 4th ed. Philadelphia: Elsevier; 2009:155-184.
2. Braveman FR, Scavone BM, Blessing ME, Wong CA. Obstetric anesthesia. In: Barash PG, Cullen BF, Stoelting RK, et al, eds. *Clinical Anesthesia.* 7th ed. Philadelphia: Lippincott William & Wilkins; 2013:1144-1177.
3. Ehrenstein V. Association of Apgar scores with death and neurological disability. *Clin Epidemiol.* 2009;9(1):45-53.

47. Correct answer: D

FHR tracing has not demonstrated a consistent correlation between abnormal patterns and newborn outcomes. Apgar scores do have a role in neonatal assessment for resuscitation and may collectively contribute to the evidence of an intrapartum hypoxic event; however, they do not reliably predict neurologic outcomes on an individual level. The 5-minute Apgar score may be a better predictor of neonatal death than umbilical artery pH; however, a score of 3 or less is associated with a higher risk, not a score of 6.

An analysis from the ACOG Committee on Obstetric Practice suggests that a pH less than 7 and a base deficit equal to or greater than 12 mmol/L at delivery are associated with acute intrapartum hypoxia that has the potential to result in cerebral palsy. The Committee recommends that venous and arterial cord blood gas measurements be obtained in cesarean deliveries for fetal compromise, low 5-minute Apgar scores, severe growth restriction, abnormal FHR tracing, maternal thyroid disease, intrapartum fever, or multifetal gestation. Hypoxic-ischemic encephalopathy is staged by assessing various physical signs similar to the Apgar score including irritability, tone, respiration, reflexes, and seizure activity. These assessments are associated with different outcomes from good (stage I) to poor (stage III).

References:

1. ACOG Committee on Obstetric Practice. ACOG Committee Opinion No. 348, November 2006. Umbilical cord blood gas and acid-base analysis. *Obstet Gynecol.* 2006;108(5):1319-1322.
2. Braveman FR, Scavone BM, Blessing ME, Wong CA. Obstetric anesthesia. In: Barash PG, Cullen BF, Stoelting RK, et al, eds. *Clinical Anesthesia.* 7th ed. Philadelphia: Lippincott William & Wilkins; 2013:1144-1177.
3. Aucott SW, Zuckerman RL. Neonatal assessment and resuscitation. In: Chestnut DH, Polley LS, Tsen LC, Wong CA, eds. *Chestnut's Obstetric Anesthesia Principles and Practice.* 4th ed. Philadelphia: Elsevier; 2009:155-184.

48. Correct answer: B

Immediately following delivery, the neonate should be evaluated and placed under radiant heat source in a position that facilitates adequate ventilation. In addition, the airway should be cleared, skin dried, and the infant should be stimulated. Assessment of vital signs including color and heart and respiratory rate is crucial to evaluate a potential need for intervention. The algorithm below provides recommendations for interventions based on the status of the infant.

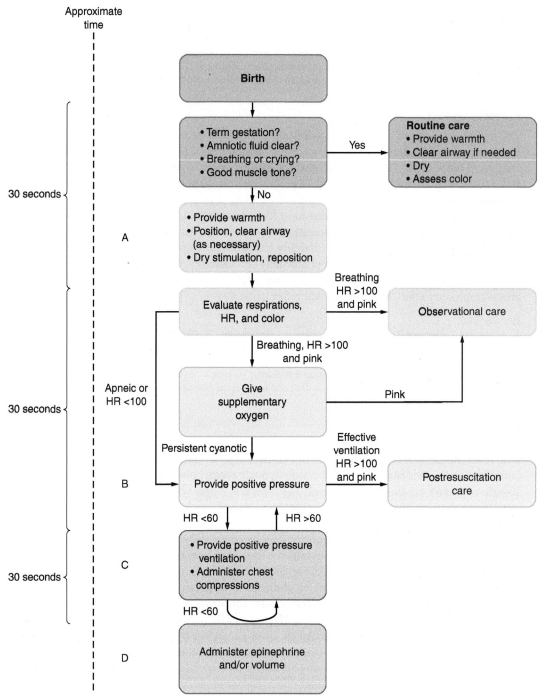

Approximate time

Birth

• Term gestation?
• Amniotic fluid clear?
• Breathing or crying?
• Good muscle tone?

→ Yes →

Routine care
• Provide warmth
• Clear airway if needed
• Dry
• Assess color

↓ No

A

• Provide warmth
• Position, clear airway (as necessary)
• Dry stimulation, reposition

30 seconds

Evaluate respirations, HR, and color

Breathing HR >100 and pink →

Observational care

Breathing, HR >100 and pink

Give supplementary oxygen

Pink →

Apneic or HR <100

30 seconds

Persistent cyanotic ↓

B

Provide positive pressure

Effective ventilation HR >100 and pink →

Postresuscitation care

HR <60 ↓   ↑ HR >60

C

• Provide positive pressure ventilation
• Administer chest compressions

30 seconds

HR <60

D

Administer epinephrine and/or volume

(From Kattwinkel J, Perlman JM, Aziz K, et al. Special report – Neonatal resuscitation: 2010 American Heart Association Guidelines for Cardiopulmonary Resuscitation and Emergency Cardiovascular Care. *Circulation.* 2010;122:S9, with permission.)

References:
1. Braveman FR, Scavone BM, Blessing ME, Wong CA. Obstetric anesthesia. In: Barash PG, Cullen BF, Stoelting RK, et al, eds. *Clinical Anesthesia.* 7th ed. Philadelphia: Lippincott William & Wilkins; 2013:1144–1177.
2. Aucott SW, Zuckerman RL. Neonatal assessment and resuscitation. In: Chestnut DH, Polley LS, Tsen LC, Wong CA, eds. *Chestnut's Obstetric Anesthesia Principles and Practice.* 4th ed. Philadelphia: Elsevier; 2009:155–184.
3. Perlman JM, Wyllie J, Kattwinkel J, et al. Part 11: Neonatal resuscitation: 2010 International Consensus on Cardiopulmonary Resuscitation and Emergency Cardiovascular Care Science with Treatment Recommendations. *Circulation.* 2010;122(16 Suppl 2):S516-S538.

49. **Correct answer: C**

Intrauterine surgery for fetal conditions is performed for a number of indications including sacrococcygeal teratoma, myelomeningocele, twin-to-twin transfusion syndrome, obstructive uropathy, congenital diaphragmatic hernia, and cystic hygroma. These procedures can range from minimally invasive to open hysterotomy, and therefore, the anesthetic management varies. Volatile agents provide a dose-dependent depression of uterine myometrial contractility and provide uterine relaxation necessary to perform the procedure. Magnesium and nitroglycerin are also frequently used for relaxation and tocolysis. Preterm labor following intrauterine surgical intervention is a legitimate concern. Patients require close monitoring and uterine activity monitoring postoperatively for 1-3 days. Given the high dose of volatile agent required for uterine relaxation, vasopressors including ephedrine and phenylephrine are often required to maintain normotension and placental perfusion to the fetus. Avoiding excessive fluid administration is important, as pulmonary edema can develop with hypervolemia and administration of tocolytic medications. It is also important to maintain normal $Paco_2$ for pregnancy (30-34 mm Hg) to avoid hypercapnia that can lead to fetal acidosis and to avoid hyperventilation that can result in placental vasoconstriction and a leftward shift of the fetal hemoglobin oxydissociation curve.

Neuromuscular blocking medications administered to the pregnant patient do not cross the placenta to the fetus, and therefore, the surgeon must inject these medications into the umbilical vessels or intramuscularly to achieve fetal paralysis. Fetal analgesia and anesthesia can be achieved by administering volatile agents and/or lipophilic anesthetic medications that will cross the placenta from maternal circulation into the fetus. Mothers who become pregnant following open intrauterine surgical procedures should be delivered via cesarean section before the initiation of labor given the risk of uterine rupture.

References:
1. Rosen MA. Anesthesia for fetal surgery and other intrauterine procedures. In: Chestnut DH, Polley LS, Tsen LC, Wong CA, eds. *Chestnut's Obstetric Anesthesia Principles and Practice*. 4th ed. Philadelphia: Elsevier; 2009:123–140.
2. Sviggum HP, Kodali BS. Maternal anesthesia for fetal surgery. *Clin Perinatal*. 2013;40(3):413-427.

50. **Correct answer: E**

Intrauterine resuscitation is aimed to maintain normal uterine blood flow to prevent fetal distress from impaired placental perfusion. Although various interventions are commonly used for intrauterine resuscitation, there is little definitive evidence regarding maternal and fetal outcomes. This mother has hypotension, and interventions such as an IV fluid bolus, positioning, and vasopressor administration are likely to correct the fetal distress if the etiology is decreased placental perfusion. Maternal position change is a very simple and low-risk intervention that frequently results in an improvement in FHR tracings. Administration of tocolytics is commonly used, and although the quality of most of the studies is somewhat poor, the results are fairly consistent in supporting the use of tocolytics. In addition, their use may "buy time" to pursue other resuscitative efforts and support the fetus while making plans for delivery.

Administration of maternal oxygen has evolved to be a somewhat controversial intervention. The data are limited but do suggest that maternal hyperoxygenation can lead to fetal acidosis, an increased need for neonatal resuscitation, and increased markers of free radial activity. It is generally accepted that maternal oxygen supplementation should be reserved for maternal hypoxia, and given that this mother is saturating 97% on room air, hypoxia is unlikely to be contributing to the fetal distress.

References:
1. Bullens LM, van Runnard Heimel PJ, va der Hout-van der Jagt MB, Oei SG. Interventions for intrauterine resuscitation in suspected fetal distress during term labor: a systematic review. *Obstet Gynecol Surv*. 2015;70(8):524-539.
2. Livingston EG. Intrapartum fetal assessment and therapy. In: Chestnut DH, Polley LS, Tsen LC, Wong CA, eds. *Chestnut's Obstetric Anesthesia Principles and Practice*. 4th ed. Philadelphia: Elsevier; 2009:141–154.
3. Hamel MS, Anderson BL, Rouse DJ. Oxygen for intrauterine resuscitation: of unproved benefit and potentially harmful. *Am J Obstet Gynecol*. 2014;211:124-127.

16

CARDIAC AND VASCULAR ANESTHESIA

Jamie L. Sparling

1. A 64-year-old former smoker with poorly controlled hypertension presents with acute pain between his scapulae. His blood pressure is noted to be 179/78 and he is diaphoretic. Transesophageal echocardiography (TEE) reveals the following image:

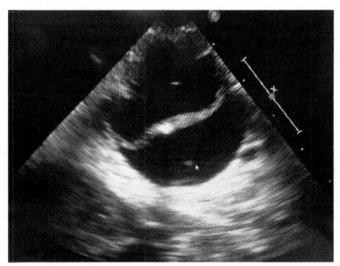

(Image courtesy of Drs Phuong Tran & Michael Andrawes.)

Which of the following is the best next step in management?

   A. Immediate surgery for open aortic root replacement
   B. Endovascular stenting
   C. Heart rate and blood pressure control
   D. It cannot be determined by the information given

2. **A 69-year-old woman presents with slowly progressive dyspnea and is found to have a diastolic decrescendo murmur. TEE shows the following images:**

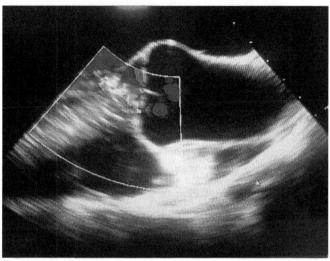

(Images courtesy of Drs Phuong Tran & Michael Andrawes.)

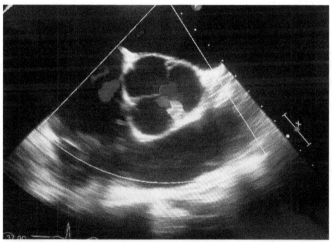

(Images courtesy of Drs Phuong Tran & Michael Andrawes.)

Which of the following statements is true regarding anesthetic management of this lesion?

    A. Atrial fibrillation is as well tolerated as sinus rhythm.
    B. It is important to maintain systemic vascular resistance (SVR) at normal to high levels.
    C. Heart rate should be maintained at a relatively high-normal rate.
    D. Patients will tolerate slight hypovolemia better than hypervolemia.

3. A 43-year-old man has had a systolic crescendo-decrescendo murmur noted for many years by his primary care physician. In the past several months, he has developed progressive angina and dyspnea on exertion. TEE shows the following image:

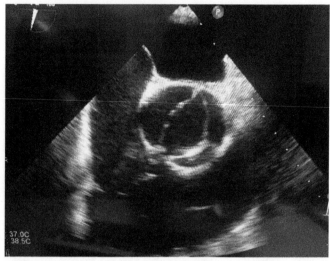

(Image courtesy of Drs Phuong Tran & Michael Andrawes.)

Which of the following is the most likely cause of this patient's valvular lesion?

    A. Rheumatic heart disease
    B. Calcific degeneration
    C. Congenital bicuspid aortic valve
    D. Infectious endocarditis

4. A 48-year-old woman presents for combined aortic root and aortic valve replacement. TEE shows the following image:

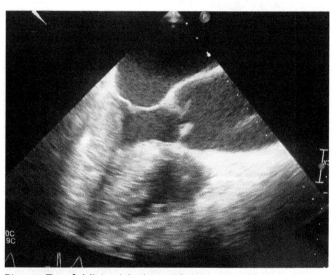

(Image courtesy of Drs Phuong Tran & Michael Andrawes.)

Which lesion is likely to accompany the aortic root pathology demonstrated here?

    A. Mitral regurgitation
    B. Bicuspid aortic valve
    C. Pericardial effusion
    D. Pulmonary hypertension

5. **A 73-year-old man presents with several episodes of presyncopal events. His exercise capacity is limited because of osteoarthritis. He has no other symptoms and no other significant medical history. Physical examination reveals a high-pitched systolic crescendo-decrescendo murmur loudest over the right second intercostal space, radiating to the bilateral carotids. What are the most appropriate hemodynamic goals for this patient?**

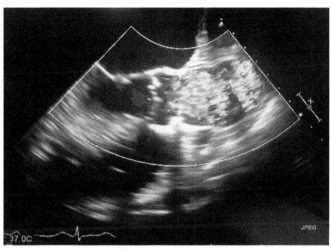

(Image courtesy of Drs Phuong Tran & Michael Andrawes.)

	PRELOAD	AFTERLOAD	HEART RATE
A.	Full	Maintain	Low normal
B.	Full	Decrease	Increase
C.	Full	Maintain	Increase
D.	Increase	Decrease	Increase

6. **A 64-year-old man with a medical history significant for Mobitz type II second-degree heart block after permanent pacemaker (PPM) placement presents for video-assisted right upper lobe wedge resection for a pulmonary nodule. Which of the following intraoperative issues is *unlikely* to occur from electromagnetic interference (EMI)?**

   A. Increase in ventricular thresholds
   B. Inhibition of pacemaker by EMI
   C. Pacemaker battery failure
   D. Transient or permanent loss of capture

7. **Which of the following codes correctly describes a pacemaker that utilizes synchronous, dual-chamber pacing and is rate-responsive?**

   A. DOOR
   B. DDDO
   C. VVIR
   D. DDIR

8. A 74-year-old man is 3 weeks after pulmonary vein isolation for atrial fibrillation and presents to the emergency department with fever, chills, and dysphagia. He is found to be hypotensive and anemic. Which of the following complications from pulmonary vein isolation commonly presents during this period?

   A. Atrial-esophageal fistula (AEF)
   B. Complete heart block
   C. Cardiac tamponade
   D. Phrenic nerve injury

9. An otherwise healthy 26-year-old woman undergoing laparoscopic myomectomy develops intraoperative narrow-complex tachycardia at a rate of 170 beats per minute, with loss of P wave. Her blood pressure quickly drops to 55/30. Which of the following is the correct next step in treatment?

   A. Diltiazem
   B. Adenosine
   C. Metoprolol
   D. Synchronized cardioversion

10. A 58-year-old woman one day after catheter ablation for atrial fibrillation complains of shortness of breath. Vital signs are as follows: 36.8°C | 74 | 134/68 | 26 | 98% on room air. ECG shows restoration of normal sinus rhythm. Chest X-ray demonstrates an elevated right hemidiaphragm. Which of the following procedural complications is the most likely source of her dyspnea?

    A. Volume overload
    B. Phrenic nerve injury
    C. Atrial-esophageal fistula
    D. Cardiac tamponade

11. Which of the following patients should undergo additional cardiac testing before proceeding for an intraoperative surgical procedure?

    A. A 71-year-old man with known untreated 3-vessel coronary disease presenting for exploratory laparotomy for perforated bowel
    B. An 81-year-old woman with chronic kidney disease (creatinine 2.3 mg/dL) and prior ischemic stroke presenting for lumpectomy for breast cancer
    C. A 68-year-old man with type 2 diabetes mellitus and prior ischemic stroke presenting for revascularization procedure for peripheral arterial disease, which limits his exercise capacity
    D. An otherwise healthy 48-year-old man presenting for median sternotomy for thymoma resection

12. A patient with type 1 diabetes mellitus and chronic kidney disease, stage III (Cr 2.5 mg/dL) presents for a video-assisted right upper lobe wedge resection for pulmonary nodule. Which of the following medications is appropriate to initiate preoperatively?

    A. Metoprolol
    B. Lisinopril
    C. Amlodipine
    D. Aspirin

13. When used alone, which ECG lead will most likely detect intraoperative myocardial ischemia?

    A. aVL
    B. II
    C. V_4
    D. V_5

14. A 59-year-old man with a suspected bowel perforation is scheduled to undergo exploratory laparotomy. His vitals are as follows: 38.2°C | 122 | 81/43 | 24 | 97% on 3 L nasal cannula. Laboratory analysis is notable for troponin of 0.12 ng/mL, and ECG shows ST depressions in leads V_4-V_6. Which of the following is the most appropriate diagnosis?

   A. Unstable angina
   B. Non-ST elevation myocardial infarction (MI), type I
   C. Non-ST elevation MI, type II
   D. ST elevation MI

15. A 49-year-old man is undergoing retroperitoneal sarcoma resection, which has been complicated by an injury to the inferior vena cava (IVC) and substantial blood loss. You note ST depressions in lead II and send an arterial blood gas revealing the following information:

pH	7.24
$Paco_2$	34 mm Hg
Pao_2	174 mm Hg
$[HCO_3^-]$	14 mEq/L
Hemoglobin	4.3 g/dL

Which of the following is most likely to resolve the ST depressions?

   A. Increasing Fio_2
   B. Transfusion of 2 units of packed red blood cells
   C. Administering rectal aspirin
   D. Increasing phenylephrine infusion

16. Which of the following statements is true concerning patients with ventricular assist devices (VADs) presenting for noncardiac surgery?

   A. Noninvasive blood pressure cuffs will not function correctly in a patient with a VAD.
   B. Anticoagulation should be held for at least 48 hours before proceeding to the operating room (OR).
   C. Implantation of a VAD may delay gastric emptying and necessitate a rapid sequence induction.
   D. Regional anesthesia should be utilized whenever possible for VAD patients.

17. Which of the following statements is true with respect to extracorporeal membrane oxygenation (ECMO) as compared with cardiopulmonary bypass (CPB)?

   A. Arterial line tracing for both ECMO and CPB will lack pulsatility.
   B. The membrane oxygenator in CPB is designed for longer-term use compared with ECMO.
   C. The heart is stopped in both ECMO and CPB.
   D. Lower flow rates are used in CPB, necessitating a greater degree of anticoagulation.

18. Which of the following factors places a patient at increased risk of anaphylaxis to protamine during reversal of heparin following CPB?

   A. Prior exposure to protamine
   B. Diabetes treated with metformin
   C. History of atopy (asthma, eczema)
   D. Prolonged heparin time

19. **Which of the following is an advantage of traditional, on-pump coronary artery bypass grafting (CABG) as compared with off-pump coronary artery bypass grafting (OPCABG)?**

    A. Lower intraoperative blood loss
    B. Reduced risk of postoperative cognitive dysfunction
    C. Higher rates of graft patency
    D. Reduced risk of thrombotic events

20. **Which of the following correctly describes the appropriate timing of inflation of an intra-aortic balloon pump?**

    A. Just after the dicrotic notch
    B. At the onset of ventricular systole
    C. When the P wave is seen on ECG
    D. During isovolumetric contraction

21. **A patient with asymptomatic, moderate aortic stenosis (V_{max} = 3.7 m/s) is presenting for elective laparoscopic colectomy for newly diagnosed colon cancer. Within what time frame should an echocardiogram have been performed before proceeding with elective surgery?**

    A. 3 months
    B. 6-12 months
    C. 1-2 years
    D. 3-5 years

22. **A 91-year-old woman presents to the emergency department with acute onset of dyspnea and is found to have a harsh, late-peaking systolic murmur and pulmonary edema on chest X-ray. Transthoracic echocardiography is performed with the following findings:**

Aortic valve area	0.8 cm²
Peak transaortic velocity (V_{max})	3.4 m/s
Mean transaortic pressure gradient	36 mm Hg

Which of the following best describes the patient's aortic stenosis (AS)?

    A. Mild AS
    B. Moderate AS
    C. Severe high-gradient AS
    D. Severe low-flow/low-gradient AS

23. **Which one of the following patients should receive infective endocarditis (IE) prophylaxis before undergoing his/her associated procedure?**

    A. A 61-year-old man with a mechanical mitral valve presenting for root canal
    B. A 34-year-old woman with a history of repaired tetralogy of Fallot presenting for dental cleaning
    C. A 54-year-old woman after aortic valve replacement for bicuspid aortic valve presenting for elective cystoscopy
    D. A 28-year-old man with history of IE because of IV drug use presenting for esophagogastroduodenoscopy

24. A 71-year-old man is presenting for elective aortic valve replacement. His transthoracic echocardiogram (TTE) shows a hypertrophic left ventricle (LV) with preserved function and an aortic valve area = 1.4 cm², V_{max} = 3.4 m/s, and mean gradient = 37 mm Hg. He is currently asymptomatic and denies angina, syncope, and dyspnea. Which of the following statements is correct regarding his anesthetic management?

    A. Phenylephrine infusion will decrease stroke volume because of increased afterload.
    B. Atrial fibrillation will be poorly tolerated.
    C. Heart rate between 80 and 100 beats per minute is ideal.
    D. Dopamine is the inotrope of choice.

25. A 61-year-old man with moderate mitral regurgitation (MR) is presenting for emergent exploratory laparotomy secondary to perforated bowel. Which of the following goals is most critical in the anesthetic management of MR?

    A. Target heart rates at the upper limit of normal (80-100 bpm).
    B. Increase preload slightly.
    C. Maintain sinus rhythm.
    D. Reduce SVR.

26. A otherwise healthy 24-year-old man with hypertrophic cardiomyopathy (HCM) is undergoing laparoscopic cholecystectomy for symptomatic cholelithiasis. He becomes acutely hypotensive following insufflation of the abdomen and positioning in the reverse Trendelenburg position. His blood pressure is unchanged at 68/43 following a rapid bolus of IV fluids, lightening the anesthetic and leveling the bed. Administration of which of the following drugs is the most appropriate next step in management?

    A. Epinephrine 10 µg IV
    B. Ephedrine 5 mg IV
    C. Norepinephrine 4 µg IV
    D. Phenylephrine 100 µg IV

27. Which of the following statements is true with regard to anesthetic management of patients with HCM?

    A. Patients without outflow obstruction at rest are at low risk for dynamic obstruction with administration of anesthetic agents.
    B. Negative inotropic agents may be useful to attenuate sympathetic stimulation perioperatively.
    C. Hypovolemia is better tolerated than hypervolemia.
    D. Lethal arrhythmias do not occur in hypertrophic obstructive cardiomyopathy patients without signs of inducible obstruction on echocardiography.

28. A 69-year-old woman becomes hypertensive to 207/109 upon emerging from a general anesthetic for laparoscopic hysterectomy. She is subsequently hypoxic and her endotracheal tube has frothy clear secretions. Which of the following is the most likely diagnosis?

    A. Volume overload
    B. Negative pressure pulmonary edema
    C. Flash pulmonary edema
    D. Transfusion-associated circulatory overload

29. A 54-year-old woman who was previously healthy presents with severe malaise and light-headedness 2 weeks after her husband died unexpectedly. Her extremities are cool and clammy, she is found to be profoundly hypotensive, and transthoracic echocardiogram shows global LV hypokinesis with apical ballooning. Which of the following statements is correct about her condition?

    A. Postmenopausal women are at highest risk for this condition.
    B. ECG changes are uncommon at presentation.
    C. This condition is unlikely to resolve over time.
    D. Most patients affected by this condition have underlying coronary artery disease.

30. A 74-year-old man with diabetes mellitus and poorly controlled hypertension has undergone robotic prostatectomy over a course of 8 hours, during which he received 4 L of Lactated Ringer and 500 cc of 5% albumin. Blood loss was approximately 200 cc, and urine output was 320 cc. His oxygen saturation is 93%-95% despite Fio_2 of 100% and positive end-expiratory pressure of 8 cm H_2O. On auscultation, bibasilar crackles are present. Which of the following is the best next step in management?

A. Emerge the patient and extubate to noninvasive positive pressure ventilation (PPV) in the OR.
B. Keep the patient intubated and admit to the surgical intensive care unit.
C. Administer a loop diuretic.
D. Initiate therapy with inhaled nitric oxide.

31. Which of the following signs or symptoms is more likely to be a presenting feature when cardiac tamponade develops chronically, rather than acutely?

A. Hypotension
B. Edema
C. Light-headedness
D. Cough

32. Which of the following causes of cardiac tamponade is an indication for immediate surgical intervention?

A. Viral pericarditis
B. Metastatic lung cancer
C. Free wall rupture following MI
D. Systemic lupus erythematosus

33. Which of the following conditions will mask the pulsus paradoxus commonly seen in cardiac tamponade?

A. Positive pressure ventilation
B. Mucous plug
C. Stridor
D. Chronic obstructive pulmonary disease (COPD)

34. A 67-year-old man presents with progressive dyspnea on exertion and intermittent positional chest discomfort. His past medical history is significant for coronary artery disease for which he underwent a 3-vessel CABG 2 years ago. Coronary catheterization shows patent grafts. Transthoracic echocardiography demonstrates evidence of increased ventricular interdependence and dissociation of intrathoracic-intracardiac pressures. Which of the following is the most likely cause of this patient's constrictive pericarditis (CP)?

A. Tuberculosis
B. Rheumatologic
C. Postradiation
D. Postcardiac surgical

35. The presence of which of the following findings is more consistent with a diagnosis of restrictive cardiomyopathy (RCM) as compared with CP?

A. Expiratory flow reversal in the hepatic vein
B. Respirophasic septal shift
C. Moderate pulmonary hypertension
D. Elevated medial mitral annulus velocity (e') ≥ 8 cm/s

36. **Which of the following statements is true of perioperative venous thromboembolism (VTE) prophylaxis?**

    A. Novel oral anticoagulants are more effective than once-daily enoxaparin in VTE prophylaxis without increased rates of postoperative bleeding.
    B. Major trauma increases VTE risk to a greater degree than postpartum status.
    C. The VTE prophylactic effects of aspirin and warfarin are synergistic.
    D. Neuraxial anesthesia initiated before surgical incision reduces rates of perioperative VTE.

37. **A 48-year-old man presents for retroperitoneal sarcoma resection. Pharmacologic VTE prophylaxis should be continued postoperatively for what length of time?**

    A. 3 days
    B. 14 days
    C. 28 days
    D. 60 days

38. **Which of the following pathophysiologic changes occurs with a pulmonary embolism?**

    A. Increased dead space
    B. Increased shunt
    C. Reduced pulmonary vascular resistance
    D. Reflex bronchodilation

39. **Which of the following arterial blood gas results, on an FIO_2 of 0.4, is most consistent with a diagnosis of acute, submassive pulmonary embolism?**

	pH	$PaCO_2$	PaO_2	$[HCO_3^-]$
A.	7.39	44	90	26
B.	7.47	40	74	28
C.	7.59	28	90	26
D.	7.50	32	74	24

40. **Which of the following ECG findings is most *sensitive* for acute pulmonary embolus?**

    A. Incomplete right bundle branch block
    B. Rightward axis
    C. Sinus tachycardia
    D. Large S wave in lead I, combined with Q wave and inverted T wave in lead III

41. **A 59-year-old woman with a history of hypertension presents for total abdominal hysterectomy for endometrial cancer. She has continued her home amlodipine and metoprolol up until the day of surgery but has held her lisinopril for 2 days. In the preoperative day, she is very anxious and her blood pressure is 179/88. Which of the following is the most appropriate next step?**

    A. Cancel the case.
    B. Administer home lisinopril dose.
    C. Proceed with the case and maintain blood pressure within high-normal range.
    D. Administer appropriate anxiolysis and reassess.

42. **Which of the following statements is true with respect to essential hypertension?**

    A. Systolic dysfunction will precede diastolic dysfunction in the progression.
    B. LV eccentric hypertrophy is likely to occur.
    C. Essential hypertension accounts for >80% of all hypertension diagnoses.
    D. Cerebral autoregulation is unchanged with long-standing essential hypertension.

43. **Which of the following antihypertensives should be held for 12-24 hours preoperatively?**

    A. Captopril
    B. Labetalol
    C. Amlodipine
    D. Clonidine

44. **In which of the following scenarios should a β-blocker be initiated preoperatively?**

    A. A 60-year-old woman presenting for bilateral mastectomy with poorly controlled hypertension on lisinopril, amlodipine, and hydrochlorothiazide
    B. A 48-year-old man with 100-pack-year smoking history presenting for thoracoscopic lobectomy
    C. A 74-year-old man with coronary artery disease presenting for endovascular aortic aneurysm repair (EVAR)
    D. A 65-year-old woman with hypertension and hyperlipidemia presenting for laparoscopic cholecystectomy for acute cholecystitis

45. **Administration of which of the following drugs is most likely to resolve intraoperative hypotension refractory to phenylephrine in a patient who took lisinopril the morning of surgery?**

    A. Ephedrine
    B. Methylene blue
    C. Norepinephrine
    D. Vasopressin

46. **Which of the following monitoring modalities is the gold standard with which to assess cerebral ischemia during carotid cross-clamp for carotid endarterectomy (CEA) under general anesthesia?**

    A. Somatosensory evoked potentials (SSEPs)
    B. Electroencephalography (EEG)
    C. Transcranial Dopplers (TCDs)
    D. Near-infrared spectroscopy

47. **Which of the following is a class I recommendation for spinal cord protection during open and endovascular thoracic aortic aneurysm repair for patients at high risk of spinal cord ischemia?**

    A. Cerebrospinal fluid drainage
    B. Systemic hypothermia
    C. Hyperventilation
    D. Hyperosmotic agents

48. **Which of the following is true regarding the physiologic changes that ensue following release of the aortic cross-clamp during aortic surgery?**

    A. Cardiac output increases.
    B. Venous return increases.
    C. Mixed venous oxygen saturation rapidly falls.
    D. $Paco_2$ abruptly falls.

49. **Which of the following statements is true with respect to EVAR compared with open abdominal aortic aneurysm repair?**

    A. Lower rate of operative survival with EVAR
    B. Increased hemodynamic shifts with EVAR
    C. Worsened intraoperative acid-base status with EVAR
    D. Higher rate of secondary interventions with EVAR at 6 years

50. **A 69-year-old man with type 2 diabetes mellitus, coronary artery disease after drug-eluting stent (28 months ago), COPD, and atrial fibrillation presents for lower limb revascularization for claudication. Which of the following is true with respect to timing of epidural placement as the primary anesthetic?**

    A. Clopidogrel should be held for 5 days before epidural placement.
    B. The case should be canceled if the epidural placement is bloody.
    C. It is unnecessary to check platelet count before epidural removal.
    D. Systemic heparin may be administered 1 hour after epidural placement.

Chapter 16 ▪ Answers

1. Correct answer: D

The TEE image depicted above demonstrates the midesophageal descending aortic short-axis view. The presence of an intimal flap is indicative of a descending aortic dissection. Without color Doppler, it is not clear which is the true lumen versus the false lumen. We cannot tell the extent of the dissection by this view alone, and thus the appropriate management strategy remains unclear at this time.

Stanford type A dissections involve the ascending aorta with or without the descending aorta, whereas Stanford type B dissections involve only the aorta distal to the left subclavian artery. Management varies depending on the location of the dissection.

Type A dissections are surgical emergencies and involve replacement of the aortic root, ascending aorta, or aortic arch together with atrioventricular repair or replacement.

Type B dissections are generally managed medically unless there is aortic rupture or evidence of malperfusion through one of the splanchnic or renal arteries. Medical management goals are detailed in the table below.

Endovascular stenting is an emerging therapy for uncomplicated type B dissections to prevent aneurysm formation and other complications.

Acute Aortic Dissection: Hemodynamic Goals

Preload	May be increased if acute AI, increase further in tamponade
Afterload	Decrease with anesthetics, analgesics, arterial dilators (nitroprusside, nicardipine): keep systolic BP <100-120 mm Hg
Contractility	May be depressed; titrate myocardial depressants carefully
Rate	Decrease to <60-80 bpm: use β-blocker; ensure contractility is adequate
Rhythm	If atrial fibrillation is present: control ventricular response
MVo$_2$	Compromised if aortic dissection involves coronary vessels
CPB	Alternate site of inflow (arterial) cannulation; deep hypothermic circulatory arrest is possible if cerebral vessels are involved

AI, aortic insufficiency; BP, blood pressure; bpm, beats per minute; CPB, cardiopulmonary bypass; MVo$_2$, myocardial oxygen consumption.
From Skubas NJ, Lichtman AD, Sharma A, et al. Anesthesia for cardiac surgery. In: Barash PG, Cullen BF, Stoelting RK, et al, eds. Clinical Anesthesia. 7th ed. Philadelphia: Wolters Kluwer Health/Lippincott Williams & Wilkins; 2013, with permission.

References:
1. Chaney MA, Zvara DA, Kolarczyk LM, et al. Cardiac anesthesia. In: Longnecker DE, Newman MF, Zapol WM, Mackey SC, Sandberg WS, eds. *Anesthesiology.* New York: McGraw-Hill; 2017:834-866.
2. Mackensen GB, Schuler A. Intraoperative transesophageal echocardiography: a systematic approach. In: Longnecker DE, Newman MF, Zapol WM, Mackey SC, Sandberg WS, eds. *Anesthesiology.* New York: McGraw-Hill; 2017:382-410.
3. Montzingo CR, Shillcutt S. Cardiac anesthesia. In: Barash PG, Cullen BF, Stoelting RK, et al, eds. *Clinical Anesthesia Fundamentals.* Philadelphia: Wolters Kluwer Health; 2015:669-686.

2. Correct answer: C

These images show the midesophageal aortic valve long axis and short axis, respectively. The aortic valve is closed in both images; thus they represent diastole and have regurgitant jets obvious in both views, indicating aortic regurgitation.

Aortic regurgitation, or aortic insufficiency, causes gradual eccentric hypertrophy over a course of decades. Hemodynamic goals in aortic insufficiency include the following:

- Increased preload
- Decreased afterload to maximize forward stroke volume

- High-normal heart rate (eg, target ~90 bpm) to minimize regurgitant volume during diastole
- Sinus rhythm

These goals help to maintain the balance in favor of forward ejection while minimizing the regurgitant fraction.

References:
1. Montzingo CR, Shillcutt S. Cardiac anesthesia. In: Barash PG, Cullen BF, Stoelting RK, et al, eds. *Clinical Anesthesia Fundamentals*. Philadelphia: Wolters Kluwer Health; 2015:669-686.
2. Mackensen GB, Schuler A. Intraoperative transesophageal echocardiography: a systematic approach. In: Longnecker DE, Newman MF, Zapol WM, Mackey SC, Sandberg WS, eds. *Anesthesiology*. New York: McGraw-Hill; 2017:382-410.

3. Correct answer: C

This patient's symptoms, physical examination findings, and TEE imaging are consistent with AS. This patient is presenting in the fifth decade of life, which is most often due to congenital bicuspid aortic valve. Bicuspid aortic valve affects 2% of the population and presents in the fourth to sixth decades of life. The TEE image shows fusion of the right and left aortic valve leaflets.

Overall, the most common cause of AS is calcific degeneration, which typically presents in the sixth to seventh decades of life. It is characterized by restricted leaflet motion.

Rheumatic AS typically affects patients who had untreated streptococcal infection earlier in life. The aortic valve leaflets are thickened and calcified, and the commissures are fused. Usually, the mitral valve is also involved.

Infectious endocarditis is not consistent with this patient's subacute presentation and lack of other infectious symptoms.

Reference:
1. Mackensen GB, Schuler A. Intraoperative transesophageal echocardiography: a systematic approach. In: Longnecker DE, Newman MF, Zapol WM, Mackey SC, Sandberg WS, eds. *Anesthesiology*. New York: McGraw-Hill; 2017:382-410.

4. Correct answer: B

This TEE image shows the midesophageal aortic valve long-axis view and is notable for aortic root dilation. This lesion can occur as a poststenotic pathology, commonly seen with AS because of congenital bicuspid aortic valve. As in the prior question, this patient is presenting early in life, in the fifth decade. Aortic root dilation may also occur independently because of myxomatous degeneration with consequent aortic insufficiency.

Reference:
1. Mackensen GB, Schuler A. Intraoperative transesophageal echocardiography: a systematic approach. In: Longnecker DE, Newman MF, Zapol WM, Mackey SC, Sandberg WS, eds. *Anesthesiology*. New York: McGraw-Hill; 2017:382-410.

5. Correct answer: A

This image shows the midesophageal aortic valve long-axis view. The color Doppler demonstrates turbulent flow distal to the aortic valve, which taken together with the history demonstrates AS.

In AS, preload should be maintained, as should afterload to sustain coronary perfusion during diastole in the setting of a thick LV wall. Because there is a fixed defect at the level of the valve, increased afterload does NOT decrease stroke volume in AS. Heart rate should be kept low normal, in sinus rhythm, to allow adequate coronary perfusion during diastole and to minimize ischemia related to tachycardia.

Answer choice D describes management of aortic insufficiency and MR. A summary of anesthetic management for patients with valvular heart disease is provided below.

Hemodynamic Goals in Patients With Valvular Heart Disease

	AORTIC STENOSIS	HYPERTROPHIC CARDIOMYOPATHY	AORTIC INSUFFICIENCY	MITRAL STENOSIS	MITRAL REGURGITATION
Preload	Full	Full	Increase slightly	Maintain; avoid hypovolemia	Increase slightly
Afterload	Maintain CPP	Increase; treat hypotension aggressively	Decrease to reduce regurgitant fraction	Prevent increase	Decrease
Rate	Avoid bradycardia (decrease CO) and tachycardia (ischemia)	Normal	Increase	Low normal	Increase slightly, avoid bradycardia
Rhythm	Sinus	Sinus is critical	Sinus	Sinus or rate-controlled atrial fibrillation	Sinus or rate-controlled atrial fibrillation

CO, cardiac output; CPP, coronary perfusion pressure.
From Montzingo CR, Shillcutt S. Cardiac anesthesia. In: Barash PG, Cullen BF, Stoelting RK, et al, eds. Clinical Anesthesia Fundamentals. Philadelphia: Wolters Kluwer Health; 2015, with permission.

References:
1. Montzingo CR, Shillcutt S. Cardiac anesthesia. In: Barash PG, Cullen BF, Stoelting RK, et al, eds. *Clinical Anesthesia Fundamentals*. Philadelphia: Wolters Kluwer Health; 2015:669-686.
2. Mackensen GB, Schuler A. Intraoperative transesophageal echocardiography: a systematic approach. In: Longnecker DE, Newman MF, Zapol WM, Mackey SC, Sandberg WS, eds. *Anesthesiology*. New York: McGraw-Hill; 2017:382-410.

6. Correct answer: C

A variety of intraoperative issues may arise in a patient with a cardiac electronic implantable device undergoing any anesthetic in which EMI may occur, which includes surgical procedures utilizing electrocautery, radiofrequency ablation, and magnetic resonance imaging. Cardiac electronic implantable devices may include PPMs, implantable cardiac defibrillators, and cardiac resynchronization therapy. EMI may lead to a number of issues including the following:

- Inhibition of PPM
- Inappropriate delivery of antitachycardia therapy (implantable cardiac defibrillator)
- Changes in lead parameters (eg, atrial mode switching, inappropriate ventricular sensing, electrical reset, increase in ventricular thresholds)
- "Runaway" pacemaker—a phenomenon where the pacemaker delivers paroxysms of pacing spikes at 2000 bpm, which may provoke ventricular fibrillation
- Reprogramming to a backup mode
- Transient or permanent loss of capture
- Entry into noise reversal mode
- Pacemaker failure due to direct contact with electrocautery and cardioversion
- Myocardial burns if electrical energy travels through leads into the myocardium

Pacemaker battery failure may occur intraoperatively, but it is not related to EMI. Of note, devices that have entered their elective battery replacement period may have different backup rates or modes compared with their baseline operation, and as such it is important to note this.

References:
1. Badescu GC, Sherman BM, Zaidan JR, Barash PG. Appendix C: pacemaker and implantable cardiac defibrillator protocols. In: Barash PG, Cullen BF, Stoelting RK, et al, eds. *Clinical Anesthesia Fundamentals*. Philadelphia: Wolters Kluwer; 2015:853-865.
2. American Society of Anesthesiologists Task Force on Perioperative Management of Patients with Cardiac Implantable Electronic Devices. Practice advisory for the perioperative management of patients with cardiac implantable electronic devices: pacemakers and implantable cardioverter-defibrillators. *Anesthesiology*. 2011;114:247-261.

7. Correct answer: D

The Generic Pacemaker Code describes the basic function of a pacemaker. The 5 positions in the code designate the following information:

- *Position I* designates the chamber being paced.
- *Position II* designates the chamber being sensed. Sensing can be turned off when the pacemaker is placed into an asynchronous mode.

- *Position III* designates the pacemaker's response to what is sensed. If *position II* is turned off, then *position III* is, as well. The response to sensing may include inhibition (where the pacemaker output is withheld), triggering (used to test pacemaker function), or dual (inhibition and triggered)
- *Position IV* refers to rate responsiveness, which may be sensed via increased motion, vibration, minute ventilation, or right atrial pressure.
- *Position V* refers to the presence of multisite pacing, which can be used in cardiac resynchronization therapy.

A summary of the code system is below:

Generic Pacemaker Code: NASPE/BPEG Revised (2002)

POSITION I, PACING CHAMBER(S)	POSITION II, SENSING CHAMBER(S)	POSITION III, RESPONSE(S) TO SENSING	POSITION IV, PROGRAMMABILITY	POSITION V, MULTISITE PACING
O = none	O = none	O = none	O = none	O = none
A = atrium	A = atrium	I = inhibited	R = rate modulation	A = atrium
V = ventricle	V = ventricle	T = triggered		V = ventricle
D = dual (A + V)	D = dual (A + V)	D = dual (T + I)		D = dual (A + V)

BPEG, British Pacing and Electrophysiology Group; NASPE, North American Society of Pacing and Electrophysiology, now called the Heart Rhythm Society.
Reproduced with permission from Practice advisory for perioperative management of patients with cardiac rhythm management devices: pacemakers and implantable cardioverter-defibrillators. A report by the American Society of Anesthesiologists Task Force on Perioperative Management of Patients with Cardiac Rhythm Management Devices. Anesthesiology. 2011;114:247-261.

Answer choice A is wrong because it represents an asynchronous mode. Answer choice B is wrong because it does not have rate responsiveness. Answer choice C is wrong because it paces only 1 chamber.

References:
1. Badescu GC, Sherman BM, Zaidan JR, Barash PG. Appendix C: pacemaker and implantable cardiac defibrillator protocols. In: Barash PG, Cullen BF, Stoelting RK, et al, eds. *Clinical Anesthesia Fundamentals*. Philadelphia: Wolters Kluwer; 2015:853-865.
2. American Society of Anesthesiologists Task Force on Perioperative Management of Patients with Cardiac Implantable Electronic Devices. Practice advisory for the perioperative management of patients with cardiac implantable electronic devices: pacemakers and implantable cardioverter-defibrillators. *Anesthesiology*. 2011;114:247-261.

8. **Correct answer: A**

Electrophysiologic procedures are used to treat patients with arrhythmias refractory to medical therapy. Radiofrequency or cryotherapy ablation may be used to treat atrioventricular nodal reentrant tachycardia, atrioventricular reentrant tachycardia, Wolff-Parkinson-White (WPW) syndrome, atrial fibrillation, atrial flutter, atrial tachycardia, and ventricular tachycardia. Although less invasive than traditional cardiac surgery, patients are at risk for a number of complications when undergoing electrophysiologic procedures. There include catheter-related issues, cardiac perforation, cardiac tamponade, cerebral vascular accident (CVA), arterial embolization, esophageal injury, complete heart block, phrenic nerve injury, and pulmonary vein stenosis. Esophageal injury encompasses a range of severity from esophageal erythema to ulcerlike changes in the esophageal wall to esophageal perforation or the development of an AEF. AEF is a life-threatening complication and generally presents 2-4 weeks following a procedure involving the left atrial. Presentation is variable and may include fever, chest pain, dysphagia, hematemesis, cardiovascular collapse, and neurologic symptoms (eg, CVA, TIA, seizures, meningitis). To avoid AEF, some electrophysiologists will avoid ablation or switch to cryotherapy when working near the esophagus.

References:
1. Kwak J. Anesthesia for electrophysiology studies and catheter ablations. *Semin Cardiothorac Vasc Anesth*. 2012;17(3):195-202.
2. Yousuf T, Keshmiri H, Bulwa Z, et al. Management of atrio-esophageal fistula following left atrial ablation. *Cardiol Res*. 2016;7(1):36-45.

9. **Correct answer: D**

This patient has developed supraventricular tachycardia (SVT) with hemodynamic instability. The immediate treatment of a patient with an unstable SVT is synchronized cardioversion; with the exception of atrial fibrillation, most SVTs can be broken with 25-50 J. Adenosine may be used in a stable patient.

Most SVTs occur due to a reentrant mechanism, wherein a self-perpetuating loop of repolarization and depolarization can occur in the conduction pathways. In a stable patient without an accessory conduction pathway (eg, WPW syndrome), β-blockers or calcium channel blockers may be used. In a patient with WPW syndrome, procainamide or amiodarone can be used to treat a stable SVT.

References:

1. Butterworth JF, Mackey DC, Wasnick JD, eds. Anesthesia for patients with cardiovascular disease. In: *Morgan and Mikhail's Clinical Anesthesiology*. 5th ed. New York: McGraw-Hill Education; 2013:375-434.
2. Butterworth JF, Mackey DC, Wasnick JD, eds. Anesthesia for cardiovascular surgery. In: *Clinical Anesthesiology*. 5th ed. New York: McGraw-Hill Education; 2013:435-486.

10. Correct answer: B

This patient has recently undergone a procedure in the electrophysiology laboratory (EPL). It is important that the anesthesiologist is aware of potential complications of EPL procedures. Although all of the listed answer choices are potential complications, the presence of an elevated hemidiaphragm together with normal vital signs aside from a mild tachypnea indicate phrenic nerve injury as the most likely cause. Given its anatomical location near the superior vena cava (SVC) and the right superior pulmonary vein, the right phrenic nerve is at risk during EPL ablations, particularly those for atrial fibrillation. This is true of radiofrequency, cryotherapy, and laser ablations. To avoid this complication, electrophysiologists may perform pacing before ablations in these critical areas to evaluate for phrenic nerve activation. Most patients who experience a phrenic nerve injury will present with dyspnea, but they may also experience hiccups during the procedure or be asymptomatic with routine imaging revealing the elevated hemidiaphragm. Many injuries resolve on their own, with a mean recovery time of 7 months.

References:

1. Roberts JD. Ambulatory anesthesia for the cardiac catheterization and electrophysiology laboratories. *Anesthesiol Clin.* 2014;32:381-386.
2. Kwak J. Anesthesia for electrophysiology studies and catheter ablations. *Semin Cardiothorac Vasc Anesth.* 2012;17(3):195-202.
3. Sacher F, Jais P, Stephenson K, et al. Phrenic nerve injury after catheter ablation of atrial fibrillation. *Indian Pacing Electrophysiol J.* 2007;7(1):1-6.

11. Correct answer: C

The 2014 ACC/AHA guidelines on perioperative cardiovascular evaluation provide a stepwise framework for approaching cardiovascular assessment on patients presenting for surgery. All patients who truly require emergent surgical procedures (answer choice A) should proceed to the OR with perioperative surveillance and risk factor modification. In other patients, a validated risk prediction tool can be useful in predicting the risk of perioperative major adverse cardiac events. The Revised Cardiac Risk Index (RCRI) is one such tool that includes a point each for creatinine >2 mg/dL, heart failure, type 1 diabetes mellitus, high-risk surgery (intrathoracic, intra-abdominal, or suprainguinal vascular surgery), and history of cerebrovascular disease or TIA. In patients with elevated risk, and poor or unknown functional capacity, additional testing may be required to indicate whether it will affect decision making or perioperative care. Although the patient in answer choice B has 2 risk factors for major adverse cardiac events, she is undergoing a low-risk surgical procedure and would not warrant additional testing. The patient in answer choice D is undergoing a high-risk surgical procedure (intrathoracic) but has no other risk factors, so no additional testing is necessary. Only answer choice C describes a scenario in which additional testing may be warranted because the patient has at least 3 risk factors (diabetes, cerebrovascular disease, and peripheral arterial disease) and he is presenting for an intermediate risk surgery.

References:

1. Butterworth JF, Mackey DC, Wasnick JD, eds. Anesthesia for patients with cardiovascular disease. In: *Morgan and Mikhail's Clinical Anesthesiology*. 5th ed. New York: McGraw-Hill Education; 2013:375-434.
2. Fleisher LA, Fleischmann KE, Auerbach AD, et al. 2014 ACC/AHA guideline on perioperative cardiovascular evaluation and management of patients undergoing noncardiac surgery. *Circulation.* 2014;130:e278-e333.

12. Correct answer: A

The 2014 ACC/AHA guidelines on perioperative cardiovascular evaluation and management include a class IIB recommendation for beginning a β-blocker in patients with 3 or more RCRI risk factors.

Despite having no known cardiac history, this patient has 3 RCRI risk factors (intrathoracic surgery, type 1 diabetes mellitus, and preoperative creatinine >2 mg/dL), and as such, it is reasonable to consider initiation of a low-dose β-blocker preoperatively. The other medications listed would not be initiated in the absence of an additional compelling indication such as baseline hypertension.

1. Fleisher LA, Fleischmann KE, Auerbach AD, et al. 2014 ACC/AHA guideline on perioperative cardiovascular evaluation and management of patients undergoing noncardiac surgery. *Circulation.* 2014;130:e278-e333.

13. Correct answer: D

Intraoperative myocardial ischemia typically affects the ST and T wave portions of the ECG signal, with the T wave affected initially followed by ST segment changes as the ischemia progresses. V_5 lead alone detects 75% of ischemic episodes, whereas the addition of V_4 increases the sensitivity to 90%, and the combination of II, V_4, and V_5 detects up to 96% of ischemic episodes.

References:

1. De Silva A. Anesthetic monitoring. In: Miller RD, Pardo MC, eds. *Basics of Anesthesia.* 6th ed. Philadelphia: Elsevier Saunders; 2007:319-331.
2. Slogoff S, Keats AS. Does perioperative myocardial ischemia lead to postoperative myocardial infarction? *Anesthesiology.* 1985;73:1074-1081.

14. Correct answer: C

This patient is febrile, tachycardic, and hypotensive, likely because of sepsis from an abdominal source. The ECG changes and mild troponin elevation are due to a mismatch between myocardial oxygen supply and demand. Supply is decreased because of the hypotension, whereas demand is increased because of the tachycardia.

A new classification scheme for MI was introduced in 2007. The classifications are as follows:

- Type 1 MI occurs secondary to a primary event such as plaque rupture, erosion, or dissection.
- Type 2 MI occurs secondary to increased myocardial demand or decreased oxygen supply.
- Type 3 MI is a sudden, unexpected cardiac death with symptoms suggestive of MI, where death occurs before biomarkers could be obtained or before they appeared in the circulation because of the event.
- Type 4 MI is associated with percutaneous coronary intervention.
- Type 5 MI is associated with CABG.

Reference:

1. Makki N, Brennan TM, Girotra S. Acute coronary syndrome. *J Intensive Care Med.* 2015;30(4):186-200.

15. Correct answer: B

Myocardial ischemia occurs due to an imbalance between myocardial oxygen supply and demand. Myocardial oxygen demand is determined by systolic wall tension, contractility, and heart rate. An increase in heart rate is especially problematic because it both increases the demand directly and decreases the amount of time for oxygen delivery to the myocardium during diastole.

Myocardial oxygen supply is determined by coronary blood flow and the arterial oxygen content, described by the following equation:

$$O_2 \text{ content} = [\text{hemoglobin (g/dL)}] \times 1.34 \times [\text{oxygen saturation (\%)}] + 0.003 \times Pao_2$$

The patient mentioned in the question is severely anemic; thus the most appropriate corrective action is transfusion to improve the myocardial oxygen supply. Increasing Fio_2 would only increase the total oxygen content marginally. The most likely cause of the ischemic ECG changes is demand ischemia rather than a primary coronary thrombus, so rectal aspirin is not likely to resolve the changes. A phenylephrine infusion may raise the blood pressure, but by increasing afterload, this will also increase the myocardial oxygen demand.

Reference:

1. Montzingo CR, Shillcutt S. Cardiac anesthesia. In: Barash PG, ed. *Clinical Anesthesia Fundamentals.* Philadelphia: Wolters Kluwer Health; 2015:669-686.

16. **Correct answer: C**

The number of patients living with left or right VADs is growing, and these patients are increasingly presenting for noncardiac surgery. A number of specific considerations are relevant. VAD patients must be maintained on long-term anticoagulation to avoid thromboembolic complications. Generally, this anticoagulation must be continued throughout the perioperative period; however, small amounts of fresh frozen plasma may be given to achieve lower limits of anticoagulation in the setting of excessive bleeding. Furthermore, because of anticoagulation, most VAD patients are not candidates for regional anesthetics. The VAD console will continuously display the device output, so invasive monitoring is not typically required and a noninvasive blood pressure will usually suffice in the absence of another indication (eg, frequent laboratory tests, large expected blood loss). Finally, many patients with VADs suffer from delayed gastric emptying and early satiety because of the location of the device in close proximity to the stomach. In these patients, rapid sequence induction may be indicated.

Reference:
1. Chaney MA, Cheung AT, Troianos CA, et al. Cardiac anesthesia. In: Longnecker DE, Brown DL, Newman MF, Zapol WM, eds. *Anesthesiology*. New York: McGraw-Hill; 2012:898-927.

17. **Correct answer: D**

Both ECMO and CPB provide temporary mechanical cardiopulmonary support. They differ in both the purpose and the time course for which they provide this support. ECMO is used as a bridge to recovery or transplant and may be used for days to weeks. CPB, on the other hand, is used over the course of hours to allow cardiac surgery to proceed. In CPB, cardioplegia is applied to stop the heart, and low flow rates are used to maintain systemic perfusion. Thus, a higher degree of anticoagulation is necessary for CPB, and the arterial line will lack pulsatility. In ECMO, however, the heart continues to contract and higher flow rates are used, reducing the risk of thrombus formation. The arterial line in V-A ECMO may have artifact but will show some pulsatility, and in V-V ECMO, the arterial line will be normal.

Reference:
1. Allen S, Holena D, McCunn M, Kohl B, Sarani B. A review of the fundamental principles and evidence base in the use of extracorporeal membrane oxygenation (ECMO) in critically ill adult patients. *J Intensive Care Med*. 2011;26(1):13-26.

18. **Correct answer: A**

Protamine is administered following separation from CPB to reverse heparinization. Life-threatening anaphylactic reactions to protamine may occur, and several important risk factors have been identified, including type 1 diabetes mellitus (specifically those taking NPH insulin), prior vasectomy, fish allergy, and prior exposure to protamine sulfate. Other common reactions include hypotension and pulmonary hypertension, the risk of which can be partially mitigated by administering protamine slowly.

References:
1. Chaney MA, Cheung AT, Troianos CA, et al. Cardiac anesthesia. In: Longnecker DE, Brown DL, Newman MF, Zapol WM, eds. *Anesthesiology*. New York: McGraw-Hill; 2012:898-927.
2. Porsche R, Brenner ZR. Allergy to protamine sulfate. *Heart Lung*. 1999;28(6):418-428.

19. **Correct answer: C**

Off-pump CABG can be performed, utilizing epicardial stabilization devices, where the cardiac surgeon performs distal graft anastomoses on a beating heart, then partially clamps the ascending aorta to perform the proximal anastomoses. OPCABG was thought to reduce postoperative complications associated with the use of CPB, including generalized systemic inflammatory response, cerebral dysfunction, myocardial depression, and hemodynamic instability. However, randomized controlled trials have demonstrated no difference in neurocognitive testing between patients undergoing CABG and those undergoing OPCABG. There are, however, higher rates of 1-year graft patency in the traditional CABG groups.

References:

1. Butterworth JF, Mackey DC, Wasnick JD, eds. Anesthesia for cardiovascular surgery. In: *Clinical Anesthesiology*. 5th ed. New York: McGraw-Hill Education; 2013:435-486.
2. Chaney MA, Cheung AT, Troianos CA, et al. Cardiac anesthesia. In: Longnecker DE, Brown DL, Newman MF, Zapol WM, eds. *Anesthesiology*. New York: McGraw-Hill; 2012:898-927.
3. Shroyer AL, Grover FL, Hattler B, et al. On-pump versus off-pump coronary-artery bypass surgery. *N Engl J Med*. 2009;361: 1827-1837.

20. Correct answer: A

The success of an intra-aortic balloon pump depends on proper timing, just after the dicrotic notch, indicating closure of the aortic valve. This helps to augment aortic diastolic pressure and thus improve coronary perfusion. Early inflation increases afterload, making the LV work harder to eject forward. Late inflation reduces the amount of diastolic augmentation. Deflation should occur just before LV ejection to reduce afterload.

Reference:

1. Butterworth JF, Mackey DC, Wasnick JD, eds. Anesthesia for cardiovascular surgery. In: *Clinical Anesthesiology*. 5th ed. New York: McGraw-Hill Education; 2013:435-486.

21. Correct answer: C

Patients with known valvular heart disease who remain asymptomatic should undergo regular monitoring with transthoracic echocardiography, depending on valve lesion, severity, ventricular size, and ventricular function, as shown in the table below.

Because this patient is asymptomatic and has moderate AS, she should undergo TTE evaluation every 1-2 years. TTE is also indicated in any patient with known valvular disease who has any change in symptoms or physical examination findings.

Recommended Frequency of Echocardiography in Asymptomatic Patients with Valvular Heart Disease and Normal Left Ventricular Function

SEVERITY		AORTIC STENOSIS	AORTIC REGURGITATION	MITRAL STENOSIS	MITRAL REGURGITATION
Progressive	Mild	3-5 years (V_{max} 2.0-2.9 m/s)	3-5 years	Every 3-5 years (MVA >1.5 cm²)	Every 3-5 years
	Moderate	1-2 years (V_{max} 3.0-3.9 m/s)	1-2 years		Every 1-2 years
Severe		6-12 months (V_{max} ≥ 4.0 m/s)	6-12 months (more frequently if dilating LV)	Every 1-2 years (MVA 1.0-1.5 cm²) Once per year (MVA <1.0 cm²)	6-12 months (more frequently if dilating LV)

References:

1. Nishimura RA, Otto CM, Bonow RO, et al. 2014 AHA/ACC guideline for the management of patients with valvular heart disease. *Circulation*. 2014;129(23):2440-2492.
2. Nishimura RA, Otto CM, Bonow RO, et al. 2017 AHA/ACC focused update of the 2014 AHA/ACC guideline for the management of patients with valvular heart disease: a report of the American College of Cardiology/American Heart Association task force on clinical practice guidelines. *J Am Coll Cardiol*. 2017;70(2):252-289.

22. Correct answer: D

The stages of AS are defined by valve anatomy, valve hemodynamics, the consequences of valve obstruction on the LV and vasculature, as well as by patient symptoms. In general, the transaortic maximum velocity (V_{max}) best characterizes the hemodynamic severity of a lesion; this measure is limited to scenarios where transaortic volume flow is normal. Patients with LV dysfunction may have an artificially low V_{max} and/or mean transaortic pressure gradient. In these patients, the aortic valve area should be used to classify the severity, recognizing that a low-flow state worsens the prognosis of a stenotic lesion.

Classification of Severity of Aortic Stenosis

CLASSIFICATION	AORTIC VALVE AREA (cm²)	PEAK TRANSAORTIC VELOCITY (V_{max}) (m/s)	MEAN TRANSAORTIC PRESSURE GRADIENT (mm Hg)
Mild		2.0-2.9	<20
Moderate		3.0-3.9	20-39
Severe, high-gradient	<1.0	≥4	≥40
Severe, low-flow/low-gradient	<1.0	<4	<40

References:

1. Nishimura RA, Otto CM, Bonow RO, et al. 2014 AHA/ACC guideline for the management of patients with valvular heart disease. *Circulation*. 2014;129(23):2440-2492.
2. Nishimura RA, Otto CM, Bonow RO, et al. 2017 AHA/ACC focused update of the 2014 AHA/ACC guideline for the management of patients with valvular heart disease: a report of the American College of Cardiology/American Heart Association task force on clinical practice guidelines. *J Am Coll Cardiol*. 2017;70(2):252-289.

23. Correct answer: A

According to the 2017 ACC/AHA guidelines, there is no evidence for IE prophylaxis for patients undergoing gastrointestinal or genitourinary procedures in the absence of known infection. Although there is no clear evidence for or against IE prophylaxis, the guidelines state that it is reasonable for dental procedures that require manipulation of the gingival tissue, the periapical region of the teeth, or perforation of the oral mucosa in the following patients:

- Patients with prosthetic heart valves (bioprosthetic or mechanical)
- Patients with repaired heart valves using prosthetic material (eg, annuloplasty rings and chords)
- Patients with a history of previous IE
- Patients with unrepaired cyanotic congenital heart disease or repaired congenital heart disease with residual shunts or valvular regurgitation at the site of prosthetic material
- Cardiac transplant recipients with valve regurgitation because of a structurally abnormal valve

Reference:

1. Nishimura RA, Otto CM, Bonow RO, et al. 2017 AHA/ACC focused update of the 2014 AHA/ACC guideline for the management of patients with valvular heart disease: a report of the American College of Cardiology/American Heart Association task force on clinical practice guidelines. *J Am Coll Cardiol*. 2017;70(2):252-289.

24. Correct answer: B

Patients with AS have an increased myocardial oxygen demand because of concentric hypertrophy, which develops in response to the need for increased intraventricular pressure. The diastolic filling pressure is also increased, which heightens the need for sufficient diastolic filling time, and it is therefore of utmost importance to maintain a slower rate (eg, 50-70 bpm) and, if possible, to maintain sinus rhythm because these patients are quite dependent on the atrial kick. Atrial fibrillation with fast rates will be poorly tolerated in AS. Similarly, one must maintain afterload for adequate coronary perfusion, usually through a phenylephrine or vasopressin infusion that will increase SVR without inotropy and concomitant increase in myocardial oxygen demand. Given the fixed lesion at the valve, stroke volume does not depend on afterload and thus will not be adversely affected by the use of a pure vasoconstrictor.

Reference:

1. Montzingo CR, Shillcutt S. Cardiac anesthesia. In: Barash PG, Cullen BF, Stoelting RK, et al, eds. *Clinical Anesthesia Fundamentals*. Philadelphia: Wolters Kluwer Health; 2015:669-686.

25. Correct answer: D

In MR the LV stroke volume comprises both the volume ejected into the systemic circulation, as well as that regurgitated into the left atrium. Therefore, it is important to reduce SVR to maximize the portion that is ejected forward. Secondarily, heart rates on the higher side will limit diastolic filling and thus ventricular dilatation. Preload must be maintained or increased slightly to ensure an adequate forward stroke volume. A mnemonic to remember for management of MR is "full, fast, and forward."

A summary of anesthetic management for patients with valvular heart disease is provided below.

Hemodynamic Goals in Patients with Valvular Heart Disease

	AORTIC STENOSIS	HYPERTROPHIC CARDIOMYOPATHY	AORTIC INSUFFICIENCY	MITRAL STENOSIS	MITRAL REGURGITATION
Preload	Full	Full	Increase slightly	Maintain; avoid hypovolemia	Increase slightly
Afterload	Maintain CPP	Increase; treat hypotension aggressively	Decrease to reduce regurgitant fraction	Prevent increase	Decrease
Rate	Avoid bradycardia (decrease CO) and tachycardia (ischemia)	Normal	Increase	Low normal	Increase slightly, avoid bradycardia
Rhythm	Sinus	Sinus is critical	Sinus	Sinus or rate-controlled atrial fibrillation	Sinus or rate-controlled atrial fibrillation

CO, cardiac output; CPP, coronary perfusion pressure.
From Montzingo CR, Shillcutt S. Cardiac anesthesia. In: Barash PG, Cullen BF, Stoelting RK, et al, eds. Clinical Anesthesia Fundamentals. Philadelphia: Wolters Kluwer Health; 2015, with permission.

Reference:
1. Montzingo CR, Shillcutt S. Cardiac anesthesia. In: Barash PG, ed. *Clinical Anesthesia Fundamentals*. Philadelphia: Wolters Kluwer Health; 2015:669-686.

26. Correct answer: D

In HCM, one-third of patients will have hypertrophy of the interventricular septum, which leads to dynamic left ventricular outflow tract (LVOT) obstruction. The pressure gradient created by this obstruction increases during systole and further increases with a decrease in LV size.

In this scenario, the patient likely experienced a rapid decrease in preload following insufflation of the abdomen and position change. Despite the IV fluid bolus, he continues to have LVOT obstruction and should be treated with an α-adrenergic drug such as phenylephrine to improve afterload and stent open the LVOT. Inotropic agents such as epinephrine and ephedrine are contraindicated and will worsen the dynamic obstruction.

References:
1. Montzingo CR, Shillcutt S. Cardiac anesthesia. In: Barash PG, Cullen BF, Stoelting RK, et al, eds. *Clinical Anesthesia Fundamentals*. Philadelphia: Wolters Kluwer Health; 2015:669-686.
2. Poliac LC, Barron ME, Maron BJ. Hypertrophic cardiomyopathy. *Anesthesiology*. 2006;104:183-192.

27. Correct answer: B

HCM is a genetic cardiac disorder, which is the most common cause of sudden cardiac death in the young and a significant comorbidity at any age. Patients with HCM are at risk for both lethal arrhythmias and hypertrophy of the interventricular septum, leading to dynamic LVOT obstruction.

LVOT obstruction in HCM is characteristically dynamic, so most patients do not demonstrate obstruction under resting conditions, yet are still at risk for obstruction when both preload and afterload drop when under an anesthetic (answer choice A).

Negative inotropic drugs, such as esmolol or metoprolol, are useful perioperatively in mitigating sympathetic stimulation and reducing the potential for dynamic obstruction (answer choice B).

Both hypovolemia and hypervolemia may be poorly tolerated in patients with HCM; however, it is hypovolemia that can be especially devastating because the LV cavity can be effectively obliterated with decreased preload and worsen LVOT obstruction (answer choice C).

Even in the absence of septal hypertrophy, patients with HCM are still at risk for arrhythmia (answer choice D) and furthermore may suffer sudden cardiac death with or without evidence of LV hypertrophy on echocardiography.

References:
1. Montzingo CR, Shillcutt S. Cardiac anesthesia. In: Barash PG, Cullen BF, Stoelting RK, et al, eds. *Clinical Anesthesia Fundamentals*. Philadelphia: Wolters Kluwer Health; 2015:669-686.
2. Poliac LC, Barron ME, Maron BJ. Hypertrophic cardiomyopathy. *Anesthesiology*. 2006;104:183-192.

28. **Correct answer: C**

"Flash pulmonary edema" is a general clinical term used to describe an acute and severe manifestation of acute decompensated heart failure, wherein there is a rapid accumulation of fluid within the lung's interstitial and alveolar spaces, as a result of acutely elevated cardiac filling pressures. The pathophysiology of flash pulmonary edema involves abnormal vasoconstriction and endothelial dysfunction because of sympathetic activation, renin-angiotensin-aldosterone activation, and impaired nitric oxide production. It is associated with renal artery stenosis. The mainstay of treatment is a loop diuretic, such as furosemide, as this group of diuretics also possesses potent antivasoconstrictor effects.

Given the acute onset of pulmonary edema in the setting of severe hypertension, the most likely diagnosis here is flash pulmonary edema. Volume overload would more likely have developed gradually over the course of the anesthetic, assuming fluids were given throughout. As the patient was still intubated, negative pressure pulmonary edema, which develops due to negative pressure against a closed glottis, is unlikely. Finally, there is no mention of transfusion to suggest transfusion-associated circulatory overload.

Reference:

1. Rimoldi SF, Yuzefpolskaya M, Allemann Y, Messerli F. Flash pulmonary edema. *Prog Cardiovasc Dis.* 2009;52(3):249-259.

29. **Correct answer: A**

LV hypokinesis with apical ballooning is pathognomonic for Tako-tsubo cardiomyopathy. This condition is a reversible cardiomyopathy, often triggered by an acute emotional trigger, but can also occur after an acute medical illness or surgery. Postmenopausal women are disproportionately affected and often lack coronary artery disease upon diagnostic catheterization. ECG changes are common (perhaps >90%), particularly ST elevation in the precordial leads; however, the magnitude of ST elevation is generally less than with an ST elevation MI in the distribution of the left anterior descending artery. LV dysfunction tends to resolve over a course of 1-3 months. Recurrence is uncommon, affecting 2%-10% of patients diagnosed with Tako-tsubo cardiomyopathy.

References:

1. Sharkey SW, Windenburg DC, Lesser JR, et al. Natural history and expansive clinical profile of stress (Tako-Tsubo) cardiomyopathy. *JACC.* 2010;55(4):333-341.
2. Bybee KA, Prasad A. Stress-related cardiomyopathy syndromes. *Circulation.* 2008;118:397-409.

30. **Correct answer: C**

This patient shows signs of diastolic dysfunction and fluid overload following a prolonged surgical case with administration of large amounts of IV fluids. Major risk factors for diastolic dysfunction include age, hypertension, diabetes mellitus, and LV hypertrophy. The appropriate next step would be to treat the fluid overload with a loop diuretic. It would not be appropriate to extubate a patient who shows signs of heart failure despite optimal ventilation. There are no signs of pulmonary hypertension or right ventricular failure, so inhaled nitric oxide would not be an appropriate treatment. Although keeping the patient intubated and admitting the patient to the SICU might also be appropriate, the most important immediate step is to treat the fluid overload.

Reference:

1. Jeong EM, Dudley SC. Diastolic dysfunction: potential new diagnostics and therapies. *Circ J.* 2015;79(3):470-477.

31. **Correct answer: B**

Cardiac tamponade is a life-threatening condition that develops when the pressure of the pericardial fluid exceeds that of the central venous pressure, leading to jugular venous distension, visceral organ engorgement, edema, and elevated pulmonary venous pressure that leads to dyspnea. Cardiac tamponade may develop acutely or chronically, which influences the clinical presentation. Rapid accumulation will cause hypotension because of the heart's inability to fill, while chronic cardiac tamponade allows the patient to drink enough liquid to keep the central venous pressure above that of the rising pericardial fluid pressure. Therefore, edema is more prominent with a slow development of tamponade.

Reference:

1. Schiavone WA. Cardiac tamponade: 12 pearls in diagnosis and management. *Cleve Clin J Med.* 2013;80(2):109-116.

32. Correct answer: C

Sudden, painful onset of cardiac tamponade because of cardiac or aortic rupture is an indication for surgical treatment. These may occur due to aortic dissection, recent MI, or iatrogenically following any number of interventional cardiac procedures. Often, the pressure that has built up in the pericardium is opposing further bleeding; a needle decompression will permit bleeding to recur, which may be life-threatening. Thus, a free wall rupture in the setting of recent MI would be an indication for surgery. Less acute development of tamponade is associated with medical causes, such as infectious disease, metastatic cancer, connective tissue disease, endocrine disease, or drug side effects. If the patient is hemodynamically stable, pericardiocentesis is not an emergency for tamponade associated with medical causes.

Reference:
1. Schiavone WA. Cardiac tamponade: 12 pearls in diagnosis and management. *Cleve Clin J Med.* 2013;80(2):109-116.

33. Correct answer: A

Pulsus paradoxus refers to an inspiratory fall in the systolic blood pressure of greater than 10 mm Hg. In cardiac tamponade, the pericardial fluid pressure exceeds the central venous pressure, so passive filling of the right atrium from the SVC and IVC does not occur in the absence of variations of intrathoracic pressure with respiration. During inspiration, the intrathoracic pressure drops, drawing blood from the right ventricle into the pulmonary vasculature and thus from the SVC and IVC into the right atrium. Additionally, the negative intrathoracic pressure prevents blood from within the pulmonary veins from returning to the left side of the heart. The interventricular septum bows from the right to the underfilled LV, the stroke volume drops, and systolic blood pressure is reduced.

PPV removes the negative intrathoracic pressure that occurs in spontaneous inspiration from the respiratory cycle, so pulsus paradoxus no longer occurs. Indeed, with the initiation of PPV, there may be no filling of the right side of the heart, resulting in hemodynamic collapse.

The other answer choices (mucous plug, stridor, and COPD) are all causes of increased negative inspiratory pressure and may cause pulsus paradoxus in the absence of cardiac tamponade.

Reference:
1. Schiavone WA. Cardiac tamponade: 12 pearls in diagnosis and management. *Cleve Clin J Med.* 2013;80(2):109-116.

34. Correct answer: D

CP is a form of diastolic dysfunction because of a poorly compliant pericardium. Although tuberculous pericarditis was once the most common cause of CP, this cause is now rare in the United States. The 2 most common causes currently are idiopathic and postcardiac surgical. Other causes include rheumatologic, postradiation, malignancy, and trauma. Given the preceding history of cardiac surgery, this patient's most likely cause is postsurgical. CP presents, on average, 2 years after cardiac surgery, and it affects 0.2%-0.4% of patients.

Reference:
1. Miranda WR, Oh JK. Constrictive pericarditis: a practical clinical approach. *Prog Cardiovasc Dis.* 2017;59(4):369-379.

35. Correct answer: C

RCM may mimic the presentation of CP, but several specific echocardiographic findings will help distinguish the 2 clinical entities:
- RCM represents restriction because of the myocardium itself. On echo, RCM manifests with biatrial enlargement, moderate or severe pulmonary hypertension, and preserved systolic function.
- Hepatic vein Doppler shows inspiratory flow reversal with RCM versus expiratory flow reversal with CP.
- RCM patients will have decreased medial mitral annulus velocity (e') because of their cardiomyopathy, whereas in CP, tissue Doppler of the medial mitral annulus typically reveals elevated early diastolic velocities.
- RCM will have ventricular concordance, whereas in CP, patients will have respirophasic septal shift because of increased ventricular interdependence.

Answer choices A, B, and D are therefore more characteristic of CP than of RCM.

Reference:
1. Miranda WR, Oh JK. Constrictive pericarditis: a practical clinical approach. *Prog Cardiovasc Dis.* 2017;59(4):369-379.

36. Correct answer: D

VTE is one of the leading causes of perioperative morbidity and mortality and one of the most preventable surgical and anesthetic complications. Several mechanical and pharmacologic interventions have been recommended for VTE prophylaxis.

Anesthetic technique may also effect VTE risk. Placement of neuraxial anesthetic before surgical incision reduces the perioperative stress response and decreases cytokine release, as well as improves total venous blood flow (answer choice D).

In a recent meta-analysis, novel oral anticoagulants were found to lower VTE risk compared with enoxaparin 40 mg daily but with an *increased* risk of postoperative bleeding (answer choice A).

Postpartum status and major trauma are both major risk factors for VTE, but postpartum status carries a higher relative risk, 20 versus 13 (answer choice B).

Aspirin is thought to carry less bleeding and infectious risk compared with heparin or warfarin, and when used with mechanical prophylaxis, aspirin may be as effective in preventing VTE. However, the prophylactic effect of aspirin is the same with or without other pharmacologic methods, ie, its effects are *neither* additive nor synergistic (answer choice C).

Reference:
1. Gordon RJ, Lombard FW. Perioperative venous thromboembolism: a review. *Anesth Analg.* 2017;125(2):403-412.

37. Correct answer: C

Both the perioperative period and the presence of an underlying malignancy place patients at a high risk for VTE. The American College of Chest Surgeons recommends that patients at high risk for VTE undergoing abdominal or pelvic surgery for cancer receive extended duration of postoperative, pharmacologic prophylaxis for 4 weeks with low-molecular-weight heparin.

Reference:
1. Gould MK, Garcia DA, Wren SM, et al. Prevention of VTE in nonorthopedic surgical patients antithrombotic therapy and prevention of thrombosis, 9th ed: American College of Chest Physicians Evidence-Based Clinical Practice Guidelines. *Chest.* 2012;141(2):e227S-e277S.

38. Correct answer: A

Pulmonary embolus, whether from thromboembolic phenomena, air, or fat, causes an increase in dead space because there is a portion of the lung that continues to be ventilated but is no longer perfused because of the vascular occlusion. This results in V/Q mismatching but does not increase shunt. The pulmonary vascular resistance is increased because there is a reduced cross-sectional area through which the pulmonary blood flow passes. Occlusion of >50% of the pulmonary circulation is generally required in otherwise healthy patients before sustained pulmonary hypertension develops. Localized bronchoconstriction, not bronchodilation, occurs as a result of local inflammation. This further increases V/Q mismatch.

Reference:
1. Butterworth JF, Mackey DC, Wasnick JD, eds. Anesthesia for patients with respiratory disease. In: *Clinical Anesthesiology.* 5th ed. New York: McGraw-Hill Education; 2013:527-544.

39. Correct answer: D

The most common acid-base disturbance in acute pulmonary embolism is a respiratory alkalosis with mild hypoxemia because of hyperventilation with a small decrease in gas exchange. Acutely, renal compensation will not yet be active, so bicarbonate remains normal. The blood gas analysis that is most consistent with these findings is answer choice D.

Reference:
1. Butterworth JF, Mackey DC, Wasnick JD, eds. Anesthesia for patients with respiratory disease. In: *Clinical Anesthesiology.* 5th ed. New York: McGraw-Hill Education; 2013:527-544.

40. Correct answer: C

In acute pulmonary embolus (PE), the ECG may show a number of abnormalities. The most common finding is sinus tachycardia, seen in 67% of patients with an acute PE who survive compared with 77%

of patients with an acute PE who do not survive. Other findings of acute cor pulmonale are less common and include complete or incomplete right bundle branch block, right-axis deviation, tall peaked T waves, and peripheral low voltage.

References:
1. Geibel A, Zehender M, Kasper W, et al. Prognostic value of the ECG on admission in patients with acute major pulmonary embolism. *Eur Respir J.* 2005;25:843-848.
2. Butterworth JF, Mackey DC, Wasnick JD, eds. Anesthesia for patients with respiratory disease. In: *Clinical Anesthesiology.* 5th ed. New York: McGraw-Hill Education; 2013:527-544.

41. Correct answer: D

Ideally, patients should only undergo elective surgery when normotensive. Most clinicians continue antihypertensives up until the day of surgery, with the exception of diuretics and angiotensin-converting enzyme inhibitors (ACEis)/angiotensin receptor antagonists, yet many patients still present with preoperative hypertension. Although there are no clear guidelines on what degree of hypertension should prompt case delay or cancellation, it is very reasonable to treat preoperative anxiety and reassess. It is generally agreed that a patient with a blood pressure <180/110 may proceed with surgery. Moreover, although not usually urgent or emergent, cancer surgery should proceed as soon as possible to minimize the risk of progression.

References:
1. Butterworth JF, Mackey DC, Wasnick JD, eds. Anesthesia for patients with cardiovascular disease. In: *Morgan and Mikhail's Clinical Anesthesiology.* 5th ed. New York: McGraw-Hill Education; 2013:375-434.
2. Olson RP, Rawlings R. Evaluation of the patient with cardiovascular disease. In: Longnecker DE, Brown DL, Newman MK, Zapol WM, eds. *Anesthesiology.* 2nd ed. New York; 2012:95-118.

42. Correct answer: C

Essential, or idiopathic, hypertension is the most common cause of hypertension and accounts for 80%-95% of all cases. Essential hypertension may occur secondary to elevations of cardiac output, SVR, or both. Over time, cardiac output returns to normal, whereas SVR is increased. The result of this chronically increased afterload is *concentric* (not eccentric) hypertrophy, accompanied by *diastolic* dysfunction. With chronically elevated blood pressures, the cerebral autoregulation curve shifts to the right, maintaining normal cerebral blood flow with mean arterial pressures as high as 110-180 mm Hg. Thus, it is imperative to maintain perioperative blood pressure near a patient's baseline.

Reference:
1. Butterworth JF, Mackey DC, Wasnick JD, eds. Anesthesia for patients with cardiovascular disease. In: *Morgan and Mikhail's Clinical Anesthesiology.* 5th ed. New York: McGraw-Hill Education; 2013:375-434.

43. Correct answer: A

Although it is optimal for a patient with hypertension to arrive for surgery with adequate blood pressure control, it is important to consider intraoperative blood pressure management as well. Several drugs, including β-blockers (eg, labetalol, metoprolol) and clonidine, an α_2-agonist, can have reflex tachycardia upon abrupt discontinuation and should thus be continued perioperatively. Calcium channel blockers are also continued perioperatively. Many studies have shown an association between ACEis and angiotensin receptor blockers (ARBs) and intraoperative hypertension, and it is known that angiotensin is important in maintaining perfusion during volume-depleted states. Thus, it is recommended to discontinue ACEis and ARBs 12-24 hours preoperatively. Diuretics are generally handled on a case-by-case basis; although it is important to avoid hypovolemia preoperatively, they should be continued in patients whose heart failure optimization is tenuous.

Reference:
1. Olson RP, Rawlings R. Evaluation of the patient with cardiovascular disease. In: Longnecker DE, Brown DL, Newman MK, Zapol WM, eds. *Anesthesiology.* 2nd ed. New York; 2012:95-118.

44. Correct answer: C

Initiation of β-blockers is indicated in patients with CAD or 2 or more cardiac risk factors undergoing vascular or intermediate-risk surgical procedures. Thus, the patient described in answer choice C would benefit from new initiation of a β-blocker. Answer choice A describes a patient with poorly controlled hypertension undergoing a low-risk surgery, so new initiation of a β-blocker should be deferred to her primary care physician should she not be able to achieve control with titration of her current medications. The patient in answer choice B has only 1 risk factor (smoking), and although the patient in answer choice D has 2 risk factors, she is undergoing low-risk surgery and it is urgent, so there is not time to titrate a β-blocker preoperatively.

References:
1. Olson RP, Rawlings R. Evaluation of the patient with cardiovascular disease. In: Longnecker DE, Brown DL, Newman MK, Zapol WM, eds. *Anesthesiology*. 2nd ed. New York; 2012:95-118.
2. Fleisher LA, Fleischmann KE, Auerbach AD, et al. 2014 ACC/AHA guideline on perioperative cardiovascular evaluation and management of patients undergoing noncardiac surgery: a report of the American College of Cardiology/American Heart Association Task Force on Practice Guidelines. *J Am Coll Cardiol*. 2014;64(22):e77-e137.

45. Correct answer: D

ACEis and ARBs block the renin-angiotensin-aldosterone system, which is responsible for release of antidiuretic hormone or vasopressin. Thus, patients on ACEis and ARBs are in a relatively vasopressin-depleted state, which may be refractory to catecholamines. In these cases, vasopressin is the treatment of choice to treat refractory intraoperative hypotension.

Reference:
1. Olson RP, Rawlings R. Evaluation of the patient with cardiovascular disease. In: Longnecker DE, Brown DL, Newman MK, Zapol WM, eds. *Anesthesiology*. 2nd ed. New York; 2012:95-118.

46. Correct answer: B

Although an awake patient with local anesthesia is the true gold standard for detecting clinically important cerebral ischemia during CEA, general anesthesia is widely used. It is obviously of utmost importance to monitor for signs and symptoms of ischemia during the period of carotid cross-clamping and often influences changes in hemodynamic management or placement of a carotid shunt to minimize ischemia. Monitoring can be accomplished through several modalities, either alone or in combination.

EEG is considered the gold standard for ischemia *while under general anesthesia*. In a study, EEG identified 99.92% of patients who may undergo CEA without a shunt. However, surface EEG monitors only cortical activity and is less reliable for subcortical structures. Combined EEG and SSEP may perform even better because it will monitor both cortical and subcortical tracts.

Other modalities include SSEP alone, which is less sensitive, because it only monitors sensory pathways. TCD is valuable in that it may detect emboli during dissection, shunting, and unclamping and postoperatively, which is the most common source of CVA surrounding CEA. However, technical difficulties make TCD difficult to interpret in 15%-20% of cases, and the size and location can make its use challenging for both surgeons and anesthesiologists. Near-infrared spectroscopy is simple and noninvasive; however, it measures only venous oxygen saturation and has shown to have lower sensitivity and specificity compared with EEG.

Reference:
1. Lemm J, Nicoara A, Swaminathan M. Anesthesia for major vascular surgery. In: Longnecker DE, Newman MF, Zapol WM, Mackey SC, Sandberg WS, eds. *Anesthesiology*. New York: McGraw-Hill; 2017:939-961.

47. Correct answer: A

The anterior two-thirds of the spinal cord are supplied by the single anterior spinal artery, which is supplied by the spinal branches of the vertebral arteries, as well as radicular arteries from the aorta. The most developed of these is known as the artery of Adamkiewicz, or the arteria radicularis magna, and most commonly arises from T9 to T12. Because of tenuous collateral blood flow to this segment of the spinal cord, it is at risk for ischemic injury during aortic occlusion or during periods of hypotension.

In 2010, the ASA, together with the ACCF, AHA, AATS, ACR, SCA, SCAI, SIR, STS, and SVM issued guidelines on the care of patients with thoracic aortic disease. Their recommendations include the following:

Class I

Cerebrospinal fluid drainage is recommended as a spinal cord protective strategy in open and endovascular thoracic aortic repair for patients at high risk of spinal cord ischemic injury.

Class IIa

Spinal cord perfusion pressure optimization using techniques, such as proximal aortic pressure maintenance and distal aortic perfusion, is reasonable as an integral part of the surgical, anesthetic, and perfusion strategy in open and endovascular thoracic aortic repair for patients at high risk of spinal cord ischemic injury. Institutional experience is an important factor in selecting these techniques.

Moderate systemic hypothermia is reasonable for protection of the spinal cord during open repairs of the descending thoracic aorta.

Class IIb

Adjunctive techniques to increase the tolerance of the spinal cord to impaired perfusion may be considered during open and endovascular thoracic aortic repair for patients at high risk of spinal cord injury. These include distal perfusion, epidural irrigation with hypothermic solutions, high-dose systemic glucocorticoids, osmotic diuresis with mannitol, intrathecal papaverine, and cellular metabolic suppression with anesthetic agents.

Neurophysiological monitoring of the spinal cord (SSEPs or motor evoked potentials) may be considered as a strategy to detect spinal cord ischemia and to guide reimplantation of intercostal arteries and/or hemodynamic optimization to prevent or treat spinal cord ischemia.

References:

1. Lemm J, Nicoara A, Swaminathan M. Anesthesia for major vascular surgery. In: Longnecker DE, Brown DL, Newman MK, Zapol WM, eds. *Anesthesiology*. 3rd ed. New York: McGraw-Hill; 2017:939-961.
2. Hiratzka LF, Bakris GL, Beckman JA, et al. 2010 ACCF/AHA/AATS/ACR/ASA/SCA/SCAI/SIR/STS/SVM guidelines for the diagnosis and management of patients with thoracic aortic disease: executive summary: a report of the American College of Cardiology Foundation/American Heart Association Task Force on Practice Guidelines, American Association for Thoracic Surgery, American College of Radiology, American Stroke Association, Society of Cardiovascular Anesthesiologists, Society for Cardiovascular Angiography and Interventions, Society of Interventional Radiology, Society of Thoracic Surgeons, and Society for Vascular Medicine. *Anesth Analg*. 2010;111(2):279-315.

48. **Correct answer: C**

Release of the aortic cross-clamp causes a number of hemodynamic and metabolic changes, which will vary depending on the level of clamping, the duration of clamping, the use of shunts or bypasses, and the administration of fluids and medications during and following clamping.

With perfusion of the lower extremities and other below-clamp tissues, total body oxygen consumption increases substantially as the hemoglobin, myoglobin, and cytochromes in the distal tissues are "reloaded." The result is a greater oxygen extraction and thus a lower $S_{MV}O_2$.

Venous return decreases for 2 reasons: (1) there is a distal shift of blood volume as the distal tissues are reperfused and (2) there is loss of intravascular fluid because of increased vascular permeability from inflammatory mediator release.

Cardiac output is decreased as a consequence of decreased venous return, in addition to impaired cardiac contractility from inflammatory mediator release.

$Paco_2$ rises with reperfusion because of circulation of blood from the distal tissues, which are rich with end products of aerobic metabolism.

Reference:

1. Lemm J, Nicoara A, Swaminathan M. Anesthesia for major vascular surgery. In: Longnecker DE, Newman MF, Zapol WM, Mackey SC, Sandberg WS, eds. *Anesthesiology*. New York: McGraw-Hill; 2017:939-961.

49. **Correct answer: D**

EVAR is an alternative to open abdominal aortic aneurysm repair, and it has the advantages of less hemodynamic lability because of aortic clamping and unclamping, decreased metabolic stress, improved acid-base status, and less catecholamine changes. A number of studies have compared outcomes for open repair versus EVAR. The EVAR 1 trial showed lower 30-day mortality with EVAR but higher costs and higher rates of graft-related complications and reinterventions. Similarly, the DREAM trial showed lower operative mortality with EVAR, with no survival difference at 2 years or 6 years. DREAM also showed a significantly higher rate of secondary interventions.

References:

1. Lemm J, Nicoara A, Swaminathan M. Anesthesia for major vascular surgery. In: Longnecker DE, Newman MF, Zapol WM, Mackey SC, Sandberg WS, eds. *Anesthesiology*. New York: McGraw-Hill; 2017:939-961.
2. Greenhalgh RM, Brown LC, Powell JT, et al. Endovascular versus open repair of abdominal aortic aneurysm. *N Engl J Med*. 2010;362(20):1863-1871.
3. Prinssen M, Verhoeven EL, Buth J, et al. A randomized trial comparing conventional and endovascular repair of abdominal aortic aneurysms. *N Engl J Med*. 2004;351(16):1607-1618.

50. **Correct answer: D**

Epidural anesthesia for lower-extremity revascularization procedures offers a number of benefits, including lower risk of postoperative pulmonary complications and a reduced surgical stress response, evidenced by attenuation of the plasminogen activator inhibitor-1 rise. This medically complex patient would likely benefit from such an anesthetic, yet has a number of comorbidities, which may indicate antiplatelet agents or anticoagulation.

Clopidogrel should be held for 7-days before epidural placement; if it has been held for 5-7 days, normal platelet function should be documented before proceeding.

Although risk of epidural hematoma may be increased in patients with a bloody neuraxial placement, there are no data to suggest that the case must be mandatorily canceled. Rather, a discussion with the anesthesiologist and surgeon should inform whether to proceed.

Patients receiving heparin for more than 4 days should have platelet levels checked before catheter removal because they are at risk for heparin-induced thrombocytopenia. Similarly, platelet levels should be checked in patients known to be thrombocytopenic or experiencing a fall in platelets.

Unfractionated heparin should not be administered for 1 hour following neuraxial placement. An epidural catheter may be removed up until 1 hour before a dose or at least 2-4 hours after a dose, once normalization of the PTT is documented.

References:

1. Lemm J, Nicoara A, Swaminathan M. Anesthesia for major vascular surgery. In: Longnecker DE, Newman MF, Zapol WM, Mackey SC, Sandberg WS, eds. *Anesthesiology*. New York: McGraw-Hill; 2017:939-961.
2. Horlocker TT, Wedel DJ, Rowlingson JC, et al. Regional anesthesia in the patient receiving antithrombotic or thrombolytic therapy: American Society of Regional Anesthesia and Pain Medicine evidence-based guidelines (third edition). *Reg Anesth Pain Med*. 2010;35(1):64-101.

17

THORACIC ANESTHESIA

Jerome Crowley

1. **To decrease the risk of postoperative pulmonary complications associated with smoking, when should the patient stop smoking?**

   A. 48 hours
   B. 1-2 weeks
   C. 2-4 weeks
   D. 4-6 weeks

2. **Which one of the following is a risk for acute lung injury (ALI) postoperatively?**

   A. Active ethanol abuse
   B. History of myocardial infarction
   C. History of peripheral vascular disease
   D. History of stroke

3. **A 67-year-old woman presents for right lower lobe lobectomy. Which of the following results obtained via spirometry testing would place her at an increased risk for postoperative complications?**

   A. Forced expiratory volume in 1 second (FEV1) of 1300 mL
   B. Predicted postoperative FEV1 70% of normal
   C. Maximum voluntary ventilation of 62% or predicted value
   D. Reserve volume (RV)/total lung capacity (TLC) of 57%

4. **Which of the following symptoms is most consistent with theophylline toxicity?**

   A. Tinnitus
   B. Itching
   C. Tachyarrhythmia
   D. Heart block

5. **Which of the following patients would have a low probability of developing postoperative respiratory complications?**

   A. A 56-year-old man whose oxygen saturation drops 6% during exercise
   B. A 58-year-old woman who has a 6-minute walk distance of 610 m
   C. A 54-year-old woman who can climb 2 flights of stairs
   D. A 55-year-old man with a Vo_2 max of 12 mL/kg/min

6. **Which of the following is a predictor of desaturation during one-lung ventilation (OLV)?**

   A. Left-sided thoracotomy
   B. Lateral position during surgery
   C. Normal preoperative spirometry
   D. Balanced perfusion on ventilation/perfusion (V/Q) imaging

7. **Which patient is most likely to desaturate during OLV?**

   A. A 68-year-old woman with a history of moderate chronic obstructive pulmonary disease (COPD) with a Pao_2: 481 mm Hg on 100% O_2 before OLV
   B. A 72-year-old man undergoing thoracotomy for left lower lobe adenocarcinoma
   C. A 59-year-old man undergoing video-assisted thoracoscopic (VAT) resection of left upper lobe adenocarcinoma
   D. A 61-year-old man with a Pao_2 of 187 mm Hg on 100% O_2 before OLV

8. **For which of the following surgical procedures is a right-sided double-lumen tube (DLT) most likely indicated?**

   A. Left lower lobectomy
   B. Bilateral lung transplantation
   C. Open thoracic aortic aneurysm repair
   D. Left sleeve resection with involvement of left mainstem

9. **During a routine right thoracotomy for tumor resection with peak airway pressures in the mid 40s cm H_2O during OLV, the patient suddenly becomes hypotensive and hypoxic. End-tidal carbon dioxide drops precipitously. Which of the following is the next best step in management?**

   A. Bronchoscopy
   B. Needle decompression of dependent lung
   C. Resumption of two-lung ventilation
   D. Application of continuous positive airway pressure (CPAP) to operative lung

10. **Which of the following is an absolute indication for OLV with a DLT as opposed to a bronchial blocker?**

    A. Need for independent lung ventilation in a patient with severe unilateral rib fractures
    B. Wedge resection
    C. Pneumonectomy
    D. Lobectomy

11. **During VAT wedge resection for a right lower lobe tumor with a bronchial blocker, the patient develops increased peak airway pressures, hypoxia, and a decreased end-tidal carbon dioxide. The surgeon reports good lung isolation in the field. Which of the following is the appropriate next step?**

    A. Fiberoptic evaluation of the bronchial blocker
    B. Deflation of the bronchial blocker and ventilation of both lungs
    C. Needle decompression of dependent lung
    D. Application of CPAP to operative lung

12. **During right middle lobe resection for adenocarcinoma, you notice that your patient appears to be developing a mild acidosis on arterial blood gas. pH is 7.22, lactic acid is mildly elevated, hemoglobin is 10.1, urine output has been 0.5 mL/kg/h for the past 3 hours, and estimated blood loss is 150 mL. Which of the following is the best next step?**

    A. Start low-dose inotropes.
    B. Give a fluid bolus of 10 mL/kg.
    C. Transfuse 1 unit of packed red blood cells.
    D. Increase minute ventilation to correct the acidosis.

13. **Which level of oxygen saturation (Spo$_2$) is acceptable for a patient undergoing OLV?**

    A. 92%
    B. 90%
    C. 80%
    D. 76%

14. **Which gas mixture is associated with the highest incidence of postthoracotomy atelectasis?**

    A. 98% O$_2$/2% sevoflurane
    B. 60% O$_2$/33% air/7% desflurane
    C. 50% O$_2$/49% air/2% isoflurane
    D. 28% O$_2$/70% nitrous oxide/2% sevoflurane

15. **A patient who has a history of bleomycin chemotherapy for testicular cancer is undergoing a left VAT surgery for metastasis. The patient begins to desaturate to 88% with stable hemodynamics. Which of the following is the most appropriate next step?**

    A. Attempt recruitment maneuver of dependent lung.
    B. Resume two-lung ventilation.
    C. Increase the fraction of inspired oxygen.
    D. Increase positive end-expiratory pressure (PEEP) of the dependent lung.

16. **A patient is undergoing surgery for correction of a bronchopleural fistula. A DLT has been placed without difficulty. During the procedure, the patient's oxygen saturation decreases to 85%. Which of the following is the most appropriate next step?**

    A. Apply CPAP to the operative lung.
    B. Increase the fraction of inspired oxygen.
    C. Fiberoptic confirmation of DLT placement.
    D. Resume two-lung ventilation.

17. **A patient is scheduled to undergo a bilateral thoracoscopic MAZE procedure for chronic atrial fibrillation. The procedure is to be performed in the supine position. Which of the following interventions will reduce the likelihood of desaturation during OLV?**

    A. Operating on the right side first
    B. Use of a total intravenous anesthetic
    C. Use of a right-sided DLT
    D. Use of a tidal volume of 10 mL/kg to maintain lung inflation

18. **A patient has persistent pain in the posterior and lateral aspects of the shoulder 10 days following thoracotomy. Which of the following positioning errors that can occur during the surgery is the most likely mechanism for this patient's pain?**

    A. Inadequate padding of the dependent chest wall
    B. Lateral flexion of the cervical spine
    C. Placement of the axillary roll in the axilla
    D. Oversupination of the suspended arm

19. **In which of the following patients would the administration of PEEP be expected to improve oxygenation during OLV?**

    A. A 68-year-old man with severe emphysema on tiotropium undergoing lobectomy
    B. A 34-year-old man with α1 antitrypsin deficiency undergoing wedge resection
    C. A 51-year-old woman with moderate COPD on pulmonary function tests (PFTs) undergoing pleurectomy for mesothelioma
    D. A 42-year-old woman with interstitial lung disease undergoing VAT wedge resection

20. A 70-kg, 1.8-m tall man is scheduled for open thoracotomy/sleeve resection for adenocarcinoma of the lung. Preoperative PFTs are within normal limits, and the patient denies any smoking history. A right-sided DLT is placed uneventfully after induction of anesthesia. Which of the following ventilation strategies is most appropriate?

    A. Volume control with a tidal volume of 700 mL, respiratory rate of 10, PEEP of 0
    B. Volume control with a tidal volume of 800 mL, respiratory rate of 8, PEEP of 5
    C. Volume control with a tidal volume of 450 mL, respiratory rate of 14, PEEP of 5
    D. Volume control with a tidal volume of 750 mL, respiratory rate of 12, PEEP of 8

21. A 61-year-old man with a history of COPD, 40-pack-year smoking history, and hypertension is undergoing right lower lobe resection for primary lung cancer. While under OLV, he is ventilated with the following settings: assist control/pressure control inspiratory pressure: 20 cm H_2O, PEEP: 5 cm H_2O, inspiratory time: 0.8 seconds, and inspired oxygen: 70%. During the return to two-lung ventilation, which of the following parameters needs to be monitored very closely for sudden changes?

    A. Peak airway pressure
    B. Systolic blood pressure variability
    C. Tidal volume
    D. Heart rate

22. A 47-year-old woman who is status post bilateral lung transplant is undergoing laparoscopic cholecystectomy. Which of the following is the benefit of pressure control ventilation in this patient?

    A. Reduced risk of lung injury from high airway pressures
    B. Better oxygenation
    C. Decreased risk of pulmonary edema
    D. Decreased risk of rejection

23. For which of the following patients might pressure control ventilation be a better ventilation strategy for OLV?

    A. A 67-year-old man having VAT bullae resection
    B. A 38-year-old man having VAT sympathectomy for hyperhidrosis
    C. A 71-year-old woman with coronary artery disease having thoracotomy for empyema decortication
    D. A 51-year-old woman undergoing thoracotomy for right lower lobe resection for adenocarcinoma

24. A 67-year-old woman with normal PFT (ideal body weight of 60 kg) is scheduled to undergo VAT lobectomy for adenocarcinoma. Which of the following ventilator settings is most optimal for lung ventilation in this patient?

    A. Tidal volume: 600 mL, PEEP: 0 cm H_2O, respiratory rate: 13 breaths per minute, Fio_2: 0.8
    B. Tidal volume: 350 mL, PEEP: 0 cm H_2O, respiratory rate: 12 breaths per minute, Fio_2: 0.8
    C. Tidal volume: 350 mL, PEEP: 5 cm H_2O, respiratory rate: 14 breaths per minute, Fio_2: 0.8
    D. Tidal volume: 600 mL, PEEP: 5 cm H_2O, respiratory rate: 11 breaths per minute, Fio_2: 0.8

25. A 28-year-old, 60-kg man with no significant medical history is undergoing VAT pleurodesis for spontaneous pneumothorax. While transitioning to OLV with a DLT, the peak airway pressure is noted to be 41 cm H_2O. Current ventilator settings are as follows: tidal volume: 600 mL, PEEP: 5 cm H_2O, respiratory rate: 14, Fio_2: 0.8. Bronchoscopy confirms proper tube position. Which of the following is the next most appropriate step?

    A. Decrease the PEEP from 5 cm H_2O to 0 cm H_2O.
    B. Increase the fraction of inspired oxygen to 100%.
    C. Decrease tidal volume.
    D. Increase the respiratory rate.

26. A 47-year-old woman is undergoing rigid bronchoscopy with jet ventilation. Which of the following most likely represents the best anesthetic choice?

    A. Inhaled anesthetic with sevoflurane.
    B. Intravenous anesthetic using only propofol.
    C. Intravenous anesthetic using propofol and remifentanil.
    D. Inhaled anesthetic with desflurane.

27. A 26-year-old man with no known medical history is status post an uneventful rigid bronchoscopy and recovering in the postanesthesia care unit when he begins to complain of pleuritic chest pain. Which of the following is the next best step in evaluation of this patient?

    A. Administration of an albuterol nebulizer
    B. Chest X-ray
    C. Electrocardiogram and cardiac enzymes
    D. Transthoracic echocardiogram

28. High-frequency jet ventilation provides which of the following benefits when compared with traditional mechanical ventilation?

    A. Decreased risk of pneumothorax
    B. Faster onset of inhaled anesthetic
    C. Decreased diaphragmatic movement
    D. Improved postoperative pain scores

29. Which of the following is the most efficient way to reduce the incidence of airway fires?

    A. Handheld jet ventilation
    B. Lowest inspired oxygen level tolerated by the patient
    C. Use of a total intravenous anesthetic
    D. Preoperative administration of bronchodilators

30. Which of the following is a drawback when utilizing jet ventilation?

    A. Inability to monitor oxygenation
    B. Difficulty in monitoring adequacy of ventilation
    C. Poor surgical access to the airway because of extra equipment
    D. Increased risk of airway fires during laser procedures

31. A patient is scheduled to undergo right upper lobectomy. What is the predicted postoperative forced expired volume in 1 second (FEV1)? Preoperative FEV1 is 80% of predicted.

    A. 69%
    B. 64%
    C. 59%
    D. 72%

32. During a double-lung transplant a patient has a saturation of 85% during OLV despite aggressive pulmonary toilet, 100% oxygen, and optimal recruitment maneuvers. Transesophageal echocardiography shows worsening right ventricular function, and pulmonary artery catheterization demonstrates decreasing pulmonary artery pressures and rising central venous pressures (CVPs). Which of the following is the next best step in management?

    A. CPAP to the operative lung
    B. Initiation of inotropes
    C. Immediate initiation of cardiopulmonary bypass or extracorporeal membrane oxygenation
    D. Diuresis to improve fluid status

33. **A patient presents for lobectomy for small cell lung cancer. He has a history of Lambert-Eaton syndrome. Which of the following symptoms would be expected on review of systems?**

    A. Weakness in the distal muscles that worsens throughout the day
    B. Improvement in muscle function with repeated use
    C. Urinary incontinence
    D. Delayed gastric emptying

34. **A patient is undergoing left sleeve lobectomy for adenocarcinoma which is subsequently causing significant narrowing of the left mainstem bronchus. Which of the following lung isolation devices is most appropriate?**

    A. Right-sided DLT
    B. Left-sided DLT
    C. EZ-Blocker
    D. Arndt bronchial blocker

35. **A patient post pneumonectomy is recovering in the surgical intensive care unit (ICU) when she suddenly develops hypotension and cardiovascular collapse. Pulmonary artery catheter demonstrates a pulmonary artery systolic pressure of 20 mm Hg (previously 42 mm Hg) and a CVP of 22 mm Hg (previously 8 mm Hg). Which of the following is the most likely cause of her acute event?**

    A. Volume overload
    B. Right ventricular failure
    C. Postpneumonectomy herniation syndrome
    D. Mucous plugging

36. **A 19-year-old man with no known medical history presents with a gunshot wound to the right chest. His vital signs are stable and he is brought to the operating room for repair of an open tibia fracture. After intubation and initiation of positive pressure ventilation, his blood pressure acutely drops and he loses his pulse. Which of the following is the next step in management?**

    A. Transcutaneous pacing
    B. Needle thoracostomy
    C. Chest X-ray
    D. Initiation of dopamine infusion

37. **A 68-year-old woman with a history of pulmonary embolism on therapeutic anticoagulation is admitted to the surgical ICU in profound shock. To guide management a pulmonary artery catheter is placed uneventfully. Four hours later you are called urgently to the bedside because the patient has had acutely worsening blood pressure and there is blood noted in the endotracheal tube. Which of the following is the next most appropriate step?**

    A. Chest tube placement
    B. Isolation of the bleeding lung and emergent transport to endovascular therapy
    C. Inflation of the pulmonary catheter balloon and advancement to the wedge position
    D. Emergent bedside thoracotomy

38. **A 47-year-old man who is status post left thoracotomy for esophageal rupture is doing well immediately postoperatively. On postoperative day 5 the patient is tolerating a regular diet when he develops progressive shortness of breath. Chest X-ray reveals a large left pleural effusion. A chest tube is placed, which drains white fluid. Which of the following is the most likely cause?**

    A. Chylothorax
    B. Esophageal perforation
    C. Empyema
    D. Reactive effusion from esophageal rupture

39. A patient with a large left upper lobe abscess is scheduled for thoracotomy and drainage. Which of the following is the optimal lung isolation system?

    A. Left-sided DLT
    B. EZ-Blocker
    C. Mainstem intubation with a single-lumen tube
    D. Arndt bronchial blocker

40. A patient is 6 days post right pneumonectomy for adenocarcinoma and is doing well on the ward. She develops progressive dyspnea and an increased oxygen requirement. Chest X-ray reveals a decreased fluid level on the right side. Which of the following is the most likely diagnosis?

    A. Mediastinal herniation
    B. Pneumonia
    C. Bronchopleural fistula
    D. Mucous plug

41. A 34-year-old, 140-kg, 160-cm woman is scheduled to undergo VAT resection of a hamartoma. Which of the following maneuvers is most effective at prolonging the time to desaturation in obese patients?

    A. Applying CPAP or PEEP during induction
    B. Applying cricoid pressure to reduce the chance of aspiration
    C. Using a video laryngoscope
    D. Using 50% Fio_2 during induction to prevent absorption atelectasis

42. A patient with severe idiopathic pulmonary fibrosis is being evaluated before undergoing elective surgery. Which of the following clinical findings reflects impaired oxygen diffusion?

    A. Elevated Pco_2 at rest
    B. Decreased Po_2 with exercise
    C. Chronic respiratory acidosis with renal compensation
    D. Improved symptoms with inhaled bronchodilators

43. A 76-year-old woman with a history of COPD presents for preoperative evaluation before shoulder surgery. Which of the following tests is best able to identify CO_2 retention?

    A. PFTs showing improvement in symptoms with bronchodilators
    B. PFTs showing a decreased diffusion capacity
    C. Arterial blood gas
    D. Exercise tolerance

44. A 68-year-old man with a history of severe COPD presents for urgent exploratory laparotomy for small bowel obstruction. A room air arterial blood gas reveals a Pao_2 of 51 mm Hg, and brief history reveals noncompliance with prescribed oxygen therapy. On induction of anesthesia, the CVP rises from 14 to 26 mm Hg, and the patient becomes progressively hypotensive. Airway pressures are normal, ECG shows sinus bradycardia, and oxygen saturation is >90%. Which of the following is the most likely mechanism of this patient's hypotension?

    A. Right ventricular dysfunction
    B. Tension pneumothorax
    C. Acute blood loss
    D. Severe bronchospasm

45. A 58-year-old woman with a 20-pack-year smoking history and severe obstructive lung disease on PFT is brought to the operating room for washout of an infected hip. She has been intubated in the ICU for several days and is on SIMV/PS with a set rate of 10 and a measured rate of 14. Because her end-tidal CO_2 is elevated, her set rate is increased to 24. She is no longer overbreathing the ventilator. Fifteen minutes later, the patient becomes acutely hypotensive, terminating into cardiac arrest. Which of the following interventions may have prevented the arrest?

   A. Decreasing the respiratory rate
   B. Increasing the PEEP
   C. Administering IV fluid bolus
   D. Initiating a vasopressin infusion

46. A 36-year-old man with severe scoliosis is scheduled to undergo operative repair. Which of the following best predicts postoperative ventilation need?

   A. A vital capacity <40% of normal
   B. A decreased DLCO
   C. A Cobb angle of 42°
   D. A lack of response to bronchodilators on PFT

47. A 48-year-old woman with small cell lung cancer presents for urgent angle incision and drainage after being bitten by a dog. In an abbreviated history, she describes increased fatigue in the mornings that improves as the day progresses. She denies any cardiac or neurologic history. Her preoperative coagulation panel, basic metabolic panel, and liver function panel are all normal. Before progression of her cancer, she had been very active. Her anesthetic is unremarkable with neuromuscular relaxation maintained with rocuronium. Despite appropriate reversal of neuromuscular blockade, she remains weak and requires postoperative mechanical ventilation. Which of the following is the most likely cause?

   A. Hypocalcemia
   B. Impaired acetylcholine release from nerve terminals
   C. Impaired pseudocholinesterase function
   D. Antibodies to acetylcholine receptors at the neuromuscular junction

48. A 27-year-old woman with a history of mild asthma is undergoing arthroscopic anterior cruciate ligament repair with a laryngeal mask airway. During incision, airway pressures increase significantly and bilateral wheezes are appreciated. Which of the following is the next step in management?

   A. Administer bolus propofol to deepen the anesthetic.
   B. Administer intravenous nitroglycerin.
   C. Increase the concentration of inhaled sevoflurane.
   D. Switch the patient to a volume-controlled mode of ventilation.

49. A 34-year-old woman with a history of chronic bronchiectasis is scheduled for partial lung resection for recurrent pneumonia. Which of the following is an important consideration for patients with chronically infected lung tissue?

   A. Preincision coverage with cefazolin
   B. Ensuring there is adequate lung isolation before positioning
   C. Place a thoracic epidural for pain control
   D. Use of high PEEP to recruit bronchiectatic lung

50. Which of the following is most concerning for vascular compression in a patient with a mediastinal mass?

   A. Supine presyncope
   B. Size of mass on chest X-ray
   C. Tachyarrhythmia
   D. Recent weight loss

Chapter 17 ■ Answers

1. Correct answer: D

Smoking is associated with significant perioperative complications, which include increased risks of infection, delayed wound healing, and increased pulmonary complications. Stopping smoking at least 4 weeks before surgery is associated with a decreased risk of pulmonary complications. It was previously thought that stopping smoking too close to surgery was associated with an increased risk of complications; however, the overall health benefits of quitting smoking are too great to ignore, and all patients should be counseled to stop smoking.

References:
1. Eisenkraft JB, Cohen E, Neustein SM. Anesthesia for thoracic surgery. In: Barash PG, Cullen BF, Stoelting RK, et al, eds. *Clinical Anesthesia*. 8th ed. Philadelphia: Lippincott; 2017:1030-1076.
2. Slinger PD, Campos JH. Anesthesia for thoracic surgery. In: Miller RD, Eriksson LI, Fleisher LA, et al, eds. *Miller's Anesthesia*. 8th ed. Philadelphia: Elsevier; 2015:1942-2006.

2. Correct answer: A

ALI is a serious postoperative concern in thoracic surgery. This can lead to prolonged mechanical ventilation, delayed time to discharge, and increased risk of infection. Perioperative risk factors include alcohol abuse. Patients with pneumonectomy are at higher risk than other thoracic surgery patients. Other factors include a positive fluid balance on postoperative day 1, poor preoperative lung function, and high ventilator pressures intraoperatively. The other comorbidities listed in the question may lead to complications but are not necessarily associated with ALI.

References:
1. Eisenkraft JB, Cohen E, Neustein SM. Anesthesia for thoracic surgery. In: Barash PG, Cullen BF, Stoelting RK, et al, eds. *Clinical Anesthesia*. 8th ed. Philadelphia: Lippincott; 2017:1030-1076.
2. Slinger PD, Campos JH. Anesthesia for thoracic surgery. In: Miller RD, Eriksson LI, Fleisher LA, et al, eds. *Miller's Anesthesia*. 8th ed. Philadelphia: Elsevier; 2015:1942-2006.

3. Correct answer: D

Preoperative spirometry is helpful in delineating the risk of thoracic surgery. Of particular note, the forced vital capacity, FEV1, maximum voluntary ventilation, and RV/TLC ratio correlate with postoperative outcomes. In particular, a FEV1 of <800 mL in a 70-kg patient, a maximum voluntary ventilation <50% of the predicted value, a predicted postoperative FEV1 <30% of normal, and a RV/TLC ratio of >50% are all associated with increased postoperative risk for lung resection procedures.

References:
1. Eisenkraft JB, Cohen E, Neustein SM. Anesthesia for thoracic surgery. In: Barash PG, Cullen BF, Stoelting RK, et al, eds. *Clinical Anesthesia*. 8th ed. Philadelphia: Lippincott; 2017:1030-1076.
2. Slinger PD, Campos JH. Anesthesia for thoracic surgery. In: Miller RD, Eriksson LI, Fleisher LA, et al, eds. *Miller's Anesthesia*. 8th ed. Philadelphia: Elsevier; 2015:1942-2006.

4. Correct answer: C

Theophylline is a methylated xanthine derivate that is used to treat difficult-to-control COPD and asthma via reducing bronchospasm in patients with reactive airway disease. Its use is limited because of the fact that it has very narrow therapeutic window and is often poorly tolerated. Of its myriad of side effects including nausea, insomnia, and dizziness, most relevant to anesthesia is its predisposition of the heart to tachyarrhythmia. It is primarily metabolized by the liver; therefore, extra concern needs to be given in patients with liver injury.

References:
1. Eisenkraft JB, Cohen E, Neustein SM. Anesthesia for thoracic surgery. In: Barash PG, Cullen BF, Stoelting RK, et al, eds. *Clinical Anesthesia*. 8th ed. Philadelphia: Lippincott; 2017:1030-1076.
2. Slinger PD, Campos JH. Anesthesia for thoracic surgery. In: Miller RD, Eriksson LI, Fleisher LA, et al, eds. *Miller's Anesthesia*. 8th ed. Philadelphia: Elsevier; 2015:1942-2006.

5. **Correct answer: B**

Preoperative functional status can be helpful in predicting patients who are likely to have postoperative pulmonary complications. It is important to note that no quality-of-life measure correlates well with quantitative measurements done via spirometry and patients undergoing elective thoracic surgery should all undergo spirometric testing. Patients who can climb 3 or more flights of stairs are at reduced risk of complications. The Vo_2 max correlates well with risk of complications; patients having a Vo_2 max > 20 mL/kg/min have a very low risk of postoperative complications. A patient's Vo_2 max can be estimated by dividing his/her 6-minute walk test distance by 30. In this case 610/30 is greater than 20 implying that the patient would be at low risk for postoperative pulmonary complications. Finally, patients with a decrease in arterial oxygen saturation of >4% during exercise are at increased risk of postoperative pulmonary complications.

References:
1. Eisenkraft JB, Cohen E, Neustein SM. Anesthesia for thoracic surgery. In: Barash PG, Cullen BF, Stoelting RK, et al, eds. *Clinical Anesthesia*. 8th ed. Philadelphia: Lippincott; 2017:1030-1076.
2. Slinger PD, Campos JH. Anesthesia for thoracic surgery. In: Miller RD, Eriksson LI, Fleisher LA, et al, eds. *Miller's Anesthesia*. 8th ed. Philadelphia: Elsevier; 2015:1942-2006.

6. **Correct answer: C**

It is usually possible to predict patients who will be at **high risk for desaturation during OLV**. Risk factors include a high percentage of ventilation or perfusion to the operative lung on V/Q scan, right-side lung surgery, poor arterial oxygen concentration during two-lung ventilation, supine position, and normal preoperative spirometry. A high percentage of ventilation or perfusion to the operative lung implies poorly functioning or poorly perfused nonoperative lung, which may not be able to generate adequate oxygen exchange during OLV. In patients with normal lung parenchyma, left-sided surgery is better tolerated by the simple fact that the right lung is larger and so isolated right lung ventilation preserves more functional lung than isolated left lung ventilation. Poor oxygenation during two-lung ventilation is a risk factor for desaturation because it may represent significant underlying lung pathology such as acute respiratory distress syndrome; however, it is important to note that if the poor oxygenation is due primarily to poor function of the operative lung, then oxygenation may improve with lung isolation. Supine position is associated with an increased risk of desaturation because the ventilated lung does not benefit from improved V/Q matching owing to gravity that is present in the lateral position. Finally, normal preoperative spirometry in patients with obstructive lung disease denotes higher risk of desaturation during OLV.

References:
1. Eisenkraft JB, Cohen E, Neustein SM. Anesthesia for thoracic surgery. In: Barash PG, Cullen BF, Stoelting RK, et al, eds. *Clinical Anesthesia*. 8th ed. Philadelphia: Lippincott; 2017:1030-1076.
2. Slinger PD, Campos JH. Anesthesia for thoracic surgery. In: Miller RD, Eriksson LI, Fleisher LA, et al, eds. *Miller's Anesthesia*. 8th ed. Philadelphia: Elsevier; 2015:1942-2006.

7. **Correct answer: D**

Poor oxygenation during two-lung ventilation is the strongest predictor of desaturation during OLV. The patient in choice D is showing a significantly decreased Pao_2/Fio_2 ratio implying the potential for significant lung parenchymal disease. Choices B and C are for surgery on the left lung, which is associated with lower risk of desaturation than surgery on the right lung. Using video-assisted techniques versus open techniques does not directly correlate with risk of desaturation, although it should be noted that VAT surgical techniques usually are more rigorous in their requirement of complete lung deflation and may limit certain rescue techniques if hypoxemia develops. Choice A involves a patient with intact oxygenation on two-lung ventilation.

References:
1. Eisenkraft JB, Cohen E, Neustein SM. Anesthesia for thoracic surgery. In: Barash PG, Cullen BF, Stoelting RK, et al, eds. *Clinical Anesthesia*. 8th ed. Philadelphia: Lippincott; 2017:1030-1076.
2. Slinger PD, Campos JH. Anesthesia for thoracic surgery. In: Miller RD, Eriksson LI, Fleisher LA, et al, eds. *Miller's Anesthesia*. 8th ed. Philadelphia: Elsevier; 2015:1942-2006.

8.   **Correct answer: D**

The most common DLT used is a left-sided DLT because of its ease of placement and suitability for the vast majority of thoracic procedures. There are, however, several circumstances where a right-sided DLT is preferred or even required and some are more intuitive than others. Any procedure where the left mainstem anatomy is significantly distorted will benefit from a right-sided DLT because it may be difficult or even impossible to place a left-sided DLT successfully. For left pneumonectomy, a right-sided DLT may be easier to use. It is possible to use a left-sided DLT; however, tube position will need to be adjusted during stapling! For a left-sided sleeve resection involving the left mainstem, a right-sided DLT is practically required because of direct surgical manipulation of the left mainstem precluding the use of a left-sided DLT.

References:

1. Eisenkraft JB, Cohen E, Neustein SM. Anesthesia for thoracic surgery. In: Barash PG, Cullen BF, Stoelting RK, et al, eds. *Clinical Anesthesia*. 8th ed. Philadelphia: Lippincott; 2017:1030-1076.
2. Slinger PD, Campos JH. Anesthesia for thoracic surgery. In: Miller RD, Eriksson LI, Fleisher LA, et al, eds. *Miller's Anesthesia*. 8th ed. Philadelphia: Elsevier; 2015:1942-2006.

9.   **Correct answer: B**

One of the challenges of OLV is the maintenance of adequate ventilation and oxygenation while having less lung parenchyma available for gas exchange. Usually, lower tidal volumes are necessary to maintain a safe airway pressure. Sudden elevations in airway pressure may be mechanical, involving the anesthetic circuit or tube migration. In this case where the tube is correctly positioned, the diagnosis for pneumothorax must be entertained. Here, with hemodynamic instability and a drop in end-tidal carbon dioxide, the most likely cause is tension pneumothorax. This is incredibly problematic in the setting of OLV because there is significantly less pulmonary reserve. Emergent needle decompression is indicated, as chest tube placement is difficult in the dependent lateral position and will likely take too long.

References:

1. Eisenkraft JB, Cohen E, Neustein SM. Anesthesia for thoracic surgery. In: Barash PG, Cullen BF, Stoelting RK, et al, eds. *Clinical Anesthesia*. 8th ed. Philadelphia: Lippincott; 2017:1030-1076.
2. Slinger PD, Campos JH. Anesthesia for thoracic surgery. In: Miller RD, Eriksson LI, Fleisher LA, et al, eds. *Miller's Anesthesia*. 8th ed. Philadelphia: Elsevier; 2015:1942-2006.

10.   **Correct answer: A**

Lung isolation is possible through several different techniques, and for most thoracic cases, multiple strategies are adequate. However, it is important to recognize based on which scenarios one technique is preferred or required. For example, bronchial blockers allow for selective lobar isolation, which may be beneficial in patients who have had prior lung resection. Most bronchial blockers also only require a single-lumen endotracheal tube, which is attractive in patients who have a difficult airway or are likely to be intubated at the conclusion of the case (no need for tube exchange at the conclusion of the case). One of the major benefits of the DLT is that it allows for intervention via bronchoscopy to both lungs. Thus, for lung lavage a DLT is an absolute requirement. In this case, ventilation of both lungs is required, albeit with different settings and ventilators. The only method to do this is with a DLT.

References:

1. Eisenkraft JB, Cohen E, Neustein SM. Anesthesia for thoracic surgery. In: Barash PG, Cullen BF, Stoelting RK, et al, eds. *Clinical Anesthesia*. 8th ed. Philadelphia: Lippincott; 2017:1030-1076.
2. Slinger PD, Campos JH. Anesthesia for thoracic surgery. In: Miller RD, Eriksson LI, Fleisher LA, et al, eds. *Miller's Anesthesia*. 8th ed. Philadelphia: Elsevier; 2015:1942-2006.

11.   **Correct answer: B**

Loss of end-tidal carbon dioxide is a significant finding intraoperatively that implies either a complete loss of ventilation (circuit disconnect, mechanical obstruction of circuit) or loss of perfusion (cardiac arrest). In this case where the operative lung is still deflated and airway pressures are elevated, mechanical causes of obstruction should be investigated. A common malposition of the bronchial blocker is migration into the trachea, causing complete occlusion of the endotracheal tube. As the patient is showing signs of clinical instability, the most appropriate next step is to communicate with the surgical team and resume two-lung ventilation with the blocker deflated. Once the patient is stable, the blocker can be repositioned with bronchoscopic guidance. The other remaining answers are incorrect because it is very difficult to apply CPAP to the operative lung with a bronchial blocker and pneumothorax is not the most likely diagnosis in this case.

References:
1. Eisenkraft JB, Cohen E, Neustein SM. Anesthesia for thoracic surgery. In: Barash PG, Cullen BF, Stoelting RK, et al, eds. *Clinical Anesthesia*. 8th ed. Philadelphia: Lippincott; 2017:1030-1076.
2. Slinger PD, Campos JH. Anesthesia for thoracic surgery. In: Miller RD, Eriksson LI, Fleisher LA, et al, eds. *Miller's Anesthesia*. 8th ed. Philadelphia: Elsevier; 2015:1942-2006.

12. Correct answer: A

Excessive fluid administration is associated with poor outcomes in thoracic surgery, and fluid boluses should only be considered when there is significant evidence of organ hypoperfusion related to hypovolemia. In this case, it is reasonable to start a low-dose inotrope to counteract the effects of general anesthesia rather than aggressively bolus with fluids because fluids will increase the risk of postoperative pulmonary edema. Blood transfusion is unlikely to be indicated in a patient who has a hemoglobin >10. Mild acidosis is usually well tolerated, and increasing ventilation will likely serve only to increase airway pressures and subsequently the risk of lung injury.

References:
1. Eisenkraft JB, Cohen E, Neustein SM. Anesthesia for thoracic surgery. In: Barash PG, Cullen BF, Stoelting RK, et al, eds. *Clinical Anesthesia*. 8th ed. Philadelphia: Lippincott; 2017:1030-1076.
2. Slinger PD, Campos JH. Anesthesia for thoracic surgery. In: Miller RD, Eriksson LI, Fleisher LA, et al, eds. *Miller's Anesthesia*. 8th ed. Philadelphia: Elsevier; 2015:1942-2006.

13. Correct answer: B

Although there are no randomized controlled trials to guide decision making on the lowest acceptable oxygen saturation during OLV, the most commonly accepted goal is 90%. Most patients without significant comorbidities will tolerate a saturation in the high 80s without negative sequelae; however, it is important to recognize that such a low saturation implies very little reserve and further insult will result in profound desaturation. The oxygen saturation goal may need to be adjusted in patients with significant comorbidities, particularly if there is evidence of impaired oxygen delivery to tissues.

References:
1. Eisenkraft JB, Cohen E, Neustein SM. Anesthesia for thoracic surgery. In: Barash PG, Cullen BF, Stoelting RK, et al, eds. *Clinical Anesthesia*. 8th ed. Philadelphia: Lippincott; 2017:1030-1076.
2. Slinger PD, Campos JH. Anesthesia for thoracic surgery. In: Miller RD, Eriksson LI, Fleisher LA, et al, eds. *Miller's Anesthesia*. 8th ed. Philadelphia: Elsevier; 2015:1942-2006.

14. Correct answer: D

Postthoracotomy atelectasis is a common finding in patients undergoing thoracic surgery. Its incidence further supports the need for aggressive pulmonary toilet and encouragement of deep breathing postoperatively. None of the modern inhaled agents differ significantly in their incidence of atelectasis (such as isoflurane, sevoflurane, or desflurane). High inspired oxygen concentrations likely contribute to the formation of absorption atelectasis. However, nitrous oxide is associated with a significantly increased risk of postthoracotomy atelectasis, and most sources recommend avoiding nitrous oxide during thoracic surgery. It should be noted, however, that there may be clinical scenarios where nitrous oxide may have more benefits than risks in thoracic surgery.

References:
1. Eisenkraft JB, Cohen E, Neustein SM. Anesthesia for thoracic surgery. In: Barash PG, Cullen BF, Stoelting RK, et al, eds. *Clinical Anesthesia*. 8th ed. Philadelphia: Lippincott; 2017:1030-1076.
2. Slinger PD, Campos JH. Anesthesia for thoracic surgery. In: Miller RD, Eriksson LI, Fleisher LA, et al, eds. *Miller's Anesthesia*. 8th ed. Philadelphia: Elsevier; 2015:1942-2006.

15. Correct answer: A

Desaturation during OLV is a common occurrence and can be treated in multiple ways. This case presents several unique challenges that preclude several common algorithms. Bleomycin causes a fibrotic lung injury that is exacerbated with elevated oxygen concentrations, and all efforts to avoid increased oxygen should be attempted. Two-lung ventilation is always an option in an emergency, barring a surgical contraindication; however, in this case with stable vital signs and a reasonable oxygen saturation, it is acceptable to trial other interventions before interrupting lung isolation. A simple but often effective intervention is to attempt a recruitment maneuver of the dependent lung to improve V/Q matching. Increasing the PEEP alone is unlikely to have much benefit in the absence of an antecedent recruitment maneuver.

References:

1. Eisenkraft JB, Cohen E, Neustein SM. Anesthesia for thoracic surgery. In: Barash PG, Cullen BF, Stoelting RK, et al, eds. *Clinical Anesthesia*. 8th ed. Philadelphia: Lippincott; 2017:1030-1076.
2. Slinger PD, Campos JH. Anesthesia for thoracic surgery. In: Miller RD, Eriksson LI, Fleisher LA, et al, eds. *Miller's Anesthesia*. 8th ed. Philadelphia: Elsevier; 2015:1942-2006.

16. Correct answer: B

Desaturation during OLV can happen for many reasons. It is important to always support the patient's vital signs first and to tailor your interventions based on the severity of the desaturation. In this case the desaturation is significant but not immediately life-threatening. It is reasonable to increase the inspired oxygen to improve the saturation while other diagnostic procedures are undertaken. Applying CPAP to the operative lung is not an option for a patient with a bronchopleural fistula. Likewise, two-lung ventilation may not improve things if the fistula is severe. Bronchoscopic confirmation of the DLT is reasonable, but increasing the oxygen first to increase safety is the correct first step.

References:

1. Eisenkraft JB, Cohen E, Neustein SM. Anesthesia for thoracic surgery. In: Barash PG, Cullen BF, Stoelting RK, et al, eds. *Clinical Anesthesia*. 8th ed. Philadelphia: Lippincott; 2017:1030-1076.
2. Slinger PD, Campos JH. Anesthesia for thoracic surgery. In: Miller RD, Eriksson LI, Fleisher LA, et al, eds. *Miller's Anesthesia*. 8th ed. Philadelphia: Elsevier; 2015:1942-2006.

17. Correct answer: A

OLV in the supine position presents a unique set of challenges because the ventilated lung will not benefit from the improved V/Q matching owing to gravity in the lateral position. Bilateral surgery also comes with its own complications, namely that the reinflated lung will have some intrinsic injury and will not be as effective as it was before deflation (at least during the operative period). To minimize the risk of desaturation, it is reasonable to start on the right side because the large right lung will be better able to support the oxygenation/ventilation requirements postreinflation than the left lung. Although a total intravenous anesthetic will reduce the alteration of hypoxic pulmonary vasoconstriction, the clinical significance of this compared with modern inhaled agents is minimal. The technique for lung isolation will not affect desaturation risk in this case. Large tidal volumes are *more* likely to increase lung injury and consequently desaturation when using the reinflated lung.

References:

1. Eisenkraft JB, Cohen E, Neustein SM. Anesthesia for thoracic surgery. In: Barash PG, Cullen BF, Stoelting RK, et al, eds. *Clinical Anesthesia*. 8th ed. Philadelphia: Lippincott; 2017:1030-1076.
2. Slinger PD, Campos JH. Anesthesia for thoracic surgery. In: Miller RD, Eriksson LI, Fleisher LA, et al, eds. *Miller's Anesthesia*. 8th ed. Philadelphia: Elsevier; 2015:1942-2006.

18. Correct answer: C

Persistent shoulder pain following thoracic surgery should be suspicious for suprascapular nerve injury. The most common cause of this injury is either anterior flexion of the arm across the chest wall or lateral over extension of the cervical spine. The other positioning problems described here do not cause suprascapular injury. Of note, it is important to remember that the axillary roll does NOT go in the axilla, as placement in the axilla increases the likelihood of brachial plexus injury.

References:

1. Eisenkraft JB, Cohen E, Neustein SM. Anesthesia for thoracic surgery. In: Barash PG, Cullen BF, Stoelting RK, et al, eds. *Clinical Anesthesia*. 8th ed. Philadelphia: Lippincott; 2017:1030-1076.
2. Slinger PD, Campos JH. Anesthesia for thoracic surgery. In: Miller RD, Eriksson LI, Fleisher LA, et al, eds. *Miller's Anesthesia*. 8th ed. Philadelphia: Elsevier; 2015:1942-2006.

19. **Correct answer: D**

Patients with severe obstructive lung disease often have large emphysematous changes that involve alveolar destruction and large dilated airspaces. Increased PEEP only serves to distend these damaged airspaces further and is not usually helpful in isolated obstructive disease. Conversely, in fibrotic lung disease there may be a component of recruitable lung and it is reasonable to trial some PEEP to improve oxygenation.

References:
1. Eisenkraft JB, Cohen E, Neustein SM. Anesthesia for thoracic surgery. In: Barash PG, Cullen BF, Stoelting RK, et al, eds. *Clinical Anesthesia*. 8th ed. Philadelphia: Lippincott; 2017:1030-1076.
2. Slinger PD, Campos JH. Anesthesia for thoracic surgery. In: Miller RD, Eriksson LI, Fleisher LA, et al, eds. *Miller's Anesthesia*. 8th ed. Philadelphia: Elsevier; 2015:1942-2006.

20. **Correct answer: C**

Initial ventilation strategy for patients undergoing OLV requires an understanding of the underlying mechanisms of injury to lung parenchyma during mechanical ventilation. These include barotrauma from elevated airway pressures and volutrauma, which results from repetitive opening and closing of alveoli during ventilation. It is reasonable to choose a low level of PEEP to start to aid in preventing derecruitment and the subsequent alveolar trauma. Extrapolating from studies in the ICU, a tidal volume of 6-8 mL/kg is a reasonable starting point, titrated down based on airway pressures. Of the answer choices, only C has a reasonable starting tidal volume.

References:
1. Eisenkraft JB, Cohen E, Neustein SM. Anesthesia for thoracic surgery. In: Barash PG, Cullen BF, Stoelting RK, et al, eds. *Clinical Anesthesia*. 8th ed. Philadelphia: Lippincott; 2017:1030-1076.
2. Slinger PD, Campos JH. Anesthesia for thoracic surgery. In: Miller RD, Eriksson LI, Fleisher LA, et al, eds. *Miller's Anesthesia*. 8th ed. Philadelphia: Elsevier; 2015:1942-2006.

21. **Correct answer: C**

There are no trials suggesting that either pressure or volume control is superior in thoracic anesthesia. Instead, the choice depends on the individual case and an important understanding of the 2 different modes of ventilation. Pressure control ventilation offers several attractive benefits, namely the avoidance of unnecessarily high airway pressures. However, this necessitates close monitoring of the tidal volume to prevent overdistension of the lung and consequent volutrauma, which is well known to be detrimental from studies on acute respiratory distress syndrome. A critical part of the case involves the restoration of two-lung ventilation. When using pressure control ventilation, it is possible to see a significant increase in tidal volumes, as the compliance of the respiratory circuit is abruptly changed by the readdition of the second lung. Although the other parameters listed are important to monitor, tidal volume is uniquely susceptible to variation when using pressure control ventilation.

References:
1. Eisenkraft JB, Cohen E, Neustein SM. Anesthesia for thoracic surgery. In: Barash PG, Cullen BF, Stoelting RK, et al, eds. *Clinical Anesthesia*. 8th ed. Philadelphia: Lippincott; 2017:1030-1076.
2. Slinger PD, Campos JH. Anesthesia for thoracic surgery. In: Miller RD, Eriksson LI, Fleisher LA, et al, eds. *Miller's Anesthesia*. 8th ed. Philadelphia: Elsevier; 2015:1942-2006.

22. **Correct answer: A**

Patients who have undergone lung transplantation present multiple challenges to the anesthesiologist. In addition to complications from immunosuppression, extreme care must be taken in managing mechanical ventilation, as transplanted lungs are at a higher risk of injury than native lungs. For this reason, pressure control ventilation is sometimes advocated for in order to avoid high airway pressures and reduce the consequent barotrauma. There are no data suggesting that pressure control is associated with decreased risk of rejection. Similarly, the risk of pulmonary edema is not any different based on mode of ventilation. Pressure control may lead to better oxygenation because of a higher mean airway pressure for a given tidal volume, but there is no guarantee.

References:
1. Eisenkraft JB, Cohen E, Neustein SM. Anesthesia for thoracic surgery. In: Barash PG, Cullen BF, Stoelting RK, et al, eds. *Clinical Anesthesia*. 8th ed. Philadelphia: Lippincott; 2017:1030-1076.
2. Slinger PD, Campos JH. Anesthesia for thoracic surgery. In: Miller RD, Eriksson LI, Fleisher LA, et al, eds. *Miller's Anesthesia*. 8th ed. Philadelphia: Elsevier; 2015:1942-2006.
3. Murray AW, Quinlan JJ, Blasiole B, Adams P. Anesthesia for heart, lung, and heart-lung transplantation. In: Kaplan JA, Augoustides JGT, Manecke GR, Maus T, Reich DL, eds. *Kaplan's Cardiac Anesthesia*. 7th ed. Philadelphia: Elsevier; 2017:974-993.

23. Correct answer: A

The hallmark of pressure control ventilation, namely the ability to control the peak airway pressure, is attractive in certain patient populations. A patient having bullae resected would likely benefit from pressure-controlled ventilation as an initial strategy to reduce the risk of bullae rupture and subsequent pneumothorax. The other patients listed are not at elevated risk of pneumothorax from high airway pressures, and therefore either pressure or volume control ventilation is a reasonable strategy.

References:
1. Eisenkraft JB, Cohen E, Neustein SM. Anesthesia for thoracic surgery. In: Barash PG, Cullen BF, Stoelting RK, et al, eds. *Clinical Anesthesia*. 8th ed. Philadelphia: Lippincott; 2017:1030-1076.
2. Slinger PD, Campos JH. Anesthesia for thoracic surgery. In: Miller RD, Eriksson LI, Fleisher LA, et al, eds. *Miller's Anesthesia*. 8th ed. Philadelphia: Elsevier; 2015:1942-2006.

24. Correct answer: C

Initial ventilation strategy for patients undergoing OLV requires an understanding of the underlying mechanisms of injury to lung parenchyma during mechanical ventilation. These include barotrauma from elevated airway pressures and volutrauma that results from repetitive opening and closing of alveoli during ventilation. It is reasonable to choose a low level of PEEP to start to aid in preventing derecruitment and the subsequent alveolar trauma. Extrapolating from studies in the ICU, a tidal volume of 6-8 mL/kg is a reasonable starting point, titrated based on airway pressures. Of the choices listed, only choice C has both a reasonable level of PEEP and a tidal volume in the appropriate range. The absence of PEEP will likely lead to increased atelectasis, both impairing oxygenation and increasing the likelihood of alveolar trauma.

References:
1. Eisenkraft JB, Cohen E, Neustein SM. Anesthesia for thoracic surgery. In: Barash PG, Cullen BF, Stoelting RK, et al, eds. *Clinical Anesthesia*. 8th ed. Philadelphia: Lippincott; 2017:1030-1076.
2. Slinger PD, Campos JH. Anesthesia for thoracic surgery. In: Miller RD, Eriksson LI, Fleisher LA, et al, eds. *Miller's Anesthesia*. 8th ed. Philadelphia: Elsevier; 2015:1942-2006.

25. Correct answer: C

Elevated airway pressures can be due to a variety of reasons. One of the most common is mechanical obstruction, which can result from mucous plugging or tube malposition. Once these are ruled out, it is reasonable to decrease the tidal volume to reduce the peak airway pressure. This needs to be balanced with the need for adequate ventilation although it should be noted that mild hypercapnia is very well tolerated in the absence of significant intracranial pathology. Increasing the respiratory rate will likely increase the peak airway pressure further. Decreasing the PEEP may lower the airway pressure; however, this can lead to increased atelectasis and may cause more harm than benefit. Finally, adjusting the inspired oxygen concentration is unlikely to significantly affect the airway pressure.

References:
1. Eisenkraft JB, Cohen E, Neustein SM. Anesthesia for thoracic surgery. In: Barash PG, Cullen BF, Stoelting RK, et al, eds. *Clinical Anesthesia*. 8th ed. Philadelphia: Lippincott; 2017:1030-1076.
2. Slinger PD, Campos JH. Anesthesia for thoracic surgery. In: Miller RD, Eriksson LI, Fleisher LA, et al, eds. *Miller's Anesthesia*. 8th ed. Philadelphia: Elsevier; 2015:1942-2006.

26. Correct answer: C

Patients undergoing rigid bronchoscopy present several challenges to the anesthesia team. One of these is the challenge in delivery of inhaled anesthetics. Because of the lack of reliable gas sampling as well as no airway seal, any delivered inhaled agent will be unreliable as well as potentially contaminating the operating room (choices A and D). Rigid bronchoscopy is very stimulating, and the dose of propofol to maintain an adequate depth of anesthesia would be very high; therefore, propofol is usually combined with another agent to attenuate the response. Of the choices listed a balanced anesthetic with propofol and remifentanil would be the best choice.

References:

1. Eisenkraft JB, Cohen E, Neustein SM. Anesthesia for thoracic surgery. In: Barash PG, Cullen BF, Stoelting RK, et al, eds. *Clinical Anesthesia*. 8th ed. Philadelphia: Lippincott; 2017:1030-1076.
2. Slinger PD, Campos JH. Anesthesia for thoracic surgery. In: Miller RD, Eriksson LI, Fleisher LA, et al, eds. *Miller's Anesthesia*. 8th ed. Philadelphia: Elsevier; 2015:1942-2006.
3. Modest VE, Alfille PH. Anesthesia for laser surgery. In: Miller RD, Eriksson LI, Fleisher LA, et al, eds. *Miller's Anesthesia*. 8th ed. Philadelphia: Elsevier; 2015:2598-2611.

27. Correct answer: B

Because of the high pressures of the jet ventilation system used in rigid bronchoscopy, airway trauma should always be high on the differential when presented with postoperative complications. Pneumothorax is a potential complication and should always be entertained in a patient complaining of shortness of breath or pain post bronchoscopy. Although it is not unreasonable to pursue a cardiovascular work-up, in a patient with no cardiac history, pneumothorax is more likely and it is reasonable to start with a chest X-ray first.

References:

1. Eisenkraft JB, Cohen E, Neustein SM. Anesthesia for thoracic surgery. In: Barash PG, Cullen BF, Stoelting RK, et al, eds. *Clinical Anesthesia*. 8th ed. Philadelphia: Lippincott; 2017:1030-1076.
2. Slinger PD, Campos JH. Anesthesia for thoracic surgery. In: Miller RD, Eriksson LI, Fleisher LA, et al, eds. *Miller's Anesthesia*. 8th ed. Philadelphia: Elsevier; 2015:1942-2006.
3. Modest VE, Alfille PH. Anesthesia for laser surgery. In: Miller RD, Eriksson LI, Fleisher LA, et al, eds. *Miller's Anesthesia*. 8th ed. Philadelphia: Elsevier; 2015:2598-2611.

28. Correct answer: C

Jet ventilation can complicate an anesthetic plan because of the difficulty in measuring ventilation, inability to utilize inhaled anesthetics, and additional equipment required. However, it offers several benefits, namely easier access to the airway for upper airway surgery as well as decreased diaphragmatic movement for procedures necessitating minimal movement of nearby structures. It is not associated with lower pain scores and is associated with an *increased* risk of pneumothorax.

References:

1. Eisenkraft JB, Cohen E, Neustein SM. Anesthesia for thoracic surgery. In: Barash PG, Cullen BF, Stoelting RK, et al, eds. *Clinical Anesthesia*. 8th ed. Philadelphia: Lippincott; 2017:1030-1076.
2. Slinger PD, Campos JH. Anesthesia for thoracic surgery. In: Miller RD, Eriksson LI, Fleisher LA, et al, eds. *Miller's Anesthesia*. 8th ed. Philadelphia: Elsevier; 2015:1942-2006.
3. Modest VE, Alfille PH. Anesthesia for laser surgery. In: Miller RD, Eriksson LI, Fleisher LA, et al, eds. *Miller's Anesthesia*. 8th ed. Philadelphia: Elsevier; 2015:2598-2611.

29. Correct answer: B

Airway fires are a devastating complication that require solid protocols to mitigate risk. One of the strategies is to use the lowest possible concentration of oxygen to reduce the flammability of surrounding equipment. Jet ventilation is not associated with a lower risk of fire, neither is TIVA nor is the use of inhaled bronchodilators. Other mitigation strategies include clear closed-loop communication between the anesthesia and surgical teams and minimizing flammable substances in the operative field when the laser is being used.

References:

1. Eisenkraft JB, Cohen E, Neustein SM. Anesthesia for thoracic surgery. In: Barash PG, Cullen BF, Stoelting RK, et al, eds. *Clinical Anesthesia*. 8th ed. Philadelphia: Lippincott; 2017:1030-1076.
2. Slinger PD, Campos JH. Anesthesia for thoracic surgery. In: Miller RD, Eriksson LI, Fleisher LA, et al, eds. *Miller's Anesthesia*. 8th ed. Philadelphia: Elsevier; 2015:1942-2006.
3. Modest VE, Alfille PH. Anesthesia for laser surgery. In: Miller RD, Eriksson LI, Fleisher LA, et al, eds. *Miller's Anesthesia*. 8th ed. Philadelphia: Elsevier; 2015:2598-2611.

30. Correct answer: B

Jet ventilation provides numerous benefits, namely ease of access to upper airway structures for the surgical team. Perhaps the biggest drawback compared with conventional endotracheal anesthesia is the difficulty in measuring the adequacy of ventilation because end-tidal carbon dioxide cannot be easily measured. Arterial blood gas sampling is often necessary if significant concern exists, which can be time-consuming and challenging to obtain depending on patient factors. Jet ventilation is not associated with altered risk of airway fires. Oxygenation is still easily measured using pulse oximetry.

References:
1. Eisenkraft JB, Cohen E, Neustein SM. Anesthesia for thoracic surgery. In: Barash PG, Cullen BF, Stoelting RK, et al, eds. *Clinical Anesthesia*. 8th ed. Philadelphia: Lippincott; 2017:1030-1076.
2. Slinger PD, Campos JH. Anesthesia for thoracic surgery. In: Miller RD, Eriksson LI, Fleisher LA, et al, eds. *Miller's Anesthesia*. 8th ed. Philadelphia: Elsevier; 2015:1942-2006.
3. Modest VE, Alfille PH. Anesthesia for laser surgery. In: Miller RD, Eriksson LI, Fleisher LA, et al, eds. *Miller's Anesthesia*. 8th ed. Philadelphia: Elsevier; 2015:2598-2611.

31. Correct answer: A

The predicted postoperative spirometry can be calculated by knowing the amount of lung to be resected as well as preoperative lung function testing. There are 42 total lung segments divided as follows: right upper lobe: 6, right middle lobe: 4, right lower lobe: 12, left upper lobe: 10, and left lower lobe: 10. Therefore, the predicted postoperative FEV1 can be calculated using the following formula:

$$ppoFEV1 = (1 - segments\ resected/total\ segments) \times preFEV1$$

Here,

$$ppoFEV1 = (1 - 6/42) \times 0.8 = 69\%\ normal$$

References:
1. Eisenkraft JB, Cohen E, Neustein SM. Anesthesia for thoracic surgery. In: Barash PG, Cullen BF, Stoelting RK, et al, eds. *Clinical Anesthesia*. 8th ed. Philadelphia: Lippincott; 2017:1030-1076.
2. Slinger PD, Campos JH. Anesthesia for thoracic surgery. In: Miller RD, Eriksson LI, Fleisher LA, et al, eds. *Miller's Anesthesia*. 8th ed. Philadelphia: Elsevier; 2015:1942-2006.

32. Correct answer: C

Double-lung transplantation presents multiple challenges for the anesthesiologist. One of these is the support of the patient on OLV while the ventilated lung either will have very poor parenchyma (often true of pretransplant lungs) or will be a freshly transplanted lung that has restrictions on airway pressure and oxygen because of the interest of graft function. Patients undergoing lung transplant also will commonly have a history of pulmonary hypertension because of chronic hypoxia. This patient is showing signs of acute right ventricular failure, which if not immediately treated will lead to death. CPAP to the operative lung is not an option because the operative lung is not necessarily able to participate in oxygen and ventilation (the anastomoses are not complete). Diuresis is unlikely to improve the situation fast enough even if volume overload is a significant contributor. Inhaled pulmonary vasodilators may offer some benefits in the acute setting. However, for this patient, who is acutely failing, this intervention may not be enough and is likely only a temporizing measure. Most likely this patient will require extracorporeal support in the form of extracorporeal membrane oxygenation or full cardiac bypass. Inotropes and pulmonary vasodilators may be needed to support the patient until extracorporeal support can be initiated.

References:
1. Eisenkraft JB, Cohen E, Neustein SM. Anesthesia for thoracic surgery. In: Barash PG, Cullen BF, Stoelting RK, et al, eds. *Clinical Anesthesia*. 8th ed. Philadelphia: Lippincott; 2017:1030-1076.
2. Slinger PD, Campos JH. Anesthesia for thoracic surgery. In: Miller RD, Eriksson LI, Fleisher LA, et al, eds. *Miller's Anesthesia*. 8th ed. Philadelphia: Elsevier; 2015:1942-2006.

33. Correct answer: B

Lambert-Eaton myasthenic syndrome is a rare paraneoplastic syndrome commonly associated with small cell lung cancer. It results from the formation of antibodies against *presynaptic* calcium channels, resulting in muscle weakness. Classically the weakness improves with repetitive muscle use. This is in contrast to classic myasthenia, which is due to antibodies directed against postsynaptic acetylcholine receptors and does not show improvement with repetitive use but rather worsens with exertion.

References:
1. Eisenkraft JB, Cohen E, Neustein SM. Anesthesia for thoracic surgery. In: Barash PG, Cullen BF, Stoelting RK, et al, eds. *Clinical Anesthesia*. 8th ed. Philadelphia: Lippincott; 2017:1030-1076.
2. Slinger PD, Campos JH. Anesthesia for thoracic surgery. In: Miller RD, Eriksson LI, Fleisher LA, et al, eds. *Miller's Anesthesia*. 8th ed. Philadelphia: Elsevier; 2015:1942-2006.

34. Correct answer: A

Surgery involving the mainstem bronchi introduces additional challenges for lung isolation. More distal surgery is easily accomplished with a variety of strategies, and when a DLT is used most commonly, a left-sided tube is chosen because of ease of placement. This is not acceptable for left sleeve lobectomy because surgical manipulation of the left mainstem will lead to tube movement or worse suturing of the tube into the reconstructed bronchus. For similar reasons, bronchial blockers are not practical either. In this case a right-sided tube is the most elegant and reliable method of lung isolation. Although theoretically it may be possible to use a left-sided tube depending on how high the anastomosis is, this will require more communication and the feasibility is not guaranteed. Therefore, a right-sided DLT is recommended for sleeve resection involving the left mainstem.

References:
1. Eisenkraft JB, Cohen E, Neustein SM. Anesthesia for thoracic surgery. In: Barash PG, Cullen BF, Stoelting RK, et al, eds. *Clinical Anesthesia*. 8th ed. Philadelphia: Lippincott; 2017:1030-1076.
2. Slinger PD, Campos JH. Anesthesia for thoracic surgery. In: Miller RD, Eriksson LI, Fleisher LA, et al, eds. *Miller's Anesthesia*. 8th ed. Philadelphia: Elsevier; 2015:1942-2006.

35. Correct answer: B

Pneumonectomies are high-risk surgeries requiring careful patient selection and appropriate intraoperative and postoperative management. Of particular concern is the function of the right ventricle and how it will handle what is effectively the loss of half the pulmonary circulation. Depending on the state of the diseased lung, this can lead to significantly increased pulmonary vascular resistance postoperatively. It is critical to remember that the right ventricle does not have the functional reserve of the left ventricle and will not tolerate significant increases in afterload. In this case the decreasing pulmonary pressures combined with increasing CVPs are highly concerning for impending right ventricular collapse and should be immediately addressed.

References:
1. Eisenkraft JB, Cohen E, Neustein SM. Anesthesia for thoracic surgery. In: Barash PG, Cullen BF, Stoelting RK, et al, eds. *Clinical Anesthesia*. 8th ed. Philadelphia: Lippincott; 2017:1030-1076.
2. Slinger PD, Campos JH. Anesthesia for thoracic surgery. In: Miller RD, Eriksson LI, Fleisher LA, et al, eds. *Miller's Anesthesia*. 8th ed. Philadelphia: Elsevier; 2015:1942-2006.

36. Correct answer: B

Penetrating chest trauma should have a very low threshold for placement of a chest tube. Because of the injury from the bullet, it is easy for a tension pneumothorax to develop after the induction of positive pressure ventilation. Management of acute tension pneumothorax involves immediate needle decompression followed by chest tube placement. Anesthesiologists should be aware of the high risk for pneumothorax following penetrating chest trauma, especially when the surgical team is not the trauma surgical team.

References:
1. Eisenkraft JB, Cohen E, Neustein SM. Anesthesia for thoracic surgery. In: Barash PG, Cullen BF, Stoelting RK, et al, eds. *Clinical Anesthesia*. 8th ed. Philadelphia: Lippincott; 2017:1030-1076.
2. Slinger PD, Campos JH. Anesthesia for thoracic surgery. In: Miller RD, Eriksson LI, Fleisher LA, et al, eds. *Miller's Anesthesia*. 8th ed. Philadelphia: Elsevier; 2015:1942-2006.

37. Correct answer: B

Acute pulmonary artery rupture from a pulmonary artery catheter unsurprisingly has a high mortality rate. The standard management is endovascular therapy. The patient must be stabilized as best as possible for transport, and this is usually accomplished by lung isolation with ventilation of the noneffected lung. Further inflation of the pulmonary artery catheter should only be attempted with fluoroscopy and not blindly. Chest tube placement may be indicated, but it is not the first step. Emergent thoracotomy is unlikely to be successful.

References:

1. Eisenkraft JB, Cohen E, Neustein SM. Anesthesia for thoracic surgery. In: Barash PG, Cullen BF, Stoelting RK, et al, eds. *Clinical Anesthesia*. 8th ed. Philadelphia: Lippincott; 2017:1030-1076.
2. Slinger PD, Campos JH. Anesthesia for thoracic surgery. In: Miller RD, Eriksson LI, Fleisher LA, et al, eds. *Miller's Anesthesia*. 8th ed. Philadelphia: Elsevier; 2015:1942-2006.

38. Correct answer: A

Chylothorax that involves the accumulation of lymphatic fluid in the chest cavity most commonly from injury to the thoracic duct during left thoracotomy should be suspected in a patient with a lymphatic predominant pleural effusion. A reactive effusion would likely be transudative and not be milky-white. Although both perforation and empyema can also have purulent-appearing drainage, they are usually associated with signs of sepsis. Finally, in this case the association with advancement of the diet, which stimulates lymphatic drainage, increases the likelihood of thoracic duct injury and resultant chylothorax.

References:

1. Eisenkraft JB, Cohen E, Neustein SM. Anesthesia for thoracic surgery. In: Barash PG, Cullen BF, Stoelting RK, et al, eds. *Clinical Anesthesia*. 8th ed. Philadelphia: Lippincott; 2017:1030-1076.
2. Slinger PD, Campos JH. Anesthesia for thoracic surgery. In: Miller RD, Eriksson LI, Fleisher LA, et al, eds. *Miller's Anesthesia*. 8th ed. Philadelphia: Elsevier; 2015:1942-2006.

39. Correct answer: A

Patients with pulmonary abscesses requiring surgery require careful planning when devising a strategy for lung isolation. In addition to the normal requirements for thoracic surgery, these patients have 2 additional considerations. The first is that there is a strong desire to avoid contamination of the other lung, necessitating adequate lung isolation before any new positioning changes are done. Second, bronchoscopic intervention is often necessary on the operative lung, necessitating DLT placement rather than a bronchial blocker or simple mainstem intubation.

References:

1. Eisenkraft JB, Cohen E, Neustein SM. Anesthesia for thoracic surgery. In: Barash PG, Cullen BF, Stoelting RK, et al, eds. *Clinical Anesthesia*. 8th ed. Philadelphia: Lippincott; 2017:1030-1076.
2. Slinger PD, Campos JH. Anesthesia for thoracic surgery. In: Miller RD, Eriksson LI, Fleisher LA, et al, eds. *Miller's Anesthesia*. 8th ed. Philadelphia: Elsevier; 2015:1942-2006.

40. Correct answer: C

There are multiple complications following a pneumonectomy that a provider needs to be aware of. Postoperative shortness of breath is an ominous sign that mandates aggressive and urgent work-up. Causes include postpneumonectomy herniation, worsening right ventricular performance, and pulmonary edema. A rarer cause involves the formation of a bronchopleural fistula because of a leak in the stump from the side of the pneumonectomy. In this case, suspicion for a leak should be high because of a decrease in the fluid level, implying increasing air in the side of the chest status post lung resection. Although the temptation may be to place a chest tube to relieve the air, this will likely worsen the fistula by providing a low-resistance pathway and consequently "steal" ventilation from the normal lung. In addition, in a pneumonectomy patient, suction on the resected side will lead to herniation and cardiovascular collapse and should be avoided.

References:

1. Eisenkraft JB, Cohen E, Neustein SM. Anesthesia for thoracic surgery. In: Barash PG, Cullen BF, Stoelting RK, et al, eds. *Clinical Anesthesia*. 8th ed. Philadelphia: Lippincott; 2017:1030-1076.
2. Slinger PD, Campos JH. Anesthesia for thoracic surgery. In: Miller RD, Eriksson LI, Fleisher LA, et al, eds. *Miller's Anesthesia*. 8th ed. Philadelphia: Elsevier; 2015:1942-2006.

41. Correct answer: A

Obese patients present multiple challenges to the anesthesia care team. From an airway standpoint, they often demonstrate challenging anatomy that may make mask ventilation and endotracheal intubation challenging. To safely induce anesthesia, it is important to optimize preoxygenation as much as possible. In obese patients, the application of CPAP will aid in maintaining lung recruitment and prolong the time to desaturation. Obese patients have lower functional residual capacity and will not have the same pulmonary reserve as nonobese patients. The use of video laryngoscope may be helpful in intubating the patient, but it will not prolong the time to desaturation. Cricoid pressure has debatable utility in preventing aspiration but will not affect the time to desaturation. Although breathing 100% oxygen can lead to absorption atelectasis, this is not significant enough that benefit is seen from preoxygenation with 50% oxygen mixtures.

References:

1. Eisenkraft JB, Cohen E, Neustein SM. Anesthesia for thoracic surgery. In: Barash PG, Cullen BF, Stoelting RK, et al, eds. *Clinical Anesthesia*. 8th ed. Philadelphia: Lippincott; 2017:1030-1076.
2. Slinger PD, Campos JH. Anesthesia for thoracic surgery. In: Miller RD, Eriksson LI, Fleisher LA, et al, eds. *Miller's Anesthesia*. 8th ed. Philadelphia: Elsevier; 2015:1942-2006.

---

42. **Correct answer: B**

Impaired oxygen diffusion is a reflection of the severity of injury to the alveolar-capillary interface. Although spirometry can quantitatively measure this, it is important to be aware of other symptoms when caring for patients who may or may not have a full pulmonary work-up. Increased partial pressure of arterial CO_2 at rest implies a problem with ventilation, commonly seen in obesity hypoventilation syndrome. Chronic respiratory acidosis is a symptom of severe COPD. Improvement with bronchodilators reflects the obstructive component of disease, not the diffusion component. Decreased partial pressure of arterial oxygen at exercise is reflective of severely impaired oxygen diffusion. This can be understood that the diffusion of oxygen in these patients is already maximal at rest, and increased blood flow dose not lead to better oxygen diffusion because of impairment of the alveolar-capillary interface.

References:

1. Eisenkraft JB, Cohen E, Neustein SM. Anesthesia for thoracic surgery. In: Barash PG, Cullen BF, Stoelting RK, et al, eds. *Clinical Anesthesia*. 8th ed. Philadelphia: Lippincott; 2017:1030-1076.
2. Slinger PD, Campos JH. Anesthesia for thoracic surgery. In: Miller RD, Eriksson LI, Fleisher LA, et al, eds. *Miller's Anesthesia*. 8th ed. Philadelphia: Elsevier; 2015:1954-2006.

---

43. **Correct answer: C**

Although severe COPD often shares multiple characteristics, including reversibility with bronchodilators, decreased diffusion with emphysema, and poor exercise tolerance, not all of these are required. Carbon dioxide retention, a characteristic of severe obstructive disease, can only be diagnosed on arterial blood gas, showing an elevated partial pressure of carbon dioxide and metabolic compensation. Knowledge of chronic retention is critical because it allows for the provider to minimize the changes of overventilating the patient and causing a subsequent severe respiratory alkalosis. Worsening carbon dioxide retention also may imply an acute exacerbation, which would necessitate postponing elective surgery to allow for better optimization.

References:

1. Eisenkraft JB, Cohen E, Neustein SM. Anesthesia for thoracic surgery. In: Barash PG, Cullen BF, Stoelting RK, et al, eds. *Clinical Anesthesia*. 8th ed. Philadelphia: Lippincott; 2017:1030-1076.
2. Slinger PD, Campos JH. Anesthesia for thoracic surgery. In: Miller RD, Eriksson LI, Fleisher LA, et al, eds. *Miller's Anesthesia*. 8th ed. Philadelphia: Elsevier; 2015:1942-2006.

---

44. **Correct answer: A**

Patients with severe COPD who develop chronic hypoxia are at high risk to develop pulmonary hypertension. Home oxygen therapy is often prescribed to reduce the progression of pulmonary hypertension. This therapy is usually appreciated by the patients, as it improves exercise tolerance; however, it is critical that the anesthesia provider is aware of the utility in reducing the progression of pulmonary hypertension. In this noncompliant patient, the acute vital sign changes are concerning for impending right ventricular collapse, which is often exacerbated by the induction of general anesthesia, particularly in the patient in whom the pulmonary hypertension is unexpected. These patients will benefit from an anesthetic strategy that minimizes interruptions in ventilation, avoids acidosis, avoids hypoxia, and maintains coronary perfusion because of the sensitivity of the right ventricle. Patients with severe enough disease may warrant additional invasive monitoring such as transesophageal echocardiography and/or pulmonary artery catheterization.

References:
1. Eisenkraft JB, Cohen E, Neustein SM. Anesthesia for thoracic surgery. In: Barash PG, Cullen BF, Stoelting RK, et al, eds. *Clinical Anesthesia*. 8th ed. Philadelphia: Lippincott; 2017:1030-1076.
2. Slinger PD, Campos JH. Anesthesia for thoracic surgery. In: Miller RD, Eriksson LI, Fleisher LA, et al, eds. *Miller's Anesthesia*. 8th ed. Philadelphia: Elsevier; 2015:1942-2006.

45. Correct answer: A

Patients with severe obstructive lung disease often require a prolonged expiratory phase to adequately exhale the large volume of air trapped in the lungs. When placed on mechanical ventilation, these patients are susceptible to the development of occult or auto-PEEP. This can have several negative consequences. One is that spontaneously breathing patients will require additional effort to trigger the ventilator. For patients with a controlled rate, this can lead to the generation of significant intrathoracic pressure, leading to decreased venous return and cardiovascular collapse. The risk of auto-PEEP can be reduced by prolonging the expiratory time; the easiest way to do this is to decrease the respiratory rate and tolerate mild elevations in carbon dioxide. Auto-PEEP can be detected by measuring the end-expiratory pressure during an expiratory hold on the mechanical ventilator.

References:
1. Eisenkraft JB, Cohen E, Neustein SM. Anesthesia for thoracic surgery. In: Barash PG, Cullen BF, Stoelting RK, et al, eds. *Clinical Anesthesia*. 8th ed. Philadelphia: Lippincott; 2017:1030-1076.
2. Slinger PD, Campos JH. Anesthesia for thoracic surgery. In: Miller RD, Eriksson LI, Fleisher LA, et al, eds. *Miller's Anesthesia*. 8th ed. Philadelphia: Elsevier; 2015:1942-2006.

46. Correct answer: A

Patients with severe scoliosis require a well-thought-out anesthetic plan for safe management during what can be a complicated surgery. Commonly encountered issues include blood loss, nerve injury, and postoperative pain control. Depending on the degree of scoliosis, the patient may also present with significant pulmonary compromise. Scoliosis-induced pulmonary dysfunction does not affect the carbon monoxide diffusing capacity (choice B) or show reversibility with bronchodilators (choice D). A Cobb angle (the angle formed by a line drawn perpendicular from the top of the first vertebra of the scoliotic curve and a perpendicular line drawn from the bottom of the last vertebra of the scoliotic curve) of greater than 65° or a vital capacity less than 40% normal is predictive of the need for postoperative ventilation.

References:
1. Eisenkraft JB, Cohen E, Neustein SM. Anesthesia for thoracic surgery. In: Barash PG, Cullen BF, Stoelting RK, et al, eds. *Clinical Anesthesia*. 8th ed. Philadelphia: Lippincott; 2017:1030-1076.
2. Slinger PD, Campos JH. Anesthesia for thoracic surgery. In: Miller RD, Eriksson LI, Fleisher LA, et al, eds. *Miller's Anesthesia*. 8th ed. Philadelphia: Elsevier; 2015:1942-2006.
3. Urban M. Anesthesia for orthopedic surgery. In: Miller RD, Eriksson LI, Fleisher LA, et al, eds. *Miller's Anesthesia*. 8th ed. Philadelphia: Elsevier; 2015:2386-2406.

47. Correct answer: B

The patient's presentation is most consistent with Lambert-Eaton myasthenic syndrome. Lambert-Eaton is a rare paraneoplastic syndrome commonly associated with small cell lung cancer. It results from the formation of antibodies against *presynaptic* calcium channels, resulting in muscle weakness. Because of the impaired calcium release, muscle weakness can persist despite adequate reversal of nondepolarizing muscle relaxants, and these patients may require prolonged ventilatory support. Although Lambert-Eaton is a rare disorder, patients with a history of small cell lung cancer should have a detailed history to determine if there are any suspicious findings of a neuromuscular disorder present.

References:
1. Eisenkraft JB, Cohen E, Neustein SM. Anesthesia for thoracic surgery. In: Barash PG, Cullen BF, Stoelting RK, et al, eds. *Clinical Anesthesia*. 8th ed. Philadelphia: Lippincott; 2017:1030-1076.
2. Slinger PD, Campos JH. Anesthesia for thoracic surgery. In: Miller RD, Eriksson LI, Fleisher LA, et al, eds. *Miller's Anesthesia*. 8th ed. Philadelphia: Elsevier; 2015:1942-2006.

48. Correct answer: A

Bronchospasm while under anesthesia can occur for many reasons. Management targets toward maintaining patient stability and reversing the bronchoconstriction. In a patient with mild reactive airway disease, the most likely culprit in this case is light anesthesia. Deepening the plane of anesthesia is likely sufficient to treat the bronchospasm. Because of impaired gas flow, inhaled agents may not be effective; in addition, a laryngeal mask airway may limit the amount of positive pressure that can be delivered and ventilation may be impaired while the bronchospasm persists; therefore, an intravenous agent is most appropriate. Changing the ventilation mode will not treat the bronchospasm. Intravenous epinephrine can be helpful in treating severe or refractory bronchospasm but is not a first-line therapy.

References:

1. Eisenkraft JB, Cohen E, Neustein SM. Anesthesia for thoracic surgery. In: Barash PG, Cullen BF, Stoelting RK, et al, eds. *Clinical Anesthesia*. 8th ed. Philadelphia: Lippincott; 2017:1030-1076.
2. Slinger PD, Campos JH. Anesthesia for thoracic surgery. In: Miller RD, Eriksson LI, Fleisher LA, et al, eds. *Miller's Anesthesia*. 8th ed. Philadelphia: Elsevier; 2015:1942-2006.

49. **Correct answer: B**

Patients with chronic/recurrent pulmonary infections may require thoracic surgery for definitive therapy because prolonged antibiotics may not be effective. It is important to recognize several factors common to this patient population. One is that they are often colonized with resistant organisms and normal antibiotic prophylaxis may not be sufficient; consultation with infectious disease specialists is often advised. Second, it is ideal to avoid contaminating the other lung with infected material, which can then lead to additional abscess formation. Although it is impossible to fully avoid this, it is ideal to first achieve lung isolation and confirm good separation before turning the patient to the lateral position. A thoracic epidural will likely help with postoperative pain control but will not affect the risk of lung contamination. Bronchiectatic lung is not as amenable to recruitment, and increased PEEP may be of little benefit.

References:

1. Eisenkraft JB, Cohen E, Neustein SM. Anesthesia for thoracic surgery. In: Barash PG, Cullen BF, Stoelting RK, et al, eds. *Clinical Anesthesia*. 8th ed. Philadelphia: Lippincott; 2017:1030-1076.
2. Slinger PD, Campos JH. Anesthesia for thoracic surgery. In: Miller RD, Eriksson LI, Fleisher LA, et al, eds. *Miller's Anesthesia*. 8th ed. Philadelphia: Elsevier; 2015:1942-2006.

50. **Correct answer: A**

Mediastinal masses present some of the most difficult challenges to the anesthesia care team. They are high risk for significant complications during induction, including loss of airway and cardiovascular collapse due to vascular compression. A patient who presents with symptoms concerning for presyncope when supine is at very high risk and may lose venous return upon induction of anesthesia. Adequate plans must be in place before the procedure, which may include the presence of cardiac surgery to enable extracorporeal support should cardiovascular collapse ensue.

References:

1. Eisenkraft JB, Cohen E, Neustein SM. Anesthesia for thoracic surgery. In: Barash PG, Cullen BF, Stoelting RK, et al, eds. *Clinical Anesthesia*. 8th ed. Philadelphia: Lippincott; 2017:1030-1076.
2. Slinger PD, Campos JH. Anesthesia for thoracic surgery. In: Miller RD, Eriksson LI, Fleisher LA, et al, eds. *Miller's Anesthesia*. 8th ed. Philadelphia: Elsevier; 2015:1942-2006.

18

EAR, NOSE, AND THROAT (ENT)/ OPHTHALMOLOGY SURGERY

Ryan Joseph Horvath

1. **Which of the following features of the infant airway compared with the adult airway is *correct*?**

   A. Infants are obligate mouth breathers through the first several months of life.
   B. The infant larynx is more cephalad in the neck than the adult larynx.
   C. The infant epiglottis is shorter and broader than the adult epiglottis.
   D. The narrowest part of the upper airway in the infant is at the level of the vocal cords.
   E. The larger occiput of the infant requires extra elevation of the head to achieve an optimal "sniffing" position.

2. **Which of the following statements is *correct* concerning airway innervation?**

   A. The recurrent laryngeal nerve innervates all the intrinsic muscles of the larynx save the cricothyroid, which is innervated by the external branch of the superior laryngeal nerve.
   B. To numb sensation to the posterior third of the tongue and oropharynx, local anesthetic can be infiltrated into the base of the palatoglossal arch to block the lingual nerve.
   C. An inferior laryngeal nerve block is completed by injecting local anesthetic 1 cm below the greater cornu of the hyoid bone bilaterally.
   D. A transtracheal block, achieved by injecting local anesthetic through the cricoid membrane into the trachea, can serve as the sole anesthetic needed for an awake fiberoptic intubation.
   E. Numbing of the oropharynx through topical approaches is rarely effective, and direct injection of local anesthetics is usually required to achieve adequate numbing for an awake fiberoptic intubation.

3. **In the postanesthesia care unit (PACU), a patient develops hoarseness following surgical removal of the left lobe of the thyroid (without violation of the right neck), and you suspect a unilateral recurrent laryngeal nerve injury. You consult your ENT colleagues to help evaluate recurrent laryngeal nerve function. Which of the following appearances of the vocal cords would be expected from this proposed mechanism of injury?**

   A. Immobile bilateral vocal cords, with an adequate glottic opening and no change during vocalization
   B. Immobile bilateral vocal cords, with a very small glottic opening
   C. Immobile left vocal cord and movement of the right vocal cord across midline during phonation
   D. Immobile right vocal cord and movement of the left vocal cord across midline during phonation
   E. Bilateral flaccid, partially abducted, immobile vocal cords

4. A 26-year-old professional singer is in your operating room (OR) undergoing suspension microlaryngoscopy for vocal cord polyps. Soon after induction and just after the surgeon places the patient into suspension, the heart rate drops from 85 to 30 beats per minute. Which of the following is the *best* initial course of action?

A. Increase the depth of anesthetic.
B. Administer an opioid.
C. Administer glycopyrrolate.
D. Continue to monitor the heart rate and cycle the blood pressure cuff with the knowledge that these parameters should recover, as the patient becomes accustomed to the positioning.
E. Direct the surgeon to take the patient out of suspension and before proceeding with additional measures.

5. An ENT surgeon is planning microlaryngoscopy for laser ablation of vocal cord hemangiomas and asks that low-frequency jet ventilation be used so that "the smallest tube possible can be used." Which of the following is NOT an important consideration when using jet ventilation?

A. Care must be taken to allow passive exhalation and avoid breath stacking to limit the possibility of barotrauma.
B. Reliable pulse oximetry is essential because jet ventilation relies on the venture effect and entrainment of room air, making the exact Fio_2 challenging to measure.
C. Total intravenous anesthesia is required.
D. Pressure monitoring at the distal tip of the jet ventilation catheter is essential.
E. The trigger pressure must be preset at a level to allow adequate synchronization between the jet ventilator and the patient's spontaneous breaths.

6. When considering the anesthetic management for a patient undergoing suspension microlaryngoscopy, which of the following is MOST important?

A. Complete immobility during surgical manipulation of the larynx
B. Light sedation so that the surgeon may observe vocal cord mobility during phonation
C. Permissive hypotension to limit surgical bleeding
D. Generous β-blockade to limit sympathetic discharge with suspension
E. Long-acting opioids are the best agents to manage postoperative pain

7. You are caring for a patient in the intensive care unit (ICU) who remains intubated overnight following oromaxillofacial surgery procedure for irrigation and debridement of a submandibular abscess. The patient has a nasotracheal tube sutured in place and still has significant external facial swelling as well as discharge from the surgically placed drains. The patient has passed a spontaneous breathing trial and has a fully intact neurologic exam. Which of the following evaluations is likely to provide the *best* information regarding the patient's readiness for extubation?

A. Upright X-ray of the neck
B. CT of the neck
C. Bedside cuff leak test
D. Fiberoptic evaluation around the endotracheal tube (ETT) to visualize the posterior pharynx, larynx, and glottic aperture
E. Fiberoptic evaluation through the ETT to visualize the trachea and proximal bronchi

8. A 35-year-old man with no significant medical history, with the exception of morbid obesity, is currently undergoing elective laparoscopic cholecystectomy for biliary cholic. Five minutes after a routine induction and a smooth intubation, the peak airway pressures rise precipitously and the patient becomes acutely tachycardic and hypotensive. You also note audible wheezes as well as blotchy erythema on his body. Which medication is MOST likely driving these symptoms?

A. Rocuronium
B. Fentanyl
C. Propofol
D. Midazolam
E. Lidocaine

9. **A 24-year-old woman with a medical history of exercise-induced asthma and subsequent use of an albuterol inhaler several times a week is currently undergoing urgent laparoscopic appendectomy. Several minutes after induction, you note increased peak inspiratory pressures and observe diffuse bilateral wheezes and a falling blood pressure. Which of the following is the _best initial_ treatment?**

A. Spray albuterol into the breathing circuit with inspiration.
B. Administer a corticosteroid such as hydrocortisone.
C. Administer IV epinephrine 1 mg.
D. Administer histamine blockers such as Benadryl and ranitidine.
E. Administer IV epinephrine in 50-100 μg divided doses.

10. **A patient undergoing a routine elective inguinal hernia repair suffers from a suspected anaphylactic reaction, which is successfully treated with epinephrine, corticosteroids, and histamine blockers. However, at the end of the case, airway pressures remain elevated, there is evidence of swelling of the oral mucosa, and the decision is made to bring the patient into the ICU intubated. Upon admission to the ICU, the patient appears to be euvolemic by examination but remains hypotensive. After an additional dose of epinephrine, corticosteroids, and histamine blockers, which of the following would be the MOST appropriate next step?**

A. Proceed to extubation, as anaphylaxis rarely requires more than 2 treatments.
B. Trend tryptase levels until they begin to downtrend, then consider extubation.
C. Transition from crystalloid infusion to albumin, as capillary leak is likely to lead to pulmonary edema, which could delay extubation.
D. Begin a low-dose epinephrine infusion and titrate to blood pressure and bronchospasm.
E. Begin a low-dose norepinephrine infusion, as the continued symptoms demonstrate that they are refractory to epinephrine therapy.

11. **Which of the following statements about anaphylaxis is MOST true?**

A. Elevated tryptase levels are pathognomonic of anaphylaxis.
B. The level of severity of cutaneous reaction correlates with the severity of shock with anaphylaxis.
C. The most common causes of intraoperative anaphylaxis are opioids and inhalational anesthetics.
D. Patients suffering from an intraoperative anaphylactic reaction should be monitored in an inpatient unit for 24 hours.
E. Prophylaxis against anaphylaxis allows for the repeated safe use of the offending agent.

12. **A 3-year-old child with fever, dysphagia, and drooling is brought to the emergency department (ED) by the caregiver. Lateral neck X-ray films reveal evidence of a "thumbprint" sign. Which of the following disorders is _highest_ on your differential?**

A. Epiglottitis
B. Croup
C. Tracheal stenosis
D. Tracheoesophageal fistula
E. Tonsillitis

13. **Which organism is MOST associated with epiglottitis?**

    A. Parainfluenza
    B. *Haemophilus influenza*
    C. Group A *Streptococcus*
    D. Group B *Streptococcus*
    E. *Candida albicans*

14. **The 3-year-old patient from question 12, suffering from dysphagia and drooling, is now "tripoding" with increased work of breathing, and the decision is made to proceed to intubation. Which of the following is the *safest* method of securing the airway?**

    A. Proceed to an immediate rapid sequence intubation in the ED via direct laryngoscopy.
    B. Proceed to an intravenous induction in the semirecumbent position in the ED via video laryngoscopy with fiberoptic backup.
    C. Move to an OR for emergent surgical airway.
    D. Proceed to an OR for an emergent rapid sequence intubation with surgeons at the bedside for possible rigid bronchoscopy or surgical airway.
    E. Proceed to an OR for an urgent inhalational induction in the seated position followed by laryngoscopy with surgeons at the bedside for possible rigid bronchoscopy or surgical airway.

15. **You are called to the ED to evaluate an 18-month-old child suffering from a suspected aspiration. The child's parents describe coughing, choking, and a slight bluish tinge to the lips after a meal, including pieces of corn and carrots, rushing to the hospital. The child is now quietly lying down without any outward signs of respiratory distress but with an O_2 saturation of 92%. Which of the following is the MOST appropriate method of caring for this patient?**

    A. Reassure the parents of the child that because it was only small pieces of vegetable and not a larger piece of meat or other protein, and the child is no longer actively coughing, no intervention is required and should simply be monitored in the ED until the O_2 saturation normalizes.
    B. Advise that you are booking an OR for emergent bronchoscopic removal of the aspirate and oral midazolam should be administered immediately to ensure that the child remains calm and does not dislodge the aspirated material.
    C. Ask that antibiotics and steroids be started in the emergency department to be continued for only a 4-day course because this has been shown to be noninferior to a 7-day course.
    D. Take the patient to the OR emergently and complete a gentle inhaled induction to maintain spontaneous ventilation, place a laryngeal mask airway (LMA), and allow a surgeon to pass a flexible fiberoptic bronchoscope through the LMA to remove the aspirated particles.
    E. Take the child to the OR emergently, and after placing a peripheral IV under topical anesthesia with the child on the OR table, proceed with a rapid sequence intubation, securing the airway with an ETT before allowing the surgeon to proceed with flexible or rigid bronchoscopy.

16. **You are called emergently to the bedside of a patient in the ICU after his nurse observed an acute desaturation event. You note the patient had a tracheostomy placed 6 days ago for chronic respiratory failure after a prolonged course of acute respiratory distress syndrome. You arrive at the patient's bedside to find an O_2 saturation of 88%, the trach collar seated against the skin with the pilot balloon inflated, and the patient moving air very noisily through his mouth. The nurse describes that during a coughing fit his trach "fell out," but she was able to push it back in. Which of the following would be the most *inappropriate* next move?**

    A. Place an oxygen mask over the patient's mouth and nose.
    B. Attach an Ambu bag to the trach and support the patient's ventilation.
    C. Remove the trach and cover the ostomy site with a bandage.
    D. Call for a fiberoptic bronchoscope to interrogate the tracheostomy track.
    E. Attach an Ambu bag to a mask, place over the mouth and nose, and support the patient's ventilation.

17. According to the ASA Practice Guidelines for Management of the Difficult Airway, which of the following is the *correct* definition of a difficult airway?

    A. A clinical situation where a physician experiences difficulty with ventilation, intubation, or both.

    B. A clinical situation in which a conventionally trained anesthesiologist requires adjuncts for ventilation and/or advanced airway equipment for intubation.

    C. A clinical situation in which a conventionally trained anesthesiologist fails to ventilate and/or intubate a patient.

    D. A clinical situation in which a conventionally trained anesthesiologist experiences difficulty with facemask ventilation of the upper airway, difficulty with tracheal intubation, or both.

    E. A clinical situation in which a conventionally trained physician experiences difficulty with facemask ventilation, tracheal intubation, or both.

18. Which of the following has NOT been independently associated with challenging mask ventilation?

    A. Edentulousness

    B. Neck circumference >19 cm

    C. BMI >36 kg/m^2

    D. Presence of a beard

    E. Snoring/obstructive sleep apnea (OSA) history

19. According to the ASA Practice Guidelines for Management of the Difficult Airway, which of the following components of the preoperative airway physical examination is *correctly* paired with a nonreassuring finding, as it relates to a potential difficult intubation?

    A. Relationship of maxillary and mandibular incisors during voluntary protrusion of the mandible: inability to bring mandibular incisors anterior to maxillary incisors

    B. Thyromental distance: four ordinary finger breaths

    C. Visibility of uvula: only upper third of uvula visible

    D. Range of motion of the head and neck: inability to rotate chin to each shoulder

    E. Interincisor distance: 5 cm

20. According to the Mallampati classification, if you are able to view the fauces, then the score must be at least which of the following?

    A. Class 0

    B. Class I

    C. Class II

    D. Class III

    E. Class IV

21. Which of the following is MOST correct regarding the Mallampati classification system?

    A. The Mallampati score correlates well with difficulty of mask ventilation.

    B. Phonation increases the specificity of the Mallampati test.

    C. A Mallampati IV classification has a high positive predictive value of difficult direct laryngoscopy.

    D. Ability to visualize lingual tonsils requires a Mallampati IV score.

    E. Partial view of the glottis or arytenoids defines a Mallampati II score.

22. According to the ASA Difficult Airway Algorithm, which of the following is NOT included in the assessment of the likelihood of basic management problems?

    A. Difficulty with patient cooperation

    B. Difficult mask ventilation

    C. Difficult laryngoscopy

    D. Difficult intubation

    E. Difficult extubation

23. **According to the ASA Difficult Airway Algorithm, which of the following *correctly* describes the pathway through the "Awake Intubation" Algorithm?**

   A. The first decision to make is to determine whether invasive airway access or noninvasive intubation will be attempted.
   B. If noninvasive intubation fails, then progress to facemask ventilation.
   C. If noninvasive intubation fails, then consider waking the patient up and canceling the case.
   D. If invasive airway access fails, then consider canceling the case.
   E. If noninvasive intubation is successful, then the patient should be provided with a difficult airway note following the case.

24. **According to the ASA Practice Guidelines for Management of the Difficult Airway, which of the following definitions is MOST correct?**

   A. Failed intubation: inability to place an ETT after a single attempt
   B. Difficult laryngoscopy: failure of direct laryngoscopy and required use of video laryngoscopy or fiberoptic bronchoscopy for successful intubation
   C. Difficult supraglottic airway placement: tracheal pathology making a supraglottic airway seal inadequate
   D. Difficult tracheal intubation: tracheal intubation requiring multiple attempts, with or without tracheal pathology
   E. Difficult facemask ventilation: use of airway adjuncts, including 2-handed mask and oral/nasal airways to achieve adequate ventilation

25. **According to the ASA Difficult Airway Algorithm for intubation after induction of general anesthesia, if initial intubation is unsuccessful and facemask ventilation is not adequate, then which of the following would be the *best* next step?**

   A. Awaken the patient.
   B. Proceed to emergency invasive airway access.
   C. Proceed video-assisted or fiberoptic intubation.
   D. Cancel the case.
   E. Attempt supraglottic airway placement.

26. **According to the ASA Difficult Airway Algorithm, which of the following is NOT considered a noninvasive alternative in the difficult intubation approach?**

   A. Light wand
   B. Intubating LMA
   C. Video-assisted laryngoscopy
   D. Percutaneous jet ventilation
   E. Blind nasal intubation

27. **According to the ASA Practice Guidelines for Management of the Difficult Airway, which of the following is NOT a recommended preformulated strategy for extubation of the difficult airway?**

   A. Long-term intubation until the perioperative period is completed
   B. Short-term use of an airway exchange catheter
   C. Consideration of fully awake extubation
   D. Preparation for postextubation noninvasive ventilation or high-flow oxygen
   E. Extubation to an LMA

28. **Which of the following symptoms is a major indication for tonsillectomy?**

   A. Initial presentation with tonsillitis
   B. Children with valvular cardiac disease at first presentation with tonsillitis
   C. Severe OSA
   D. Recurrent step pharyngitis
   E. Presence of tonsillar stones

29. According to the ASA Practice Guidelines for the Perioperative Management of Patients with OSA, which of the following is recommended for children undergoing tonsillectomy for OSA?

   A. Codeine is superior to nonsteroidal anti-inflammatory drugs for postoperative pain relief.
   B. Sleep studies should be obtained on all children undergoing elective tonsillectomy and/or adenoidectomy.
   C. For children undergoing tonsillectomy for OSA, the task force advises that opioid dosing should be decreased because repeated hypoxemia increases the sensitivity of μ-opioid receptors.
   D. All children undergoing tonsillectomy and/or adenoidectomy for OSA should be watched in a monitored setting for at least 24 hours following surgery.
   E. The ASA Practice Guidelines require the use of noninvasive CPAP in the immediate postoperative setting for all children undergoing tonsillectomy and/or adenoidectomy for OSA.

30. Recent studies have shown that a single intraoperative dose of dexamethasone is associated with all the following EXCEPT which one?

   A. Decreased postoperative pain
   B. Decreased postoperative bleeding
   C. Decreased time to first oral intake
   D. Decreased postoperative nausea and vomiting in the immediate postoperative period
   E. Decreased postoperative nausea and vomiting in the first 24 hours

31. Which of the following is MOST correct regarding posttonsillectomy hemorrhage?

   A. Primary hemorrhage occurs during the tonsillectomy surgery itself, whereas secondary hemorrhage occurs within the first 24 hours.
   B. Posttonsillectomy hemorrhage is a common occurrence and should be treated with maintenance of NPO status and "watchful waiting."
   C. Nearly half of patients suffering from posttonsillectomy hemorrhage have an undiagnosed coagulation disorder.
   D. Posttonsillectomy hemorrhage usually presents as brisk bleeding.
   E. Because of the friable nature of the tonsillar tissue, take-back surgeries for bleeding should be completed under moderate sedation.

32. A 5-year-old child presents to the ED 12 hours posttonsillectomy with bleeding and he appears pale and weak. Which of the following is the next *best* course of action?

   A. Proceed directly to the OR, induce via inhalation, secure IV access, and intubate.
   B. IV access should be secured in the ED with fluid resuscitation before proceeding to the OR.
   C. Proceed directly to the OR, secure IV access, and proceed with the least sedation necessary to allow for hemostasis through electrocautery.
   D. Consult interventional radiology for embolization of the external carotid artery on the side of bleeding.
   E. Manage the patient medically with volume resuscitation and reversal of coagulopathy.

33. Which of the following blocks is correctly matched with the anatomic location of injection of local anesthetic?

   A. Retrobulbar block: extraconal block outside the muscle cone formed by 4 recti muscles
   B. Peribulbar block: intraconal block in the middle of the muscle cone
   C. Median orbital block: in the space between the medial rectus muscle and the medial orbital wall
   D. Superior orbital block: medial to the supraorbital notch and advanced intraconal
   E. Subtenon block: in the space between the conjunctiva and subtenon capsule

34. **Which of the following correctly describes the pathway involved with the oculocardiac reflex?**

    Afferent Nerve → Center → Efferent Nerve

    A. Cranial nerve V → medulla → cranial nerve X
    B. Cranial nerve V → medulla → cardiac accelerator fibers
    C. Cranial nerve VII → midbrain → cervical parasympathetics
    D. Cranial nerve VII → medulla → cranial nerve V
    E. Cranial nerve V → pons → cervical parasympathetics

35. **Which of the following complications of ophthalmic regional anesthesia is *correctly* paired?**

    A. Optic nerve sheath injection: retinal detachment/loss of vision
    B. Intra-arterial injection: loss of vision
    C. Globe penetration/injection: epidural injection
    D. Extraocular muscle injury: diplopia
    E. Trauma to the optic nerve: local anesthetic toxicity, seizure activity

36. **Which of the following ophthalmic medications is *correctly* paired with its side effect or anesthetic complication?**

    A. Epinephrine topical solution: reflex bradycardia
    B. Echothiophate: increased longevity of succinylcholine
    C. Cyclopentolate: sedation
    D. Acetazolamide: metabolic alkalosis
    E. Sulfur hexafluoride: nitrous oxide is not contraindicated

37. **Which of the following ophthalmic medications is *correctly* paired with its side effect or anesthetic complication?**

    A. Dipivefrin hydrochloride: trigger angle-closure glaucoma attack
    B. Phenylephrine topical solution: reflex tachycardia
    C. Timolol: meiosis
    D. Apraclonidine: agitation
    E. Scopolamine topical solution: sedation in the elderly

38. **Which of the following medications, when administered intravenously, is MOST associated with increased ocular pressure?**

    A. Midazolam
    B. Ketamine
    C. Propofol
    D. Dexmedetomidine
    E. Etomidate

39. **Which of the following can *increase* intraocular pressure (IOP)?**

    A. Hypoxia
    B. Hypotension
    C. Hypothermia
    D. Hyperventilation
    E. Enhanced venous outflow

40. **A 17-year-old boy presents to the ED with an open globe injury after being hit in the eye by a line drive while playing baseball. He had a hot dog just before sustaining his injury. Which of the following statements is MOST correct with regard to attempting to prevent increased ocular pressure with the induction of general anesthesia?**

A. Benzodiazepine premedication is contraindicated.

B. Succinylcholine should be avoided at all cost.

C. Awake fiberoptic intubation with minimal sedation or topicalization is the "gold standard" approach.

D. Direct pressure to the globe by an assistant should be provided during direct laryngoscopy to limit any extrusion of vitreal contents.

E. Every effort should be made to limit Valsalva or coughing during intubation.

41. **Which of the following statements is MOST correct concerning the anesthetic implication of sulfur hexafluoride injection for retinal detachment?**

A. Nitrous oxide is contraindicated following injection with sulfur hexafluoride; however, it is safe to use with octafluoropropane.

B. Nitrous oxide should be discontinued 15-20 minutes before injection of gas into the globe.

C. At least a 30-day safety margin should be given before nitrous oxide is used for a patient who received an unknown intraocular gas injection.

D. The worst complication of nitrous oxide use with an intraocular gas bubble is transient diplopia.

E. At least a 15-day safety margin should be given before nitrous oxide is used for a patient who received an intraocular air injection.

42. **When considering surgical placement of a cochlear implant, which of the following is MOST important regarding the anesthetic management?**

A. Nitrous oxide is absolutely contraindicated.

B. Conscious sedation is the preferred technique.

C. Regional block and local anesthetic infiltration provide superior surgical outcomes.

D. Patient immobility is paramount.

E. Mean arterial pressures should be maintained at greater than 65 mm Hg to ensure middle ear perfusion during mastoidotomy.

43. **A 55-year-old woman is in the second hour of a middle ear exploration with eventual stapedotomy. Current vital signs are as follows: HR 85, BP 145/83, RR 16, Spo_2 99%, and $ETco_2$ 40 mm Hg. The current anesthetic is a propofol/remifentanil total IV anesthetic. The surgeon reports "more bleeding" than she expected and asks for your assistance in reducing the blood loss. Which of the following strategies is MOST likely to be effective in limiting surgical bleeding?**

A. Increase the respiratory rate on the ventilator to reduce $Paco_2$.

B. Add nitrous oxide to the anesthetic.

C. Add paralytic to the anesthetic.

D. Lower BP through deepening the plane of propofol anesthesia or adding an antihypertensive agent.

E. Place the patient in Trendelenburg position.

44. **You are giving a lunch break for a fellow anesthesiologist who has been taking care of a 32-year-old otherwise healthy man who is undergoing functional endoscopic sinus surgery. About 10 minutes into the break, the surgeon notes that "there is too much bleeding" and places some fluid-saturated sponges into the nasal passage. Several minutes later, you note that the blood pressure cuff cycles several times before reading 220/110, the patient's heart rate has increased to 130 beats per minute, and there are depressions of the ST segments on the intraoperative ECG. Which of the following treatments is MOST likely to improve the patient's condition?**

A. Administration of Dantrolene 1 mg/kg bolus followed by 0/25 mg/kg/h infusion

B. Administration of an intralipid 2.5 mg/kg bolus

C. Transition from a propofol/remifentanil total IV anesthetic to inhalational anesthesia

D. Administration of an intravenous β-blocker

E. Deepening the plane of anesthesia

45. Which of the following is an advantage of a deep extubation versus a normal emergence and extubation following fiberoptic endoscopic sinus surgery?

   A. There is a lower incidence of laryngospasm.
   B. Time to discharge is decreased.
   C. It is associated with decreased postoperative opioid use.
   D. It can facilitate extubation with minimal movement or bucking.
   E. It allows for less intensive postoperative nursing care.

46. You are assigned to give a break to another anesthesiologist just beginning a routine tonsillectomy for a 4-year-old child under general anesthesia with a cuff-less polyvinyl chloride (PVC) ETT. The surgeon is utilizing electrocautery, and you note that the Fio_2 is still 95%. Which of the following is the *best* action to take?

   A. Immediately reduce the fresh gas flow to 2 L and turn off the sevoflurane inhalational anesthetic.
   B. Ask the surgeon to turn down the intensity of the electrocautery until the Fio_2 is below 30%.
   C. Immediately tell the surgeon to cease using electrocautery until the Fio_2 is below 30%.
   D. Allow the surgeon to continue, but turn the oxygen dial to 0 and increase the air dial to maximum, disconnect the circuit from the ETT, occlude the end of the circuit, and "flush" it with multiple manual compressions of the reservoir bag.
   E. Remove the PVC ETT and exchange it for an armored ETT.

47. According to the American Society of Anesthesiologists Practice Advisory for the Prevention and Management of Operating Room Fires, the proper management of a *nonairway* fire includes all of the following EXCEPT which one?

   A. Remove the drapes and all burning and flammable materials from the patient.
   B. Stop the flow of all airway gases immediately.
   C. Remove the ETT.
   D. Extinguish flames by pouring saline or smothering.
   E. If burning persists, utilize a CO_2 fire extinguisher.

48. An airway fire has just occurred in an adjacent OR where 100% O_2 was being used for laser surgery of the vocal cords with a normal PVC ETT, and you are asked to provide assistance. When you arrive, the fire has been put out, there is a burnt and mangled ETT by the anesthesia machine, and the patient is being bag masked on room air. Which of the following describes the *best* immediate management for this patient?

   A. Order a STAT chest X-ray (CXR) in the OR to assess for inhalational injury.
   B. Travel to the CT scanner to assess for ETT remnants in the airway.
   C. Begin high-volume saline lavage of the lungs.
   D. Immediately switch to low Fio_2 to avoid further oxygen toxicity.
   E. Proceed to rigid or flexible bronchoscopy to assess for plastic remnants and thermal or smoke injury.

49. Which of the following is MOST closely linked to OR fires caused by inhalational anesthetics?

   A. Use of xenon inhalational anesthesia
   B. Use of high Fio_2
   C. A preceding period of ventilator inactivity
   D. High humidity in the breathing circuit
   E. Concomitant use of nitrous oxide

50. **According to the American Society of Anesthesiologists: "Practice advisory for the prevention and management of operating room fires," which of the following is considered a *best* practice?**

A. For every case the entire OR team should take part in determining whether a significant fire risk exists and should jointly take active roles in mitigating the risk of fire.

B. High Fio_2 at high flows should be used for sedation procedures to lessen the risk of oxygen accumulation under the drapes.

C. Nitrous oxide should be used as an anesthetic adjunct to mitigate the fire risk of 100% Fio_2.

D. Unipolar electrocautery should be used ahead of bipolar electrocautery to mitigate the risk of fire.

E. If an airway fire is suspected, the ETT should be left in place until rigid bronchoscopy can be used to ensure that the tube is removed intact.

Chapter 18 ▪ Answers

1. Correct answer: B

The infant larynx is located around C3-C4 in the neck, whereas the adult larynx is located around C5-C6 in the neck, making B the correct answer.

Answer choice A is incorrect because of the increased tongue to mouth ratio in infants that causes them to breathe mainly through their nose for the first few months of life.

Answer choice C is incorrect because the infant's epiglottis is narrower, longer, and more "omegoid" shaped compared with the adult's epiglottis.

The narrowest portion of the upper airway in an adult is at the level of the vocal cords. There is some controversy about the narrowest portion of the upper airway in infants; however, the most commonly accepted historical studies and dogma name the cricoid ring as the narrowest portion of the upper airway. These same studies describe the infant airway as conically shaped, although this too has been questioned in more recent studies. For these reasons, and for the purposes of the boards, answer choice D is incorrect.

The head to body ratio of infants is larger than that of adults, meaning that they do not require elevation of the head but rather sometime elevation of the shoulders to achieve an optimal "sniffing" position. For this reason, answer choice E is incorrect.

References:

1. Lerman J. Pediatric anesthesia. In: Barash PG, Cullen BF, Stoelting RK, et al, eds. Clinical Anesthesia. 7th ed. Philadelphia: Lippincott; 2013:1216–1256.
2. Everett LL. Anesthesia for children. In: Longnecker DE, Brown DL, Newman MF, et al, eds. Anesthesiology. 2nd ed. New York: McGraw Hill; 2012:1182–1193.

2. Correct answer: A

Answer choice B is incorrect because infiltration of local anesthetic into the base of the palatoglossal arch will block the lingual and pharyngeal branches of the glossopharyngeal nerve, which innervate the posterior third of the tongue and oropharynx. The lingual nerve is a branch of the trigeminal nerve and has no sensory branches to the airway.

Answer choice C is incorrect because injection of local anesthetic 1 cm below the greater cornu of the hyoid bone would block the superior laryngeal nerve, not the inferior laryngeal nerve.

Answer choice D is incorrect because a transtracheal block only reliably numbs sensation below the level of the epiglottis, as only a small amount of local anesthetic can be coughed into the supraglottic space, which is not enough to provide adequate numbing of the oropharynx for an awake fiberoptic intubation.

Innervation of the oropharynx is complex, relying on branches of the facial, vagus, and glossopharyngeal nerves. Because of this complex innervation, blockade through injection of local anesthetic is challenging. Topicalization through aerosolized, gargled, or sprayed on local anesthetic is usually an easier method of numbing the oropharynx. For these reasons, answer choice E is incorrect.

References:

1. Rosenblatt WH, Sukhupragarn W. Airway management. In: Barash PG, Cullen BF, Stoelting RK, et al, eds. Clinical Anesthesia. 7th ed. Philadelphia: Lippincott; 2013:762–802.
2. Klock PA, Hernandez M, Seraphin S. Airway management. In: Longnecker DE, Brown DL, Newman MF, et al, eds. Anesthesiology. 2nd ed. New York: McGraw Hill; 2012:546–576.
3. Larson CP. Airway management. In: Morgan GE, Mikhail MS, Murray MJ, eds. Morgan & Mikhail's Clinical Anesthesiology. 4th ed. New York: McGraw Hill; 2006:104–147

3. Correct answer: C

Answer choice A is incorrect because this description is consistent with complete bilateral recurrent laryngeal nerve injury, which is unlikely, given the description of the surgery performed. A complete bilateral recurrent laryngeal nerve injury causes loss of both abduction and adduction; therefore this rarely causes difficult ventilation.

Answer choice B is incorrect because this description is consistent with incomplete bilateral recurrent laryngeal nerve injury, which is also unlikely, given the description of the surgery performed. An incomplete bilateral recurrent laryngeal nerve injury can cause unopposed adduction and is thus potentially an emergent surgical airway situation.

Answer choice D is the opposite examination as would be expected from a suspected left recurrent laryngeal nerve injury.

Answer choice E is incorrect because this description is consistent with a central process such as a cerebral infarct or complete vagus nerve injury.

References:
1. Rosenblatt WH, Sukhupragarn W. Airway management. In: Barash PG, Cullen BF, Stoelting RK, et al, eds. Clinical Anesthesia. 7th ed. Philadelphia: Lippincott; 2013:762–802.
2. Klock PA, Hernandez M, Seraphin S. Airway management. In: Longnecker DE, Brown DL, Newman MF, et al, eds. Anesthesiology. 2nd ed. New York: McGraw Hill; 2012:546–576.

4. Correct answer: E

In this question, the patient has just been induced and becomes profoundly bradycardic after microlaryngoscopy and suspension by an ENT surgeon. This phenomenon is usually attributable to laryngeal manipulation in a lightly anesthetized patient, leading to a reflex arc between the superior laryngeal nerve and vagal cardioinhibitory fibers.

Increasing the depth of the anesthesia (answer choice A) and administration of a β-blocker or opioid (answer choice B) could blunt the response to suspension microlaryngoscopy, and administering glycopyrrolate (answer choice C) could inhibit vagal tone, leading to recovery from bradycardia; however, none of these choices are very fast acting.

Only answer choice E, directing the surgeon to take the patient out of suspension, would quickly eliminate the stimulation driving the reflex arc and give time to administer medications as discussed above before proceeding with further attempts at suspension.

Answer choice D is incorrect because, although the reflex arc mediating the bradycardia should lessen with time, the immediate effects of bradycardia and likely hypotension must be immediately intervened upon.

Reference:
1. Ragan B. Anesthesia for otorhinolaryngologic (ear, nose, and throat) surgery. In: Longnecker DE, Brown DL, Newman MF, et al, eds. Anesthesiology. 2nd ed. New York: McGraw Hill; 2012:1226–1247.

5. Correct answer: E

Answer choices A, B, C, and D are incorrect because each has very important consideration for low-frequency jet ventilation.

Answer choice E is correct because low-frequency jet ventilation is typically not used as an "assist" form of ventilation and has no ability to synchronize with a patient's ventilatory efforts. Additionally, suspension microlaryngoscopy requires precise surgical movement, which typically requires minimal movements and immobility of the respiratory muscles.

Reference:
1. Weiss SJ, Ochroch EA. Thoracic anesthesia. In: Longnecker DE, Brown DL, Newman MF, et al, eds. Anesthesiology. 2nd ed. New York: McGraw Hill; 2012:950–1008.

6. Correct answer: A

Answer choice A is correct because immobility is essential during microlaryngoscopy to ensure that surgical micromanipulation does not lead to iatrogenic injury.

Answer choice B is incorrect because, contrary to video nasal fiberoptic visualization of the glottis during phonation where light sedation is necessary to allow patient interaction, suspension microlaryngoscopy is extremely stimulating and requires a full anesthetic.

Answer choice C is incorrect because microlaryngoscopy is rarely a bloody procedure and permissive hypotension is not necessary.

Answer choice D is incorrect because suspension microlaryngoscopy often leads to vagal discharge and bradycardia. Additional β-blockade could be detrimental.

Answer choice E is incorrect because microlaryngoscopy, while stimulating intraoperatively, rarely produces significant pain postoperatively.

Reference:

1. Ragan B. Anesthesia for otorhinolaryngologic (ear, nose, and throat) surgery. In: Longnecker DE, Brown DL, Newman MF, et al, eds. Anesthesiology. 2nd ed. New York: McGraw Hill; 2012:1226–1247.

7. Correct answer: D

Answer choice A is incorrect because, although an upright X-ray of the neck can be helpful in determining tracheal patency, it is unlikely to be helpful in assessing swelling at the level of the epiglottis and above.

Answer choice B is incorrect because, although a CT of the neck could provide information on the patency of the airway around the ETT and allow for assessment of the status of submandibular abscess, it is a large expenditure of resources, requires travel outside of the ICU, and is impractical for serial assessment over hours to days.

Answer choice B is incorrect because, although a cuff leak provides some assurance that the airway is not so edematous as to be closed around the ETT, the lack of a cuff leak does not necessarily mean that there would be occlusive airway edema following removal of the ETT because of the low specificity of the test.

Fiberoptic evaluation of the posterior pharynx, larynx, and glottic aperture allows for direct visualization of the airway, assessment of any edema present, and assessment of airspace around the ETT at the level of the glottis. Fiberoptic evaluation is also cost-effective, can be readily done at the bedside, and can be repeated serially.

Although answer choice E would allow for assessment of the airway distal to the ETT (only marginal views through the ETT are usually possible because the fiberoptic scope is advanced down the tube), the area of interest for this patient is in the upper airway.

Reference:

1. Klock PA, Hernandez M, Seraphin S. Airway management. In: Longnecker DE, Brown DL, Newman MF, et al, eds. Anesthesiology. 2nd ed. New York: McGraw Hill; 2012:546–576.

8. Correct answer: A

This question describes a patient suffering from a suspected anaphylactic reaction, with symptoms including bronchospasm, rash, tachycardia, and hypotension. Neuromuscular blockading agents, especially the aminosteroids, are historically the worst offending medication for inducing allergic reactions during anesthesia.

Although there are case reports supporting almost all anesthetic medications inducing anaphylaxis, neuromuscular blocking agents and antibiotics are the most likely offending agents. In addition, although fentanyl has been associated with chest wall rigidity, decreased pulmonary compliance, and increased peak inspiratory pressures, it is less likely that rocuronium produce an allergic reaction.

References:

1. Levy JH. The allergic response. In: Barash PG, Cullen BF, Stoelting RK, et al, eds. Clinical Anesthesia. 7th ed. Philadelphia: Lippincott; 2013:287–303.
2. Holzman RS. Anaphylactic reactions and anesthesia. In: Longnecker DE, Brown DL, Newman MF, et al, eds. Anesthesiology. 2nd ed. New York: McGraw Hill; 2012:1478–1490.

9. Correct answer: E

The constellation of symptoms including increased airway pressures, wheezes, and hypotension support the diagnosis of anaphylaxis. Epinephrine, in addition to corticosteroids and histamine blockers, is the gold standard treatment for anaphylaxis because it has efficacy across multiple fronts.

The mechanism of action of epinephrine includes the following:

α1-Receptor agonism: increased peripheral vasoconstriction and decreased mucosal edema

β1-Receptor agonism: increased inotropy and chronotropy

β2-Receptor agonism: decreased bronchoconstriction and stabilization of mast cells and basophils, which are responsible for the symptoms generated by anaphylactic (IgE-mediated) and anaphylactoid (non-IgE-mediated) reactions

Answer choice A is incorrect because, although albuterol might transiently improve airway constriction, epinephrine is far more potent and can also treat the other symptoms associated with anaphylaxis including hypotension.

Answer choice B is incorrect because, although corticosteroids are one of the pillars of anaphylaxis treatment, they can take hours to reach full effect and are aimed at preventing protracted reactions or biphasic reactions.

Answer choice C is incorrect because epinephrine 1 mg is the ACLS "code" dose and is inappropriately high for the treatment of hypotension and airway constriction. A more appropriate starting dose would be in the range of 50-100 µg to treat these symptoms.

Answer choice D is incorrect because, although histamine blockers are a pillar of anaphylaxis treatment, they will do little to resolve bronchospasm and hypotension.

References:
1. Levy JH. The allergic response. In: Barash PG, Cullen BF, Stoelting RK, et al, eds. Clinical Anesthesia. 7th ed. Philadelphia: Lippincott; 2013:287–303.
2. Holzman RS. Anaphylactic reactions and anesthesia. In: Longnecker DE, Brown DL, Newman MF, et al, eds. Anesthesiology. 2nd ed. New York: McGraw Hill; 2012:1478–1490.
3. Campbell RL, Kelso JM. Anaphylaxis: Emergency Treatment. 2017. www.UpToDate.com.

10. Correct answer: D

This patient is displaying symptoms of continued anaphylaxis, sometimes referred to as recrudescence or a biphasic response.

Answer choice A is incorrect because symptoms of anaphylaxis can continue for a prolonged period, and extubation should not be entertained until there is no longer any risk of airway edema.

Answer choice B is incorrect because, although drawing a tryptase level within 4 hours of suspected anaphylaxis can be helpful in retrospectively diagnosing anaphylaxis, there is no proven utility in trending tryptase levels to monitor for resolution.

Answer choice C is incorrect because, although volume repletion is an important aspect in the early treatment of anaphylaxis, the patient appears euvolemic on examination and continued epinephrine therapy would be more appropriate.

Answer choice E is incorrect because continued epinephrine therapy is the most appropriate treatment for refractory anaphylaxis. Norepinephrine would likely produce less effective inotropy and peripheral vasoconstriction and none of the mast cell and basophil stabilization effects of epinephrine.

References:
1. Levy JH. The allergic response. In: Barash PG, Cullen BF, Stoelting RK, et al, eds. Clinical Anesthesia. 7th ed. Philadelphia: Lippincott; 2013:287–303.
2. Holzman RS. Anaphylactic reactions and anesthesia. In: Longnecker DE, Brown DL, Newman MF, et al, eds. Anesthesiology. 2nd ed. New York: McGraw Hill; 2012:1478–1490.
3. Campbell RL, Kelso JM. Anaphylaxis: Emergency Treatment. 2017. www.UpToDate.com.

11. Correct answer: D

Answer choice A is incorrect because, although elevated tryptase levels are associated with anaphylaxis and support its diagnosis, tryptase in itself is a nonspecific enzyme marker of mast cell activation and degranulation.

Answer choice B is incorrect because anaphylaxis can occur without cutaneous manifestations. Severe anaphylactic shock is often associated without any rash or wheals.

Answer choice C is incorrect because the most common causes of intraoperative anaphylaxis (in approximate order of descending occurrence) include latex, neuromuscular blockers, antibiotics, transfusion, local anesthetics, and opioids. Of note, although inhalational anesthetics can induce malignant hyperthermia, they rarely are the cause of anaphylaxis.

Answer choice D is correct because even after anaphylaxis is treated, there is a risk of recrudescence or second phase of symptoms, making monitoring essential.

Answer choice E is incorrect because, although prophylaxis against lower-level allergic reactions (as with isolated rashes against IV contrast dye) can allow for the subsequent safe use of the agent, there is no safe prophylaxis against anaphylaxis save avoiding the offending agent.

References:
1. Levy JH. The allergic response. In: Barash PG, Cullen BF, Stoelting RK, et al, eds. Clinical Anesthesia. 7th ed. Philadelphia: Lippincott; 2013:287–303.

2. Holzman RS. Anaphylactic reactions and anesthesia. In: Longnecker DE, Brown DL, Newman MF, et al, eds. Anesthesiology. 2nd ed. New York: McGraw Hill; 2012:1478–1490.

3. Kemp SF. *Pathophysiology of Anaphylaxis*. 2017. www.UpToDate.com.

12. Correct answer: A

The "thumbprint" sign is a radiographic finding of a flattened, thickened epiglottis on lateral neck X-ray suggestive of epiglottitis. Dysphagia, drooling, and "tripoding" (leaning forward on knees with arms extended, allowing gravity to help pull the inflamed and edematous epiglottis away from the glottic aperture) are classic signs and symptoms of epiglottitis.

Answer choice B is incorrect because croup is usually associated with a "barking" cough and can readily be distinguished clinically from epiglottitis. In addition, a lateral neck X-ray would be of limited value in this diagnosis.

Answer choice C is incorrect because tracheal stenosis would more likely present with stridor and CXR would show tracheal narrowing in the subglottic region.

Answer choice D is incorrect because tracheoesophageal fistula is usually suggested by clinical findings of difficult feeding or breathing early in life and is better assessed through fiberoptic evaluation or CT scan.

Answer choice E is incorrect because the symptoms of tonsillitis, including pain and upper airway obstruction, do not fit the signs and symptoms presented here.

References:

1. Ferrari LR, Nargozian C. Anesthesia for otolaryngologic surgery. In: Barash PG, Cullen BF, Stoelting RK, et al, eds. Clinical Anesthesia. 7th ed. Philadelphia: Lippincott; 2013:1356–1372.

2. Ragan B. Anesthesia for otorhinolaryngologic (ear, nose, and throat) surgery. In: Longnecker DE, Brown DL, Newman MF, et al, eds. Anesthesiology. 2nd ed. New York: McGraw Hill; 2012:1226–1247.

13. Correct answer: B

Answer choice A is incorrect because parainfluenza is mostly associated with croup.

Answer choice B is correct because *Haemophilus influenzae* is mostly associated with epiglottitis.

Answer choice C is incorrect because group A *Streptococcus* is mostly associated with strep pharyngitis.

Answer choice D is incorrect because group B *Streptococcus* is mostly associated with vaginal flora and is an infection risk for an infant during delivery.

Answer choice E is incorrect because *Candida albicans* is mostly associated with thrush when found in the oral cavity.

References:

1. Ferrari LR, Nargozian C. Anesthesia for otolaryngologic surgery. In: Barash PG, Cullen BF, Stoelting RK, et al, eds. Clinical Anesthesia. 7th ed. Philadelphia: Lippincott; 2013:1356–1372.

2. Ragan B. Anesthesia for otorhinolaryngologic (ear, nose, and throat) surgery. In: Longnecker DE, Brown DL, Newman MF, et al, eds. Anesthesiology. 2nd ed. New York: McGraw Hill; 2012:1226–1247.

14. Correct answer: E

This patient, suffering from suspected epiglottitis, has increased work of breathing and is at imminent threat of complete airway obstruction. The patient requires urgent intubation; however, the question of where the safest place for this to occur is at the heart of the question.

Answer choice A is incorrect because for the moment the patient has a patent airway and proceeding to a rapid sequence induction intubation in the ED, without the advanced airway equipment and surgical backup present in the OR, represents an undue risk.

Answer choice B is similarly incorrect because it does not address the critical need of surgical backup.

Answer choice C is incorrect because, although it calls for the patient to be transported to an OR, it calls for the immediate progression to a surgical airway, which is not necessarily required at this time.

Answer choices D and E depict very similar sequences of events and only differ in their method of induction. Answer choice E is the better answer because it allows for induction through spontaneous ventilation and maintenance of a patent airway for as long as possible.

References:

1. Ferrari LR, Nargozian C. Anesthesia for otolaryngologic surgery. In: Barash PG, Cullen BF, Stoelting RK, et al, eds. Clinical Anesthesia. 7th ed. Philadelphia: Lippincott; 2013:1356–1372.

2. Ragan B. Anesthesia for otorhinolaryngologic (ear, nose, and throat) surgery. In: Longnecker DE, Brown DL, Newman MF, et al, eds. Anesthesiology. 2nd ed. New York: McGraw Hill; 2012:1226–1247.

15. Correct answer: D

Answer choice A is incorrect for several reasons. Vegetable aspirates can increase in volume because they absorb moisture from the respiratory tract, thus leading to higher levels of occlusion over time. Vegetable aspirates can also break apart with coughing and thus lead to multiple occlusions. Leaving foreign bodies in the airway also predisposes the patient to postobstructive pneumonias. In addition, although the child is no longer coughing and choking, the O_2 saturation of 92% suggests that oxygenation is impaired. For these reasons, it is important to remove vegetable aspirates as soon as possible.

Although it may seem like sedating a child to lessen the risk of agitation, which can lead to dislodging, and migration of the aspirate sounds like an appropriate plan, it is potentially contraindicated. No sedating medication should be given to a patient with aspiration before being in a controlled environment with full airway and surgical instrumentation present. For these reasons, answer choice B is incorrect.

Answer choice C is incorrect because no further routine medical therapy, including antibiotics and steroids, after removal of the aspirated material has been shown to have benefit. A few caveats to this exist, however: If there is evidence of a postobstructive pneumonia, then antibiotic therapy is appropriate; and if there is evidence of airway mucosal inflammation and edema from the aspiration event or bronchoscopic removal, then steroid therapy has a role.

Answer choice D is the correct answer because the sequence of events allows for maintenance of spontaneous ventilation for as long as possible until the aspirate can be removed.

Answer choice E is incorrect because most pediatric anesthesiologists advocate for an inhalational induction in a cooperative patient and avoidance of positive pressure ventilation, which might convert a partial obstruction to a complete obstruction.

References:
1. Ferrari LR, Nargozian C. Anesthesia for otolaryngologic surgery. In: Barash PG, Cullen BF, Stoelting RK, et al, eds. Clinical Anesthesia. 7th ed. Philadelphia: Lippincott; 2013:1356–1372.
2. Ragan B. Anesthesia for otorhinolaryngologic (ear, nose, and throat) surgery. In: Longnecker DE, Brown DL, Newman MF, et al, eds. Anesthesiology. 2nd ed. New York: McGraw Hill; 2012:1226–1247.

16. Correct answer: B

In this question, the patient has a tracheostomy tube in place, which has acutely come partially (or completely) out of the airway during a coughing fit. The nurse was able to push the trach back in; however, there is concern that it might be malpositioned. Evidence for this is that the patient is noted to be moving air through his mouth, which should not be possible if the trach were properly positioned in the trachea with the cuff inflated. It should be noted that when a patient has a "fresh" tracheostomy tube (0-72 h) and it becomes dislodged, or falls out, it should not be "pushed back in" blindly, given the risk of creating a false passage.

Answer choice A is a possible correct move (and thus an incorrect answer to this question), given that the patient is only moving air through the upper airway, and thus providing supplemental oxygen via this route would be supportive.

Answer choice B would be an incorrect move (and thus the correct answer to this question), given that there is concern for trach malposition. If the trach was not in the trachea, then ventilating through the Ambu bag could push air into the mediastinum, causing tension physiology.

Answer choice C is a possible correct move (and thus an incorrect answer to this question) because removing the trach from its malpositioned site could allow for better air movement through the larynx and trachea.

Answer choice D is a possible correct move (and thus an incorrect answer to this question) because a fiberoptic bronchoscope could be used to interrogate the tracheostomy track and aid in successful repositioning into the tracheal lumen.

Answer choice E is a possible correct move (and thus an incorrect answer to this question) because supporting ventilation through the patent upper airway could improve oxygenation.

Reference:
1. Ragan B. Anesthesia for otorhinolaryngologic (ear, nose, and throat) surgery. In: Longnecker DE, Brown DL, Newman MF, et al, eds. Anesthesiology. 2nd ed. New York: McGraw Hill; 2012:1226–1247.

Planning for a difficult airway/Difficult Airway Algorithm (17-27)

17. Correct answer: D

The ASA Practice Guidelines for Management of the Difficult Airway: An Updated Report by the American Society of Anesthesiologists Task Force on Management of the Difficult Airway defines difficult airway as a clinical situation in which a conventionally trained anesthesiologist experiences difficulty with facemask ventilation of the upper airway, difficulty with tracheal intubation, or both (answer choice D).

Reference:

1. Apfelbaum JL, Hagberg CA, Caplan RA, et al. Practice guidelines for management of the difficult airway: an updated report by the American Society of Anesthesiologists Task Force on Management of the Difficult Airway. *Anesthesiology*. 2013;118(2).

18. Correct answer: B

Patient characteristics associated with challenging mask ventilation have been extensively studied. Lack of teeth (answer choice A), obesity (answer choice C), facial hair (answer choice D), and snoring/OSA history (answer choice E) have all been associated with challenging mask ventilation.

Answer choice B is incorrect because, although increased neck circumference is associated with challenging intubation, it has not been shown to be independently associated with challenging mask ventilation.

References:

1. Apfelbaum JL, Hagberg CA, Caplan RA, et al. Practice guidelines for management of the difficult airway: an updated report by the American Society of Anesthesiologists Task Force on Management of the Difficult Airway. *Anesthesiology*. 2013;118(2).
2. Sweitzer BJ, Pilla M. Overview of preoperative assessment and management. In: Longnecker DE, Brown DL, Newman MF, et al, eds. Anesthesiology. 2nd ed. New York: McGraw Hill; 2012:52–75.

19. Correct answer: A

Answer choice A is correct because an inability to prognath the lower jaw is associated with possible difficult intubation.

Answer choice B is incorrect because a thyromental distance of less than 3 ordinary finger breaths would be a nonreassuring finding.

Answer choice C is incorrect because ability to view the uvula is at least a Mallampati II. A nonreassuring finding would be inability to visualize any portion of the uvula (Mallampati > II).

Answer choice D is incorrect because flexion/extension of the head and neck is far more correlated with difficult intubations compared with rotation. A nonreassuring finding on physical examination would be that patients cannot extend their neck or touch their chin to their chest.

Answer choice E is incorrect because smaller mouth openings are associated with difficult intubations. A nonreassuring finding would be an interincisor distance of less than 3 cm.

References:

1. Apfelbaum JL, Hagberg CA, Caplan RA, et al. Practice guidelines for management of the difficult airway: an updated report by the American Society of Anesthesiologists Task Force on Management of the Difficult Airway. *Anesthesiology*. 2013;118(2).
2. Sweitzer BJ, Pilla M. Overview of preoperative assessment and management. In: Longnecker DE, Brown DL, Newman MF, et al, eds. Anesthesiology. 2nd ed. New York: McGraw Hill; 2012:52–75.

20. Correct answer: C

The Mallampati classification system was originally proposed by Mallampati and Samsoon to describe visual examination of the upper airway and correlate these findings with difficulty of rigid bronchoscopy. This classification system has been extended to correlate with the difficulty of laryngoscopy. To perform the visual examination for this classification system, patients are asked to maximally open their mouth and protrude their tongue. Of note, although the visual recognition of Mallampati classifications is well known to anesthesiologists, their written descriptions are sometime challenging. The classification system is described below:

- Class 0 (not in original classification): ability to visualize any portion of the epiglottis
- Class I: ability to visualize the soft palate, uvula, fauces, and pillars
- Class II: ability to visualize the soft palate, fauces, and pillars
- Class III: ability to visualize only the soft palate
- Class IV (not in original classification): soft palate not visible

References:
1. Hata TM, Hata JS. Preoperative patient assessment and management. In: Barash PG, Cullen BF, Stoelting RK, et al, eds. Clinical Anesthesia. 7th ed. Philadelphia: Lippincott; 2013:583–611.
2. Phero JC, Patil YJ, Hurford WE. Evaluation of the patient with a difficult airway. In: Longnecker DE, Brown DL, Newman MF, et al, eds. Anesthesiology. 2nd ed. New York: McGraw Hill; 2012:118–129.

21. Correct answer: B

Answer choice A is incorrect because, although the Mallampati score correlates with difficulty of direct laryngoscopy and intubation, it does not correlate with ability to mask ventilate.

Answer choice B is correct because subsequent studies have shown that the Mallampati test is effort-dependent and phonation improves both mouth opening and tongue protrusion.

Answer choice C is incorrect because, although increasing Mallampati scores are correlated with increased relative risks of difficult intubation (>11 times greater risk for Mallampati IV compared with Mallampati I), difficult intubations remain relatively rare events. In retrospective studies, only approximately 6% of Mallampati IV scores turned out to be difficult intubations.

Answer choice D is incorrect because lingual tonsils are not part of the Mallampati classification, as they cannot be seen by simple external visual examination of the airway. Lingual tonsils have been associated with "cannot ventilate, cannot intubate" scenarios, making their discovery on direct laryngoscopy a potential airway emergency.

Answer choice E is incorrect because a partial view of the glottis or arytenoids describes a Cormack and Lehane laryngoscopic view, not a Mallampati external visual examination view.

References:
1. Hata TM, Hata JS. Preoperative patient assessment and management. In: Barash PG, Cullen BF, Stoelting RK, et al, eds. Clinical Anesthesia. 7th ed. Philadelphia: Lippincott; 2013:583–611.
2. Phero JC, Patil YJ, Hurford WE. Evaluation of the patient with a difficult airway. In: Longnecker DE, Brown DL, Newman MF, et al, eds. Anesthesiology. 2nd ed. New York: McGraw Hill; 2012:118–129.

22. Correct answer: E

The ASA Difficult Airway Algorithm outlines assessment of the likelihood and clinical impact of basic management of the following problems: difficulty with patient cooperation or consent (answer choice A); difficult mask ventilation (answer choice B), difficult supraglottic airway placement; difficult laryngoscopy (answer choice C); difficult intubation (answer choice D); and difficult surgical airway access. Difficult extubation (answer choice E) is not included in the Difficult Airway Algorithm; however, it is addressed in the ASA Practice Guidelines for Management of the Difficult Airway.

Reference:
1. Apfelbaum JL, Hagberg CA, Caplan RA, et al. Practice guidelines for management of the difficult airway: an updated report by the American Society of Anesthesiologists Task Force on Management of the Difficult Airway. Anesthesiology. 2013;118(2).

23. Correct answer: A

Answer choice A is correct because the first step in the Awake Intubation Algorithm is to determine if the airway is to be approached by noninvasive intubation or by invasive airway access (surgical airway, percutaneous jet ventilation, and retrograde intubation).

Answer choice B is incorrect because by definition the patient is awake and spontaneously breathing; therefore, mask ventilation should not be necessary.

Answer choice C is incorrect because by definition the patient is already awake; however, canceling the case could be considered if awake noninvasive intubation fails.

Answer choice D is incorrect because, once the decision is made for awake invasive airway access, the ASA Difficult Airway Algorithm has been excited.

Answer choice E is incorrect because the decision to perform an awake intubation is based on multiple basic management choices. Factors influencing these decisions include potentially modifiable factors (ie, trauma with cervical spine instability, airway edema, tumor, abscess, etc) and more persistent factors (ie, degenerative arthritis, lingual thyroid, tonsillar hypertrophy, or syndromic/dysmorphic facial features). A difficult airway note should be given only to patients with persistent factors that will likely make any future intubation challenging.

Reference:
1. Apfelbaum JL, Hagberg CA, Caplan RA, et al. Practice guidelines for management of the difficult airway: an updated report by the American Society of Anesthesiologists Task Force on Management of the Difficult Airway. Anesthesiology. 2013;118(2).

24. **Correct answer: D**

Answer choice A is incorrect because failed intubation is defined as an inability to place an ETT after multiple attempts.

Answer choice B is incorrect because difficult laryngoscopy is defined as an inability to visualize any portion of the vocal cords after multiple attempts at conventional laryngoscopy. It does not refer to any advanced techniques or how intubation was achieved.

Answer choice C is incorrect because difficult supraglottic airway placement is defined as supraglottic placement requiring multiple attempts, with or without tracheal pathology.

Answer choice E is incorrect because the difficult facemask ventilation is defined as an inability of an adequately trained anesthesiologist to provide adequate ventilation. It does not contain any requirements regarding the use of airway adjuncts or advanced maneuvers.

Reference:

1. Apfelbaum JL, Hagberg CA, Caplan RA, et al. Practice guidelines for management of the difficult airway: an updated report by the American Society of Anesthesiologists Task Force on Management of the Difficult Airway. *Anesthesiology*. 2013;118(2).

25. **Correct answer: E**

Answer choice A is incorrect because, although awakening the patient might be a subsequent step if further attempts at ventilation fail, supraglottic airway placement (answer choice E) should be attempted first.

Answer choice B is incorrect because, although emergency invasive airway access is the final step in the inadequate ventilation pathway, supraglottic airway placement (answer choice E) should be attempted first.

Answer choice C is incorrect because, although these advanced airway techniques might be needed for final intubation, adequate ventilation via a supraglottic airway (answer choice E) should be attempted first.

Answer choice D is incorrect because, although the case might need to ultimately be canceled, adequate ventilation, through a noninvasive or invasive approach, should be attempted.

Reference:

1. Apfelbaum JL, Hagberg CA, Caplan RA, et al. Practice guidelines for management of the difficult airway: an updated report by the American Society of Anesthesiologists Task Force on Management of the Difficult Airway. *Anesthesiology*. 2013;118(2).

26. **Correct answer: D**

The ASA Difficult Airway Algorithm describes noninvasive alternative difficult intubation approaches including (but not limited to) light wand (answer choice A), supraglottic airways (LMAs, intubating LMAs) as an intubating conduit (answer choice B), alternative laryngoscope blades, video-assisted laryngoscopy (answer choice C), fiberoptic intubation, tube changers, or intubating stylets (bougie), and blind oral or nasal intubation (answer choice E).

Percutaneous jet ventilation (answer choice D) is considered invasive airway access.

Reference:

1. Apfelbaum JL, Hagberg CA, Caplan RA, et al. Practice guidelines for management of the difficult airway: an updated report by the American Society of Anesthesiologists Task Force on Management of the Difficult Airway. *Anesthesiology*. 2013;118(2).

27. **Correct answer: A**

Answer choice A is correct because the ASA Practice Guidelines for Management of the Difficult Airway recommendations for extubation for the difficult airway do not advise maintenance of intubation for any specific period. Extubation of the difficult airway would likely be challenging and require preparation and a preformulated strategy even if delayed for some period of time.

The ASA Practice Guidelines for Management of the Difficult Airway recommendations for extubation for the difficult airway include consideration of the merits of awake versus deep extubation (answer choice C); a postextubation ventilation plan (noninvasive ventilation and high-flow oxygenation, answer choice D); and short-term use of stylets, intubating bougies, airway exchange catheters (answer choice B), LMAs (answer choice E), etc.

Reference:

1. Apfelbaum JL, Hagberg CA, Caplan RA, et al. Practice guidelines for management of the difficult airway: an updated report by the American Society of Anesthesiologists Task Force on Management of the Difficult Airway. *Anesthesiology*. 2013;118(2).

28. **Correct answer: C**

Tonsillectomy and adenoidectomy are the most common surgical procedures performed on children and adolescents, with greater than 300 000 surgical procedures performed annually in North America. Major indications for tonsillectomy include hypertrophied tonsils, peritonsillar abscess, children with valvular cardiac disease at risk for seeding of cardiac valves from recurrent streptococcal bacteremia for infected tonsils, and OSA (answer choice C).

Answer choices A and B are incorrect because tonsillectomy is only indicated with recurrent disease even in children with valvular heart disease at risk for bacteremic seeding.

Answer choices D and E are incorrect because recurrent strep pharyngitis and presence of tonsillar stones are not indications for tonsillectomy.

References:
1. Ferrari LR, Nargozian C. Anesthesia for otolaryngologic surgery. In: Barash PG, Cullen BF, Stoelting RK, et al, eds. Clinical Anesthesia. 7th ed. Philadelphia: Lippincott; 2013:1356–1372.
2. Ragan B. Anesthesia for otorhinolaryngologic (ear, nose, and throat) surgery. In: Longnecker DE, Brown DL, Newman MF, et al, eds. Anesthesiology. 2nd ed. New York: McGraw Hill; 2012:1226–1247.

29. **Correct answer: C**

Answer choice A is incorrect because the US Food and Drug Administration has issued a black box warning in 2012 for the use of codeine in postoperative pain management in children after tonsillectomy and/or adenoidectomy.

Answer choice B is incorrect because, although sleep studies can be helpful in diagnosing OSA, they are expensive, labor-intensive, and challenging to complete in children. Therefore, it is impractical to complete these studies on all children undergoing tonsillectomy and/or adenoidectomy.

Answer choice C is correct. The ASA task force guidelines advise that "repeated hypoxemia may alter μ-opioid receptors, making these children sensitive to opioids and therefore requiring a reduced opioid dose (ie, approximately half the usual dose)."

Answer choice D is incorrect because, although some children undergoing tonsillectomy and/or adenoidectomy for OSA will require 24 hours of monitoring, the ASA task force guidelines advise that children should first be monitored breathing room air in an unstimulated environment, "preferably while asleep," before a decision is made concerning discharge. There is no formally specified timeframe for postoperative observation.

Answer choice E is incorrect because, although noninvasive CPAP might be helpful for some children following tonsillectomy and/or adenoidectomy, ASA Practice Guidelines are advisories and are not considered standards or requirements.

Reference:
1. Gross JB, Apfelbaum JL, Caplan RA, et al. Practice guidelines for the perioperative management of patients with obstructive sleep apnea: an updated report by the American Society of Anesthesiologists Task Force on Perioperative Management of Patient's with Obstructive Sleep Apnea. Anesthesiology. 2014;120(2).

30. **Correct answer: B**

A series of recent randomized controlled trials and meta-analyses have shown an association between intraoperative intravenous dexamethasone and decreased postoperative pain (answer choice A), decreased time to first oral intake (answer choice C), and decreased postoperative nausea and vomiting in the immediate postoperative period through the first 24 hours (answer choices D and E).

Answer choice B is incorrect because some small trials have shown increased bleeding associated with dexamethasone use, whereas several larger studies have shown equivocal results.

References:
1. Ferrari LR, Nargozian C. Anesthesia for otolaryngologic surgery. In: Barash PG, Cullen BF, Stoelting RK, et al, eds. Clinical Anesthesia. 7th ed. Philadelphia: Lippincott; 2013:1356–1372.
2. Ragan B. Anesthesia for otorhinolaryngologic (ear, nose, and throat) surgery. In: Longnecker DE, Brown DL, Newman MF, et al, eds. Anesthesiology. 2nd ed. New York: McGraw Hill; 2012:1226–1247.
3. Sadhasivam S. Anesthesia for Tonsillectomy With or Without Adenoidectomy in Children. 2017. www.UpToDate.com.

31. **Correct answer: C**

Answer choice A is incorrect because primary hemorrhage is defined as bleeding within the first 24 hours, whereas secondary hemorrhage is defined as bleeding anytime thereafter.

Answer choice B is incorrect because posttonsillectomy bleeding is considered a surgical emergency and requires immediate intervention.

Answer choice C is correct because research studies have shown that posttonsillectomy bleeding occurs in nearly 5% of cases and nearly half of these patients have an undiagnosed coagulation disorder.

Answer choice D is incorrect because posttonsillectomy hemorrhage usually presents as slow oozing; however, it can progress to brisk bleeding.

Answer choice E is incorrect because patients suffering from posttonsillectomy bleeding should be considered full stomachs because of swallowed blood. Therefore, a rapid sequence intubation should be performed.

References:
1. Ferrari LR, Nargozian C. Anesthesia for otolaryngologic surgery. In: Barash PG, Cullen BF, Stoelting RK, et al, eds. Clinical Anesthesia. 7th ed. Philadelphia: Lippincott; 2013:1356–1372.
2. Ragan B. Anesthesia for otorhinolaryngologic (ear, nose, and throat) surgery. In: Longnecker DE, Brown DL, Newman MF, et al, eds. Anesthesiology. 2nd ed. New York: McGraw Hill; 2012:1226–1247.

32. **Correct answer: B**

Answer choice A is incorrect because posttonsillectomy bleeding is a surgical emergency; however, proceeding to the OR under resuscitated has been associated with increased mortality. Additionally, these patients should be considered full stomachs and require rapid sequence intubation.

Answer choice B is correct because posttonsillectomy bleeding patients should be volume-resuscitated before going to the OR to prevent morbidity and mortality on induction.

Answer choice C is incorrect because these patients should be treated as full stomachs, requiring rapid sequence intubations followed by gastric decompression.

Answer choice D is incorrect because hemostasis can usually be achieved surgically in posttonsillectomy hemorrhage patients. Only if they develop repeated bouts of secondary bleeding should interventional radiology embolization be contemplated.

Answer choice E is incorrect because posttonsillectomy is a surgical emergency and requires intervention. Although nearly half of patients were found to have an undiagnosed coagulation disorder, there is rarely a clinically significant coagulopathy that can be reversed in the acute setting.

References:
1. Ferrari LR, Nargozian C. Anesthesia for otolaryngologic surgery. In: Barash PG, Cullen BF, Stoelting RK, et al, eds. Clinical Anesthesia. 7th ed. Philadelphia: Lippincott; 2013:1356–1372.
2. Ragan B. Anesthesia for otorhinolaryngologic (ear, nose, and throat) surgery. In: Longnecker DE, Brown DL, Newman MF, et al, eds. Anesthesiology. 2nd ed. New York: McGraw Hill; 2012:1226–1247.

33. **Correct answer: C**

Answer choice A is incorrect because a retrobulbar block is also known as an intraconal block and involves injection of local anesthetic into the fatty tissue of the orbit in the middle of the muscle cone formed by the recti muscles.

Answer choice B is incorrect because a peribulbar block is also known as an extraconal block and involves injection outside the muscle cone, allowing diffusion of local anesthetics into the structure in the middle of the muscle cone.

Answer choice C is correct because a median orbital block involves injection of local anesthetic into the space between the medial rectus muscle and the medial orbital wall and can be used to augment both retrobulbar and peribulbar blocks by increasing anesthesia to the medial orbital structures.

Answer choice D is incorrect because a superior orbital block involves injection of local anesthetic lateral to the supraorbital notch; however, this technique is complicated by the proximity of the globe to the superior orbit and increased vascularity compared with the inferior orbit.

Answer choice E is incorrect because a subtenon block involves injection of local anesthetic into the episcleral space, defined as the space between the sclera and the subtenon capsule.

References:
1. McGoldrick KE, Gayern SI. Anesthesia for ophthalmic surgery. In: Barash PG, Cullen BF, Stoelting RK, et al, eds. Clinical Anesthesia. 7th ed. Philadelphia: Lippincott; 2013:1373–1399.
2. Bayes J, Basta SJ. Anesthesia for ophthalmic surgery. In: Longnecker DE, Brown DL, Newman MF, et al, eds. Anesthesiology. 2nd ed. New York: McGraw Hill; 2012:1206–1225.

34. Correct answer: A

The oculocardiac reflex is produced when direct pressure is applied to the globe or surgical traction is applied to the extraorbital muscles. It commonly presents as bradycardia but can progress to atrioventricular block or even asystole. The oculocardiac reflex involves sensory input from cranial nerve V, which is directed through the medulla and effects the heart rate through cranial nerve X. The oculocardiac reflex is fatigable (ie, with repeated stimulation, the bradycardic effect on the heart generally lessens); however, pharmacologic intervention with atropine or glycopyrrolate is often necessary.

References:
1. McGoldrick KE, Gayern SI. Anesthesia for ophthalmic surgery. In: Barash PG, Cullen BF, Stoelting RK, et al, eds. Clinical Anesthesia. 7th ed. Philadelphia: Lippincott; 2013:1373–1399.
2. Bayes J, Basta SJ. Anesthesia for ophthalmic surgery. In: Longnecker DE, Brown DL, Newman MF, et al, eds. Anesthesiology. 2nd ed. New York: McGraw Hill; 2012:1206–1225.

35. Correct answer: D

Answer choice A is incorrect because the major complication of optic nerve sheath injection is epidural propagation of the local anesthetic and CNS effects.

Answer choice B is incorrect because the major complication of intra-arterial injection is local anesthetic toxicity and seizure activity.

Answer choice C is incorrect because the major complication of globe penetration and injection is retinal detachment and possible loss of vision.

Answer choice D is correct because extraocular muscle injury can cause diplopia through loss on conjugate gaze.

Answer choice E is incorrect because the major complication of trauma to the optic nerve can be loss of vision.

References:
1. McGoldrick KE, Gayern SI. Anesthesia for ophthalmic surgery. In: Barash PG, Cullen BF, Stoelting RK, et al, eds. Clinical Anesthesia. 7th ed. Philadelphia: Lippincott; 2013:1373–1399.
2. Bayes J, Basta SJ. Anesthesia for ophthalmic surgery. In: Longnecker DE, Brown DL, Newman MF, et al, eds. Anesthesiology. 2nd ed. New York: McGraw Hill; 2012:1206–1225.

36. Correct answer: B

Answer choice A is incorrect because epinephrine is typically dosed as a 2% topical solution. Each drop contains between 0.5 and 1.0 mg of epinephrine, which when absorbed can cause systemic affects including tachycardia and hypertension.

Answer choice B is correct because echothiophate is a long-acting anticholinesterase, which historically had been used to treat glaucoma. Even after cessation of therapy, plasma cholinesterase levels can be reduced by approximately 50%. Therefore, succinylcholine can have up to 3 times the normal duration.

Answer choice C is incorrect because cyclopentolate, a mydriatic medication, at doses above a 1% solution can be associated with psychosis.

Answer choice D is incorrect because acetazolamide, a carbonic anhydrase inhibitor used to decrease intraocular pressures in glaucoma, can be associated with metabolic acidosis and electrolyte abnormalities including hyponatremia and hypokalemia.

Answer choice E is incorrect because sulfur hexafluoride, a gas injected into the globe for the treatment of retinal detachment, can increase in size with use of nitrous oxide and cause dangerously high IOPs.

References:
1. McGoldrick KE, Gayern SI. Anesthesia for ophthalmic surgery. In: Barash PG, Cullen BF, Stoelting RK, et al, eds. Clinical Anesthesia. 7th ed. Philadelphia: Lippincott; 2013:1373–1399.
2. Bayes J, Basta SJ. Anesthesia for ophthalmic surgery. In: Longnecker DE, Brown DL, Newman MF, et al, eds. Anesthesiology. 2nd ed. New York: McGraw Hill; 2012:1206–1225.

37. Correct answer: A

Answer choice B is incorrect because a single drop of phenylephrine ophthalmic solution can contain 5 mg phenylephrine, which can cause systemic effects including hypertension, cardiac dysrhythmias, and reflex bradycardia.

Answer choice C is incorrect because timolol, a β-blocker used to treat glaucoma, has no effect on pupil size. Systemic uptake of ophthalmic β-blockers can lead to bradycardia, light-headedness, heart block, syncope, and in rare cases, asthma attacks.

Answer choice D is incorrect because apraclonidine, a topical α2-adrenergic agent used to treat glaucoma, can cause sedation and drowsiness when absorbed systemically.

Answer choice E is incorrect because scopolamine ophthalmic solution can cause CNS excitement and agitation in the elderly. Agitation in the elderly can be treated through intravenous physostigmine.

References:
1. McGoldrick KE, Gayern SI. Anesthesia for ophthalmic surgery. In: Barash PG, Cullen BF, Stoelting RK, et al, eds. Clinical Anesthesia. 7th ed. Philadelphia: Lippincott; 2013:1373–1399.
2. Bayes J, Basta SJ. Anesthesia for ophthalmic surgery. In: Longnecker DE, Brown DL, Newman MF, et al, eds. Anesthesiology. 2nd ed. New York: McGraw Hill; 2012:1206–1225.

38. Correct answer: B

Although many medications can increase IOP through decreased vitreous humor drainage, most anesthetic agents have no effect or slightly reduce IOP. Inhalational and inhalational anesthetics in addition to sedatives have a dose-related effect on decreasing IOPs. Of the listed medications, only ketamine is associated with increased IOPs.

References:
1. McGoldrick KE, Gayern SI. Anesthesia for ophthalmic surgery. In: Barash PG, Cullen BF, Stoelting RK, et al, eds. Clinical Anesthesia. 7th ed. Philadelphia: Lippincott; 2013:1373–1399.
2. Bayes J, Basta SJ. Anesthesia for ophthalmic surgery. In: Longnecker DE, Brown DL, Newman MF, et al, eds. Anesthesiology. 2nd ed. New York: McGraw Hill; 2012:1206–1225.

39. Correct answer: A

Answer choice A is correct because hypoxia can cause mild increases in IOP.

Hypotension (answer choice B), hypothermia (answer choice C), hyperventilation (answer choice D), and enhanced venous outflow (answer choice E) are all associated with decreased IOPs.

References:
1. McGoldrick KE, Gayern SI. Anesthesia for ophthalmic surgery. In: Barash PG, Cullen BF, Stoelting RK, et al, eds. Clinical Anesthesia. 7th ed. Philadelphia: Lippincott; 2013:1373–1399.
2. Bayes J, Basta SJ. Anesthesia for ophthalmic surgery. In: Longnecker DE, Brown DL, Newman MF, et al, eds. Anesthesiology. 2nd ed. New York: McGraw Hill; 2012:1206–1225.

40. Correct answer: E

Induction of general anesthesia for emergent open globe injuries is a commonly tested topic on many Board Examinations. Often, cases are presented that require rapid sequence intubation with the goal of increasing IOP as little as possible. Of note, Valsalva and coughing can increase IOPs by more than 40 mm Hg.

Answer choice A is incorrect because benzodiazepines can slightly decrease IOP and could help avoid patient agitation, breath holding, and Valsalva, thus avoiding increases in IOP.

Answer choice B is incorrect because, although succinylcholine has been shown to increase IOP by approximately 6-12 mm Hg, this effect is transient, lasting only 7-10 minutes. If succinylcholine is deemed necessary for rapid sequence intubation, then its use is allowable.

Answer choice C is incorrect because awake fiberoptic intubation with minimal sedation or topicalization would almost certainly lead to coughing and Valsalva, which has been shown to increase IOP by greater that 40 mm Hg.

Answer choice D is incorrect because direct pressure to the globe can itself lead to extrusion of vitreal contents. Much care must be taken to avoid direct contact with fingers, mask, etc during induction.

References:
1. McGoldrick KE, Gayern SI. Anesthesia for ophthalmic surgery. In: Barash PG, Cullen BF, Stoelting RK, et al, eds. Clinical Anesthesia. 7th ed. Philadelphia: Lippincott; 2013:1373–1399.
2. Bayes J, Basta SJ. Anesthesia for ophthalmic surgery. In: Longnecker DE, Brown DL, Newman MF, et al, eds. Anesthesiology. 2nd ed. New York: McGraw Hill; 2012:1206–1225.

41. Correct answer: B

Answer choice A is incorrect because both sulfur hexafluoride and octafluoropropane are perfluorocarbon gases, which can expand up to 3 times in size with nitrous oxide use.

Answer choice B is correct because adequate time must be given for nitrous oxide dissolved in the blood to be fully dissipated via ventilation before injection.

Answer choice C is incorrect because various forms of perfluorocarbon gases, including octafluoropropane and perfluoropropane, have been developed to maintain a stable gas bubble for up to 70 days before being absorbed. For this reason, a safety margin of 90 days is suggested before use of nitrous oxide after an unknown intraocular gas injection.

Answer choice D is incorrect because several cases of blindness have been reported after nitrous oxide use following intraocular perfluorocarbon gas bubble injection.

Answer choice E is incorrect because air is more readily soluble than perfluorocarbons, and therefore only a 5-day safety margin need to be adhered to before subsequent nitrous oxide use.

References:
1. McGoldrick KE, Gayern SI. Anesthesia for ophthalmic surgery. In: Barash PG, Cullen BF, Stoelting RK, et al, eds. Clinical Anesthesia. 7th ed. Philadelphia: Lippincott; 2013:1373–1399.
2. Bayes J, Basta SJ. Anesthesia for ophthalmic surgery. In: Longnecker DE, Brown DL, Newman MF, et al, eds. Anesthesiology. 2nd ed. New York: McGraw Hill; 2012:1206–1225.

42. Correct answer: D

Answer choice A is incorrect because nitrous oxide is not contraindicated as part of the anesthetic for cochlear implant surgery; however, it is often avoided to lessen the possibility of postoperative nausea and vomiting.

Answer choice B is incorrect because conscious sedation is not an adequate anesthetic for this type of surgery.

Answer choice C is incorrect because, although regional blocks and infiltration of local anesthetics provide for some improvement in postoperative pain, they do not affect surgical outcomes.

Answer choice D is correct because the surgical approach, with placement of electrodes, necessitates complete patient immobility.

Answer choice E is incorrect because permissive hypotension is preferred during mastoidotomy to limit blood loss.

Reference:
1. Bayes J, Basta SJ. Anesthesia for ophthalmic surgery. In: Longnecker DE, Brown DL, Newman MF, et al, eds. Anesthesiology. 2nd ed. New York: McGraw Hill; 2012:1206–1225.

43. Correct answer: D

Answer choice A is incorrect because, although increasing the respiratory rate on the ventilator would reduce the $Paco_2$, which would lead to cerebral vasoconstriction and slightly reduce the cerebral blood volume, this would not have a significant effect on blood flow to the middle ear.

Answer choice B is incorrect because, although the addition of nitrous oxide could deepen the plane of anesthesia, it would be unlikely to affect middle ear perfusion.

Answer choice C is incorrect because the addition of paralytic would be unlikely to affect bleeding during this case.

Answer choice D is correct because deepening the plane of propofol anesthesia or adding an antihypertensive agent would lower the blood pressure and thus could limit surgical bleeding.

Answer choice E is incorrect because moving the patient into Trendelenburg position would increase blood flow to the head and could thus increase surgical bleeding.

References:

1. Ferrari LR, Nargozian C. Anesthesia for otolaryngologic surgery. In: Barash PG, Cullen BF, Stoelting RK, et al, eds. Clinical Anesthesia. 7th ed. Philadelphia: Lippincott; 2013:1356–1372.
2. Ragan B. Anesthesia for otorhinolaryngologic (ear, nose, and throat) surgery. In: Longnecker DE, Brown DL, Newman MF, et al, eds. Anesthesiology. 2nd ed. New York: McGraw Hill; 2012:1226–1247.

44. Correct answer: D

Answer choice A is incorrect because this is the treatment for malignant hypertension. Although hypertension and tachycardia are 2 of the signs associated with malignant hypertension, there is no mention of any of the signs including heightened Pco_2 or hyperthermia and acute change in vital signs does not fit this scenario.

Answer choice B is incorrect because this is the treatment for local anesthetic toxicity. If local anesthetic was the fluid lavaged by the surgeon and it were at doses high enough to cause cardiac toxicity, we would expect a reduction in blood pressure and heart rate.

Answer choice C is incorrect because switching from a total IV anesthetic to an inhalational anesthetic would not be expected to significantly change the patient's vital signs unless a new plane of anesthesia is achieved.

Answer choice D is correct because β-blockade would be the most likely intervention to reduce the patient's heart rate and blood pressure acutely. Phenylephrine (a potent α-agonist) and epinephrine (a potent β- and α-agonist) can be used to cause local vasoconstriction through transdermal uptake. Given the increase in both heart rate and blood pressure, it is likely that the surgeon place epinephrine-soaked sponges in the nasal passage allowing for significant systemic uptake.

Answer choice E is incorrect because, although deepening the plane of anesthesia could reduce the patient's blood pressure, it would less likely reduce the tachycardia and would likely be slower than administration of a β-blocker.

Reference:

1. Ragan B. Anesthesia for otorhinolaryngologic (ear, nose, and throat) surgery. In: Longnecker DE, Brown DL, Newman MF, et al, eds. Anesthesiology. 2nd ed. New York: McGraw Hill; 2012:1226–1247.

45. Correct answer: D

Answer choice A is incorrect because deep extubation is associated with a higher incidence of laryngospasm, especially as the anesthesia lightens in the PACU.

Answer choice B is incorrect because, although deep extubation can allow for earlier exit from the OR, this time saving is usually taken up by longer stays in the PACU, as the patient emerges.

Answer choice C is incorrect because there are no differences in postoperative pain between deep-extubated patients and normally emerged and extubated patients.

Answer choice D is correct because removal of the ETT, while the patient is still anesthetized, can decrease movement and bucking.

Answer choice E is incorrect because deep extubation requires more intensive PACU nursing, as emergence and its potential complications take place in the PACU and not the OR.

Reference:

1. Ragan B. Anesthesia for otorhinolaryngologic (ear, nose, and throat) surgery. In: Longnecker DE, Brown DL, Newman MF, et al, eds. Anesthesiology. 2nd ed. New York: McGraw Hill; 2012:1226–1247.

46. Correct answer: C

In this surgery, a cuff-less ETT is being utilized and can be assumed to have some amount of leak around the cords. The patient's oropharynx will then become filled with an admixture of the inspired gas and room air. At the beginning of this case, the Fio_2 was not turned down from 95%; therefore this admixture most certainly would support combustion with electrocautery.

Reducing the fresh gas flow (answer choice A) would not alter the Fio_2 ratio, and turning off the fluorinated inhalational anesthetic would have no effect because these gases do not support combustion. Of note, nitrous oxide serves equally well as oxygen as an oxidizing source to support combustion.

Answer choice B is not the best answer because any ignition source, even "low-intensity" electrocautery, is dangerous in a rich oxidizing atmosphere of 95% O_2.

Answer choice C is the correct answer because it accomplishes fire prevention by not allowing all 3 elements of the fire triad to come together: fuel (tissue, ETT, cotton packing in the mouth), oxidizer (high Fio_2 oxygen), and ignition source (electrocautery).

The steps outlined in answer choice D would lower the Fio_2 in the anesthesia circuit but would not reduce the expired O_2 concentration coming from the patient's lungs. Additionally, allowing the surgeon to continue with electrocautery would be extremely dangerous with a now-disconnected ETT with a patient expiring high concentrations of oxygen.

Answer choice E is incorrect because it does not address removing an ignition source from the oxygen-rich environment. Additionally, the term "armored" can mean several things, including a metal ETT, which will not ignite; a "laser-safe" ETT that has a protective coating, which will not ignite from direct contact with the laser beam but can still burn internally; and a PVC ETT with a wire embedded in the wall, which helps prevent kinking but is still flammable.

References:

1. Ehrenwerth J, Seifert HA. Electrical and fire safety. In: Barash PG, Cullen BF, Stoelting RK, et al, eds. Clinical Anesthesia. 7th ed. Philadelphia: Lippincott; 2013:189–218.
2. Ragan B. Anesthesia for otorhinolaryngologic (ear, nose, and throat) surgery. In: Longnecker DE, Brown DL, Newman MF, et al, eds. Anesthesiology. 2nd ed. New York: McGraw Hill; 2012:1226–1247.

47. Correct answer: C

All the above answers are included in the American Society of Anesthesiologists Practice Advisory for the Prevention and Management of Operating Room Fires the proper management of a nonairway fire except answer choice C, which is only included in the airway fire algorithm. Without suspicion of an airway fire, expert opinion states ventilation should be maintained with a minimally oxidizing gas (ie, air).

Reference:

1. Apefelbaum JL, Caplan RA, Barker SJ, et al. Practice advisory for the prevention and management of operating room fires: an updated report by the American Society of Anesthesiologists Task Force on Operating Room Fires. *Anesthesiology*. 2013;118(2).

48. Correct answer: E

Answer choice A is incorrect because a CXR is unlikely to provide any immediate information about the extent of the inhalational injury.

Answer choice B is incorrect because direct visualization of the airway (answer choice E) would be superior to CT scan.

Answer choice C is incorrect because saline lavage of the lungs has not been shown to improve inhalational injury and could disseminate inhaled particles throughout the lung.

Answer choice D is incorrect because, although limiting the possibility of iatrogenic oxygen toxicity is a good idea, it is more of a chronic concern and not of immediate importance.

Answer choice E is correct because rigid bronchoscopy allows for visual assessment of the airway for plastic remnants and thermal/smoke injury and provides a means to remove any remnant pieces of the ETT.

References:

1. Ehrenwerth J, Seifert HA. Electrical and fire safety. In: Barash PG, Cullen BF, Stoelting RK, et al, eds. Clinical Anesthesia. 7th ed. Philadelphia: Lippincott; 2013:189–218.
2. Ragan B. Anesthesia for otorhinolaryngologic (ear, nose, and throat) surgery. In: Longnecker DE, Brown DL, Newman MF, et al, eds. Anesthesiology. 2nd ed. New York: McGraw Hill; 2012:1226–1247.

49. Correct answer: C

Answer choice A is incorrect because xenon is an inert gas and does not react with CO_2 absorbents.

Answer choices B and E are incorrect because, although oxygen and nitrous oxide are oxidizing agents and support combustion, they are not associated with an increased risk of inhalational anesthetic-induced fires.

Answer choice C is correct because inhalational anesthetic (eg, sevoflurane and isoflurane)-induced fires are associated with desiccated CO_2 absorbers and anesthesia machines that have been idle for some time (first case of the day or after a weekend).

Answer choice D is incorrect because low-humidity and desiccated CO_2 absorbers and not high humidity is associated with OR fires.

References:

1. Ehrenwerth J, Seifert HA. Electrical and fire safety. In: Barash PG, Cullen BF, Stoelting RK, et al, eds. Clinical Anesthesia. 7th ed. Philadelphia: Lippincott; 2013:189–218.
2. Ragan B. Anesthesia for otorhinolaryngologic (ear, nose, and throat) surgery. In: Longnecker DE, Brown DL, Newman MF, et al, eds. Anesthesiology. 2nd ed. New York: McGraw Hill; 2012:1226–1247.

50. Correct answer: A

Answer choice B is incorrect because it is best practice to use low Fio_2 (<30%) whenever possible when there is high risk of fire.

Answer choice C is incorrect because nitrous oxide is itself an oxidizing agent and will support ignition and fire.

Answer choice D is incorrect because bipolar is considered a safer fire risk than unipolar electrocautery because of its lower power and more direct route of current flow.

Answer choice E is incorrect because it is considered best practice to immediately remove the ETT; if an airway fire is suspected, then investigate the airway via bronchoscopy.

Reference:

1. Apfelbaum JL, Caplan RA, Barker SJ, et al. Practice advisory for the prevention and management of operating room fires: an updated report by the American Society of Anesthesiologists Task Force on Operating Room Fires. Anesthesiology. 2013;118(2).

ANESTHESIA FOR SPECIAL INDICATIONS

Rebecca I. Kalman and Maricela Schnur

1. **All of the following qualities make carbon dioxide a suitable gas for intraperitoneal insufflation EXCEPT which one?**

   A. Noncombustible
   B. High blood solubility
   C. Clear and colorless
   D. Lack of cardiopulmonary effects

2. **A 70-year-old woman is scheduled for total abdominal hysterectomy for endometrial cancer. Her medical history is significant ischemic cardiomyopathy with an ejection fraction of 25% and severe mitral regurgitation. Which of the following is a common effect of pneumoperitoneum seen with laparoscopic surgical procedures that would be least deleterious for her?**

   A. Pneumoperitoneum-induced increase in systemic vascular resistance (SVR)
   B. Release of pneumoperitoneum-related decrease in SVR
   C. Hypercapnia-related decrease in arrhythmia threshold
   D. Hypercapnia-related increase in pulmonary vascular resistance (PVR)

3. **Which of the following patients is likely to be the most negatively affected by the effects of carbon dioxide insufflation?**

   A. A 78-year-old with severe COPD undergoing extraperitoneal laparoscopic inguinal lymph node dissection
   B. A 32-year-old with morbid obesity undergoing laparoscopic gastric bypass
   C. A 52-year-old with asthma undergoing laparoscopic appendectomy
   D. A 72-year-old with congestive heart failure undergoing laparoscopic Nissen fundoplication

4. **A 62-year-old man is undergoing laparoscopic Nissen fundoplication. During the procedure, the patient becomes progressively hypoxemic with an oxygenation saturation that falls to 82%. You note a significant rise in end-tidal CO_2 despite hyperventilation, increased peak inspiratory pressure, and unequal chest expansion with ventilation. What should your first action be?**

   A. Suction the endotracheal tube.
   B. Give albuterol.
   C. Change the CO_2 absorbent.
   D. Stop the surgery and deflate the pneumoperitoneum.

5. A 65-year-old woman with a history of hypertension and chronic kidney disease is undergoing a laparoscopic liver resection for hepatocellular carcinoma. You record 100 cc of urine output after positioning at the beginning of the case. Three hours into the procedure, you note the patient has not had any further urine output. The patient is hemodynamically stable, oxygenating and ventilating well, and has no pulse pressure variation in her arterial line tracing. Which of the following is most likely contributing to her low urine output?

   A. High central venous pressure
   B. Elevated intra-abdominal pressure (IAP) of 22 mm Hg
   C. Kinked foley catheter
   D. Reverse Trendelenburg position

6. A 24-year-old woman is scheduled to undergo a laparoscopic appendectomy. The surgeon inserts the Veress needle and insufflates the abdomen to an IAP of 15 mm Hg without incident. As the surgeon proceeds with insertion of the other ports, you note the patients' blood pressure drops precipitously. The end-tidal CO_2 remains stable at 38 mm Hg. Given this clinical scenario, what is the most likely cause of the hypotension?

   A. CO_2 embolism
   B. Positioning
   C. Deep anesthesia
   D. Hemorrhage

7. All of the following are benefits of laparoscopic versus open surgical procedures EXCEPT which one?

   A. Decrease in hypothermia
   B. Decrease in postoperative pain
   C. Decrease in time to ambulation
   D. Minimize surgical incision and stress response

8. A 64-year-old woman with obesity and obstructive sleep apnea is undergoing a laparoscopic low anterior resection for colon cancer. Your anesthetic consists of 1.2 minimum alveolar concentration of sevoflurane. Three hours into the procedure, you note her blood pressure and heart rate start to rise. You treat this with 2 mg of hydromorphone. Thirty minutes later they are still elevated and you administer another 2 mg of hydromorphone. You are relieved for a lunch break, and when you return, your colleague tells you he gave another 2 mg of hydromorphone. The heart rate and blood pressure are not improved. Which of the following is the next best step?

   A. Increase the sevoflurane.
   B. Start a propofol infusion.
   C. Give 200 μg of fentanyl.
   D. Ensure adequate ventilation to maximize CO_2 removal.

9. Changes in pulmonary function during laparoscopic procedures include all of the following EXCEPT which one?

   A. Reduction in lung volume
   B. Reduction in lung compliance
   C. Reduction in ventilation-perfusion mismatch
   D. Increase in airway pressures

10. A 64-year-old woman with a medical history significant for COPD, coronary artery disease, and diastolic congestive heart failure is undergoing laparoscopic lysis of adhesions and partial colectomy for recurrent colon cancer. You are assigned to take over the case, which has been going for over 8 hours. You find a woman in steep Trendelenburg position covered by drapes. Your colleague signs out that the patient developed a low-dose vasopressor requirement a half hour ago. Over the next hour, the patient becomes more hypotensive requiring increasing dose of vasopressor, and you note the end-tidal CO_2 has continued to rise despite maximizing your ventilation strategy. Upon examination of the patient's chest and neck under the drapes, you note extensive subcutaneous emphysema. Which of the following statements is true regarding this clinical situation?

   A. Treatment with sodium bicarbonate is appropriate.
   B. Prolonged operative times is a risk factor for developing subcutaneous emphysema.
   C. Subcutaneous emphysema does not have postoperative implications.
   D. Subcutaneous emphysema is assumed to be isolated to the chest and neck.

11. Regarding robotic surgery, which of the following statements is false?

   A. Robotic surgery improves depth perception.
   B. One advantage of robotic surgery is that it broadens the application of minimally invasive surgery.
   C. Studies have shown that robotic surgery tends to have shorter operative times when compared with laparoscopic surgery.
   D. Robotic surgery enhances a surgeon's skills and can be utilized for technically challenging procedures.

12. The da Vinci robotic surgical system is composed of which of the following?

   A. A control console, an equipment tower with an optical system, and a side cart with robotic arms
   B. A control console and a robotic platform
   C. An equipment tower, which includes equipment that allows the physician to control the robot utilizing any computer and a side car with robotic arms
   D. An equipment tower, which includes technology that allows the physician to control the robot utilizing any computer, a control console, and an anesthesia unit

13. A healthy 52-year-old man is scheduled for a robotic prostatectomy. He tells you that he read on the Internet that robotic surgery can have negative impacts on his "cardiac" system and he is clearly concerned. Which of the following would be your most appropriate response?

   A. The Trendelenburg/head down tilt required for robotic prostatectomies does cause increased strain on the heart.
   B. Cardiac performance measures in healthy patients are maintained despite steep Trendelenburg position and pneumoperitoneum.
   C. Increased cardiac output in healthy patients has not been shown to increase overall cardiac risk.
   D. Increases in SVR can cause an increased cardiac risk even in healthy patients.

14. During a robotic surgical procedure, the surgeon tells you the patient is "tight and likely no longer adequately paralyzed" and requests the administration of additional paralytic. Which of the following would be your reply?

   A. Additional paralytic is not needed for robotic surgical procedures.
   B. You will give additional paralytic, as muscle paralysis reduced IAP needed for the same degree of abdominal distension.
   C. Additional paralytic is not needed, as studies have not shown a correlation between the degree of muscle paralysis and surgeons' ability to perform the surgical procedure.
   D. You will give additional paralytic, as patient movement during robotic surgery can result in displacement of robotic arms, which can cause potential patient harm.

15. Following a laparoscopic cholecystectomy, a 67-year-old patient states that he can feel crackling when he touches his stomach and chest area. Which of the following is a risk for this specific complication following a laparoscopic procedure?

    A. Short surgery duration
    B. Patient age above 65 years
    C. Use of fewer surgical ports
    D. Laparoscopic cholecystectomy

16. A 36-year-old man is undergoing a laparoscopic appendectomy. Your anesthetic consists of isoflurane, oxygen, and air. You chose to avoid nitrous oxide secondary to which of the following?

    A. The ability of nitrous oxide to contribute significantly to postoperative nausea and vomiting
    B. The potential of nitrous oxide to build up in the lumen of bowel, causing distension and obscuring the view of the surgeon
    C. The increase in postoperative opioid requirements
    D. The increase in IAPs

17. A 63-year-old woman is undergoing a robotic hysterectomy for uterine cancer. The duration of the surgery is 6 hours, and despite aggressive warming maneuvers at the end of the procedure, the patient's core temperature is 35.8°C. Which of the following statements is true regarding the incidence of hypothermia following laparoscopic or robotic surgery?

    A. Extra heat loss is thought to occur via convection of cold gas in laparoscopic/robotic surgical procedures.
    B. Cold CO_2 gas makes esophageal temperature probes inaccurate following laparoscopic/robotic procedures.
    C. Additional heat loss is thought to occur via radiation, as forced warming blankets can only be placed on a small percentage of body area in laparoscopic/robotic surgical procedures.
    D. Heat loss is transient and drastically improves upon cessation of the laparoscopic procedure without the use of additional heating equipment.

18. A 61-year-old obese man is undergoing a robotic prostatectomy for prostate cancer. The surgery is technically difficult and lasts approximately 7 hours, most of which the patient is in a steep head down position. Which of the following positioning complications is not attributable to patient positioning in a robotic prostatectomy?

    A. Upper airway obstruction because of pharyngeal and laryngeal edema
    B. Blindness
    C. Numbness and burning of the lower ear lobe
    D. Corneal abrasions

19. A 22-year-old man is complaining of pain in both the right upper quadrant and right lower quadrant of his abdomen which he states is a 6/10 upon his arrival to the postoperative anesthesia recovery unit (PACU) following a laparoscopic appendectomy. Given the procedure that the patient underwent, the pain is likely classified as which type of pain?

    A. Parietal
    B. Referred
    C. Visceral
    D. Neuropathic

20. You are providing anesthesia for an in-office liposuction procedure that is utilizing a tumescent lidocaine technique. What is the maximum dose of lidocaine that can be safely utilized for this procedure?

A. 5-7 mg/kg
B. 3-5 mg/kg
C. 15-25 mg/kg
D. 35-55 mg/kg

21. During a liposuction procedure that is utilizing the tumescent lidocaine technique, the patient begins to desaturate and reports feeling anxious. She begins to cough and you note she has almost pink, frothy sputum. You begin to suspect that the cause of her symptoms originates from which of the following?

A. Pulmonary edema
B. Pulmonary embolism
C. Hemorrhage
D. Abdominal viscous perforation

22. A 28-year-old woman is undergoing a blepharoplasty under minimum alveolar concentration anesthesia. Before the start of the procedure, you give her a small amount of midazolam and place a nasal cannula with an Fio_2 of 60%. After the surgeon injects a local anesthetic, it will be important for you to communicate the timing of which part of the procedure to prevent an adverse intraoperative event?

A. Scalpel usage
B. Need for additional local anesthetic
C. Tissue removal
D. Use of electrocautery

23. You are performing a preoperative interview with a 38-year-old woman just before the start of her planned procedure of a tissue graft to her right thigh for a scald injury. Which of the following is not considered to be a risk factor associated with poor wound healing?

A. Smoking
B. Marijuana use
C. Poor nutrition
D. Obesity

24. You are performing a laparoscopic cholecystectomy on a 49-year-old obese woman with a past medical/surgical history of a right-sided mastectomy and lymph node dissection for breast cancer, hepatitis C, and a remote history of IV drug abuse. As you attempt to place the IV, you note that the patient does not have many sites where an IV can be placed. Even after utilizing ultrasound, you can only see the median cubital vein clearly on the right. The patient tells you she has always been told to never let anyone place an IV on her right arm. Which of the following do you inform the patient?

A. She may need central vascular access if no superficial cite can be found.
B. The median cubital vein on the ipsilateral side of her previous surgical procedure should be utilized because there is poor evidence that needlesticks on the same side as a previous lymph node dissection contribute to lymphedema.
C. Venous access on the ipsilateral side of her mastectomy and lymph node dissection is unlikely to cause lymphedema if good skin hygiene is utilized following the procedure.
D. She should have a peripherally inserted central catheter line placed under fluoroscopy.

25. A 25-year-old man is brought to the emergency department after being involved in an accident. All of his fingers have been amputated from his right hand, and digital reimplantation is planned. After a successful surgical procedure, the patient is brought to the PACU. Which of the following has not been shown to influence the viability of the reimplantation?

A. Room temperature
B. Pain control
C. Hydration status
D. Secure dressing

Chapter 19 ▪ Answers

1. Correct answer: D

Carbon dioxide is used for intraperitoneal insufflation because it is noncombustible, highly soluble in blood (decreasing the consequences of gas embolism), naturally excreted from the body during ventilation, and clear and colorless. Carbon dioxide is readily absorbed from the peritoneum, leading to increased $Paco_2$. In healthy individuals, this is rarely hemodynamically significant. However, in those with limited cardiopulmonary reserve, CO_2 elimination may be affected, and hypercarbia-induced tachycardia and pulmonary vascular constriction may not be tolerated.

Reference:

1. Joshi GP, Cunningham A. Anesthesia for laparoscopic and robotic surgeries. In: Barash PG, Cullen BF, Stoelting RK, et al., eds. *Clinical Anesthesia.* 7th ed. Philadelphia: Lippincott; 2013:1257-1273.

2. Correct answer: B

The cardiovascular effects of laparoscopy are due to the mechanical and neuroendocrine effects of pneumoperitoneum, the effects of absorbed CO_2, and the patient positioning required for some procedures. Increased SVR in this setting is multifactorial. SVR increases as a result of increased sympathetic output related to CO_2 absorption. A pneumoperitoneum-related increase in IAP results in activation of the renin-angiotensin system and vasopressin release. This also contributes to an increase in SVR. For patients with coronary artery disease and reduced systolic function, increases in SVR can lead to worsening heart failure and increased myocardial oxygen demand. In addition, increases in SVR can reduce cardiac output in the setting of mitral regurgitation. For these reasons, a pneumoperitoneum-related increase in SVR is likely to be particularly harmful to this patient and answer A is incorrect.

The release of pneumoperitoneum can lead to reversal of this process and decreased SVR. This would be favorable for this patient in the setting of both her low ejection fraction and severe mitral regurgitation. Thus, answer choice B is correct.

Hypercapnia related to CO_2 absorption can lead to many deleterious effects, including reduced arrhythmia threshold, tachycardia, increases in SVR and PVR, and increased intracranial pressure. Given this patient's cardiopulmonary disease, neither arrhythmia (answer choice C) nor increase pulmonary vascular resistance (answer choice D) is favorable.

Rapid peritoneal distension with the establishment of pneumoperitoneum can lead to vagal response and bradycardia. Bradycardia can worsen severe mitral regurgitation; thus, answer choice E is particularly deleterious for this patient.

References:

1. Yong J, Hibbert P, Runciman WB, Coventry BJ. Bradycardia as an early warning sign for cardiac arrest during routine laparoscopic surgery. *Int J Qual Health Care.* 2015;27(6):473-478.
2. Joshi GP, Cunningham A. Anesthesia for laparoscopic and robotic surgeries. In: Barash PG, Cullen BF, Stoelting RK, et al., eds. *Clinical Anesthesia.* 7th ed. Philadelphia: Lippincott; 2013:1257-1273.

3. Correct answer: A

Carbon dioxide absorption is greater during extraperitoneal insufflation than during intraperitoneal insufflation. Although healthy patients may tolerate this well, a patient with severe lung disease and reduced CO_2 elimination at baseline may not. Thus, answer choice A is correct.

Although morbid obesity may have negative impacts on lung function including diminished compliance and reduced functional residual capacity (FRC), laparoscopic gastric bypass is performed in the reverse Trendelenburg position, which can improve respiratory compliance, FRC, and alveoli recruitment. Thus, carbon dioxide insufflation is usually tolerated relatively well in this setting. Asthma in itself is not exacerbated by hypercapnia, and these procedures involve intraperitoneal insufflation.

References:

1. Joshi GP, Cunningham A. Anesthesia for laparoscopic and robotic surgeries. In: Barash PG, Cullen BF, Stoelting RK, et al., eds. *Clinical Anesthesia.* 7th ed. Philadelphia: Lippincott; 2013:1257-1273.
2. Sabharwal A. Christelis N. Anaesthesia for bariatric surgery. *Contin Educ Anaesth Crit Care Pain.* 2010;10(4):99-103.

4. **Correct answer: D**

This clinical scenario is consistent with capnothorax. Capnothorax is most likely to develop in procedures that involve dissection around the diaphragm and retroperitoneum. One should have a high index of suspicion during such procedures in the setting of increased end-tidal carbon dioxide, decreased oxygen saturation, increased peak airway pressures, hypotension, and unequal chest expansion. The diagnosis can be confirmed with chest X-ray, ultrasonography, or observation of a bulging hemidiaphragm through the endoscope. If capnothorax is suspected, the surgery should be stopped and pneumoperitoneum should be desufflated. Supportive treatment is with oxygen, hyperventilation, positive end expiratory pressure, and hemodynamic management. In cases of minimal compromise, these conservative measures may be adequate. In cases of moderate to severe compromise, a chest tube or drain may be placed.

Reference:
1. Joshi GP, Cunningham A. Anesthesia for laparoscopic and robotic surgeries. In: Barash PG, Cullen BF, Stoelting RK, et al., eds. *Clinical Anesthesia*. 7th ed. Philadelphia: Lippincott; 2013:1257-1273.

5. **Correct answer: B**

Blood flow to the kidneys and the liver can be compromised with increasing IAP and is an important consideration in patients with preexisting disease. Raised IAP is an independent risk factor for acute kidney injury. IAP of 20 mm Hg can reduce glomerular filtration rate by 25%. The mechanism is likely related to the combined effect of reduced renal afferent flow from decreased cardiac output and reduced efferent flow from increases in renal venous pressure.

High CVP would not cause decreased urine output. Although both fluoride ions and compound A have been described in nephrotoxicity secondary to sevoflurane usage, neither is thought to be clinically relevant. A kinked foley could cause lack of urine output although mechanical failure should not be assumed and the foley was working after positioning at the beginning of the case. The reverse Trendelenburg position could result in decreased preload and low urine output although this patient is hemodynamically stable without pulse pressure variation in her arterial line tracing, indicating she is not intravascularly depleted.

Reference:
1. Hayden P, Cowman S. Anaesthesia for laparoscopic surgery. *Contin Educ Anaesth Crit Care Pain*. 2011;11(5):177-180.

6. **Correct answer: D**

Hemorrhage can occur due to inadvertent insertion of the Veress needle or trocar into a vessel such as the aorta, common iliac vessels, inferior vena cava, or abdominal wall vasculature. Initial access for CO_2 insufflation is usually achieved via one of the 2 methods: the Veress needle inserted blindly or a trocar inserted under direct vision. As the Veress needle is inserted blindly, hemorrhage may not be immediately identified. Although CO_2 embolism can also occur with vessel injury, the fact that the end-tidal CO_2 did not decrease puts hemorrhage higher up on the differential; thus, answer choice D is more likely than A in this clinical scenario. In reality, it may be difficult to differentiate massive hemorrhage from large CO_2 embolism because a decrease in preload and cardiac output can lead to both abrupt hypotension and a drop in end-tidal CO_2.

Laparoscopic appendectomy is performed in steep Trendelenburg position, which is more likely to lead to increased blood pressure than hypotension. Deep anesthesia is less likely than hemorrhage or CO_2 embolism in this clinical scenario. Answer choice C is incorrect.

Reference:
1. Joshi GP, Cunningham A. Anesthesia for laparoscopic and robotic surgeries. In: Barash PG, Cullen BF, Stoelting RK, et al., eds. *Clinical Anesthesia*. 7th ed. Philadelphia: Lippincott; 2013:1257-1273.

7. **Correct answer: A**

Although one might expect a lower degree of hypothermia with a closed procedure such as laparoscopy, the incidence is similar to that of open procedures. This is likely related to heat loss by convection because of the flow of the CO_2, which exits the cylinder at 21°C and is exposed to the large surface area of the much warmer peritoneal cavity.

Compared with open surgery, minimally invasive procedures have been shown to decrease postoperative pain and opioid requirements, allow more rapid ambulation and shorter hospital stays, have smaller incisions, diminish stress response, and lead to fewer wound complications.

Reference:
1. Joshi GP, Cunningham A. Anesthesia for laparoscopic and robotic surgeries. In: Barash PG, Cullen BF, Stoelting RK, et al., eds. *Clinical Anesthesia*. 7th ed. Philadelphia: Lippincott; 2013:1257-1273.

8. Correct answer: D

Hypertension during laparoscopic procedures may be related to increased sympathetic output from CO_2 absorption and the neuroendocrine response to pneumoperitoneum. Although opiates can be used as a part of a balanced general anesthetic, treating pneumoperitoneum-induced hypertension with opioids can lead to a relative opioid dose. This patient with obstructive sleep apnea is particularly sensitive to the effects of opiates, and continuing to administer them can only lead to a further decrease in the respiratory drive. Deepening the anesthetic with propofol or halogenated agents also may lead to prolonged emergence because she already has adequate depth of anesthesia.

Appropriate treatment includes ensuring adequate CO_2 removal via safe and effective ventilation strategies to mitigate the sympathetic effects of hypercarbia as well as treating hypertension and tachycardia with appropriate short-acting agents.

Reference:
1. Joshi GP, Cunningham A. Anesthesia for laparoscopic and robotic surgeries. In: Barash PG, Cullen BF, Stoelting RK, et al., eds. *Clinical Anesthesia*. 7th ed. Philadelphia: Lippincott; 2013:1257-1273.

9. Correct answer: C

Reduction in lung volume and compliance is due to the cephalad displacement of the diaphragm caused by increased IAP. This also results in reduced FRC, reduced total lung compliance, and increased airway pressure. These changes result in an increase in ventilation-perfusion mismatch.

Reference:
1. Joshi GP, Cunningham A. Anesthesia for laparoscopic and robotic surgeries. In: Barash PG, Cullen BF, Stoelting RK, et al., eds. *Clinical Anesthesia*. 7th ed. Philadelphia: Lippincott; 2013:1257-1273.

10. Correct answer: B

Risk factors for the development of subcutaneous emphysema include operative times greater than 200 minutes and use of 6 or more surgical ports.

Subcutaneous emphysema in this setting is due to extravasation of CO_2 and can result in severe hypercapnia. A blood gas would reveal a respiratory (hypercarbic) acidosis, and treatment with sodium bicarbonate is inappropriate because sodium bicarbonate is metabolized to CO_2 and H_2O. In the setting of a respiratory acidosis, administering sodium bicarbonate worsens the acidosis because of inability to ventilate off CO_2.

Patients who develop subcutaneous emphysema during laparoscopy can develop late hypercarbia because the CO_2 is absorbed into the bloodstream. They may present with somnolence, tachycardia, and other adverse effects in the postoperative period. Patients with underlying pulmonary disease are at higher risk for this complication.

Subcutaneous emphysema tracks up to the chest, neck, and head via a continuum of fascial planes. If it tracks up to the chest and neck, it must be assumed that the emphysema may extend to the thorax and mediastinum, which can result in capnothorax and or capnomediastinum. Thus, in this clinical situation a chest X-ray should be obtained to investigate these potential complications.

Reference:
1. Joshi GP, Cunningham A. Anesthesia for laparoscopic and robotic surgeries. In: Barash PG, Cullen BF, Stoelting RK, et al., eds. *Clinical Anesthesia*. 7th ed. Philadelphia: Lippincott; 2013:1257-1273.

11. Correct answer: C

In terms of benefits, robotic surgeries are believed to enhance a surgeon's skills and thus increase the ability to perform technical challenging cases. In particular, robotic surgery appears to aid in depth perception and provides better instrument control that more similarly mimics natural hand and wrist movement and can also eliminate surgeon tremor.

Recent studies have shown that robotic surgeries are associated with an increased duration as compared with laparoscopic surgeries despite a similar percentage of adverse outcomes. In a recent randomized controlled trial performed by Jayne and colleagues, 471 patients with rectal cancer underwent either laparoscopic or robotic resection. In this study, the mean operative time was approximately 37.5 minutes longer for the robotic procedure than for the laparoscopic procedure, and the cost of robotic surgeries was approximately $1000 more expensive. Additionally, in another observational study comparing laparoscopic and robotic resection for radical nephrectomy performed by Jeong and colleagues, there was no difference in adverse outcomes found between the 2 techniques; however, the robotic procedures were significantly longer and costlier. For these reasons, answer choice C is correct.

References:

1. Joshi GP, Cunningham A. Anesthesia for laparoscopic and robotic surgeries. In: Barash PG, Cullen BF, Stoelting RK, et al., eds. *Clinical Anesthesia*. 7th ed. Philadelphia: Lippincott; 2013:1257-1273.
2. Wright JD. Robotic-assisted surgery: balancing evidence and implementation. *JAMA*. 2017;318(16):1545-1547.

12. Correct answer: A

The most common robotic surgical unit is the da Vinci Surgical System, which consists of 3 components:
1. A control console where the surgeon sits to operate the robotic arms and camera
2. An equipment tower
3. The patient side cart that includes the robotic arms

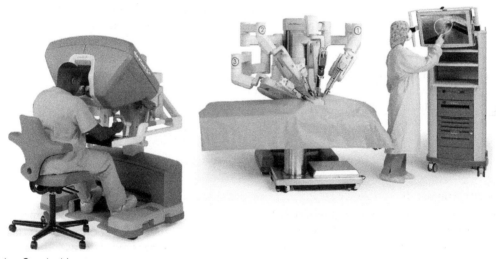

© Intuitive Surgical Inc.

Reference:

1. Joshi GP, Cunningham A. Anesthesia for laparoscopic and robotic surgeries. In: Barash PG, Cullen BF, Stoelting RK, et al., eds. *Clinical Anesthesia*. 7th ed. Philadelphia: Lippincott; 2013:1257-1273.

13. Correct answer: B

In abdominal robotic surgeries, cardiac performance is maintained despite an increase in systemic vascular resistance and MAP. The hemodynamic changes that occur in robotic surgery appear to be similar to that of laparoscopic surgery with the majority of studies performed on men undergoing prostatectomies. Conditions in these studies involved patients in a 45° head down position and pneumoperitoneum, with an IAP of 12 mm Hg. Despite noting an increase in cardiac filling pressures, stroke volume, cardiac output, mixed venous oxygen saturation, and cardiac dimensions as measured by echocardiography were maintained.

Benefits of laparoscopic and robotic surgery include improved arterial oxygenation and gas exchange, which has been shown to occur following pneumoperitoneum. This is likely due to a decrease in ventilation-perfusion mismatching secondary to redistribution of blood away from collapsed areas of the lungs. As robotic surgery can be safely performed in a healthy patient without fear of cardiac compromise, the correct answer choice for this question is B.

Reference:

1. Joshi GP, Cunningham A. Anesthesia for laparoscopic and robotic surgeries. In: Barash PG, Cullen BF, Stoelting RK, et al., eds. *Clinical Anesthesia.* 7th ed. Philadelphia: Lippincott; 2013:1257-1273.

14. Correct answer: D

During robotic surgical procedures, the displacement of the robotic arms that can occur with patient movement can have detrimental effects on patient safety. Muscle paralysis is required throughout the robotic procedure. In comparison, studies involving paralysis and laparoscopic procedures have failed to demonstrate a correlation between the degree of muscle paralysis and the surgeon's ability to safely perform the procedure.

Reference:

1. Joshi GP, Cunningham A. Anesthesia for laparoscopic and robotic surgeries. In: Barash PG, Cullen BF, Stoelting RK, et al., eds. *Clinical Anesthesia.* 7th ed. Philadelphia: Lippincott; 2013:1257-1273.

15. Correct answer: B

Subcutaneous emphysema can occur during laparoscopic surgery if CO_2 tracks into subcutaneous tissues. There are several known risk factors including multiple attempts at abdominal entry, improper cannula placement, loose fitting cannula placement, torque of the laparoscope, and increased IAP. Other risk factors (as also stated in a previous question) include lengthy surgery greater than 3.5 hours, the use of 6 or more surgical ports, advanced patient age, and Nissen fundoplication surgery. Of all these risk factors, the patient in the scenario is above the age of 65 years, making answer choice B correct.

Changes seen with subcutaneous emphysema include crepitus, insufflation problems (ie, problems with flow and IAP), positive end-tidal CO_2 greater than 50 mm Hg, acidosis, changes in lung compliance, cardiac arrhythmias, sinus tachycardia, and hypertension. Currently, it is estimated that the incidence of grossly detectable subcutaneous emphysema ranges from 0.43% to 2.3%; however, in studies of subclinical subcutaneous emphysema among patients who underwent a laparoscopic cholecystectomy, the incidence was noted to be around 56%.

Reference:

1. Ott DE. Subcutaneous emphysema—beyond the pneumoperitoneum. *JSLS.* 2014;18(1):1-7.

16. Correct answer: B

Nitrous oxide is a commonly utilized inhaled anesthetic, which can reduce the requirements of other inhaled anesthetics as well as intravenous anesthetics. Use of nitrous oxide at the end of a procedure accelerates the loss of other inhaled gases and can thus increase the speed of emergence. The use of nitrous oxide during laparoscopic and robotic procedures has been controversial, given the theoretical ability of nitrous oxide to diffuse into the lumen of bowel, which in turn causes bowel distension. For this reason, it is not a preferred agent during either a laparoscopic or robotic procedure, making answer choice B correct.

Additionally, nitrous oxide has been shown to cause postoperative nausea and vomiting, but the degree to which it contributes is modest. Nitrous oxide is a known combustible gas, and studies have shown that after 2 hours the levels were high enough to support combustion; however, the clinical significance of this is unclear.

The use of nitrous oxide has not been shown to increase postoperative opioid requirements, nor has it been shown to dangerously increase IAPs as in answer choices C and D.

Reference:

1. Joshi GP, Cunningham A. Anesthesia for laparoscopic and robotic surgeries. In: Barash PG, Cullen BF, Stoelting RK, et al., eds. *Clinical Anesthesia.* 7th ed. Philadelphia: Lippincott; 2013:1257-1273.

17. Correct answer: A

Although the main mechanism for heat loss during surgical procedures is radiation, the additional heat loss observed during laparoscopic/robotic surgeries occurs mainly by convection, with CO_2 temperatures of around 21°C, exiting the containment canisters before insufflation. Logically, it is expected that the degree of hypothermia should be lessened in laparoscopic and abdominal robotic procedures because of the fact that abdominal contents are not exposed to the environment. However, the degree of hypothermia in laparoscopic/robotic procedures is similar to that of open abdominal operations, as stated above, likely because of convection. Thus, the correct answer choice is A.

New equipment has recently become available, which houses built-in heating elements to warm insufflating gas. Despite this advance, the use of heating elements without humidification may not be enough to prevent hypothermia.

Cold CO_2 gas does not cause inaccuracy in esophageal temperature probes, and despite cessation of surgery, the hypothermia is not necessarily quickly corrected. Hypothermic patients should be actively warmed in the postoperative anesthesia unit using forced air warmers and heated fluids if necessary.

Reference:

1. Joshi GP, Cunningham A. Anesthesia for laparoscopic and robotic surgeries. In: Barash PG, Cullen BF, Stoelting RK, et al., eds. *Clinical Anesthesia*. 7th ed. Philadelphia: Lippincott; 2013:1257-1273.

18. Correct answer: C

Several positioning complications have been known to occur more frequently in robotic prostatectomies as compared with other surgical procedures. Several of these complications occur secondary to the steep head down position that is often required for prolonged period. This position can lead to significant pharyngeal and laryngeal edema, which in turn can cause upper airway obstruction as well as laryngospasm following extubation.

Additionally, the steep head down position has the potential to cause postoperative blindness secondary to congestion in the optic canal, and thus, this risk must always be discussed with patients preoperatively. A common positioning complication that has been known to occur with patients undergoing robotic prostatectomies is corneal abrasions. Numbness and burning of the lower earlobe, which would indicate a potential neuropathy of the superficial cervical plexus, is not a common complication seen with positioning for this type of surgical procedure.

Reference:

1. Joshi GP, Cunningham A. Anesthesia for laparoscopic and robotic surgeries. In: Barash PG, Cullen BF, Stoelting RK, et al., eds. *Clinical Anesthesia*. 7th ed. Philadelphia: Lippincott; 2013:1257-1273.

19. Correct answer: C

In comparison with open surgical procedures, laparoscopic surgery is widely believed to facilitate less postoperative pain, which is also shorter in duration. Pain control is still an important component of postoperative patient care to facilitate recovery. In laparoscopic procedures, the main source of pain is typically visceral in nature. However, patients can suffer from parietal pain from the incision site itself and referred pain in their shoulder, which most often results from diaphragm irritation. Factors that have been known to influence pain in laparoscopic surgery include procedure duration, IAP utilized, and the residual volume of subdiaphragmatic gas. Neuropathic pain is not commonly seen directly following a laparoscopic procedure. Thus, answer choice C is correct.

In terms of treatment, multimodal therapy is often utilized with a combination of a NSAID plus a weak opioid. Infiltration of the portal sites with local anesthetic is also another method of pain control, which has been shown to provide analgesia that outlasts the duration of action of the local anesthetic. Neuraxial anesthesia is typically not utilized in these procedures because the chance of adverse events such as hemodynamic instability, urinary retention, and delay of early ambulation often does not outweigh the benefits when compared with other modes of analgesia.

Reference:

1. Joshi GP, Cunningham A. Anesthesia for laparoscopic and robotic surgeries. In: Barash PG, Cullen BF, Stoelting RK, et al., eds. *Clinical Anesthesia*. 7th ed. Philadelphia: Lippincott; 2013:1257-1273.

20. Correct answer: D

The most commonly performed cosmetic procedure is liposuction, which involves utilizing hollow rods inserted into small incisions in the skin and suctioning subcutaneous fat. One technique, known as tumescent lidocaine, involves utilizing large volumes of infiltrate solution, generally 1-4 mL, with epinephrine 1:1 000 000 and lidocaine 0.025% to 0.1%, per 1 cc of fat removed. Although it is well known, the typical dose for lidocaine is 7 mg/cc. This particular technique utilizes 35-55 mg/kg, as its clearance is similar to that of a sustained release medication. For these reasons, although it seems quite high, the correct answer is D.

Peak serum levels occur 12-14 hours after the use of tumescent lidocaine with a decline over the subsequent 6-14 hours. Patients should be monitored for delayed adverse reactions to epinephrine and/or local anesthetic toxicity.

Reference:

1. Hausman LM, Rosenblatt MA. Office Based anesthesia. In: Barash PG, Cullen BF, Stoelting RK, et al., eds. *Clinical Anesthesia.* 7th ed. Philadelphia: Lippincott; 2013:860-876.

21. Correct answer: A

Liposuction has been associated with significant morbidity and mortality. In a census survey in the year 2000, the American Society of Aesthetic Plastic Surgeons revealed a high mortality rate for liposuction of 19.1 per 100 000 liposuctions performed. Approximately 23.1% of deaths were associated with pulmonary embolisms, whereas other causes included pulmonary edema, fat embolism, infection, abdominal viscous perforation, and hemorrhage. Risk factors for morbidity included the use of multiliter solutions, mega-volume aspiration, concurrent procedures, anesthetic effects, and permissive discharge policies. Current recommendations include limiting total aspirant to 5 L and that large volume liposuction not be performed in conjunction with other procedures.

Tumescent liposuction, often thought of as outpatient liposuction, also comes with the risk of attributable to the lidocaine in the solution as well as the epinephrine. Additionally, as in the scenario described in this question, pulmonary edema should be considered particularly when large volumes of solution are utilized and the patient is also receiving intravenous hydration. Clues about the cause of this patient's symptoms are her desaturation, feelings of anxiousness, and her low hemoglobin, which without signs of hemorrhage likely represents hemodilution. The correct answer choice for this question would therefore be A.

References:

1. Hausman LM, Rosenblatt MA. Office Based anesthesia. In: Barash PG, Cullen BF, Stoelting RK, et al., eds. *Clinical Anesthesia.* 7th ed. Philadelphia: Lippincott; 2013:860-876.
2. Rao RB, Ely SF, Hoffman RS. Deaths related to liposuction. *N Engl J Med.* 1999;340(19):1471-1475.

22. Correct answer: D

Surgical fires are a major adverse event that can be associated with supplemental oxygen in the operating room environment. In fact, high Fio$_2$ was reported as a major risk factor in approximately 74% of all surgical fires, and thus during periods of electrocautery or laser, supplemental oxygen should be turned off if possible or decreased to atmospheric level (ie, 21%). Constant communication should occur between the anesthesiologist and surgeon in facial surgical procedures where supplemental oxygen must be utilized, therefore making answer choice D correct.

Additionally, if low levels of supplemental oxygen are needed, nasal cannula should be utilized because face masks have demonstrated higher flow rates in the surgical field. If a moderate or higher amount of oxygen is needed, the patient should undergo general anesthesia with a plan discussed if an operative fire were to occur. If possible, laser-resistant tracheal tubes should be utilized and the tracheal tube cuff should be filled with saline rather than air.

According to the American Society of Anesthesiology practice advisory, if an airway fire involving a patient under general anesthesia were to occur, the endotracheal tube should be removed immediately and all contributing materials (such as lasers, electrocautery, and airway gases) should be removed. The endotracheal tube should be examined for any pieces that may remain in the patient's airway, and a rigid bronchoscopy should be considered to assess the thermal injury.

References:
  1. Hausman LM, Rosenblatt MA. Office Based anesthesia. In: Barash PG, Cullen BF, Stoelting RK, et al., eds. *Clinical Anesthesia*. 7th ed. Philadelphia: Lippincott; 2013:860-876.
  2. Huddleston S, Hamadani S, Phillips ME, Fleming JC. Fire risk during ophthalmic plastic surgery. *Ophthalmology*. 2013;120(6):1309.e1.
  3. Apfelbaum JL, Caplan RA, Barker SJ, et al. Practice advisory for the prevention and management of operating room fires: an updated report by the American Society of Anesthesiologists Task Force on Operating Room Fires. *Anesthesiology*. 2013;118: 271-290.

23.   Correct answer: B

Wound healing is an important aspect of any surgical procedure, and plastic surgeons in particular pay close attention to any risk factors that may compromise the wound healing process. One such factor, smoking, is easily modifiable before most plastic surgery procedures and is often reassessed just before any surgical intervention. A recent survey of North American plastic surgeons revealed that most plastic surgeons use a period of mandatory smoking cessation before performing elective plastic surgery procedures; however, no consensus on the exact time frame currently exists with a range of smoking cessation anywhere between 2 and 4 weeks utilized. As most plastic surgeons stated in this survey that if a patient was noncompliant, they would cancel an elective procedure, and every patient should be asked about smoking status immediately preoperatively. Other modifiable risk factors for poor wound healing include poor nutrition status, obesity, hyperglycemia, hypercholesterolemia, and hypertension. Although it may also be present with nutritional deficiencies as well as tobacco use, there is currently no association between marijuana use and poor wound healing, making answer choice B correct.

Preoperative Checklist
- Assess and optimize cardiopulmonary function. Correct hypertension.
- Treat vasoconstriction. Attend to blood volume.
- Assess recent nutrition and treat as appropriate.
- Treat existing infection. Among other actions, clean and treat skin infections.
- Assess wound risk by SENIC score to decide on the extent to which prophylactic measures should be taken.
- Start vitamin A or anabolic steroids in patients taking prednisone.
- Improve or maintain blood glucose level.

From Hunt TK, Hopf HW. Wound healing and wound infection. What surgeons and anesthesiologists can do. Surg Clin North Am. *1997;77:587, with permission.*

References:
  1. Rinker B. The evils of nicotine: an evidence-based guide to smoking and plastic surgery. *Ann Plast Surg*. 2013;70(5):599-605.
  2. Hausman LM, Rosenblatt MA. Office Based anesthesia. In: Barash PG, Cullen BF, Stoelting RK, et al., eds. *Clinical Anesthesia*. 7th ed. Philadelphia: Lippincott; 2013:860-876.

24.   Correct answer: C

Avoidance of needlesticks on the ipsilateral side of lymph node removal or dissection is one of the most common preventative maneuvers to prevent lymphedema. The historical origin of this recommendation was that needlesticks on the ipsilateral side of a procedure performed on the lymph nodes were thought to potentially lead to infection, which in turn would lead to lymphedema, and thus the recommendation was made to avoid all ipsilateral needlesticks and maintain good skin hygiene. Unfortunately, the majority of evidence supporting this recommendation is levels 4 and 5 (anecdotal and/or retrospective) with generally very small sample sizes.

One level 2 study was performed by Harlow et al. in 2005, and they followed up 188 women through their treatment course for breast cancer. The study concluded that hospital skin puncture on the ipsilateral side of the procedure versus none conferred an increased risk for lymphedema with a risk ratio of 2.44. However, because the study was not randomized, it is unknown if the majority of patients seen with lymphedema also have other confounding factors such as obesity or mastectomies. Additionally, the timing between the lymphedema and the intravenous access was not mentioned, and it is unclear whether it is related. At this time, there is poor evidence to recommend against venous access on the same side of a previous mastectomy or lymph node dissection, particularly if no other superficial vascular access is available. Thus, answer choice C is correct.

LEVEL OF EVIDENCE	DESCRIPTION
1	Randomized control trials
2	Nonrandomized control studies, prospective studies
3	Well-designed observational studies
4	Retrospective observational studies
5	Expert opinion

Modified from Cemal Y, Pusic A, Mehrara BJ. Preventative measures for lymphedema: separating fact from fiction. J Am Coll Surg. 2011;213(4):543-551.

References:
1. Cemal Y, Pusic A, Mehrara BJ. Preventative measures for lymphedema: separating fact from fiction. *J Am Coll Surg.* 2011;213(4):543-551.
2. Clark B, Sitzia J, Harlow W. Incidence and risk of arm oedema following treatment for breast cancer: a three-year follow-up study. *QJM.* 2005;98:343-348.

25. **Correct answer: D**

In the postoperative period following reimplantation of digits, care should be taken to avoid vasospasm and any indication of vascular compromise in the reimplanted fingers should be addressed promptly. First and foremost, the room should be kept warm, and the patient should be well hydrated. If the patient is uncomfortable and/or anxious, he should be treated immediately to avoid any adrenergic response, which may induce vasoconstriction in the reimplanted digits. Additionally, if the patient is a smoker, he should be advised to abruptly stop to avoid hypoxia to the digits. In terms of surgical dressing, it should be loosely applied without any risk of constriction to the affected fingers. The purpose of a loose dressing is also that clinicians can regularly assess the reimplanted digits for skin color, tissue turgor, and capillary refill. As long as the reimplantation is uncomplicated, no anticoagulation is required; however, antibiotics should be continued. For these reasons, answer choice D is correct.

If vascular compromise in the form of arterial obstruction is suspected, clinicians will note a decrease in tissue turgor, coolness of the digit, and the absence of bleeding if poked with a needle. Nonsurgical interventions for this complication include placing the reimplanted digits in a dependent position as well as systemically anticoagulating the patient. In comparison, patients with venous congestions, noted by blue discoloration and swollen digits, would benefit from improved outflow provided by fingertip incision and leech therapy.

Reference:
1. Maricevich M, Carlsen B, Mardini S, Moran S. Upper extremity and digital replantation. *Hand (N Y).* 2011;6(4):356-363.

20

ORTHOPEDIC ANESTHESIA

Nicole Zaneta Spence

1. A healthy 24-year-old man fell while he was snowboarding and was found to have a complete rotator cuff tear of his left shoulder. You would like to perform a peripheral nerve block under ultrasound guidance for intraoperative and postoperative analgesia. Which of the following is the most common complication for which you should counsel the patient?

    A. Ipsilateral pneumothorax
    B. Ipsilateral phrenic nerve paresis
    C. Infection at the site of the peripheral block
    D. Peripheral nerve block failure
    E. Ipsilateral Horner syndrome

2. A 35-year-old woman was involved in a motor vehicle accident and broke her right ulna. She reports using heroin daily. You have already performed an upper-extremity brachial plexus block, but she reports anesthesia in all digits except her fifth digit. The surgeon asks you to supplement her block. Where should you inject local anesthesia?

    A. Within the coracobrachialis muscle near its point of insertion on the humerus
    B. Medial to the brachial artery in the antecubital fossa
    C. Between the humeral and ulnar heads of the flexor carpi ulnaris muscle
    D. Posterior to the axillary artery in the axilla

3. You are the anesthesiologist for a 19-year-old man who is scheduled to undergo resection of his proximal tibia Ewing sarcoma. Where should a peripheral nerve catheter be placed to provide the greatest analgesia?

    A. Between the semimembranosus and biceps femoris muscles
    B. Between the greater trochanter and the ischial tuberosity
    C. Lateral to the femoral artery in the inguinal groove
    D. Deep to the sartorius muscle and medial to the vastus medialis muscle
    E. Between the adductor longus and adductor brevis muscles

4. A 13-year-old girl fractured her right ankle during her basketball game. You decide to perform an ultrasound-guided peripheral nerve block as her primary anesthetic. She continues to deny anesthesia over her medial malleolus. To provide complete coverage, you must supplement the:

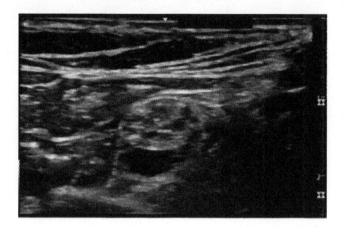

    A. Tibial nerve
    B. Deep peroneal nerve
    C. Saphenous nerve
    D. Sural nerve
    E. Superficial peroneal nerve

5. A 68-year-old patient is scheduled to undergo a left total knee replacement. He has a history of hypertension and coronary artery disease and had drug-eluting stents placed 6 months ago. His daily medications include aspirin 81 mg (last taken 1 d ago), clopidogrel 75 mg (last taken 3 d ago), metoprolol 100 mg (last taken 1 d ago), and a multivitamin (last taken 1 d ago). You are counseling him regarding his anesthetic options. You advise:

    A. Neuraxial anesthesia
    B. General anesthesia
    C. Femoral nerve block
    D. Sciatic nerve block
    E. Any are appropriate

6. An 85-year-old patient with mild dementia, hypertension, paroxysmal atrial fibrillation on Coumadin, and chronic kidney disease fell and fractured her femoral shaft. The orthopedic surgeons need to place intramedullary nails. Her health care proxy is at bedside, and you discuss the risks and benefits of regional and general anesthesia with the health care proxy. Which of the following statements is correct?

    A. Provided her international neutralized ratio (INR) is less than 1.5, a neuraxial technique is safe.
    B. Provided her INR is less than 1.8, a neuraxial technique is safe.
    C. Provided her INR is less than 2.0, a neuraxial technique is safe.
    D. Provided her INR is less than 2.0, a neuraxial technique is safe if she receives 1 unit of fresh frozen plasma.

7. A 22-year-old man severed his first and second digits. You elect to place an infraclavicular catheter for use intraoperatively and postoperatively. To provide adequate coverage, the cords that must be covered are:

    A. Lateral cord
    B. Medial cord
    C. Posterior cord
    D. A, B, and C
    E. A and B
    F. A and C

8. While snowboarding, a 33-year-old man suffered a bimalleolar ankle fracture. You are planning a regional anesthetic technique as his primary anesthetic using nerve stimulation. You elicit a foot twitch of plantar flexion. This response means that your needle must be located:

    A. Medially, within the semitendinosus muscle, and the needle should be redirected laterally
    B. Laterally, eliciting stimulation of the biceps femoris muscle, and the needle should be redirected medially
    C. Near the common peroneal nerve, eliciting a foot twitch, and the needle should not be redirected
    D. Near the tibial nerve, eliciting a foot twitch, and the needle should not be redirected

9. Before confirmation of the anatomy with ultrasonography, you anticipate that the femoral nerve is located _____ and is responsible for _____.

    A. Lateral to the femoral artery; knee extension
    B. Medial to the femoral artery; hip flexion
    C. Medial to the femoral artery; knee flexion
    D. Lateral to the femoral artery; hip flexion

10. A 73-year-old man is scheduled for a right total knee arthroplasty for severe osteoarthritis. He has a history of aortic stenosis with an aortic valve area of 1.1 cm², hypertension, and chronic obstructive pulmonary disease. He takes lisinopril daily and is not on home oxygen. The surgeons are eager for him to engage in physical therapy on postoperative day 0. Consequently, you would like to minimize weakness of the quadriceps muscle. You believe the best anesthetic and analgesic plan for this patient is to:

    A. Offer a femoral nerve block and general anesthesia
    B. Offer a femoral nerve block and spinal anesthesia
    C. Offer a saphenous nerve block and general anesthesia
    D. Offer a saphenous nerve block and spinal anesthesia
    E. Forego a peripheral nerve block given his aortic stenosis and proceed with general anesthesia

11. When performing a peripheral nerve block, the fascial layers that must be penetrated to create a successful block are 1, 2, 3, and 4 as identified by the anatomic landmarks indicated on the ultrasound shown (scanned along the inguinal crease).

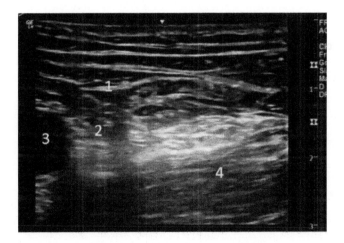

    A. 1, fascia lata; 2, fascia iliaca; 3, femoral artery; 4, fascia femoris
    B. 1, femoral nerve; 2, iliacus muscle; 3, femoral artery; 4, subcutaneous tissue
    C. 1, femoral fascia; 2, femoral nerve; 3, femoral vein; 4, psoas muscle
    D. 1, fascia iliaca; 2, fascia lata; 3, femoral nerve; 4, sartorious muscle
    E. 1, fascia lata; 2, fascia iliaca; 3, femoral artery; 4, iliacus muscle

12. **A 81-year-old man presents for an open reduction and internal fixation of his distal tibial fracture after he suffered a mechanical fall at home. He currently takes clopidogrel 75 mg daily, hydrochlorothiazide 12.5 mg daily, and omeprazole. His family is very anxious about general anesthesia. You would like to offer a regional anesthetic and counsel him and his family that:**

   A. Although there are small risks of bleeding, infection, and postdural puncture headache, you will proceed with neuraxial anesthesia.
   B. You can offer regional anesthesia if he has stopped his clopidogrel for 5 days.
   C. You can offer regional anesthesia if he has stopped his clopidogrel for 7 days.
   D. You can offer regional anesthesia if he has stopped his clopidogrel for 14 days.
   E. You can offer regional anesthesia if his INR is less than 1.5.

13. **A 22-year-old incarcerated woman was involved in a fight and subsequently suffered a distal radius fracture. The surgeon informs you that the procedure will take under an hour, and he plans to use a tourniquet. You decide to offer the patient a regional anesthetic. You can offer her:**

   A. Supraclavicular nerve block
   B. Infraclavicular nerve block with intercostobrachial nerve block
   C. Interscalene nerve block with intercostobrachial nerve block
   D. Paravertebral nerve block
   E. Regional anesthesia is inappropriate for this patient

14. **A 19-year-old baseball player is scheduled to undergo repair of his ulnar collateral ligament. He would like a peripheral nerve block. You choose to perform a(n):**

   A. Interscalene nerve block
   B. Sciatic nerve block
   C. Femoral nerve block
   D. Supraclavicular nerve block

15. **A 53-year-old woman with chronic obstructive pulmonary disease on 2 L of oxygen at baseline and end-stage renal disease is scheduled to undergo an arteriovenous fistula creation. The surgeon requests a regional anesthetic. You perform a peripheral nerve block, and intraoperatively, the surgeon complains that the patient does not have anesthesia on her lateral forearm. You fear that you may have missed the:**

   A. Intercostobrachial nerve
   B. Lateral cord
   C. Musculocutaneous nerve
   D. Posterior cord
   E. Median nerve

16. **A 23-year-old woman is in the recovery room following an exploratory laparotomy for a small bowel obstruction. Her incision is 10 cm long, midline, and below the umbilicus. To spare her opioids, you perform a block. Identify the following structures and the target for your needle:**

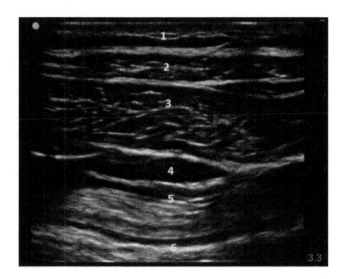

A. 1, external oblique muscle; 2, internal oblique muscle; 3, rectus muscle; 4, transversus abdominis muscle; 5, local anesthetic; 6, bowel

B. 1, external oblique muscle; 2, internal oblique muscle; 3, innermost oblique muscle; 4, local anesthetic; 5, internal oblique muscle; 6, transversus abdominis muscle

C. 1, subcutaneous tissue; 2, external oblique muscle; 3, internal oblique; 4, local anesthetic; 5, transversus abdominis muscle; 6, bowel

D. 1, subcutaneous tissue; 2, external oblique muscle; 3, transversus abdominis muscle; 4, local anesthetic; 5, internal oblique muscle; 6, bowel

E. 1, subcutaneous tissue; 2, internal oblique muscle; 3, transversus abdominis muscle; 4, bowel; 5, local anesthetic; 6, rectus sheath

17. **The block identified in the question above targets which nerves?**

A. Ilioinguinal nerve
B. Iliohypogastric nerve
C. Intercostal nerve
D. Subcostal nerve
E. All of the above
F. A and B
G. A, B, and D

18. **A 67-year-old man underwent a peripheral nerve block for his reverse total shoulder arthroplasty 1 week ago. On his follow-up visit, his wrist remains in flexion. You determine that he has suffered an injury to his:**

A. Radial nerve
B. Median nerve
C. Ulnar nerve
D. Musculocutaneous nerve
E. Axillary nerve

19. A 27-year-old man who has a history of type 1 diabetes mellitus and recent intravenous heroin use presents for an amputation of his first 3 toes. To provide adequate anesthesia and analgesia, you need to block the:

A. Femoral nerve, sural nerve, superficial peroneal nerve, deep peroneal nerve, posterior tibial nerve
B. Saphenous nerve, sural nerve, common peroneal nerve, lateral femoral cutaneous nerve
C. Femoral nerve, superficial peroneal nerve, deep peroneal nerve, posterior tibial nerve
D. Saphenous nerve, sural nerve, femoral nerve, posterior tibial nerve

20. A 16-year-old ice hockey player injured his right arm during a game. He is unable to abduct his fingers and exhibits a loss of sensation over his fourth and fifth digits. This injury may have occurred:

A. Medial to the brachial artery in the antecubital fossa
B. Medial aspect of the olecranon
C. In the humeral groove
D. Medial within the flexor retinaculum

21. A 20-kg, 5-year-old child suffered traumatic finger amputations of his left hand. You and your colleagues consent the parents for placement of an infraclavicular catheter. After the child is anesthetized, you place the catheter and bolus with 0.2% plain ropivacaine. The maximum dose of ropivacaine in this child is:

A. 40 mg
B. 60 mg
C. 100 mg
D. 120 mg
E. 140 mg

22. In the child mentioned in question 21, the first sign of local anesthetic toxicity is:

A. Bradycardia
B. Hypotension
C. Unresponsiveness
D. Seizures
E. Cardiac arrest

23. The absorption of local anesthetic, from greatest to least, is:

A. Intravenous > intercostal > supraclavicular > caudal > intrathecal
B. Intercostal > caudal > brachial plexus > lumbar plexus > Intrathecal
C. Intravenous > intercostal > caudal > epidural > brachial plexus
D. Transtracheal > intercostal > epidural > brachial plexus > subcutaneous
E. Intrathecal > epidural > sciatic > transtracheal > subcutaneous

24. Your surgical colleague inquires about performance of a nerve block for a coagulopathic gentleman with fulminant hepatic failure with a MELD score of 41. You educate your colleague that you would use _____ as it is metabolized by _____

A. Lidocaine; pseudocholinesterase
B. Chloroprocaine; pseudocholinesterase
C. Mepivacaine; pseudocholinesterase
D. Bupivacaine; pseudocholinesterase
E. Prilocaine; pseudocholinesterase

25. A patient experiences sudden restlessness, dizziness, tinnitus, and what appears to be rhythmic movements of her body following accidental release of an arm tourniquet 10 minutes after performing an intravenous Bier block. Which of the following medications is the most appropriate initial treatment?

A. Physostigmine
B. Phenytoin
C. Midazolam
D. Diphenhydramine
E. Propofol

26. A 59-year-old man is undergoing debridement of a nonhealing foot ulcer. An ankle block was performed using a landmark technique. One hour following performance of the block, the surgeon makes incision, but the patient describes pain on the plantar surface of the foot. Failure to anesthetize which of the following nerves is responsible?

A. Sural nerve
B. Deep peroneal nerve
C. Superficial peroneal nerve
D. Posterior tibial nerve
E. Saphenous nerve

27. A 66-year-old man with a history of emphysema (on 2 L nasal cannula oxygen at night) and atrial fibrillation (on warfarin) had a witnessed fall while at home. He suffered a small subdural hematoma, left proximal humerus fracture, left-sided rib fractures (ribs 6-8), and a right-sided hemothorax. He is alert and oriented. Neurology recommended monitoring his subdural hematoma. He is saturating 93% on 3 L nasal cannula. The orthopedic surgeon plans to bring him to the operating room to perform a left total shoulder arthroplasty. You would like to perform a peripheral nerve block to help with postoperative pain control. You decide to perform:

A. Axillary nerve block
B. Suprascapular nerve block
C. Interscalene nerve block
D. Paravertebral nerve block
E. Supraclavicular nerve block

28. A 31-year-old intravenous heroin user was involved in a motor vehicle accident and is scheduled for an open reduction and internal fixation of his left ankle. He has been on prophylactic enoxaparin. You should wait for how many hours before inserting a peripheral nerve catheter for postoperative pain control?

A. 2 hours
B. 8 hours
C. 12 hours
D. 24 hours
E. 72 hours

29. A 13-year-old boy is scheduled to undergo an open reduction internal fixation of his medial epicondyle fracture. You are in the process of performing a peripheral block and obtain the ultrasound shown. Suddenly, the boy complains of feeling anxious and like he cannot breathe. His heart rate increases to 112 beats per minute and his blood pressure remains hemodynamically stable. After you stop injecting, you administer:

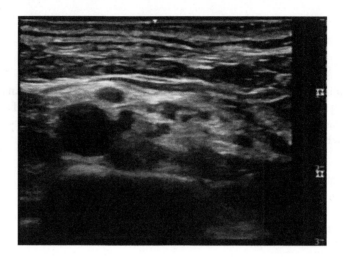

A. Propofol
B. Midazolam
C. Fentanyl
D. Intralipid

30. A 56-year-old woman is scheduled to undergo operative fixation of a left distal humerus fracture. You are performing a supraclavicular nerve block for postoperative pain. You choose to use:

A. 20 cc of 0.5% bupivacaine
B. 10 cc of 1.5% mepivacaine
C. 40 cc of 0.2% ropivacaine
D. 30 cc of 0.25% bupivacaine

31. A 14-year-old, 40-kg girl presented to the emergency department as a pedestrian struck by a vehicle. She suffered a right wrist fracture with significant articular displacement necessitating an open reduction and internal fixation. You perform a supraclavicular block using 15 mL of 0.5% bupivacaine. The patient complains of full sensation of her fifth digit. You choose to supplement your block but cannot use more than:

A. 12 cc of 0.25% bupivacaine
B. 10 cc of 0.5% bupivacaine
C. 10 cc of 0.25% bupivacaine
D. 9 cc of 0.5% bupivacaine
E. 5 cc of 0.5% bupivacaine

32. A 25-year-old man sustained a pelvic fracture during a motor vehicle accident and has been receiving 5000 units of subcutaneous heparin 3 times daily to prevent deep venous thromboses. He desires an epidural for analgesia. Which of the following laboratory tests is most valuable before epidural placement?

A. Bleeding time
B. Anti-Xa level
C. International neutralized ratio
D. PTT (partial thromboplastin time)
E. PT (prothrombin time)
F. Platelet count

33. A 36-year-old man is undergoing a lower-extremity orthopedic procedure under regional anesthesia. You note that his blood pressure continues to rise despite administration of β-blockers and intravenous opioids, and you suggest to the surgeon that the tourniquet should be deflated. You expect to observe all of the following hemodynamic responses EXCEPT a(n):

   A. Decrease in central venous pressure
   B. Increase in $ETCO_2$
   C. Decrease in minute ventilation
   D. Decrease in temperature
   E. Decrease in mean arterial pressure

34. A 35-year-old man is scheduled to undergo a cubital tunnel release of the right upper extremity. The surgeon plans to use a tourniquet. The patient desires regional anesthesia with monitored anesthesia care. To use an axillary nerve block as your primary anesthetic, you must ensure all of the following nerves are covered EXCEPT:

   A. Ulnar nerve
   B. Median nerve
   C. Intercostobrachial nerve
   D. Radial nerve
   E. Suprascapular nerve

35. A 62-year-old man is undergoing a right total hip replacement, and the surgeon mentions that the patient is continuing to "ooze." You note that all of his laboratory values and coagulation factors are within normal limits. You suggest a dose of tranexamic acid because it has been shown to reduce bleeding during orthopedic surgical procedures. The pharmacologic mechanism by which tranexamic acid works is:

   A. By potentiating the action of antithrombin II and inactivating thrombin to prevent the conversion of fibrinogen to fibrin
   B. By reversibly and noncompetitively binding the adenosine diphosphate receptor on the platelet surface to reduce platelet aggregation
   C. By forming a complex that displaces plasminogen from fibrin to block the conversion to plasmin
   D. By inhibiting vitamin K complexes and therefore reducing the synthesis of clotting factors

36. An 18-year-old man undergoes open appendectomy, and you place a postoperative truncal regional block for pain control. You believe the most effective block involves placing local anesthesia:

   A. Superficial to the iliacus muscle
   B. Deep to the superior costotransverse ligament
   C. Between the rectus abdominis muscle and the posterior rectus sheath
   D. Superficial to the transversus abdominis muscle
   E. Deep to the ligamentum flavum

37. A patient underwent an interscalene nerve block for his left total shoulder arthroplasty. Although nerve injury is uncommon, all of the following complications can occur, with the exception of:

   A. Left wrist drop
   B. Inability to abduct the left upper arm
   C. Inability to abduct the fingers of the left hand
   D. Inability to flex at the elbow joint
   E. Inability to extend at the elbow joint

38. **A 33-year-old patient with sickle cell disease is presenting for an orthopedic procedure, and the surgeon would like to use a tourniquet. You counsel the patient that:**

    A. Tourniquet use in this patient population is not associated with increased complications.
    B. The tourniquet will be placed at the proximal part of the limb at the greatest circumference of the limb.
    C. Tourniquet use of longer than 2 hours increases the risk of compression neurapraxia.
    D. All of the above.
    E. None of the above.

39. **You are taking care of an 18-year-old woman in the operating room. The tourniquet has been inflated for more than 90 minutes. The signs and symptoms that support your theory that her pain is secondary to the tourniquet inflation EXCEPT:**

    A. Hypertension
    B. Tachycardia
    C. Hypoxia
    D. Diaphoresis

40. **A 25-year-old woman elects to have spinal anesthesia for her procedure on her right lower extremity. Following placement of her neuraxial anesthesia, she can move her toes but does not have sensation around her knee. This differential block is explained by:**

    A. Sympathetic nerve fibers that are blocked at the lowest concentration of local anesthetic
    B. Motor nerve fibers that are sensitive to local anesthetic blockade
    C. An ineffective spinal anesthetic
    D. A subarachnoid block
    E. A slow-onset intrathecal block

41. **Following injection of local anesthetic, blood levels are highest for (from highest to lowest):**

    A. Caudal > epidural > sciatic > brachial plexus > subcutaneous
    B. Intercostal > epidural > sciatic > brachial plexus > subcutaneous
    C. Intercostal > epidural > caudal > brachial plexus > subcutaneous
    D. Intercostal > caudal > epidural > brachial plexus > sciatic
    E. Epidural > caudal > sciatic > brachial plexus > subcutaneous

42. **A lumbar epidural is placed for intraoperative anesthesia and postoperative analgesia. Epidurals may affect pulmonary function tests by causing a(n):**

    A. Significant decrease in forced expiratory volume in 1 second
    B. Decrease in cough strength
    C. Increase in vital capacity
    D. Increase in residual volume
    E. Decrease in tidal volumes

43. **A 46-year-old woman is presenting for a procedure on her left upper extremity. She has been on 120 mg of methadone daily for a history of opioid abuse. During her preoperative visit, you recommend:**

    A. Discontinuation of methadone as it will make managing her pain postoperatively more difficult
    B. Changing her methadone to oxycodone that she should use the morning of surgery
    C. Discontinuation of methadone and performance of a left brachial plexus block
    D. Administration of intravenous methadone in addition to her oral morning dose
    E. Continuation of methadone perioperatively

44. **A 64-year-old man is scheduled to undergo a left total shoulder arthroplasty. You are performing an interscalene block using nerve stimulation. You notice the patient begins to hiccup, so you decide to:**

A. Reposition the needle more anteriorly
B. Withdraw your needle
C. Reposition the needle more posteriorly
D. Reposition the needle deep to this point of stimulation

45. **A 33-year-old G3P1 woman who has been taking buprenorphine for a history of oxycodone abuse is scheduled to undergo a repeat cesarean section. Your colleague suggests performance of transversus abdominis plane (TAP) blocks to help with postoperative pain. Which of the following statements regarding TAP blocks is true?**

A. TAP blocks help with visceral and somatic pain.
B. TAP blocks should be performed as laterally as possible on the trunk.
C. TAP blocks involve injection of local anesthetic deep to the transversus abdominis muscle.
D. TAP blocks cannot be performed if a patient is on buprenorphine.
E. TAP block placement requires discontinuation of prophylactic heparin for at least 1 hour.

46. **A patient is undergoing surgery on her wrist and hand. Your colleague performs an axillary nerve block, but the patient can flex the wrist and has sensation over the lateral portion of the palm. To provide complete anesthesia, you need to supplement by ensuring blockade of which nerve?**

A. Ulnar nerve
B. Radial nerve
C. Median nerve
D. Musculocutaneous nerve
E. Axillary nerve

47. **In the patient mentioned in question 46, where should the supplemental nerve block be performed?**

A. Medial to the brachial artery in the antecubital fossa
B. Within the belly of the coracobrachialis muscle
C. At the medial epicondyle of the humerus
D. Within the radial groove of the humerus
E. At the lateral epicondyle of the humerus

48. **A 16-year-old man injured his ankle while skateboarding. You elect to perform a peripheral nerve block for intraoperative anesthesia and postoperative analgesia. You use a total of 18 mL of ropivacaine 0.2%, but the patient reports complete sensation of his lateral shin. You need to ensure adequate coverage of:**

A. Saphenous nerve
B. Tibial nerve
C. Common peroneal nerve
D. Sural nerve
E. Deep peroneal nerve

49. **A 35-year-old man is presenting for a procedure on his right elbow. You are deciding what type of block to perform. In discussions with your colleagues, you suggest:**

A. A supraclavicular block would be adequate for his elbow procedure and would cover the arm
B. An interscalene block would be adequate for his elbow procedure and would provide anesthesia and analgesia up to the midforearm
C. An infraclavicular block would be adequate for his elbow procedure and would provide anesthesia and analgesia up to the wrist
D. An axillary nerve block would be adequate for his elbow procedure and would provide anesthesia and analgesia of his arm
E. A targeted median and ulnar nerve block at the olecranon would be best to provide adequate anesthesia and analgesia of his elbow

50. A 35-year-old woman with *BRCA* gene mutation is presenting for an elective mastectomy and tissue expander reconstruction. You perform a peripheral nerve block to help with postoperative pain control. The paravertebral block proceeds smoothly (ultrasound image). To ensure adequate postoperative analgesia, you should ensure that she has anesthesia in which dermatomes?

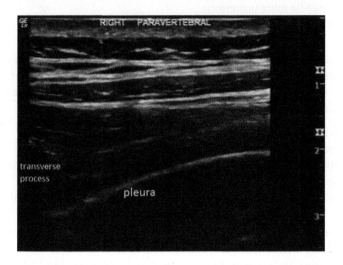

A. C6-T2
B. T2-T6
C. T3-T4
D. T6-T10
E. T10-T12

Chapter 20 ▪ Answers

1. Correct answer: B

Interscalene nerve blocks are commonly performed for shoulder surgery. Interscalene blocks target the roots or trunks of the brachial plexus. Coverage following an interscalene block is of the C5, C6, and occasionally C7 nerve distribution. Depending on the volume of local anesthetic used, hoarseness and Horner syndrome can be an expected side effect (because of palsy of the recurrent laryngeal nerve and sympathetic nerves). Nearly 100% of the time, the ipsilateral phrenic nerve also is anesthetized because it is located superficial to the anterior scalene muscle. The risk of infections following peripheral nerve blocks is small and depends on the location of the nerve block but ranges from 1 in 4000 to 1 in 200 000.

Reference:
1. Urmey WF, Talts KH, Sharrock NE. One hundred percent incidence of hemidiaphragmatic paresis associated with interscalene brachial plexus anesthesia as diagnosed by ultrasonography. *Anesth Analg.* 1991;72(4):498.

2. Correct answer: C

A supraclavicular, infraclavicular, or axillary block likely was performed. Her fifth digit is innervated by the ulnar nerve, which can be spared or missed during placement of a peripheral nerve block. The ulnar nerve courses from the medial cord of the brachial plexus and courses along the medial aspect of the upper extremity, passing between the olecranon and medial epicondyle of the humerus to continue distally to supply the fourth and fifth digits. The ulnar nerve can be supplemented anywhere along its course to provide anesthesia and analgesia to the fifth digit. The musculocutaneous nerve is located within the coracobrachialis muscle. The median nerve is located medial to the brachial artery in the antecubital fossa. The radial nerve is located posterior to the axillary artery and travels in the humeral groove.

References:
1. NYSORA: New York School of Regional Anesthesia. Available online: www.NYSORA.com.
2. Netter FH, Hansen JT, Lambert DR. *Netter's Clinical Anatomy: APA.* 6th ed. Carlstadt, NJ: Icon Learning Systems; 2005.

3. Correct answer: B

To provide the most coverage of the proximal tibia, a more proximal block is required, such as a high sciatic nerve block in either a transgluteal or subgluteal approach as described by answer choice B. Coverage of the femoral nerve (answer choice C) would provide coverage of the anterior thigh and medial lower extremity. Placing a catheter in the adductor canal (answer choice D) would also cover the medial lower extremity but usually spares motor branches to the quadriceps muscles. The obturator nerve is located between the adductor longus and brevis muscles and is responsible for adduction of the lower extremity.

Reference:
1. Netter FH, Hansen JT, Lambert DR. *Netter's Clinical Anatomy: APA.* 6th ed. Carlstadt, NJ: Icon Learning Systems; 2005.

4. Correct answer: C

The image shown is of the sciatic nerve a few centimeters proximal to the popliteal fossa. At this point, the sciatic nerve branches into the tibial nerve and the common peroneal nerve. These nerves supply a majority of the lower leg. The medial aspect of the lower leg and the medial aspect of the foot are supplied by the saphenous nerve, which is a branch of the femoral nerve.

Reference:
1. Netter FH, Hansen JT, Lambert DR. *Netter's Clinical Anatomy: APA.* 6th ed. Carlstadt, NJ: Icon Learning Systems; 2005.

5. Correct answer: B

According to American Society of Regional Anesthesia (ASRA) anticoagulation guidelines, clopidogrel should be held for at least 7 days before offering neuraxial anesthesia to a patient. These ASRA anticoagulation guidelines are generally extrapolated to apply to include peripheral nerve blocks.

Reference:

1. Horlocker TT, Wedel DJ, Rowlingson JC, et al. Regional anesthesia in the patient receiving antithrombotic or thrombolytic therapy: American Society of Regional Anesthesia and Pain Medicine Evidence-Based Guidelines (Third Edition). *Reg Anesth Pain Med.* 2010;35(1):64-101.

6. Correct answer: A

According to ASRA guidelines, neuraxial techniques have a lower risk of complications when the INR is less than 1.5.

Reference:

1. Horlocker TT, Wedel DJ, Rowlingson JC, et al. Regional anesthesia in the patient receiving antithrombotic or thrombolytic therapy: American Society of Regional Anesthesia and Pain Medicine Evidence-Based Guidelines (Third Edition). *Reg Anesth Pain Med.* 2010;35(1):64-101.

7. Correct answer: D

The first 2 digits are innervated by the radial nerve, which supplies the posterior aspect, and the median nerve, which supplies the palmar side. These nerves arise from the posterior cord and the lateral and medial cord, respectively. Therefore, for a complete block, all 3 cords must be covered.

Reference:

1. Netter FH, Hansen JT, Lambert DR. *Netter's Clinical Anatomy: APA.* 6th ed. Carlstadt, NJ: Icon Learning Systems; 2005.

8. Correct answer: D

Tibial nerve response is the preferred response when performing a sciatic nerve block in the popliteal fossa. Stimulation of the tibial nerve results in plantar flexion and inversion of the foot, whereas stimulation of the common peroneal nerve results in dorsiflexion and eversion of the foot.

References:

1. Netter FH, Hansen JT, Lambert DR. *Netter's Clinical Anatomy: APA.* 6th ed. Carlstadt, NJ: Icon Learning Systems; 2005.
2. NYSORA: New York School of Regional Anesthesia. Available online: www.NYSORA.com.

9. Correct answer: A

The femoral nerve is lateral to the femoral artery, which is lateral to the femoral vein. The femoral nerve is responsible for quadriceps muscles contraction, which guides knee extension. Clinically, it is important to counsel patients that if they have undergone a femoral nerve block, they are at risk for falling due to quadriceps muscle weakness while the block is in effect.

References:

1. NYSORA: New York School of Regional Anesthesia. Available online: www.NYSORA.com.
2. Netter FH, Hansen JT, Lambert DR. *Netter's Clinical Anatomy: APA.* 6th ed. Carlstadt, NJ: Icon Learning Systems; 2005.

10. Correct answer: C

Normal aortic valve area is 2-4 cm^2 (see below Ref [1]). Symptomatic aortic stenosis usually occurs when the aortic valve area is less than 0.8-0.9 cm^2. Critical aortic stenosis occurs when the valve area is less than 0.7 cm^2 with a transvalvular gradient of 50 mm Hg. In patients with aortic stenosis, it is important to avoid hypotension, and afterload must be maintained. Subsequently, central neuraxial anesthesia can be used with caution in mild cases but should otherwise be avoided, as it can decrease systemic vascular resistance and myocardial perfusion. Generally, epidural is preferred over spinal anesthesia. A saphenous nerve block will provide adequate analgesia for this patient with preservation of quadriceps muscle strength, whereas it would be relatively absent if a femoral nerve block is placed.

References:

1. Skubas NJ, Lichtman AD, Sharma A. Anesthesia for cardiac surgery. In: Barash PG, Cullen BF, Stoelting RK, et al., eds. *Clinical Anesthesia.* 7th ed. Philadelphia: Lippincott Williams & Wilkins; 2013:1076-1111.
2. Baumgartner H, Hung J, Bermejo J, et al. Recommendations on the echocardiographic assessment of aortic valve stenosis: a focused update from the European Association of Cardiovascular Imaging and the American Society of Echocardiography. *J Am Soc Echocardiogr.* 2017;30(4):372-292. Available online: http://asecho.org/wordpress/wp-content/uploads/2017/04/2017ValveStenosisGuideline.pdf.

11. Correct answer: E

The femoral nerve is the echogenic structure that is superficial to the iliacus muscle and lateral to the femoral nerve. The femoral nerve is located deep to the fascia lata and fascia iliaca. The femoral nerve contains sensory and motor fibers and supplies the vastus lateralis, intermedius, and medialis and the rectus femoris.

Reference:
1. Netter FH, Hansen JT, Lambert DR. *Netter's Clinical Anatomy: APA*. 6th ed. Carlstadt, NJ: Icon Learning Systems; 2005.

12. Correct answer: C

Although it is true that there are risks of bleeding, infection, and postdural puncture headache (more common in younger patients, larger needles, etc), clopidogrel should be stopped for at least 7 days before performing neuraxial procedures, which is denoted by the ASRA guidelines. Clopidogrel inhibits the binding of ADP to platelets and the subsequent ADP-mediated activation of glycoprotein GP IIb/IIIa, which inhibits platelet aggregation irreversibly. The INR is not monitored for patients on clopidogrel.

Reference:
1. Horlocker TT, Wedel DJ, Rowlingson JC, et al. Regional anesthesia in the patient receiving antithrombotic or thrombolytic therapy: American Society of Regional Anesthesia and Pain Medicine Evidence-Based Guidelines (Third Edition). *Reg Anesth Pain Med*. 2010;35(1):64-101.

13. Correct answer: B

The patient can be offered a few different types of brachial plexus nerve blocks but should also be given an intercostobrachial nerve block or superficial infiltration to provide better coverage for the tourniquet that will be placed at the upper arm.

References:
1. *Cutaneous Nerve Blocks of the Upper Extremity*. NYSORA: New York School of Regional Anesthesia. Available online: http://www.nysora.com/cutaneous-nerve-blocks-of-the-upper-extremity.
2. Netter FH, Hansen JT, Lambert DR. *Netter's Clinical Anatomy: APA*. 6th ed. Carlstadt, NJ: Icon Learning Systems; 2005.

14. Correct answer: D

For elbow surgery, a nerve block along the brachial plexus block would provide appropriate coverage. A supraclavicular block could be used for elbow surgery. If a tourniquet is to be used, then generally, an intercostobrachial or T2 nerve block should also be performed. An interscalene nerve block will not provide reliable coverage for elbow surgery because an interscalene block primarily targets the roots or trunks of C5 and C6 with occasional spread to C7.

References:
1. NYSORA: New York School of Regional Anesthesia. Available online: http://www.nysora.com/.
2. Netter FH, Hansen JT, Lambert DR. *Netter's Clinical Anatomy: APA*. 6th ed. Carlstadt, NJ: Icon Learning Systems; 2005.

15. Correct answer: C

Interscalene nerve blocks cause paresis of the ipsilateral phrenic nerve nearly 100% of the time and should therefore be used with extreme caution or avoided. In patients who have chronic obstructive pulmonary disease, diaphragmatic hemiparalysis could cause respiratory decompensation. A supraclavicular nerve block could have some local anesthetic spread to the ipsilateral phrenic nerve but less likely than an interscalene nerve block. A supraclavicular nerve block, or "spinal of the arm," would allow the surgeons anesthesia and analgesia of the arm. If the patient is lacking anesthesia of her lateral forearm, then the lateral cutaneous branch of the musculocutaneous nerve was not covered. When performing an axillary nerve block, the musculocutaneous nerve may need to be blocked separately within the coracobrachialis muscle, as it may not abut the axillary artery. The intercostobrachial, or T2, nerve supplies the medial aspect of the proximal arm.

Reference:
1. Netter FH, Hansen JT, Lambert DR. *Netter's Clinical Anatomy: APA*. 6th ed. Carlstadt, NJ: Icon Learning Systems; 2005.

16. **Correct answer: C**

The TAP block describes placement of local anesthesia between the internal oblique muscle and transversus abdominis muscle. This block interrupts the innervation to abdominal skin, muscles, and parietal peritoneum. The TAP block does not prevent dull, visceral pain. If the needle were to penetrate deep to the transversus muscle, bowel injury is a risk of this block. To perform a TAP block using ultrasound, the ultrasound probe is placed in the midaxillary line at the triangle of Petit. It is important to place local anesthesia posteriorly to attempt to cover the anterior, posterior, and lateral branches of the spinal nerve.

References:
1. Mukhtar K. Transversus Abdominis Plane (TAP) Block. *J NY Sch Reg Anesth.* 2009;12:28-33.
2. Netter FH, Hansen JT, Lambert DR. *Netter's Clinical Anatomy: APA.* 6th ed. Carlstadt, NJ: Icon Learning Systems; 2005.

17. **Correct answer: E**

Innervation of the abdominal wall below the umbilicus arises from the anterior rami of spinal nerves T10 to L1, which includes the intercostal nerves (T10-T11), subcostal nerve (T12), and iliohypogastric and ilioinguinal nerves (L1).

Reference:
1. Mukhtar K. Transversus Abdominis Plane (TAP) Block. *J NY Sch Reg Anesth.* 2009;12:28-33.

18. **Correct answer: A**

Radial nerve injury causes wrist drop. The radial nerve innervates the supinators, triceps, and extensors of the digits. A loss of the radial nerve then leaves the patient unable to extend the wrist.

Median nerve injury can lead to the inability to flex the wrist and/or turn the hand over. In addition, one may also suffer from weakness of their grip strength and inability to move the thumb across the palm.

Ulnar nerve injury can lead to decreased sensation and strength of the fourth and fifth fingers ("claw hand"), as well as a decrease in grip strength.

Musculocutaneous nerve injury can lead to decreased elbow flexion and supination.

Axillary nerve injury can lead to weakness of the shoulder/deltoid muscle and sensory loss below the shoulder.

Reference:
1. Netter FH, Hansen JT, Lambert DR. *Netter's Clinical Anatomy: APA.* 6th ed. Carlstadt, NJ: Icon Learning Systems; 2005.

19. **Correct answer: A**

The lower extremity is innervated by the lumbosacral plexus. The sciatic and femoral nerves contribute to most of the innervation of the leg. The saphenous nerve, a branch of the femoral nerve that receives contributions from L2-L4, innervates the medial aspect of the distal leg and the medial aspect of the foot.

Reference:
1. Netter FH, Hansen JT, Lambert DR. *Netter's Clinical Anatomy: APA.* 6th ed. Carlstadt, NJ: Icon Learning Systems; 2005.

20. **Correct answer: B**

The injury described affects the ulnar nerve distribution. The ulnar nerve is responsible for digit abduction and sensation over the medial fingers, or digits 4 and 5. The ulnar nerve could be injured anywhere along the brachial plexus course. Given that the deficits seem isolated to the ulnar nerve, it is likely that the nerve is injured more distally. The ulnar nerve courses from the medial cord of the brachial plexus to travel medially, along the medial aspect of the olecranon and medial epicondyle of the humerus, to enter the forearm and supply the medial hand. The median nerve traverses medial to the brachial artery within the antecubital fossa and within the flexor retinaculum. The radial nerve travels within the humeral groove and, if injured, could result in wrist drop or difficulty with wrist extension.

Reference:
1. Netter FH, Hansen JT, Lambert DR. *Netter's Clinical Anatomy: APA.* 6th ed. Carlstadt, NJ: Icon Learning Systems; 2005.

21. Correct answer: B

The maximum recommended dose of ropivacaine is 3 mg/kg. Ropivacaine 0.2% is equivalent to 2 mg/mL of ropivacaine. A child weighing 20 kg should have less than 60 mg of ropivacaine. Local anesthetic toxicity is manifested with cardiac and/or central nervous system derangements.

Reference:

1. Tsui BCH, Rosenquist RW. Peripheral nerve blockade. In: Barash PG, Cullen BF, Stoelting RK, et al., eds. *Clinical Anesthesia*. 7th ed. Philadelphia: Lippincott Williams & Wilkins; 2013:937-995.

22. Correct answer: C

Older patients may communicate sensations of perioral numbness or metallic taste as first signs of local anesthetic toxicity. Other symptoms patients may describe include tinnitus, dizziness, feelings of impending doom, and unconsciousness. Signs of systemic toxicity manifest as either central nervous system toxicity, which includes tinnitus, disorientation, and seizures, or cardiovascular toxicity, which includes hypotension, dysrhythmias, and cardiac arrest. Generally, signs of central nervous system toxicity occur before cardiovascular toxicity.

Reference:

1. Tsui BCH, Rosenquist RW. Peripheral nerve blockade. In: Barash PG, Cullen BF, Stoelting RK, et al., eds. *Clinical Anesthesia*. 7th ed. Philadelphia: Lippincott Williams & Wilkins; 2013:937-995.

23. Correct answer: C

The absorption of local anesthetic is greater in areas of greater blood flow, as described in scenario C above.

Reference:

1. Tsui BCH, Rosenquist RW. Peripheral nerve blockade. In: Barash PG, Cullen BF, Stoelting RK, et al., eds. *Clinical Anesthesia*. 7th ed. Philadelphia: Lippincott Williams & Wilkins; 2013:937-995.

24. Correct answer: B

Local anesthetics are either characterized as esters or amides, and this depends on their linkage between the benzene ring (lipophilic end) and amino group (hydrophilic end). Ester-linked local anesthetics are hydrolyzed by pseudocholinesterase. The hydrolysis of ester-linked local anesthetics leads to the formation of *para*-aminobenzoic acid. Ester-linked local anesthetics include benzocaine, procaine, tetracaine, and chloroprocaine. Amide-linked local anesthetics include lidocaine, mepivacaine, prilocaine, bupivacaine, etidocaine, ropivacaine, and levobupivacaine. (Notably, amide-linked local anesthetics have 2 "i" letters in their names.) Lidocaine, an amide local anesthetic, is metabolized by the liver, specifically CYP3A4.

Reference:

1. Tsui BCH, Rosenquist RW. Peripheral nerve blockade. In: Barash PG, Cullen BF, Stoelting RK, et al., eds. *Clinical Anesthesia*. 7th ed. Philadelphia: Lippincott Williams & Wilkins; 2013:937-995.

25. Correct answer: C

Patients who exhibit neurotoxicity, such as seizures, should be administered a benzodiazepine to mitigate the seizure activity. Ventilation with 100% oxygen is also crucial. Hypoxia, hypercarbia, and acidosis potentiate the negative inotropic and chronotropic effects of local anesthetic toxicity. Signs of cardiotoxicity include widened QRS complex, bradycardia, hypotension, ventricular fibrillation, and/or cardiovascular collapse. Although standard resuscitative measures should be instituted, patients should also be given lipid emulsion.

Reference:

1. Tsui BCH, Rosenquist RW. Peripheral nerve blockade. In: Barash PG, Cullen BF, Stoelting RK, et al., eds. *Clinical Anesthesia*. 7th ed. Philadelphia: Lippincott Williams & Wilkins; 2013:937-995.

26. Correct answer: D

The plantar aspect of the foot is innervated by the medial and lateral plantar nerves and the medial calcaneal branches over the base of the heel. These nerves all arise from the tibial nerve. Minimal contributions come from the sural nerve laterally and the saphenous nerve medially covering the arch of the foot. Therefore, almost all of the plantar aspect of the foot is innervated by the sciatic nerve.

Reference:

1. Hadzic A, New York School of regional anesthesia. *Textbook of Regional Anesthesia and Acute Pain Management*. 2nd ed. New York: McGraw-Hill Education; 2017.

---

27. **Correct answer: B**

Although interscalene nerve blocks are commonly used, they cause an ipsilateral phrenic nerve blockade with a 100% incidence. This phrenic nerve blockade causes a 25% reduction in pulmonary function, which can be intolerable in patients with respiratory insufficiency. As a result, there has been much interest in exploring diaphragm-sparing analgesic techniques. The suprascapular nerve, which is made of contributions of C5 and C6, emerges proximally from the brachial plexus at the levels of the trunks. The suprascapular nerve innervates the supraspinatus and infraspinatus muscles and provides sensory innervation to the acromioclavicular joint and glenohumeral joint. The suprascapular nerve travels with the suprascapular artery and passes through the suprascapular notch. Under ultrasound, the suprascapular groove is identified deep to the trapezius and supraspinatus muscles. The suprascapular block is usually combined with blockade of the axillary nerve, which carries sensory information from the shoulder joint as well as the skin over the deltoid muscle.

References:

1. Tran DQ, Elgueta MF, Aliste J, Finlayson RJ. Diaphragm-sparing nerve blocks for shoulder surgery. *Reg Anesth Pain Med*. 2017;42(1):32-38.
2. Netter FH, Hansen JT, Lambert DR. *Netter's Clinical Anatomy: APA*. 6th ed. Carlstadt, NJ: Icon Learning Systems; 2005.

---

28. **Correct answer: C**

According to ASRA guidelines, prophylactic enoxaparin (less than or equal to 60 mg daily) should be held for 12 hours before neuraxial anesthesia and treatment enoxaparin (usually 1 mg/kg every 12 h) should be held for 24 hours before neuraxial procedures. The ASRA guidelines are extrapolated to apply to peripheral nerve blockade.

Reference:

1. Horlocker TT, Wedel DJ, Rowlingson JC, et al. Regional anesthesia in the patient receiving antithrombotic or thrombolytic therapy: American Society of Regional Anesthesia and Pain Medicine Evidence-Based Guidelines (Third Edition). *Reg Anesth Pain Med*. 2010;35(1):64-101.

---

29. **Correct answer: B**

His description of feeling anxious or "impending doom" could be a sign of impending local anesthetic toxicity. Without impending hemodynamic changes, intralipid does not need to be administered immediately but should be accessible should the patient decompensate. A benzodiazepine should be given not only for anxiolysis but would also be given if the patient began to experience a seizure. An infraclavicular block also runs the risk of pneumothorax, so the patient should have supplemental oxygen.

Reference:

1. NYSORA: New York School of Regional Anesthesia. Available online: www.NYSORA.com.

---

30. **Correct answer: A**

To maximize the patient's postoperative analgesia, the local anesthetic with the maximal duration should be selected. A local anesthetic's duration is determined by its protein binding (specifically, to albumin and α1-acid glycoprotein). Bupivacaine lasts longer than etidocaine > ropivacaine > mepivacaine > lidocaine > procaine and 2-chloroprocaine. The speed of onset of a local anesthetic is related to its pH. The lipid solubility of local anesthetics is correlated to potency.

References:

1. Blomberg J. Distal humerus fracture. *OrthoBullets*. 2017. Available online: https://www.orthobullets.com/trauma/1017/distal-humerus-fractures?expandLeftMenu=true.
2. Tsui BCH, Rosenquist RW. Peripheral nerve blockade. In: Barash PG, Cullen BF, Stoelting RK, et al., eds. *Clinical Anesthesia*. 7th ed. Philadelphia: Lippincott Williams & Wilkins; 2013:937-995.

31. **Correct answer: D**

The toxic dose of bupivacaine, a long-acting amide local anesthetic, is 3 mg/kg. The most common nerve spared during a supraclavicular block is the ulnar nerve, which is responsible for fifth digit sensation, such as described in this patient. Given that this patient is 40 kg, she can receive no more than 120 mg of bupivacaine. She has already received 15 mL of bupivacaine 0.5%, or 5 mg/cc, which is equivalent to 75 mg of bupivacaine. Her supplemental dose, therefore, cannot exceed 45 mg of bupivacaine.

Reference:

1. Tsui BCH, Rosenquist RW. Peripheral nerve blockade. In: Barash PG, Cullen BF, Stoelting RK, et al., eds. *Clinical Anesthesia*. 7th ed. Philadelphia: Lippincott Williams & Wilkins; 2013:937-995.

32. **Correct answer: D**

According to ASRA guidelines, a PTT should be checked for a patient receiving 3 times daily prophylactic heparin. Before placement of neuraxial anesthesia, the PTT should be less than 35. The PTT laboratory value is followed for patients receiving heparin, as PTT tests the intrinsic coagulation pathway.

References:

1. Tsui BCH, Rosenquist RW. Peripheral nerve blockade. In: Barash PG, Cullen BF, Stoelting RK, et al., eds. *Clinical Anesthesia*. 7th ed. Philadelphia: Lippincott Williams & Wilkins; 2013:937-995.
2. Horlocker TT, Wedel DJ, Rowlingson JC, et al. Regional anesthesia in the patient receiving antithrombotic or thrombolytic therapy: American Society of Regional Anesthesia and Pain Medicine Evidence-Based Guidelines (Third Edition). *Reg Anesth Pain Med*. 2010;35(1):64-101.

33. **Correct answer: C**

Tourniquet pain can overcome regional anesthesia, and the best way to relieve this is to release the tourniquet. Tourniquet pain may manifest as a sympathetic nervous system response. After 2 hours of tourniquet inflation, neuropraxias may occur. Upon tourniquet deflation, the washout of metabolic by-products, including lactate and potassium, lead to a brief metabolic acidosis, increased $Paco_2$, $ETco_2$, and minute ventilation. Central venous pressure and mean arterial pressure are decreased, and temperature decreases transiently, by approximately 0.7°C.

Reference:

1. Tsui BCH, Rosenquist RW. Peripheral nerve blockade. In: Barash PG, Cullen BF, Stoelting RK, et al., eds. *Clinical Anesthesia*. 7th ed. Philadelphia: Lippincott Williams & Wilkins; 2013:937-995.

34. **Correct answer: E**

The axillary nerve block provides coverage to the branches of the brachial plexus. It covers C7-T1 and includes the radial, ulnar, median, and musculocutaneous nerves. For patients undergoing surgeries of the upper extremity in which a tourniquet will be used, the intercostobrachial nerve needs to be covered to allow adequate tourniquet analgesia. The intercostobrachial nerve block is performed superficially. The suprascapular nerve receives contributions from C5 and C6, emerges from the brachial plexus proximally, and is important in shoulder joint innervation.

Reference:

1. Netter FH, Hansen JT, Lambert DR. *Netter's Clinical Anatomy: APA*. 6th ed. Carlstadt, NJ: Icon Learning Systems; 2005.

35. **Correct answer: C**

Tranexamic acid works by forming a reversible complex that displaces plasminogen from fibrin and inhibits fibrinolysis. Aminocaproic acid competitively binds to plasminogen and is also an antifibrinolytic. Heparin potentiates the action of antithrombin III, thus inactivating thrombin (and factors IX, X, XI, and XII and plasmin) and preventing the conversion of fibrinogen to fibrin. Clopidogrel has an active metabolite that irreversibly blocks ADP receptors on the platelet surface, which prevents activation of GP IIb/IIIa receptor complex to reduce platelet aggregation. Platelets inactivated by clopidogrel are affected for the remainder of their life span, which is approximately 7-10 days. Warfarin blocks vitamin K–dependent coagulation factors (coagulation factors II, VII, IX, and X and proteins C and S require the presence of vitamin K).

Reference:

1. Bernards CM, Hostetter LS. Epidural and spinal anesthesia. In: Barash PG, Cullen BF, Stoelting RK, et al., eds. *Clinical Anesthesia*. 7th ed. Philadelphia: Lippincott Williams & Wilkins; 2013:905-937.

36. Correct answer: D

The incision for an open appendectomy is unilateral and within the T11-T12 dermatomes in the right iliac fossa. The goal of the TAP block is to block most of the lower thoracic spinal nerves, usually T7-T12 and the iliohypogastric and ilioinguinal nerves of L1. Single-shot rectus sheath blocks provide somatic analgesia for upper abdominal, midline incisions. Fascia iliaca blocks are fascial plane blocks that anesthetize the femoral and lateral femoral cutaneous nerves.

References:

1. Young MJ, Gorlin AW, Modest VE, Quraishi SA. Clinical implications of the transversus abdominis plane block in adults. *Anesthesiol Res Pract*. 2012;2012:731645.
2. Lissauer J, Mancuso K, Merritt C, Prabhakar A, Kaye AD, Urman RD. Evolution of the transversus abdominis plane block and its role in postoperative analgesia. *Best Pract Res Clin Anaesthesiol*. 2014;28(2):117-126.
3. Abrahams M, Derby R, Horn JL. Update on ultrasound for truncal blocks: a review of the evidence. *Reg Anesth Pain Med*. 2016;41(2):275-288.

37. Correct answer: C

Injury to the radial nerve causes wrist drop (contributions from C5-C8 and T1). The deltoid is responsible for arm abduction and is innervated by the axillary nerve (contributions from C5-C6). The ulnar nerve is responsible for finger abduction (contributions from C7-C8 and T1). The biceps are responsible for elbow flexion, and the musculocutaneous nerve innervates the biceps (contributions from C5-C7). Elbow extension is possible by contraction of the triceps muscle, which is innervated by the radial nerve (contributions from C5-C8 and T1). The primary targets of the interscalene nerve block are C5, C6, and occasionally C7.

References:

1. Netter FH, Hansen JT, Lambert DR. *Netter's Clinical Anatomy: APA*. 6th ed. Carlstadt, NJ: Icon Learning Systems; 2005.
2. NYSORA: New York School of Regional Anesthesia. Available online: www.NYSORA.com.

38. Correct answer: D

Some studies have shown that tourniquets have been used uneventfully in patients with sickle cell disease, whereas other studies have shown an increased complication rate (see below Refs [1-4]). The tourniquet is placed at the largest circumference, as there is the largest muscle bulk, which protects against nerve injury. Tourniquet times should be limited to less than 2 hours with pressures less than 250 mm Hg in the upper extremity and 350 mm Hg in the lower extremity to decrease the risk of nerve injury (see below Ref [5]).

References:

1. Fisher B, Roberts CS. Tourniquet use and sickle cell hemoglobinopathy: how should we proceed? *South Med J*. 2010;103:1156-1160.
2. Al-Ghamdi AA. Bilateral total knee replacement under tourniquet in a homozygous sickle cell patient. *Anesth Analg*. 2003;98:543-544.
3. Adu-Gyamfi Y, Sankarankutty M, Marwa S. Use of a tourniquet in patients with sickle-cell disease. *Can J Anaesth*. 1993;40:24-27.
4. Stein RE, Urbaniak J. Use of the tourniquet during surgery in patients with sickle cell hemoglobinopathies. *Clin Orthop*. 1980;151:231-233.
5. Horlocker TT, Hebl JR, Gali B, et al. Anesthetic, patient, and surgical risk factors for neurologic complications after prolonged total tourniquet time during total knee arthroplasty. *Anesth Analg*. 102(3):950-955.

39. Correct answer: C

Tourniquet pain is due to the activation of unmyelinated C fibers. Tourniquet pain is typically described as achy, burning, and severe and manifests with signs of progressive sympathetic activation: hypertension, tachycardia, and diaphoresis. Tourniquet pain is resistant to treatment with opioids and deepening of anesthesia.

Reference:

1. Tsui BCH, Rosenquist RW. Peripheral nerve blockade. In: Barash PG, Cullen BF, Stoelting RK, et al., eds. *Clinical Anesthesia*. 7th ed. Philadelphia: Lippincott Williams & Wilkins; 2013:937-995.

40. Correct answer: A

Differential blocks are a normal phenomenon. Sympathetic nerve fibers are blocks by the lowest concentration of local anesthetic, as these are small and unmyelinated fibers. Sympathetic nerves are most sensitive to local anesthetic agents, and their distribution is 2-4 dermatomal levels beyond motor blockade.

Motor fibers are the least sensitive to local anesthetics. The presumed etiology of a differential block is that as the local anesthetic gets further from the injection site, it is present in lesser concentrations, and sympathetic nerve fibers do not require the same concentration to be blocked as do motor fibers.

Reference:
1. Tsui BCH, Rosenquist RW. Peripheral nerve blockade. In: Barash PG, Cullen BF, Stoelting RK, et al., eds. *Clinical Anesthesia*. 7th ed. Philadelphia: Lippincott Williams & Wilkins; 2013:937-995.

41. Correct answer: D

Blood levels after injection of local anesthetic are highest for intercostal > caudal > epidural > brachial plexus > sciatic/femoral > subcutaneous.

Reference:
1. Tsui BCH, Rosenquist RW. Peripheral nerve blockade. In: Barash PG, Cullen BF, Stoelting RK, et al., eds. *Clinical Anesthesia*. 7th ed. Philadelphia: Lippincott Williams & Wilkins; 2013:937-995.

42. Correct answer: B

Epidurals can affect PFTs in that they cause a slight decrease in vital capacity and forced expiratory volume in 1 second without clinical significance. There is also a decrease in expiratory effort and cough strength because of thoracoabdominal muscle paralysis (with up to 50% reduction in intrathoracic pressures and intra-abdominal pressures has been reported).

Reference:
1. Tsui BCH, Rosenquist RW. Peripheral nerve blockade. In: Barash PG, Cullen BF, Stoelting RK, et al., eds. *Clinical Anesthesia*. 7th ed. Philadelphia: Lippincott Williams & Wilkins; 2013:937-995.

43. Correct answer: E

Patients who have been on chronic opioids should continue these medications in the perioperative period, as abrupt discontinuation can lead to withdrawal and can also potentiate hyperanalgesic pain crises. Methadone is an NMDA receptor antagonist and opioid agonist. Patients who have had substance use disorders may be on methadone, buprenorphine with or without naloxone, and naltrexone.

Reference:
1. Macres SM, Moore PG, Fishman SM. Acute pain management. In: Barash PG, Cullen BF, Stoelting RK, et al., eds. *Clinical Anesthesia*. 7th ed. Philadelphia: Lippincott Williams & Wilkins; 2013:1611-1644.

44. Correct answer: C

Hiccups likely represent twitches of the diaphragm, which would occur if the needle is stimulating the phrenic nerve. The phrenic nerve is located superficial to the anterior scalene muscle; thus the needle should be withdrawn and positioned more posterolaterally. If the needle was directed more deeply, it could cause an intravascular injection, pneumothorax, or cord injury. An appropriate response to nerve stimulation in the interscalene groove would be twitch of the pectoralis, deltoid, triceps, biceps, or forearm muscles.

References:
1. Netter FH, Hansen JT, Lambert DR. *Netter's Clinical Anatomy: APA*. 6th ed. Carlstadt, NJ: Icon Learning Systems; 2005.
2. NYSORA: New York School of Regional Anesthesia. Available online: www.NYSORA.com.

45. Correct answer: B

The rami of spinal nerves T7-L1 innervate the abdominal wall but branch into anterior and lateral divisions laterally; thus, effective TAP blocks require lateral placement of local anesthetic. Appropriate landmarks for TAP blocks are the triangle of Petit. Local anesthetic is deposited between the internal oblique and transversus abdominus muscle. If the needle descends deep to the transversus, there is risk of bowel injury and perforation. TAP blocks provide somatic analgesia but will not block visceral pain. Generally, ASRA guidelines for anticoagulants and neuraxial anesthesia are used when considering placement of nerve blocks; however, this may differ depending on the institution or type of the block.

Reference:
1. Mukhtar K. Transversus abdominis plane (TAP) block. *J NY Sch Reg Anesth*. 2009;12:28-33.

46. Correct answer: A

The axillary nerve block targets the branches of the brachial plexus. The relation of the nerves is around the axillary artery: the radial nerve is deep to the artery; the median nerve is lateral to the artery; and the ulnar nerve is medial to the artery. The musculocutaneous nerve travels away from the axillary artery and is usually found traveling to the coracobrachialis muscle. If the patient is able to flex at the wrist and also has complete sensation over the medial aspect of the palm, the ulnar nerve is implicated.

Reference:
1. Netter FH, Hansen JT, Lambert DR. *Netter's Clinical Anatomy: APA.* 6th ed. Carlstadt, NJ: Icon Learning Systems; 2005.

47. Correct answer: D

The median nerve provides sensation of the lateral aspect of the palm. An axillary nerve block blocks the nerves in their terminal branches. The median, ulnar, and radial nerves lie around the axillary artery, but the musculocutaneous nerve is lateral to the artery and travels laterally to be within the coracobrachialis muscle. The median nerve courses from the axillary artery down the arm, medial to the brachial artery in the antecubital fossa. At the wrist, the median nerve is located lateral to the palmaris longus between the palmaris longus and the flexor carpi radialis. The ulnar nerve courses medially, at the medial epicondyle of the humerus, and into the forearm. Distal branches of nerves can be blocked anywhere along their course.

References:
1. Netter FH, Hansen JT, Lambert DR. *Netter's Clinical Anatomy: APA.* 6th ed. Carlstadt, NJ: Icon Learning Systems; 2005.
2. NYSORA: New York School of Regional Anesthesia. Available online: www.NYSORA.com.

48. Correct answer: C

To provide full anesthesia and analgesia to the ankle, both the sciatic and femoral nerves need to be covered. The sciatic nerve branches into the common peroneal and tibial nerves proximal to the popliteal fossa. (The distance from the fossa is different in every patient but averages 7 cm proximal.) The common peroneal nerve is located lateral to the tibial nerve and is smaller in size. The common peroneal nerve provides coverage to the lateral aspect of the lower extremity and can also be injured while a patient is in the lithotomy position.

References:
1. Tsui BCH, Rosenquist RW. Peripheral nerve blockade. In: Barash PG, Cullen BF, Stoelting RK, et al., eds. *Clinical Anesthesia.* 7th ed. Philadelphia: Lippincott Williams & Wilkins; 2013:937-995.
2. NYSORA: New York School of Regional Anesthesia. Available online: www.NYSORA.com.

49. Correct answer: A

A supraclavicular nerve block targets the divisions of the brachial plexus. This block anesthetizes the arm. Interscalene blocks are generally used for shoulder surgery and do not cover the elbow. Infraclavicular blocks are similar to supraclavicular blocks and cover the arm below the mid-humerus. An axillary nerve block targets the branches of the brachial plexus. An axillary block is used for the distal aspect of the arm.

References:
1. Tsui BCH, Rosenquist RW. Peripheral nerve blockade. In: Barash PG, Cullen BF, Stoelting RK, et al., eds. *Clinical Anesthesia.* 7th ed. Philadelphia: Lippincott Williams & Wilkins; 2013:937-995.
2. NYSORA: New York School of Regional Anesthesia. Available online: www.NYSORA.com.

50. Correct answer: B

Paravertebral blocks are advanced blocks that provide a unilateral block of the dorsal and ventral rami of the spinal nerves and the sympathetic trunk. Anatomically, the paravertebral space is wedge-shaped and bounded by the ribs. The posterior boundary is the superior costotransverse ligament, and the antero-lateral wall is bounded by the parietal pleura with the endothoracic fascia. The medial boundary is the vertebral body or epidural space. The caudal limit of the paravertebral space is at the origin of the psoas muscle at L1. Depending on the location of the paravertebral block, the local anesthetic can spread into the epidural space and can cause side effects such as hypotension. If the block is performed too laterally, then it becomes an intercostal block. The chest wall is covered by dermatomal levels T2-T6.

References:
1. Tsui BCH, Rosenquist RW. Peripheral nerve blockade. In: Barash PG, Cullen BF, Stoelting RK, et al., eds. *Clinical Anesthesia.* 7th ed. Philadelphia: Lippincott Williams & Wilkins; 2013:937-995.
2. NYSORA: New York School of Regional Anesthesia. Available online: www.NYSORA.com.

21

TRAUMA

Jennifer Cottral, Christine Choi, Jean Kwo, Christoph Nabzdyk,
Alexander Nagrebetsky, and Kyan Safavi

1. **A 53-year-old woman victim of a high-speed motor vehicle accident has just arrived at the emergency department (ED). As the anesthesiologist, you are a member of the trauma team expected to provide initial care. First responders in the field report that the patient was an unrestrained driver in a head-on collision with a telephone pole around 25 minutes ago. The patient was the sole victim in the crash, and it is unclear whether alcohol contributed to the accident. En route, the patient's mental status steadily declined, and she remained hypotensive despite receiving 2 L of lactated ringers. Her current vital signs are: NIBP 81/53, RR 20, SPo$_2$ 96%, and T 36.2°F. What is the best initial step in the management of this patient?**

   A. Obtain a brief medical history from the patient's next of kin.
   B. Assess the patient's airway and prepare to intubate as needed.
   C. Obtain a complete blood count for suspected hemorrhagic shock.
   D. Immediately transport the patient to CT scan.
   E. Place an arterial line to assess patient's oxygenation and ventilation with an arterial blood gas.

2. **You are called to intubate a 17-year-old boy who was hit in the face with a baseball. You notice bilateral periorbital ecchymosis and swelling, a displaced nasal bridge, and a large soft tissue hematoma underneath his left maxilla. A few seconds later, the patient coughs and bright red blood can be visualized in the oropharynx. After suctioning the oropharynx, what is the best approach for tracheal intubation in this patient?**

   A. Perform an awake fiberoptic intubation.
   B. Administer a short-acting opioid to facilitate tolerance of an awake fiberoptic intubation.
   C. Induce general anesthesia followed by bag mask ventilation (BVM) with cricoid pressure with subsequent orotracheal intubation.
   D. Induce general anesthesia followed by rapid sequence orotracheal intubation.

3. **A 39-year-old man who requires intubation has a potentially unstable cervical spine and Glasgow Coma Scale (GCS) of 7. Before induction of general anesthesia, you ask your surgical colleague to perform manual in-line stabilization (MILS) and your anesthesia colleague to apply cricoid pressure. Your first 2 attempts at indirect video laryngoscopy result in visualization of the epiglottis only, and the patient begins to desaturate. What is the next appropriate step in the management of this patient?**

   A. Maintain MILS, and ask your anesthesia colleague to release cricoid pressure.
   B. Ask your surgical colleague to adjust MILS to improve airway view, and ask your anesthesia colleague to release cricoid pressure.
   C. Call for help and prepare to perform cricothyroidotomy.
   D. Wake the patient up.

4. A 68-year-old man who sustained an epidural hematoma after a fall while skiing is now being emergently taken to the operating room (OR) for decompression. Per the ED note, on physical examination the patient opens his eyes to sternal rub and grabs the hand used to perform the sternal rub. When asked where he is, the patient responds, "Take the cat to the car." What is the patient's GCS score?

   A. 5
   B. 8
   C. 10
   D. 12
   E. 15

5. A 23-year-old man is a victim of a high-speed all-terrain vehicle (ATV) accident. His vital signs in the ED are BP 80/65, HR 107, RR 14, and T 97.4°F, and he is noted to be mildly anxious with a GCS of 15. A primary survey reveals obvious swelling and ecchymosis over his bilateral thighs, and a portable plain film shows bilateral comminuted femur fractures. In resuscitating this trauma patient with suspected ongoing hemorrhage, what would be the best target blood pressure goal?

   A. A blood pressure of 80/40 mm Hg, which is tolerable in a young trauma patient who is otherwise healthy
   B. A systolic blood pressure (SBP) of >100 mm Hg
   C. A SBP of <100 mm Hg
   D. A mean arterial pressure (MAP) of >65 mm Hg
   E. Specific blood pressure goals in trauma resuscitation do not affect survival to hospital discharge

6. An 18-year-old woman is an unrestrained victim of a high-speed motor vehicle collision. In the resuscitation bay of the ED, the patient appears confused and lethargic. Her initial vitals are BP 75/50, HR 144, and RR 32. Based on the Advanced Trauma Life Support (ATLS) classification of hemorrhagic shock, approximately what is this patient's estimated blood loss?

   A. <750 cc
   B. 750-1500 cc
   C. 1500-2000 cc
   D. >2000 cc

7. A 24-year-old unseatbelted passenger who was involved in a motor vehicle collision is scheduled for an emergent exploratory laparotomy and external fixation of the pelvis. Her vitals in the ED are BP 85/60, HR 125, and RR 28 with a negative FAST exam. As you prepare the OR for her anesthesia, what should be your primary source of fluid for volume resuscitation in this patient?

   A. Hypotonic crystalloid
   B. Isotonic crystalloid
   C. 5% albumin
   D. Blood and blood components

8. You are asked to help interpret an arterial blood gas test that was obtained by your colleague on one of her patients who is hemorrhaging in the OR. The values include pH 7.23, Pao_2 415, $Paco_2$ 41, Fio_2 1.0, and base deficit 10.4. What degree of shock is this patient in?

   A. Mild shock
   B. Moderate shock
   C. Severe shock
   D. Not enough information to determine degree of shock

9. A 19-year-old man is emergently taken to the OR for an exploratory laparotomy after sustaining multiple gunshots to his chest and abdomen. The patient underwent open-chest cardiac massage in ED and received a total of 10 units of packed red blood cells and 8 units of fresh frozen plasma (FFP). The ED sends of a sample of the patient's whole blood for thromboelastography (TEG), and the results are demonstrated below:

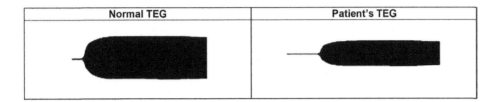

Based on this thromboelastogram, what blood product would the patient most benefit from receiving at this time?

  A. Fresh frozen plasma
  B. Platelets
  C. Cryoprecipitate
  D. Tranexamic acid

10. A 68-year-old woman with a history of hypertension, hyperlipidemia, coronary artery disease, atrial fibrillation on dabigatran, and type 2 diabetes is brought to the OR for an emergent decompressive craniectomy after sustaining a spontaneous intraparenchymal hemorrhage with midline shift. Vitals are BP 150/75, HR 72, and RR 14. The neurosurgeon asks if there is "something you can give" to reverse the anticoagulant effects of her dabigatran. You reach for which of the following?

  A. Idarucizumab
  B. Bebulin
  C. Pertuzumab
  D. Kcentra
  E. Fresh frozen plasma

11. A 29-year-old woman on warfarin for a history of an unprovoked pulmonary embolism is now undergoing an urgent open reduction and internal fixation for a right femur fracture sustained in a motorcycle crash. At the start of the case, she is transfused 2 units of FFP for significant oozing despite tourniquet use. Her anesthetic and surgical course are otherwise unremarkable. During surgical closure, the patient becomes acutely hypoxemic, febrile, and hypotensive, and pink froth is noted to be coming out of her endotracheal tube. Rales are heard on auscultation, and a chest radiograph reveals diffuse bilateral infiltrates. Laboratory test results are significant for hemoglobin 10.3 mg/dL, platelets 250 000 K/μL, INR 1.4, and BNP 150 pg/mL. Which of the following immediate interventions will be unlikely to help this patient?

  A. Increased fraction of inspired oxygen
  B. Bolus of lactated ringers
  C. Initiation of phenylephrine
  D. Diuretic therapy

12. A 32-year-old man is a helmeted victim in a car versus pole motor vehicle collision with prolonged extrication. He is found on secondary survey to have bilateral comminuted femur fractures and an open book pelvic fracture. He is brought emergently to the OR for external fixation. Before arrival to the OR, he has received 6 units of packed red blood cells and 4 units of FFP and remains hemodynamically unstable. His most recent laboratory test results include hemoglobin 6.9 mg/dL, platelets 150 000, INR 1.9, and fibrinogen 250 mg/dL. In addition to blood products, your colleague suggests administering tranexamic acid (TXA). Which of the following is your response?

    A. TXA given beyond 1 hour of injury may increase bleeding-related mortality.
    B. TXA given beyond 2 hours of injury may increase bleeding-related mortality.
    C. TXA given beyond 3 hours of injury may increase bleeding-related mortality.
    D. There is no difference in bleeding-related mortality in trauma patients given TXA.

13. A 48-year-old woman is the seatbelted driver of a high-speed motor vehicle collision. She is intubated in the ED for a GCS of 7, and as she awaits CT angiography, transesophageal echocardiography of her aorta is performed and reveals the following:

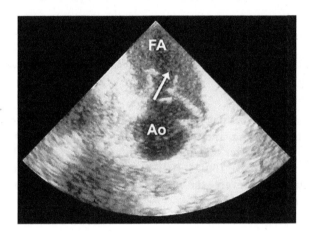

Which of the following is the grade of her blunt thoracic aorta injury?

    A. Grade 1
    B. Grade 2
    C. Grade 3
    D. Grade 4

14. A 42-year-old otherwise healthy right-handed man is brought in by helicopter after falling approximately 50 feet while hiking. He was intubated in the field for a GCS of 7, and a CT scan of his head reveals right frontal and anterior temporal cortical contusions, with punctate hemorrhages at the gray-white junctions and hypodensities in the right frontal white matter. Vital signs include BP 90/50, HR 114 (sinus), T 35.9°C, and RR = 16 on volume control ventilation. Laboratory test results are significant for a hemoglobin of 9.2 mg/dL. Which of the following is the best fluid to use for initial volume resuscitation?

    A. Normal saline 0.9%
    B. 5% dextrose in water
    C. Lactated ringers
    D. Albumin 5%
    E. Packed red blood cells

15. A bedside Codman ICP Monitor ("bolt") is placed by your neurosurgical colleague in the OR after induction of anesthesia for a patient who suffered blunt trauma to the head and had a GCS of 8. The intracranial pressure (ICP) is found to be 35 mm Hg. Other vitals include BP 90/60, HR 84, and core T 36.5°C. Jugular venous pressure is 9 cm H_2O. What is the patient's cerebral perfusion pressure (CPP) in relation to the recommended CPP for traumatic brain injury (TBI) patients?

   A. The patient's CPP is too high.
   B. The patient's CPP is too low.
   C. The patient's CPP is within the target range for TBI patients.
   D. There is no CPP target range for TBI patients.

16. Mannitol is initiated to decrease a patient's ICP. Which of the following is the target ICP in TBI?

   A. <15 mm Hg
   B. <20-25 mm Hg
   C. <25-30 mm Hg
   D. <35 mm Hg

17. A 24-year-old woman is admitted to the ICU postoperatively after surgical management of her traumatic right lower extremity amputation. To prevent venous thromboembolism (VTE), a sequential compression device is placed on her left lower extremity, and she is administered a daily prophylactic dose of low-molecular-weight heparin. On hospital day 4, she complains of left thigh pain, and a deep vein thrombosis (DVT) is found on duplex ultrasonography. All the following risk factors for VTE in blunt trauma victims have been shown to be refractory to well-established VTE prophylaxis clinical management guidelines EXCEPT which one?

   A. Pelvic ring injury
   B. Spinal cord injury
   C. Immobilization
   D. >3 days of mechanical ventilation

18. An otherwise healthy 37-year-old man weighing 100 kg has burned 40% of his total body surface area (TBSA) in a construction accident. By current guidelines, which of the following is an acceptable range of crystalloid administration in the first 24 hours?

   A. 4-8 L
   B. 5-10 L
   C. 8-16 L
   D. 10-20 L

19. A 21-year-old otherwise healthy man is being taken emergently to the OR for an exploratory laparotomy with possible thoracotomy after sustaining multiple gunshot wounds to his chest and abdomen. During placement of his arterial line, you note he appears to be "oozing" more than expected. His vitals on arrival to the OR are as follows: BP 75/40, HR 122, RR 28, and core T 33.9°C. Blood gas is pH 7.11, Pao_2 315, and $Paco_2$ 30 on Fio_2 60%. You attribute his acidosis and bleeding to hypothermia. Which of the following core body temperatures should be targeted?

   A. >34°C
   B. >35°C
   C. >36°C
   D. >37°C

20. A 20-year-old woman restrained passenger in a high-speed motor vehicle collision is brought into the OR emergently secondary to hemodynamic instability. Her vital signs on arrival are BP 70/40, HR 130, RR 30, and SPo$_2$ 92% on high-flow nasal cannula. She is confused, but is following commands, and has bruises over her chest and abdomen. A bedside transthoracic echocardiogram reveals the following:

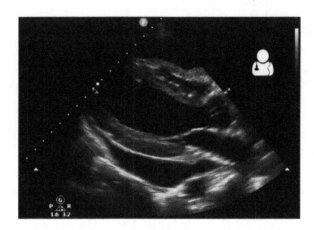

Which of the following medications would be the best choice for use during induction of endotracheal anesthesia for this patient?

A. Ketamine
B. Dexmedetomidine
C. Propofol
D. Remifentanil

21. A 56-year-old man with a history of end-stage liver disease (ESLD) presents for liver transplant evaluation. His ESLD has been complicated by esophageal varices, recurrent gastrointestinal (GI) bleeds, and hepatorenal syndrome, and the MELD (Model for End-Stage Liver Disease) score is calculated to be 32 with a Child-Pugh score of 13. Which of the following is NOT included as a component when calculating the MELD score?

A. Total bilirubin
B. International normalized ratio (INR)
C. Serum creatinine
D. Partial thromboplastin time

22. A 62-year-old woman with ESLD due to alcoholic cirrhosis is undergoing an orthotopic liver transplant. Her medical history is significant for paroxysmal atrial fibrillation, coronary artery disease, hypertension, and chronic kidney failure. The patient starts having frequent premature ventricular contractions, which progress into a sustained ventricular tachycardia causing hemodynamic instability after the surgeon releases the inferior vena cava (IVC) clamp. Of the following choices listed below, which would NOT be considered an appropriate choice for immediate therapy?

A. Sodium bicarbonate infusion
B. Low-dose epinephrine bolus
C. Immediate synchronized cardioversion
D. Calcium chloride injection

23. **A 59-year-old man with ESLD complicated by portopulmonary hypertension (PPH), hepatorenal syndrome, and hepatic encephalopathy presents for an orthotopic liver transplant. Intraoperatively, the patient becomes progressively hypoxic despite adjustments to the ventilator. Of the following choices listed below, which would NOT be considered an appropriate INITIAL choice for therapeutic intervention to improve the patient's oxygenation status?**

   A. Start milrinone.
   B. Start dobutamine.
   C. Start inhaled nitric oxide (iNO).
   D. Start dopamine.

24. **A 48-year-old woman with end-stage renal disease secondary to severe hypertension presents for a renal transplant. Intraoperatively, you notice that the patient's urine output has dropped to less than 0.5 mL/h after the allograft kidney has been transplanted. The surgeon is requesting that you intervene to increase urine output by improving renal perfusion. Of the following choices listed below, which would NOT be considered an appropriate INITIAL agent to improve renal perfusion during renal transplant?**

   A. Dopamine
   B. Mannitol
   C. Albumin
   D. Norepinephrine

25. **A 72 year old man with a history of ESLD due to hepatitis C received an orthotopic liver transplant 2 months ago and is now presenting for a ventral hernia repair. Which of the following laboratory values is the best marker in assessing the patient's liver synthetic function posttransplant?**

   A. Bilirubin
   B. AST/ALT (aspartate aminotransferase/alanine aminotransferase)
   C. International normalized ratio
   D. Albumin

26. **A 71-year-old woman with a history of rheumatoid arthritis is scheduled for a left total knee arthroplasty. She has been taking prednisone 5 mg PO daily for the last 2 weeks to control her rheumatoid arthritis. Which of the following is the most appropriate perioperative steroid plan given her chronic steroid regimen?**

   A. Recommend to the patient that she stop taking prednisone before the operation given the risk of intraoperative hyperglycemia.
   B. Recommend that she continues taking her home dose of prednisone up until the operation.
   C. Recommend that she doubles her dose of steroid on the morning of the operation.
   D. Recommend that she continue taking her home dose of prednisone up until the operation and give her an additional dose of hydrocortisone during the operation.

27. **A 64-year-old woman with a 70-pack-year smoking history and hypertension was recently admitted to the hospital with a severe COPD exacerbation and is currently receiving 40 mg of prednisone daily. On hospital day 3 she begins to complain of abdominal pain and spikes a fever. Imaging demonstrates evidence of appendicitis, and she is scheduled for an urgent appendectomy. Throughout the procedure, you note that she is becoming gradually more hypotensive. You place a radial arterial catheter, and she is consistently in the 80s-90s/40s-50s. You decide to do which of the following?**

   A. Start peripheral phenylephrine, place an nasogastric tube (NGT), and administer 40 mg prednisone.
   B. Place a central venous catheter, and start norepinephrine.
   C. Administer 100 mg hydrocortisone IV (intravenously) in addition to placing an NGT and administering 40 mg prednisone.
   D. Administer 100 mg hydrocortisone IV, and start peripheral phenylephrine.

28. A 46-year-old man, with a history of IV drug use on chronic methadone therapy and hepatitis C, is 1 year post orthotopic liver transplant and is now scheduled for a ventral hernia repair. In an attempt to address his anticipated postoperative pain with nonopioid analgesia, you plan to give him IV ketorolac. Which of the following immunosuppressive agents, in combination with ketorolac, increases the risk for potential postoperative renal dysfunction?

   A. Tacrolimus
   B. Mycophenolate Mofetil
   C. Azathioprine
   D. Prednisone

29. A 55-year-old woman with a history of a kidney transplant has newly diagnosed lung cancer and presents for a right-sided thoracotomy. You plan to place a preoperative epidural. Which of the following immunosuppressive agents would raise concern for a possible increased risk of epidural hematoma?

   A. Azathioprine
   B. Cyclosporine
   C. Tacrolimus
   D. Prednisone

30. Antithymocyte globulin (ATG) is given for acute rejection prevention during a kidney transplant. What is ATG's mechanism of action?

   A. Reduction in the demargination of neutrophils
   B. Depletion of B cells
   C. Inhibition of IL-1 receptors on B cells and T cells
   D. Depletion of T cells

31. Compared with pulsatile left ventricular assist devices (LVADs), continuous-flow LVAD therapy confers which of the following?

   A. Comparable risk of device-related infections
   B. A worse neurologic outcome
   C. Increased risk of GI bleeding
   D. Increased levels of circulating von Willebrand factor

32. Regarding perioperative considerations for lung transplantation (LTx), which of the following statements are true?

   A. Compared with donation-after-brain-death LTx, donation-after-circulatory-death (DCD) LTx results in decreased graft survival.
   B. Perioperative hyperglycemia is associated with increased mortality in patients undergoing LTx.
   C. Use of lung protective ventilation strategies in organ donors with brain death has not increased the number of available donor lungs.
   D. Lung transplant using cardiopulmonary bypass (CPB) provides better long-term outcomes compared with off-pump LTx.

33. A 59-year-old man with a history of mild hypertension, hyperlipidemia, and B-cell lymphoma with doxorubicin-induced cardiomyopathy requiring orthotopic heart transplantation 5 years ago is brought in by EMS to the ED. His posttransplant course was complicated by postoperative renal failure with permanent need for dialysis. He presents now in shock. He does not follow a renal diet but has undergone a routine hemodialysis 2 days ago. "He only takes tacrolimus and mycophenolate mofetil" at home per EMS report. His vitals are HR 115, BP 74/41, RR 35, and O₂ Sat 85% on 10 L FM. The patient's ECG shows ST elevations in multiple leads, his troponin I is 0.4, and serum lactate is 6. Before he can be brought to a heart catheterization laboratory, the patient passes away. Which of the following medications/intervention most likely would have helped prevent this situation?

A. Pravastatin
B. Aspirin
C. Diltiazem
D. Prophylactic coronary angioplasty with left main coronary artery stent deployment

34. Which of the statements regarding thyroid function and its impacts on cardiovascular pathophysiology is most likely true?

A. Pulmonary hypertension is linked to hyper- and hypothyroidism.
B. Hypothyroidism is associated with a slower progression of heart failure patients.
C. Triiodothyronine (T3)/thyroxin (T4) therapy to the donor increases availability of thoracic donor organs but causes increased graft rejection after transplantation.
D. T3 levels do not correlate with the presence of coronary artery disease.

35. Patients with end-stage heart failure pending heart transplantation may require temporary circulatory assist devices perioperatively. Regarding the individual devices, which of the following statements is correct?

A. Intra-aortic balloon pump (IABP) counterpulsation raises the effective cardiac output more than percutaneously inserted axial flow pumps (eg, Impella).
B. Percutaneously inserted axial flow pumps (eg, Impella) generally do not require anticoagulation while inserted.
C. Extracorporeal membrane oxygenation (ECMO) decreases left ventricular (LV) afterload less than IABP.
D. It is recommended to continue supportive catecholamine infusions with indwelling percutaneously inserted axial flow pumps to enhance cardiac output.

36. You are taking care of an otherwise healthy 35-year-old man undergoing repair of his left anterior cruciate ligament. Shortly after induction, his heart rate increased from 70 to 110 beats per minute and his blood pressure drops to 60/40 mm Hg. You also notice an increase in his peak inspiratory pressure. Which of the following is your next step?

A. Administer a 500-cc bolus of crystalloid, and turn down the concentration of volatile anesthetic.
B. Start a phenylephrine infusion to target an MAP greater than 60 mm Hg.
C. Call for help, give epinephrine 10-100 μg IV, and repeat or escalate dose every 1-2 minutes and titrate to effect.
D. Call for help, and give epinephrine 1 mg IV.

37. The following scenario applies to the next 3 questions: You are asked to evaluate a 65-year-old 80-kg man in the postanesthesia care unit (PACU). He has just undergone a laser lithotripsy of a right ureteral stone. His temperature is 38.5°C, heart rate is 100 beats per minute, blood pressure is 83/55 mm Hg, and respiratory rate is 30 breaths per minute. He is arousable but confused. He has already received 2 L of crystalloid in the perioperative period. The most appropriate next step in management is administration of which of the following?

    A. Start norepinephrine infusion, and titrate to MAP >65 mm Hg.
    B. Start dopamine infusion, and titrate to MAP >65 mm Hg.
    C. Start phenylephrine infusion, and titrate to SBP >90 mm Hg.
    D. Give 250 cc of 5% albumin.

38. The patient is now on norepinephrine at 20 µg/min, and his MAP remains less than 65 mm Hg. The next appropriate step is which of the following?

    A. Add dopamine as a second vasopressor.
    B. Add phenylephrine as a second vasopressor.
    C. Add vasopressin as a second vasopressor.
    D. Decrease your MAP goal to 60 mm Hg, as his baseline pressure is usually low.

39. The patient has already received 2 L of crystalloid, but you want to determine if he remains intravascularly volume-depleted. How is "fluid responsiveness" defined?

    A. Decrease in heart rate
    B. Urine output
    C. Increase in SBP
    D. Increase in cardiac output

40. A 55-year old man is scheduled for elective colectomy. His medical history is significant for hypertension, which is controlled on lisinopril. Shortly after induction with propofol and rocuronium, his blood pressure decreases from 130/85 to 80/50 mm Hg. Administration of ephedrine 5 mg and phenylephrine 40 µg IV has no effect. The most appropriate treatment at this time is administration of which of the following?

    A. Vasopressin
    B. Epinephrine
    C. Phenylephrine
    D. Calcium chloride

41. Which of the following treatments for catecholamine-resistant vasoplegia does NOT inhibit nitric oxide?

    A. Methylene blue
    B. Hydroxocobalamin
    C. Vitamin C
    D. Angiotensin II

42. A 70-year-old man is in the ICU after undergoing a left upper lobectomy. He develops atrial fibrillation on the second postoperative day. His heart rate is 150 beats per minute and blood pressure is 85/50 mm Hg. Which of the following is the *least* appropriate treatment of his tachycardia?

    A. Phenylephrine
    B. Amiodarone
    C. Metoprolol
    D. Verapamil

43. A 75-year-old man is admitted to the ICU with perforated diverticulitis and septic shock. He has a history of poorly controlled hypertension and chronic renal insufficiency. Which of the following is an appropriate blood pressure goal for him?

   A. Mean arterial pressure >60 mm Hg
   B. Mean arterial pressure >65 mm Hg
   C. Mean arterial pressure >70 mm Hg
   D. Mean arterial pressure >80 mm Hg

44. A 63-year old man is admitted to the ICU with sepsis after abdominal surgery for perforated diverticulitis. After fluid resuscitation, he continues to require high doses of norepinephrine. Bedside echocardiography shows a dilated left ventricle with a reduced ejection fraction. Which of the following statements is true?

   A. The recommendation for use of dobutamine in patients with evidence of persistent hypoperfusion despite adequate fluid loading and vasopressor use is based on high-quality evidence.
   B. Milrinone is a phosphodiesterase inhibitor that increases contractility independent of β-adrenergic receptors.
   C. Levosimendan increases both inotropy and blood pressure.
   D. When compared with norepinephrine and dobutamine, epinephrine is associated with increased mortality.

45. A 65-year-old man is admitted to the ICU after undergoing an uncomplicated 3-vessel coronary artery bypass graft (CABG × 3). His blood pressure is 185/95 mm Hg. Which of the following is false regarding clevidipine?

   A. It is contraindicated in patients with allergies to soybeans, soy products, eggs, or egg products.
   B. When compared with nitroprusside, clevidipine demonstrated a significant mortality advantage.
   C. Clevidipine is superior for blood pressure control when compared with nitroprusside, nitroglycerin, and nicardipine.
   D. Rebound hypertension can occur after discontinuation of clevidipine.

46. Which of the following agents is categorized as a Category A bioterrorism agent by the Centers for Disease Control and Prevention (CDC)?

   A. Ricin toxin
   B. *Vibrio cholerae*
   C. *Yersinia pestis* (plague)
   D. Hantavirus

47. You are asked to evaluate several patients who presented with symptoms of mydriasis, ptosis, diplopia, dysphagia, dysarthria, and progressive, symmetric descending flaccid paralysis. The patients are conscious and have no cardiovascular perturbations. You hear from colleagues that there are several similar cases at area hospitals as well. You recommend which of the following?

   A. Treatment with plasmapheresis or IV immunoglobulin and close respiratory and cardiovascular monitoring
   B. Supportive care, close monitoring for respiratory failure and risk of aspiration, and administration of antitoxin
   C. Treatment with atropine, pralidoxime, anticonvulsants if seizures occur, and close monitoring for respiratory failure and risk of aspiration
   D. Thorough skin examination, removal of tick, and supportive care

48. **Which of the following statements regarding smallpox is false?**

    A. The incubation period for smallpox is 10-14 days.
    B. Smallpox is highly infective requiring exposure to only 10-100 organisms to be infected.
    C. The lesions of smallpox appear over the face and trunk and progress from macule to papule to vesicle to crust within 24-48 hours, and lesions at different stages can coexist on any 1 part of the body.
    D. The World Health Organization (WHO) recommends a surveillance and containment strategy for the management of smallpox.

49. **What are the 4 properties of hazards within the biological weapon spectrum?**

    A. Toxicity, latency, persistency, and transmissibility
    B. Virulence, stability, endemic, and determination
    C. Toxicity, stability, transmissibility, and transitory
    D. Virulence, weaponization, toxicity, and transmissibility

50. **You are caring for a 35-year-old man with respiratory failure, fever, shock, and acidosis. He presented 3 days ago with nonspecific complaints of fever, cough, and malaise. His chest radiograph shows mediastinal widening and pleural effusions. Blood cultures are growing *Bacillus anthracis*. Which of the following is NOT part of his management?**

    A. He should be started on an antibiotic with bactericidal activity such as a fluoroquinolone as well as a protein synthesis inhibitor such as clindamycin to reduce toxin production.
    B. He should be placed on airborne precautions in a negative pressure room.
    C. A lumbar puncture should be performed to evaluate for meningitis.
    D. He should be treated early with an anthrax antitoxin.

Chapter 21 ▪ Answers

1. **Correct answer: B**

Trauma is classically categorized as either blunt or penetrating. Regardless of the mechanism of injury, the initial assessment and management of a trauma patient as taught by the ATLS guidelines comprises 5 actions: primary survey, resuscitation, secondary survey, continued monitoring and reevaluation, and definitive care. The aim is to provide systemic, efficient, priority-driven care.

The goal of the primary survey is to identify and manage urgently life-threatening injuries. The primary survey is specifically organized to meet this goal and should be performed in the following order: airway, breathing, circulation, disability, and exposure. Ongoing resuscitation efforts should then be directed toward any injuries discovered during the primary survey.

The goal of the secondary survey is to identify non–life-threatening injuries. It typically comprises a head-to-toe physical examination with adjuncts such as laboratory studies and radiographic imaging (if the patient's stability allows). The following algorithm has been proposed for the initial management of the major trauma patient.

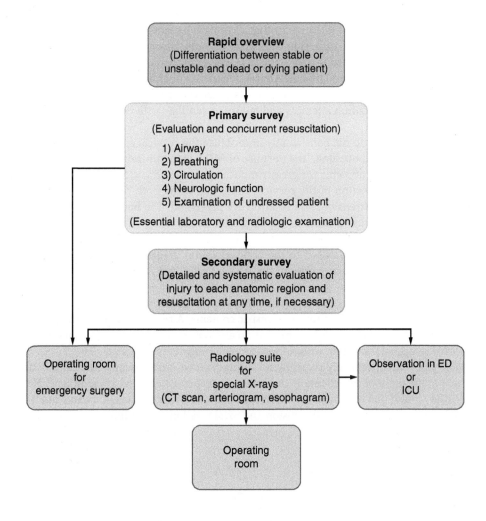

References:
1. ATLS Subcommittee. Advanced trauma life support (ATLS®): the ninth edition. *J Trauma Acute Care Surg.* 2013;74(5):1363-1366.
2. Capan LM, Miller SM, Gingrich KJ. Trauma and burns. In: Barash PG, Cullen BF, Stoelting RK, et al, eds. *Clinical Anesthesia.* 7th ed. Philadelphia: Wolters Kluwer Health/Lippincott Williams & Wilkins; 2013:1490-1534.

2. Correct Answer: D

In 2014, the ASA Committee on Trauma and Emergency Preparedness (COTEP) published modifications to the 2013 ASA Difficult Airway Algorithm to accommodate the unique issues encountered in airway management of the trauma patient. Recommendations for awake fiberoptic intubation from this committee preclude our patient, who is both hemodynamically unstable and uncooperative. COTEP recommends that appropriate candidates for awake fiberoptic intubation are awake (GCS ≥9), cooperative, hemodynamically stable, and able to maintain adequate O_2 saturation. The COTEP difficult airway algorithm recommends BVM with cricoid pressure only after initial intubation attempt is unsuccessful.

Reference:
1. Hagberg C, Kaslow O. *Difficult Airway Management Algorithm in Trauma Updated by COTEP*. Vol 78. ASA Monitor; 2014: 56-60.

3. Correct answer: B

In 2014, the ASA COTEP published modifications to the 2013 ASA Difficult Airway Algorithm to accommodate the unique issues encountered in airway management of the trauma patient. COTEP provides a stepwise formula to use in the event of an unrecognized difficult airway in a trauma patient, noted in the figure provided. MILS is recommended in a trauma patient with suspected cervical spine injury, which is the case in this patient given his risk factors for combined brain and spine injuries (MVC and GCS ≤8). COTEP recommends that all trauma patients requiring intubation receive cricoid pressure to reduce the risk of aspiration of gastric contents. However, both MILS and cricoid pressure may be altered or discontinued if they impede tracheal intubation, particularly if the patient has become hypoxemic. The modified Difficult Airway Algorithm does not include blind nasal or orotracheal intubation, and emergency invasive airway access, such as a cricothyroidotomy, is recommended only after multiple failed intubation attempts and failure to ventilate with either BVM or a supraglottic airway device.

Rigid cervical collars do not consistently immobilize the cervical spine during intubation and considerably decrease mouth opening. The purpose of MILS is to minimize any cervical spine movement during intubation, while allowing for greater mouth opening and jaw displacement. It is performed by removing the anterior portion of the cervical collar and using both hands to hold the cervical spine such that neck flexion, extension, and rotation are prevented. The benefit of MILS has been recently called into question because it tends to impair glottic visualization. This can result in a longer time to tracheal intubation, failure to secure the airway, or can cause the laryngoscopist to apply more lifting pressure (which can be transmitted to the cervical spine). Regardless, MILS is still the standard of practice, and its use is supported in both the ASA COTEP and ATLS guidelines for airway management in the trauma patient.

Of note, the application of cricoid pressure may worsen glottic visualization in up to 30% of patients without effectively preventing aspiration of gastric contents. A recent study examining the impact of cricoid pressure on success of subsequent intubation attempts revealed that discontinuing cricoid pressure often enabled tracheal intubation without worsening laryngoscopic grade of view.

COTEP does not specifically recommend indirect video laryngoscopy, although it states that this "may be a preferred tool in patients with known or suspected cervical spine injury." Notably, a 2013 cadaver study found that relative to the Macintosh blade or Fastrach, the Lightwand and Airtraq devices produced significantly less flexion-extension and axial rotation during intubation in patients with C1-2 ligamentous instability.

References:
1. ACS Committee on Trauma. *ATLS Student Course Manual: Advanced Trauma Life Support*. 9th ed. American College of Surgeons; 2012.
2. Capan LM, Miller SM, Gingrich KJ. Trauma and burns. In: Barash PG, Cullen BF, Stoelting RK, et al, eds. *Clinical Anesthesia*. 7th ed. Philadelphia: Wolters Kluwer Health/Lippincott Williams & Wilkins; 2013:1490-1534.
3. Hagberg C, Kaslow O. *Difficult Airway Management Algorithm in Trauma Updated by COTEP*. Vol 78. ASA Monitor; 2014:56-60.

4. Smith C. *Trauma Anesthesia.* 2nd ed. Cambridge, United Kingdom: Cambridge University Press; 2015.
5. Wendling A, Tighe P, Conrad B, et al. Comparison of four airway devices on cervical spine alignment in cadaver models of global ligamentous instability at c1-2. *Anesth Analg.* 2013;117(1):126-132.

4. Correct answer: C

The GCS score provides a standardized approach to evaluating a patient's neurologic status. Three parameters are tested: eye response, verbal response, and motor response. In head trauma, the sum of the individual parameters tested in the GCS has been demonstrated to correlate with the state of consciousness, the severity of the head injury, and the patient's prognosis. The GCS is scored as follows:

Glasgow Coma Scale Scoring

	6	5	4	3	2	1
Eye opening			Spontaneous, already open and blinking	To speech	To pain	None
Verbal response		Oriented	Answers, but confused	Inappropriate but recognizable words	Incomprehensible sounds	None
Motor response	Obeys verbal commands	Localizes painful stimulus	Withdraws from painful stimulus	Decorticate posturing	Decerebrate posturing	None

The patient described earlier opens eyes to pain (2), localizes painful stimulus (5), and is saying recognizable words that are inappropriate in context (3), for a GCS score of 10.

Reference:

1. Capan LM, Miller SM, Gingrich KJ. Trauma and burns. In: Barash PG, Cullen BF, Stoelting RK, et al, eds. *Clinical Anesthesia.* 7th ed. Philadelphia: Wolters Kluwer Health/Lippincott Williams & Wilkins; 2013:1490-1534.

5. Correct answer: C

Hemorrhage, the most common cause of hypotension in the setting of trauma, is a leading cause of trauma-related mortality. Other common causes of hypotension in trauma and their initial management are listed below. Life-threatening or exsanguinating hemorrhage can occur in 1 of 5 sites: chest, abdomen, retroperitoneum, long bone fractures, or "on the street" (hemorrhage outside the body). Achieving hemodynamic balance in a hemorrhaging trauma patient is challenging, as both underfluid and overfluid resuscitating a trauma patient each carry its own morbidity. However, it has become clear in recent literature that deliberate hypotensive resuscitation in trauma patients is correlated with improved morbidity and mortality. Specifically, 1 prospective study demonstrated that torso trauma patients randomized to delayed resuscitation (no fluid until patient reached the OR) had a higher survival to hospital discharge than patients randomized to standard of care (up to 2 L of crystalloid infused in the prehospital setting)—70% versus 62%, respectively ($P < .04$). In a preliminary report of another prospective study, trauma patients randomized to a target MAP around 50 mm Hg (compared with a target MAP of 65 mm Hg) had lower early postoperative mortality, lower incidence of coagulopathy, and lower mortality related to coagulopathy. In light of recent findings in the literature, most major trauma centers allow for hypotensive resuscitation, generally targeting an SBP <100 mm Hg with an MAP between 50 and 60 mm Hg. A SBP of 110 mm Hg is accepted as a prehospital triage threshold for delivery to a Level I trauma center for trauma patients older than 65 years; SBP of 90 mm Hg remains a triage threshold for young patients.

Initial Assessment and Shock Management

CONDITION	ASSESSMENT (PHYSICAL EXAMINATION)	MANAGEMENT
Tension pneumothorax	Tracheal deviation Distended neck veins Tympany Absent breath sounds	Needle decompression Tube thoracostomy
Massive hemothorax	Tracheal deviation Flat neck veins Percussion dullness Absent breath sounds	Venous access Volume replacement Surgical consultation/thoracotomy Tube thoracostomy
Cardiac tamponade	Distended neck veins Muffled heart tones Ultrasonography	Venous access Volume replacement Thoracotomy Pericardiocentesis
Intra-abdominal hemorrhage	Distended abdomen Uterine lift, if pregnant DPL/ultrasonography Vaginal examination	Venous access Volume replacement Surgical consultation Displace uterus from vena cava
Obvious external bleeding	Identify source of obvious external bleeding	Direct pressure Splints Closure of actively bleeding scalp wounds

References:
1. ACS Committee on Trauma. *ATLS Student Course Manual: Advanced Trauma Life Support.* 9th ed. American College of Surgeons; 2012.
2. Capan LM, Miller SM, Gingrich KJ. Trauma and burns. In: Barash PG, Cullen BF, Stoelting RK, et al, eds. *Clinical Anesthesia.* 7th ed. Philadelphia: Wolters Kluwer Health/Lippincott Williams & Wilkins; 2013:1490-1534.
3. Smith C. *Trauma Anesthesia.* 2nd ed. Cambridge, United Kingdom: Cambridge University Press; 2015.

6. **Correct answer: D**

Although relatively insensitive and nonspecific, initial vital signs can be used as early clinical indicators of the severity of blood loss in patients at risk for hemorrhagic shock (see table below). Per the ATLS guidelines, heart rate, blood pressure, pulse pressure, respiratory rate, urine output, and mental status can be used as early clinical indicators of the severity of hemorrhagic shock. The patient described earlier meets Class IV criteria with lethargy, a heart rate of 145 beats per minute, respiratory rate of 40 breaths per minute, and a low SBP and urine output. Thus, according to the ATLS classification of hemorrhagic shock, she has likely lost greater than 2 L of blood.

Estimated Blood Loss[a] Based on Patient's Initial Presentation

	CLASS I	CLASS II	CLASS III	CLASS IV
Blood loss (mL)	Up to 750	750-1500	1500-2000	>2000
Blood loss (% blood volume)	Up to 15%	15%-30%	30%-40%	>40%
Pulse rate (BPM)	<100	100-120	120-140	>140
Systolic blood pressure	Normal	Normal	Decreased	Decreased
Pulse pressure (mm Hg)	Normal or increased	Decreased	Decreased	Decreased
Respiratory rate	14-20	20-30	30-40	>35
Urine output (mL/h)	>30	20-30	5-15	Negligible
CNS/mental status	Slightly anxious	Mildly anxious	Anxious, confused	Confused, lethargic
Initial fluid replacement	Crystalloid	Crystalloid	Crystalloid and blood	Crystalloid and blood

[a]For a 70-kg man.

References:

1. ACS Committee on Trauma. *ATLS Student Course Manual: Advanced Trauma Life Support.* 9th ed. American College of Surgeons; 2012.
2. Capan LM, Miller SM, Gingrich KJ. Trauma and burns. In: Barash PG, Cullen BF, Stoelting RK, et al, eds. *Clinical Anesthesia.* 7th ed. Philadelphia: Wolters Kluwer Health/Lippincott Williams & Wilkins; 2013:1490-1534.

7. Correct answer: D

The Assessment of Blood Consumption (ABC) score is one of the many clinical diagnostic tools that have been developed to improve the ability to predict severe hemorrhage and therefore the need for massive transfusion (transfusion of ≥10 units of packed red blood cells during the first 24 hours of admission). There are 4 yes/no questions, where "yes" answers are assigned 1 point and "no" answers are assigned 0 points: penetrating mechanism of injury, SBP ≤90 mm Hg, heart rate ≥120 beats per minute, and a positive FAST finding. In the development and validation studies for the ABC scoring system, scores ≥2 were likely to require massive transfusion with sensitivity and specificity ranging from 75% to 90% and 67% to 88%, respectively. The patient's ABC score is 2, suggesting that she will likely require massive transfusion resuscitation.

References:

1. Capan LM, Miller SM, Gingrich KJ. Trauma and burns. In: Barash PG, Cullen BF, Stoelting RK, et al, eds. *Clinical Anesthesia.* 7th ed. Philadelphia: Wolters Kluwer Health/Lippincott Williams & Wilkins; 2013:1490-1534.
2. Cotton BA, Dossett LA, Haut ER, et al. Multicenter validation of a simplified score to predict massive transfusion in trauma. *J Trauma.* 2010;69(Suppl 1):S33-S39.
3. Nunez TC, Voskresensky IV, Dossett LA, Shinall R, Dutton WD, Cotton BA. Early prediction of massive transfusion in trauma: simple as ABC (assessment of blood consumption)? *J Trauma.* 2009;66(2):346-352.

8. Correct answer: C

Base deficit is an established index of organ perfusion and is useful to trend during all phases of shock; it is considered a better prognostic marker than arterial pH, and its normalization can be used as an accurate end point of resuscitation. In previously healthy adult and pediatric trauma patients, the base deficit accurately reflects the severity of shock, oxygen debt, disturbances in oxygen delivery, sufficiency of fluid resuscitation, likelihood of multiorgan failure, and survival. The extent of base deficit as it correlates with the degree of shock has been demonstrated, where mild, moderate, and severe shock ranges from −3 to −5 mmol/L, from −6 to −9 mmol/L, and <−10 mmol/L, respectively. It has also demonstrated that an admission base deficit below −5 to −8 mmol/L correlates with increased mortality and that initial ED base deficit predicts transfusion requirements and mortality better than ATLS classification. Elevated blood lactate is a less specific indicator of tissue hypoperfusion in trauma because it can also be produced in well-oxygenated tissues (eg, decreased hepatic clearance of lactate and mitochondrial dysfunction). However, failure to normalize within 24 hours after reversal of circulatory shock is a predictor of increased mortality and therefore serves as a useful end point of resuscitation.

Reference:
1. Capan LM, Miller SM, Gingrich KJ. Trauma and burns. In: Barash PG, Cullen BF, Stoelting RK, et al, eds. *Clinical Anesthesia*. 7th ed. Philadelphia: Wolters Kluwer Health/Lippincott Williams & Wilkins; 2013:1490-1534.

9. Correct answer: B

Thromboelastography (Haemonetics, Boston, MA) is a point-of-care device that provides a relatively rapid graphic evaluation of clotting function (see figure in question 9). It is a viscoelastic hemostatic assay that measures the viscoelastic properties of whole blood clot formation. TEG determines in sample of whole blood the time it takes for initial fibrin formation, clot consistency, the rate of clot formation, and the times required for both clot retraction and lysis. See below for further details. The patient's TEG demonstrates decreased maximal amplitude, suggesting a decrease in quality or quantity of platelets. Given the described clinical setting of massive transfusion without concomitant platelet repletion, the low maximum amplitude (MA) seen on his TEG likely represents thrombocytopenia, and therefore, he would likely benefit from (B) platelet transfusion.

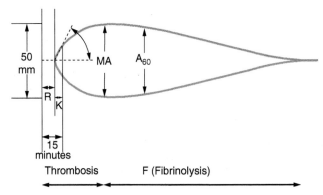

(From Capan LM, Miller SM, Gingrich KJ. Trauma and burns. In: Barash PG, Cullen BF, Stoelting RK, et al, eds. *Clinical Anesthesia*. 7th ed. Philadelphia: Wolters Kluwer Health/Lippincott Williams & Wilkins; 2013:1520, with permission.)

TEG VALUE	HEMOSTASIS ACTIVITY	BLOOD COMPONENT
R and K	Formation, buildup, and cross-linking of fibrin	Coagulation factors
Maximum amplitude	Absolute strength of the fibrin clot	Platelet function and quantity
α angle	Speed of clot formation and fibrin cross-linking	Coagulation factors and platelets
Amplitude of TEG 60 min after maximum amplitude (A_{60})	Fibrinolysis	Fibrinogen and fibrin

References:
1. Capan LM, Miller SM, Gingrich KJ. Trauma and burns. In: Barash PG, Cullen BF, Stoelting RK, et al, eds. *Clinical Anesthesia*. 7th ed. Philadelphia: Wolters Kluwer Health/Lippincott Williams & Wilkins; 2013:1490-1534.
2. Whiting D, DiNardo JA. TEG and ROTEM: technology and clinical applications. *Am J Hematol*. 2014;89(2):228-232.

10. Correct answer: A

Dabigatran belongs to a class of medications called direct oral anticoagulants. It directly binds and inhibits thrombin, which ultimately leads to inhibition of secondary hemostasis. It is clinically indicated to prevent nonhemorrhagic strokes in nonvalvular atrial fibrillation. Patients taking dabigatran are at increased risk for life-threatening bleeding, and (A) idarucizumab is the first reversal agent approved to reverse its effects. It is only approved for reversal of dabigatran and is a monoclonal antibody that works by binding to the drug compound to neutralize its effect without procoagulant effects. (B and D) There are 2 forms of prothrombin complex concentrate: Bebulin (factors II, IX, and X), and Kcentra (factors II, VII, IX, and X). They are approved for the quick reversal of vitamin K–antagonist oral anticoagulants (eg, warfarin), particularly intracranial bleeding. (E) Recent guidelines recommend against administration of FFP in direct thrombin inhibitor–related intracranial hemorrhage. (C) Pertuzumab is a monoclonal antibody used for the treatment of metastatic HER2-positive breast cancer.

References:
1. Capan LM, Miller SM, Gingrich KJ. Trauma and burns. In: Barash PG, Cullen BF, Stoelting RK, et al, eds. *Clinical Anesthesia*. 7th ed. Philadelphia: Wolters Kluwer Health/Lippincott Williams & Wilkins; 2013:1490-1534.
2. Whiting D, DiNardo JA. TEG and ROTEM: technology and clinical applications. *Am J Hematol*. 2014;89(2):228-232.
3. Gulati D, Dua D, Torbey MT. Hemostasis in intracranial hemorrhage. *Front Neurol*. 2017;8:80.
4. Pollack Jr CV, Reilly PA, Eikelboom J, et al. Idarucizumab for dabigatran reversal. *N Engl J Med*. 2015;373(6):511-520.
5. Swain SM, Baselga J, Kim SB, et al. Pertuzumab, trastuzumab, and docetaxel in HER2-positive metastatic breast cancer. *N Engl J Med*. 2015;372(8):724-734.

11. Correct answer: D

Transfusion-related acute lung injury (TRALI) and transfusion-associated circulatory overload (TACO) are both rare but potentially fatal complications of blood product transfusion. All blood products have been associated with TRALI and TACO, with plasma-rich components such as FFP and apheresis platelets being the most frequently implicated. Although there is no one distinct feature that distinguishes TRALI from TACO, both are clinical diagnoses with a constellation of clinical features (see below). The clinical features in the patient described earlier most correlate with TRALI and would be unlikely to benefit from diuretics.

FEATURE	TRALI	TACO
Respiratory symptoms	Acute dyspnea	Acute dyspnea
Hemodynamic changes	Hypotension	Hypertension
Fever	Likely	Unlikely
Jugular venous distension	Unlikely	Likely
PA occlusion pressure	Likely normal	Elevated
Pulmonary edema fluid	Exudate	Transudate
Chest radiograph	Diffuse bilateral infiltrates	Diffuse bilateral infiltrates
Plasma BNP	Likely normal	Elevated
Fluid balance	Even or negative	Positive
Response to diuretic	Minimal	Significant

References:
1. Capan LM, Miller SM, Gingrich KJ. Trauma and burns. In: Barash PG, Cullen BF, Stoelting RK, et al, eds. *Clinical Anesthesia*. 7th ed. Philadelphia: Wolters Kluwer Health/Lippincott Williams & Wilkins; 2013:1490-1534.
2. Skeate RC, Eastlund T. Distinguishing between transfusion related acute lung injury and transfusion associated circulatory overload. *Curr Opin Hematol*. 2007;14(6):682-687.

12. Correct answer: C

Hemorrhage is a leading cause of death among patients with major trauma. TXA is a synthetic derivative of the amino acid lysine and works by reversibly blocking lysine binding sites on plasminogen, thereby competitively inhibiting fibrinolysis. TXA has been shown to reduce bleeding in patients undergoing CPB, as well as other elective surgeries. The Clinical Randomization of Antifibrinolytic Therapy in Significant Haemorrhage (CRASH-2) trial demonstrated in a subgroup analysis that TXA given within 3 hours of injury (1 g in a 10-min bolus and then 1 g infused over the next 8 h) significantly reduced the risk of death due to bleeding. However, the same treatment given to trauma patients after 3 hours of injury significantly increased the risk of death due to bleeding. Though previous studies have demonstrated increased risk of VTE with the administration of TXA, in CRASH-2 there were no significant differences in the rate of vaso-occlusive events.

References:
1. Shakur H, Roberts I, Bautista R, et al. Effects of tranexamic acid on death, vascular occlusive events, and blood transfusion in trauma patients with significant haemorrhage. *Lancet*. 2010;376(9734):23-32.
2. Capan LM, Miller SM, Gingrich KJ. Trauma and burns. In: Barash PG, Cullen BF, Stoelting RK, et al, eds. *Clinical Anesthesia*. 7th ed. Philadelphia: Wolters Kluwer Health/Lippincott Williams & Wilkins; 2013:1490-1534.

13. Correct answer: C

The most commonly damaged area of the aorta in blunt trauma is the isthmus of the descending aorta, located immediately distal to the takeoff of the left subclavian artery. It is vulnerable to shearing forces because the isthmus is anchored in relation to the proximal aorta by the ligamentum arteriosum and left mainstem bronchus. The common clinical nomenclature and management are listed below. This patient has a (C) grade 3 injury with a pseudoaneurysm (FA, false aneurysm) communicating with the true lumen of the descending aorta.

Grade	Injury	Example image on TEE	Clinical management
1 GRADE I Intimal tear Intima Media Adventitia	Intimal tear		Nonoperative management: aggressive heart rate and blood pressure control
2 GRADE II Intramural hematoma	Intramural hematoma		Operative management
3 GRADE III Pseudoaneurysm	Pseudoaneurysm		Operative management
4 GRADE IV Rupture	Rupture	N/A	Operative management

(Drawings in left column redrawn after Lee WA, Matsumura JS, Mitchell RS, et al. Endovascular repair of traumatic thoracic aortic injury: clinical practice guidelines of the Society for Vascular Surgery. *J Vasc Surg*. 2011;53:187-192. Images in right column from Goarin J-P, Cluzel P, Gosgnach M, et al. Evaluation of transesophageal echocardiography for diagnosis of traumatic aortic injury. *Anesthesiology*. 2000;93:1373, with permission.)

References:
1. Azizzadeh A, Keyhani K, Miller 3rd CC, Coogan SM, Safi HJ, Estrera AL. Blunt traumatic aortic injury: initial experience with endovascular repair. *J Vasc Surg*. 2009;49(6):1403-1408.
2. Capan LM, Miller SM, Gingrich KJ. Trauma and burns. In: Barash PG, Cullen BF, Stoelting RK, et al, eds. *Clinical Anesthesia*. 7th ed. Philadelphia: Wolters Kluwer Health/Lippincott Williams & Wilkins; 2013:1490-1534.
3. Fox N, Schwartz D, Salazar JH, et al. Evaluation and management of blunt traumatic aortic injury: a practice management guideline from the Eastern Association for the Surgery of Trauma. *J Trauma Acute Care Surg*. 2015;78(1):136-146.

14. Correct answer: A

Isotonic crystalloids, such as normal saline, are the ideal choice for fluid resuscitation in most patients with TBI, as (B and C) hypotonic crystalloid solutions, such as lactated ringers and 5% dextrose in water, have been shown to facilitate cerebral edema in uninjured areas of the brain. Glucose-containing solutions and hyperglycemia should also be avoided because their anaerobic metabolites produce free water and promote acidosis, which can exacerbate cerebral edema. (D) A post hoc analysis of the SAFE Study (2004) demonstrated increased 28-day mortality in patients with TBI who were resuscitated with albumin, as compared with normal saline. (E) In a randomized control trial of patients with moderate or severe TBI, a liberal transfusion threshold (>10 g/dL) did not result in improved outcome at 6 months compared with a threshold of 7 g/dL and was associated with a higher frequency of thromboembolic events.

References:

1. Capan LM, Miller SM, Gingrich KJ. Trauma and burns. In: Barash PG, Cullen BF, Stoelting RK, et al, eds. *Clinical Anesthesia*. 7th ed. Philadelphia: Wolters Kluwer Health/Lippincott Williams & Wilkins; 2013:1490-1534.
2. Haddad S, Arabi T. Critical care management of severe traumatic brain injury in adults. *Scand J Trauma Resusc Emerg Med*. 2012;20:12.
3. Finfer S, Bellomo R, Boyce N, et al. A comparison of albumin and saline for fluid resuscitation in the intensive care unit. *N Engl J Med*. 2004;350:2247-2256.
4. Robertson CS, Hannay HJ, Yamal JM, et al. Effect of erythropoietin and transfusion threshold on neurological recovery after traumatic brain injury: a randomized clinical trial. *JAMA*. 2014;312(1):36-47.

15. Correct answer: B

With regard to brain ischemia, the primary goal in early management of TBI is preventing any secondary insults to the brain parenchyma that may decrease oxygen supply (eg, hypotension, hypoxemia, acidosis, anemia, elevated ICP, and hyperglycemia). Important initial interventions thus include establishing and maintaining normal ICP and CPP to defend oxygen delivery. The CPP is the pressure gradient that promotes cerebral blood flow (CBF) and is calculated by subtracting the MAP by either the jugular venous pressure or ICP (whichever value is higher). In this case, the patient's CPP is 80 − 35 = 45 mm Hg. Guidelines by the Brain Trauma Foundation and the American Association of Neurological Surgeons recommend that for the treatment of head-injured patients, a CPP between 50 and 70 mm Hg should be maintained. Therefore, this patient's CPP is too low (B), thus decreasing CBF and threatening adequate oxygen delivery to the brain.

Reference:

1. Capan LM, Miller SM, Gingrich KJ. Trauma and burns. In: Barash PG, Cullen BF, Stoelting RK, et al, eds. *Clinical Anesthesia*. 7th ed. Philadelphia: Wolters Kluwer Health/Lippincott Williams & Wilkins; 2013:1490-1534.

16. Correct answer: B

Patients with head injury and intracranial hypertension benefit from prompt normalization of ICP, as doing so has been shown to reduce mortality in severe TBI. Guidelines recommend a target ICP of 20-25 mm Hg (B). Mannitol is an osmotic diuretic, which when given in appropriate doses can improve CBF and oxygen delivery by reducing the hematocrit, thereby reducing blood viscosity. The initial recommended dose is 0.25-0.5 g/kg repeated every 4-6 hours as needed, though some authors suggest up to 2 mg/kg is appropriate. At higher doses, mannitol toxicity can develop, which is typically characterized by hyponatremia, high serum osmolality, and serum osmolality gap >10 mOsm/L. Mannitol can trigger renal failure and therefore should be used judiciously in patients at particular risk (eg, preexisting renal disease, hypovolemia, rhabdomyolysis, or nephrotoxic drug use).

Reference:

1. Capan LM, Miller SM, Gingrich KJ. Trauma and burns. In: Barash PG, Cullen BF, Stoelting RK, et al, eds. *Clinical Anesthesia*. 7th ed. Philadelphia: Wolters Kluwer Health/Lippincott Williams & Wilkins; 2013:1490-1534.

17. Correct answer: C

The general risk of DVT and pulmonary embolism in blunt trauma patients is 3.2%, but DVT occurs at much higher rates in a subset of injuries, despite clinical management guidelines. Specifically, 30% of major lower extremity injuries, 30% of spine injuries, 46% of major head injuries, 33% of major thoracic injuries, and 15% of serious injuries of the face or abdomen suffer from a DVT despite implementation of effective clinical management guidelines. One research group reviewed their experience of VTE in more than 10 000 blunt trauma patients over a period of 10 years, all of whom were managed using a well-established clinical management guideline. Using logistic regression, they found that independent risk factors for VTE despite guideline-managed prophylaxis include pelvic ring injuries, major lower extremity bony trauma, spinal cord injury, a higher Injury Severity Score, and >3 days of mechanical ventilation.

References:

1. Capan LM, Miller SM, Gingrich KJ. Trauma and burns. In: Barash PG, Cullen BF, Stoelting RK, et al, eds. *Clinical Anesthesia*. 7th ed. Philadelphia: Wolters Kluwer Health/Lippincott Williams & Wilkins; 2013:1490-1534.
2. Frankel H, FitzPatrick M, Gaskell S, et al. Strategies to improve compliance with evidence-based clinical management guidelines. *J Am Coll Surg*. 1999;189:533-538.

18. Correct answer: C

Microvascular permeability significantly increases after major burns, leading to large volumes of transudative fluid leaking into the interstitium. Fluid resuscitation is of utmost importance in the early care of burn patients, particularly with burn injuries over 15% of TBSA. Careful titration of fluid is exceedingly vital: Too little fluid can lead to hemodynamic instability and increase in transudative fluid extravasation, while excessive fluid resuscitation can cause life-threatening edema in the upper airway, chest wall, and abdomen. Burns ≤15% TBSA can be managed with parental or oral replacement volume 150% of the calculated maintenance rate. In burns >15% TBSA, 2 formulas are commonly used because they are best tailored to each individual patient's clinical condition. They include the Parkland (Baxter) and modified Brooke formulas. They are listed below. (D) For this patient, in the first 24 hours, it would be reasonable for him to receive between 2 * 100 * 40 = 8000 mL (8 L) and 4 * 100 * 40 = 16 000 mL (16 L).

Guidelines for Initial Fluid Resuscitation after Thermal Injury

FORMULA	FIRST 24 h	SECOND 24 h
Parkland formula	4.0 mL crystalloid * kg * % burn[a]	20%-60% of calculated plasma volume as colloid
Modified Brooke formula	2.0 mL lactated ringers * kg * % burn[a]	0.3-0.5 mL * kg * % burn[a]

[a] % burn = whole number not fraction.

Reference:

1. Barash PG. Trauma and burns. In: *Clinical Anesthesia*. 7th ed. Philadelphia: Wolters Kluwer Health; 2013:1490-1534.

19. Correct answer: B

A core body temperature below 35°C is frequently associated with acidosis, hypotension, and coagulopathy and has shown to correlate with an increased risk of severe bleeding, need for transfusion, and mortality. There is a long list of adverse effects associated with hypothermia, including: cardiac depression, myocardial ischemia, arrhythmias, peripheral vasoconstriction, impaired tissue oxygen delivery, increased oxygen consumption during rewarming, reduced response to catecholamines, increased blood viscosity, metabolic acidosis, abnormalities of potassium and calcium homeostasis, reduced drug clearance, and increased risk of infection. Both preventing hypothermia and restoring normothermia have been associated with decreased mortality rate, blood loss, fluid requirement, organ failure, and ICU length of stay. This is often achieved by using a combination of the following: convection warmer set at 43°C, circulating-water warmer, airway warming, and fluid warmer. Of note, a convection warmer can prevent but not effectively treat severe hypothermia because of (1) the often-limited body surface area outside the surgical field and (2) the low specific heat of air (less heat transferred to cold trauma patient).

Reference:

1. Capan LM, Miller SM, Scher C. Trauma and burns. In: Barash PG, Cullen BF, Stoelting RK, et al., eds. *Clinical Anesthesia*. 7th ed. Philadelphia: Wolters Kluwer Health; 2013:1486-1536.

20. Correct answer: A

The patient likely has a hemopericardium causing tamponade physiology. Patients with acute pericardial tamponade are entirely dependent on their sympathetic tone, as stroke volume is static secondary to the external compression on the heart from the pericardial fluid. Hemodynamic goals for these patients include maintenance of preload, contractility, and heart rate. Drugs that decrease heart rate, preload, or myocardial contractility should be avoided (B, C, and D) because they can precipitate cardiovascular collapse. Ketamine is an ideal induction agent for this clinical scenario because it preserves heart rate and blood pressure during the initial phase of anesthesia in non–catecholamine-depleted patients.

References:
1. Capan LM, Miller SM, Scher C. Trauma and burns. In: Barash PG, Cullen BF, Stoelting RK, et al., eds. *Clinical Anesthesia*. 7th ed. Philadelphia: Wolters Kluwer Health; 2013:1486-1536.
2. Smith B. *UOTW #78 - Ultrasound of the Week*; 2017.

21. Correct answer: D

MELD is a scoring system that was devised to assess the severity of chronic liver disease. It was originally developed with the intent of predicting mortality within 3 months of surgical procedure, and it is currently used by the United Network for Organ Sharing (UNOS) for determining priority in allocation of liver transplants. Before the development of the MELD score, Child-Pugh score was used to assess prognosis of chronic liver disease, mainly pertaining to cirrhotic patients. MELD score is calculated as follows:

$$\textbf{MELD} = 3.78 \times \ln[\text{serum bilirubin (mg/dL)}] + 11.2 \times \ln[\text{INR}] + 9.57 \times \ln[\text{serum creatinine (mg/dL)}] + 6.43$$

Based on the MELD score, the 3-month mortality of a patient is determined as the following:
- 40 or more—71.3% mortality
- 30-39—52.6% mortality
- 20-29—19.6% mortality
- 10-19—6.0% mortality
- <9—1.9% mortality

Child-Pugh score was initially developed with the intent to predict mortality during surgery; however, it is now used mostly as a prognostic tool and has been replaced largely by the MELD score. Child-Pugh score is calculated as the following:

	1 POINT	2 POINT	3 POINT
Prothrombin time	<4	4.0-6.0	>6.0
Total bilirubin (mg/dL)	<2	2-3	>3
Serum albumin	>3.5	2.8-3.5	<2.8
Ascites	None	Mild	Moderate
Hepatic encephalopathy	None	Grade 1-2	Grade 3-4

References:
1. Kamath PS, Kim WR, Advanced Liver Disease Study Group, et al. The model for end-stage liver disease (MELD). *Hepatology, U.S. National Library of Medicine*. 2007. www.ncbi.nlm.nih.gov/pubmed/17326206.
2. *ABA Keywords*. OpenAnesthesia. http://www.openanesthesia.org/child-pugh_score_factors/.

22. Correct answer: C

Orthotopic liver transplantation is divided into 3 stages: preanhepatic stage, anhepatic stage, and neohepatic phase. Prehepatic stage is from incision to cross-clamping of vascular structures surrounding the liver including IVC, hepatic artery, and portal vein. Then the anhepatic phase begins and lasts until all the vascular clamps are removed. During this time, the native liver is removed and the donor liver is implanted. Once the IVC clamp is removed and the allograft liver is reperfused, the neohepatic phase begins.

During allograft reperfusion, significant hemodynamic instability can ensue. When the IVC clamp is removed and the blood starts to flow through the portal vasculature, there is a release of inflammatory cytokines and potassium and hydrogen ions resulting from prolonged organ ischemia along with preservative solution into the systemic circulation. Microthrombi, which can form in the allograft organ, are also released into the circulation and cause significant hemodynamic instability including vasoplegia, cardiac arrhythmia, and hypotension. Hypotension can be treated with vasopressors including norepinephrine and vasopressin, and if the hypotension is refractory to these, then small boluses of epinephrine or infusion can be started. Hyperkalemia can be treated with calcium, insulin, glucose, and bicarbonate. Acidosis from reperfusion can be treated with either boluses of sodium bicarbonate or infusion. Frequent laboratory checks and assessment of acid-base status is key during the neohepatic phase.

References:
1. *ABA Keywords*. OpenAnesthesia. www.openanesthesia.org/liver-transplant-reperfusion-effect/.
2. Steadman RH, Wray CL. Anesthesia for abdominal organ transplantation. In: Miller RD, Cohen NH, Eriksson LI, et al., eds. *Miller's Anesthesia*. 8th ed. Philadelphia: Elsevier; 2015:2262-2291.

23. Correct answer: D

PPH is a severe complication in ESLD. It is present in about 2%-10% of patients awaiting a liver transplant. Although the pathophysiology of this condition is unknown, it is widely postulated that the syndrome develops due to humoral substances that are not metabolized by the liver (due to ESLD) reaching the pulmonary vasculature, resulting in vascular remodeling. The main humoral substances that are implicated are serotonin, interleukin-1, endothelin-1, thromboxane B2, and VIP. Diagnosis of PPH is made with the following criteria:

1. Presence of portal hypertension
2. Mean pulmonary artery pressure >25 mm Hg at rest
3. Pulmonary vascular resistance (PVR) > 240 dynes s/cm^5
4. Pulmonary capillary wedge pressure <15 mm Hg

The treatment of PPH intraoperatively is similar to treatment of pulmonary hypertension. Using phosphodiesterase inhibitors, such as milrinone or sildenafil, along with iNO or epoprostenol to decrease PVR is considered first-line therapy. Dobutamine when combined with iNO has been shown to have a synergistic effect in decreasing PVR, increasing cardiac index, and improvement of the Pao_2/Fio_2 ratio.

While dopamine will have similar effects as dobutamine, it is reserved for patients with severe hypotension and is not considered first-line therapy.

References:
1. Steadman RH, Wray CL. Anesthesia for abdominal organ transplantation. In: Miller RD, Cohen NH, Eriksson LI, et al., eds. *Miller's Anesthesia*. 8th ed. Philadelphia: Elsevier; 2015:2262-2291.
2. Sakai T. Liver transplantation anesthesiology. In: *Anesthesia and Perioperative Care for Organ Transplantation*. New York: Springer; 2016:353-364.

24. Correct answer: A

In this case, dopamine would not be considered a first-line therapy to improve renal perfusion during a renal transplant.

Dopamine has traditionally been known to have a renal protective effect with low-dose infusions; however, recent studies have shown conflicting results, and the use of dopamine for renal protective purposes has been fading out of practice.

Mannitol is often times used as a first-line agent to improve renal perfusion during kidney transplant (12.5-25 g). Mannitol is an osmotic agent that reduces cellular edema that can develop during ischemia and reperfusion. Mannitol has also been shown to decrease the delay in graft function. Furosemide is often administered concurrently with mannitol to encourage diuresis. Furosemide alone has not been proven to improve graft function.

During renal transplant, patients can undergo significant fluid shifts and it is important to maintain adequate intravascular volume to maintain perfusion to the newly transplanted kidney. While studies have not shown significant benefit of albumin over crystalloid solutions, nevertheless, the patient needs to be resuscitated with either crystalloid or colloid to improve perfusion.

Vasoactive medications can also be used to improve renal perfusion if need be; however, one must take into account the risk of graft failure secondary to vasoconstriction.

References:
1. Steadman RH, Wray CL. Anesthesia for abdominal organ transplantation. In: Miller RD, Cohen NH, Eriksson LI, et al., eds. *Miller's Anesthesia*. 8th ed. Philadelphia: Elsevier; 2015:2262-2291.
2. Richards KF, Belnap LP, Rees WV, Stevens LE. Mannitol reduces ATN in cadaveric allografts. *Transplant Proc*. 1989;21(1 Pt 2): 1228-1229.

25. Correct answer: C

INR is the best marker for synthetic function in a transplanted liver.

AST/ALT are enzymes that are associated with the liver parenchymal cells. Elevation in AST and ALT is more so an inflammatory marker of liver cells, rather than indicating liver synthetic function. Bilirubin is a metabolic product of heme metabolism and comes in 2 forms: unconjugated and conjugated. Bilirubin is taken up by hepatocytes and undergoes metabolism and is excreted in the urine. Elevated bilirubin indicates a problem with the liver's metabolic functions rather than synthetic functions. Elevations in AST/ALT and bilirubin are nonspecific markers of liver dysfunction.

Albumin is the main protein of the human body and is synthesized in the liver. The normal range of albumin is around 3.5-5 g/dL. Low albumin levels are nonspecific and late indicators of a decrease in liver synthetic function, as the half-life of albumin is ~20 days.

PT/INR is the specific marker of liver synthetic function. Most coagulation factors, including factors I (fibrinogen), II (prothrombin), V, VII, VIII, IX, X, XI, XIII, and protein C, protein S, and antithrombin, are all synthesized in the liver. Among these coagulation factors, factor VII has the shortest half-life of 3-6 hours and therefore will demonstrate an increase in PT/INR if liver synthetic function were to decline.

References:
1. Sakai T. Liver transplantation anesthesiology. In: *Anesthesia and Perioperative Care for Organ Transplantation*. New York: Springer; 2016:353-364.
2. Steadman RH, Wray CL. Anesthesia for abdominal organ transplantation. In: Miller RD, Cohen NH, Eriksson LI, et al., eds. *Miller's Anesthesia*. 8th ed. Philadelphia: Elsevier; 2015:2262-2291.

---

26. Correct answer: B

Patients who are on chronic glucocorticoid therapy may not respond appropriately in scenarios of stress, such as surgery, as a result of suppression of their hypothalamic pituitary axis. The anesthesiologist should consider several factors when deciding whether to give the patient glucocorticoid therapy during surgery as a way to supplement the patient's response to stress: (1) the dose and duration of steroids that the patient has been taking before the operation and (2) the type and duration of surgery being performed. Surgery is a potent stimulator of cortisol secretion, and the greater the stress of the surgery, the more pronounced the cortisol response.

Although exact cutoffs are not established for the duration or dose of steroids that would warrant supplementation, several studies indicate that patients who have been taking any amount of glucocorticoids for less than 3 weeks are unlikely to require additional supplementation. In addition, patients who receive less than 5 mg per day of prednisone or its dose equivalent for any length of time are also unlikely to require supplementation.

Reference:
1. Marik PE, Varon J. Requirement of perioperative stress doses of corticosteroids: a systematic review of the literature. *Arch Surg*. 2008;143:1222.

---

27. Correct answer: D

Patients may present to the OR who are on oral steroid regimens and require repeat dosing during surgery. This patient recently suffered an exacerbation of her COPD and has been placed on a course of oral steroids to abate the symptoms associated with her exacerbation. Given that she is becoming progressively hypotensive, one should administer "stress-dose steroids" at this time while concurrently initiating therapy with a vasoactive medication. It does appear that she would benefit from central line placement; however, that should not delay the initiation of appropriate treatment. It is unnecessary to give the patient her daily prednisone in addition to the hydrocortisone, and it is inappropriate to solely give her prednisone given her rapidly declining clinical picture.

Reference:
1. Kelly KN, Domajnko B. Perioperative stress-dose steroids. *Clin Colon Rectal Surg*. 2013;26(3):163-167.

---

28. Correct answer: A

It is important to be aware of the side effects of immunosuppressive therapies that are common in patients who have received a solid organ transplant. These patients need to be maintained on their immunosuppressive therapy usually up until the day of operation. Of the listed agents, tacrolimus is the only one with known nephrotoxicity. Tacrolimus can cause renal vasoconstriction, resulting in a dose-dependent reduction in renal blood flow and GFR. It would be less than ideal to give the patient 2 nephrotoxic agents in the setting of his operation. Another immunosuppressive agent that has nephrotoxic potential is cyclosporine.

Reference:

1. Kostopanagiotou G, Smyrniotis V, Arkadopoulos N, et al. Anesthetic and perioperative management of adult transplant recipients in nontransplant surgery. *Anesth Analg.* 1999;89(3):613-622.

29. Correct answer: A

Of the agents listed, azathioprine is associated with thrombocytopenia. Other immunosuppressive agents that could cause thrombocytopenia include ATG. Another consideration occurs in patients on warfarin and azathioprine in which azathioprine withdrawal has been associated with bleeding. The mechanism of this drug interaction is not well established. It has been postulated that 6-mercaptopurine, the primary metabolite of azathioprine, may induce the hepatic enzyme responsible for warfarin's metabolism.

References:

1. Csete M, Sipher MJ. Management of the transplant patient for nontransplant procedures. *Adv Anesth.* 1994;11:407-431.
2. Johnston TD, Katz SM. Special considerations in the transplant patient requiring other surgery. *Surg Clin N Am.* 1994;74: 1211-1221.

30. Correct answer: D

ATG is a polyclonal antibody that is used in the prophylaxis and treatment of acute rejection in patients receiving renal transplantation. Its efficacy relies on its ability to specifically target T cells and deplete their numbers. T cells are depleted in the blood and peripheral lymphoid tissues through apoptosis and complement-mediated lysis. Patients on ATG in the immediate posttransplant period are profoundly immunosuppressed and require prophylaxis against viral infections such as CMV infection.

References:

1. Deeks ED, Keating GM. Rabbit anti-thymocyte globulin (thymoglobulin): a review of its use in the prevention and treatment of acute renal allograft rejection. *Drugs.* 2009;69(11):1483-1512.
2. Guttmann RD, Caudrelier P, Alberici G, Touraine JL. Pharmacokinetics, foreign protein immune response, cytokine release, and lymphocyte subsets in patients receiving thymoglobulin and immunosuppression. *Transplant Proc.* 1997;29(7A):24S-26S.

31. Correct answer: C

Patients with pulsatile devices are more likely to develop LVAD-related infections, specifically pocket and wound infections.

There are no known differences in neurologic outcomes when comparing continuous-flow with pulsatile LVAD therapy. Owing to the higher rate of device failure in the pulsatile LVAD treatment group, only limited data at 24 months were available in that group.

Patients with continuous-flow LVAD therapy appear to have a higher rate of GI bleeding events than pulsatile LVAD recipients. GI angiodysplastic lesions (AVM) are the most common source of bleeding.

Acquired von Willebrand syndrome with decreased von Willebrand factor levels appears to occur immediately after continuous-flow LVAD implantation and persists up to 12 months.

References:

1. Schulman AR, Martens TP, Christos PJ, et al. Comparisons of infection complications between continuous flow and pulsatile flow left ventricular assist devices. *J Thorac Cardiovasc Surg*; 2007;133(3):841-842.
2. Maniar S, Kondareddy S, Topkara VK. Left ventricular assist device-related infections: past, present and future. *Expert Rev Med Devices.* 2011;8(5):627-634.
3. Loor G, Gonzalez-Stawinski G. Pulsatile vs. continuous flow in ventricular assist device therapy. *Best Pract Res Clin Anaesthesiol.* 2012;26(2):105-115.
4. Petrucci RJ, Rogers JG, Blue L, et al. Neurocognitive function in destination therapy patients receiving continuous-flow vs pulsatile-flow left ventricular assist device support. *J Heart Lung Transplant.* 2012;31(1):27-36.

32. Correct answer: B

Long-term results after lung transplant with organs procured following DCD are comparable with those obtained after donation-after-brain-death LTx. However, patients transplanted using organs from DCD donors appear to have a predisposition for development of bronchiolitis obliterans syndrome.

Diabetes mellitus is associated with increased mortality after transplantation, and degree of glycemic control correlates with survival. Patients with cystic fibrosis are at particular risk.

Use of a lung protective ventilation strategy in potential organ donors with brain death increased the number of eligible and harvested lungs compared with a conventional strategy.

Off-pump strategy may lead to better early postoperative outcomes and, possibly, an improved early survival. Intraoperative conversion from off-pump to CPB in high-risk patients appears to confer worse outcomes.

References:
1. Sabashnikov A, Patil NP, Popov AF, et al. Long-term results after lung transplantation using organs from circulatory death donors: a propensity score-matched analysis. *Eur J Cardiothorac Surg*. 2016;49(1):46-53.
2. van Suylen V, Luijk B, Hoek RAS, et al. A multicenter study on long-term outcomes after lung transplantation comparing donation after circulatory death and donation after brain death. *Am J Transplant*. 2017;17(10):2679-2686.
3. Ruttens D, Martens A, Ordies S, et al. Short- and long-term outcome after lung transplantation from circulatory-dead donors: a single-center experience. *Transplantation*. 2017;101(11):2691-2694.
4. Krutsinger D, Reed RM, Blevins A, et al. Lung transplantation from donation after cardiocirculatory death: a systematic review and meta-analysis. *J Heart Lung Transplant*. 2015;34(5):675-684.

33. Correct answer: A

The patient presents in cardiogenic shock secondary to ST-elevation myocardial infarction in the setting of advanced cardiac allograft vasculopathy (CAV).

CAV can be found in ≥50% of transplant recipients and is largely refractory to standard atherosclerosis medication. It is believed to result in ≈5% graft loss per year. Alloimmunity is considered the primary mechanism, although the pathogenesis appears multifactorial.

Classically, luminal narrowing in CAV is diffuse, extending with comparable severity along the entire coronary vasculature. In contrast, native atherosclerosis tends to be more focal, involving more proximal coronary vessels. Although percutaneous coronary angioplasty with stenting may achieve good temporary local effects in CAV, CAV's diffuse and progressive nature contributes to mixed results with regard to long-term patency and survival benefits.

Pravastatin use after heart transplantation leads to a decreased incidence of rejection causing hemodynamic compromise, a decreased onset of CAV, and improved 1-year survival. In a retrospective study, HMG-CoA reductase inhibitor use was associated with an increased 5-year survival rate following heart transplantation.

Diltiazem is commonly prescribed to prevent CAV and decrease heart rate. Although there is radiologic evidence that diltiazem may inhibit early CAV development, there is limited evidence that diltiazem improves survival.

Aspirin, though often routinely prescribed as prophylactic agent, has not yet been shown to significantly improve outcomes in a randomized controlled trial. In fact, there is evidence that platelets of heart transplant recipients may be resistant to the inhibitory effect of aspirin. However, one retrospective observational study suggests that early aspirin may be associated with reduced CAV development.

References:
1. Pober JS, Jane-wit D, Qin L, et al. Interacting mechanisms in the pathogenesis of cardiac allograft vasculopathy. *Arterioscler Thromb Vasc Biol*. 2014;34(8):1609-1614.
2. Rahmani M, Cruz RP, Granville DJ, et al. Allograft vasculopathy versus atherosclerosis. *Circ Res*. 2006;99(8):801-815.
3. Beygui F, Varnous S, Montalescot G, et al. Long-term outcome after bare-metal or drug-eluting stenting for allograft coronary artery disease. *J Heart Lung Transplant*. 2010;29(3):316-322.
4. Dasari TW, Hennebry TA, Hanna EB, et al. Drug eluting versus bare metal stents in cardiac allograft vasculopathy: a systematic review of literature. *Catheter Cardiovasc Interv*. 2011;77(7):962-969.
5. Lee MS, Finch W, Weisz G, et al. Cardiac allograft vasculopathy. *Rev Cardiovasc Med*. 2011;12(3):143-152.

34. Correct answer: A

Hypothyroidism and hyperthyroidism are both associated with pulmonary arterial hypertension. Thus far, the mechanisms are not fully understood.

In a cohort of euthyroid patients, free T3 levels inversely correlated with the presence of CAD and low T3 syndrome conferred a worse prognosis.

T3/T4 therapy to the brain-dead organ donor results in more transplantable hearts and lungs, with no detriment to posttransplant graft or recipient survival.

Even mildly elevated thyroid-stimulating hormone levels in congestive heart failure patients are associated with heart failure progression. One meta-analysis suggested that hypothyroidism increased all-cause mortality in patients with heart failure.

References:

1. Frazier SK, Diagnosing and treating primary pulmonary hypertension. *Nurse Pract.* 1999;24(9):18, 21-2, 25-6 passim; quiz 42-4.
2. Scicchitano P, Dentamaro I, Tunzi F, et al. Pulmonary hypertension in thyroid diseases. *Endocrine.* 2016;54(3):578-587.
3. Ferris A, Jacobs T, Widlitz A, et al. Pulmonary arterial hypertension and thyroid disease. *Chest.* 2001;119(6):1980-1981.
4. Gerdes AM, Iervasi G. Thyroid replacement therapy and heart failure. *Circulation.* 2010;122(4):385-393.
5. Coceani M, Iervasi G, Pingitore A, et al. Thyroid hormone and coronary artery disease: from clinical correlations to prognostic implications. *Clin Cardiol.* 2009;32(7):380-385.

35. Correct answer: C

IABP raises the cardiac output to a lesser degree (~0.5 L/min) than percutaneously inserted axial flow pumps (eg, Impella 5.0 = 5 L/min).

IABP, not percutaneously inserted axial flow pumps, may be safely used without heparin anticoagulation in select cases. Percutaneously inserted axial flow pumps generally require heparin or anti-Xa–based anticoagulation protocols.

IABP therapy alone in cardiogenic shock complicating acute myocardial infarction did not improve 30-day mortality. When compared directly with percutaneously inserted axial flow pumps, IABP did not change in hospital mortality. IABP improves coronary perfusion pressure and decreases LV afterload, while ECMO increases LV afterload, putting the patient at risk for pulmonary edema. In antegrade flow states, addition of IABP to ECMO can improve coronary perfusion and decrease LV afterload. ECMO + IABP may improve mortality when compared with ECMO or IABP alone, though data are not consistent.

It is recommended to minimize catecholamine use with indwelling percutaneously inserted axial flow pumps to rest the myocardium.

References:

1. Myat A, Patel N, Tehrani S, et al. Percutaneous circulatory assist devices for high-risk coronary intervention. *JACC Cardiovasc Interv.* 2015;8(2):229-244.
2. Kogan A, Preisman S, Sternik L, et al. Heparin-free management of intra-aortic balloon pump after cardiac surgery. *J Card Surg.* 2012;27(4):434-437.
3. Pucher PH, Cummings IG, Shipolini AR, et al. Is heparin needed for patients with an intra-aortic balloon pump? *Interact Cardiovasc Thorac Surg.* 2012;15(1):136-139.
4. Cooper HA, Thompson E, Panza JA. The role of heparin anticoagulation during intra-aortic balloon counterpulsation in the coronary care unit. *Acute Card Care.* 2008;10(4):214-220.
5. Jiang CY, Zhao LL, Wang JA, et al. Anticoagulation therapy in intra-aortic balloon counterpulsation: does IABP really need anti-coagulation? *J Zhejiang Univ Sci.* 2003;4(5):607-611.

36. Correct answer: C

Intraoperative anaphylaxis can be hard to recognize, and its incidence under general anesthesia is 1:10 000 to 1:20 000. Mortality is higher when anaphylaxis occurs under general anesthesia than in the general population because early symptoms such as itching or shortness of breath are masked by general anesthesia. Therefore, most cases of anaphylaxis are not recognized until the patient develops cardiovascular or respiratory collapse.

The cornerstone of treatment of anaphylaxis is epinephrine. Epinephrine's effects on α-adrenergic receptors cause peripheral vasoconstriction, treating hypotension, and also reduce erythema, urticaria, and angioedema. Epinephrine's effects on β-adrenergic receptors cause bronchodilation, increase myocardial contractility and cardiac output, and suppress mediator release from mast cells and basophils. However, large doses of epinephrine have been associated with severe hypertension, cardiac arrhythmias, and myocardial infarction. Recommended dosing of epinephrine for anaphylaxis is 10-100 μg IV every 1-2 minutes. The dose can be increased to effect. If no pulse can be palpated, then give fluid bolus and initiate Advanced Cardiac Life Support. An epinephrine infusion can be started for persistent hypotension or bronchospasm.

References:

1. Fisher MM, Baldo BA. The incidence and clinical features of anaphylactic reactions during anesthesia in Australia. *Ann Fr Anesth Reanim.* 1993;12:97.
2. Kemp SSF, Lockey RF, Simons FER, et al. Epinephrine: The drug of choice for anaphylaxis – A statement of the World Allergy Organization. *World Allergy Organ J.* 2008;1:S18-S26.
3. Mali S. Anaphylaxis during the perioperative period. *Anesth Essays Res.* 2012;6:124-133.
4. McLean-Tooke APC, Bethune CA, Fay AC, et al. Adrenaline in the treatment of anaphylaxis: what is the evidence? *BMJ.* 2003;327:1332-1335.

37. Correct answer: A

This patient likely has sepsis with fever, low blood pressure, altered mental status, and tachypnea. The first-choice vasopressor for adults with septic shock is norepinephrine. Norepinephrine increases MAP through its α-adrenergic effects. However, it also has β-adrenergic effects and, thus, maintains cardiac output and heart rate. One large multicenter trial randomized patients with shock (septic, cardiogenic, or hypovolemic) to receive either dopamine or norepinephrine to restore and maintain blood pressure. Of the 1679 patients in the study, 62% had septic shock. There was no difference between the 2 groups in the primary end point of 28-day mortality. However, there were arrhythmias, notably atrial fibrillation, in the patients who received dopamine. A meta-analysis of vasopressors for the treatment of septic shock found that norepinephrine was associated with decreased mortality and decreased risk of arrhythmias when compared with dopamine. Dopamine may have a role in septic patients with absolute or relative bradycardia.

The data on use of phenylephrine in sepsis are limited. Current guidelines recommend its use when serious tachyarrhythmias occur with norepinephrine or epinephrine or if MAP goal is not met despite norepinephrine, vasopressin, and epinephrine use.

While additional fluid may be indicated in this patient, vasopressors should be started to maintain tissue perfusion.

References:

1. De Backer D, Biston P, Devriendt J, et al. Comparison of dopamine and norepinephrine in the treatment of shock. *N Engl J Med.* 2010;362:779-789.
2. Avni T, Lador A, Lev S, et al. Vasopressors for the treatment of septic shock: a systematic review and meta-analysis. *PLoS One.* 2015;10:e0129305.
3. Pollard S, Edwin SB, Alaniz C. Vasopressor and inotropic management of patients with septic shock. *P T.* 2015;40:438-442, 449-450.
4. Rhodes A, Evans LE, Alhazzani W, et al. Surviving Sepsis Campaign: International Guidelines for Management of Sepsis and Septic Shock: 2016. *Crit Care Med.* 2017;45:486-552.

38. Correct answer: C

Septic shock is a state of relative vasopressin deficiency; vasopressin levels are not as high as expected given degree of hypotension. Thus, it is hypothesized that administration of exogenous vasopressin can increase vascular tone and decrease the need for catecholamines. Current guidelines recommend adding low-dose vasopressin (0.03 U/min) to norepinephrine to raise the MAP to target or adding vasopressin with the intent to decrease norepinephrine dosage. In the Vasopressin versus Norepinephrine infusion in Patients with Septic Shock (VASST) trial, there was no difference in mortality at 28 and at 90 days between the patients who received norepinephrine and those who received norepinephrine and vasopressin. There were no differences in the rates of organ dysfunction or serious adverse events in the 2 groups. The patients who received vasopressin were on significantly lower doses of norepinephrine and had heart rates that were significantly lower than the patients who received norepinephrine alone.

References:

1. Russell JA, Walley KR, Singer J, et al. Vasopressin versus norepinephrine infusion in patients with septic shock. *N Engl J Med.* 2008;358:877-887.
2. Rhodes A, Evans LE, Alhazzani W, et al. Surviving Sepsis Campaign: International Guidelines for Management of Sepsis and Septic Shock: 2016. *Crit Care Med.* 2017;45:486-552.

39. Correct answer: D

Although fluid administration is the standard for resuscitation, fluid overload is associated with detrimental consequences. Fluid overload is associated with increased mortality in critically ill patients with acute respiratory distress syndrome and sepsis. Use of fluid resuscitation and vasopressors should be balanced to maintain tissue perfusion and minimize tissue edema. Fluid responsiveness is defined as an increase in cardiac output or stroke volume by 10%-15% in response to a fluid challenge. One recent systematic review and meta-analysis showed that fluid resuscitation guided by assessment of fluid responsiveness was associated with reduced mortality, ICU length of stay, and duration of mechanical ventilation.

References:

1. Monnet X, Marik PE, Teboul JL. Prediction of fluid responsiveness: an update. *Ann Intensive Care.* 2016;6:111.
2. Bednarczyk JM, Fridfinnson JA, Kumar A, et al. Incorporating dynamic assessment of fluid responsiveness into goal-directed therapy: a systematic review and meta-analysis. *Crit Care Med.* 2017;45:1538-1545.

40. **Correct answer: A**

Angiotensin-converting enzyme inhibitors and angiotensin receptor blockers block the renin-angiotensin system, resulting in vasodilatation and decreased blood pressure. These agents are commonly used to treat hypertension and heart failure and to prevent diabetic nephropathy. However, perioperative use of these agents can result in severe intraoperative hypotension that can be resistant to catecholamines.

Blood pressure is regulated by 3 systems: the adrenergic nervous system, the renin-angiotensin system, and the vasopressin system. Anesthetic agents typically affect the adrenergic nervous system causing vasodilatation and hypotension. If the renin-angiotensin system is also blocked by perioperative administration of angiotensin-converting enzyme inhibitors and angiotensin receptor blockers, small doses of exogenous vasopressin (0.5-1 unit bolus) can be used to treat hypotension.

References:

1. Coriat P, Richer C, Douraki T, et al. Influence of chronic angiotensin-converting enzyme inhibition on anesthetic induction. *Anesthesiology.* 1994;81:299-307.
2. Lange M, Aken HV, Westphal M. Role of vasopressinergic V1 receptor agonists in the treatment of perioperative catecholamine-refractory arterial hypotension. *Best Pract Res Clin Anesthesiol.* 2008;22:369-381.

41. **Correct answer: D**

Nitric oxide binds to and activates guanylyl cyclase, resulting in the production of cyclic guanosine monophosphate (cGMP) and vasodilatation. Agents that inhibit nitric oxide can be used to treat vasoplegia.

Methylene blue inhibits guanylate cyclase and decreases vascular smooth muscle relaxation.

Hydroxocobalamin is a form of vitamin B12 used for the treatment of cyanide toxicity. One side effect of hydroxocobalamin infusion is hypertension due to binding of nitric oxide and inhibition of nitric oxide synthase and guanylate cyclase.

Vitamin C is a potent antioxidant and free radical scavenger. Use of high-dose vitamin C has been reported to decrease pressor requirements, reduce mortality, and decrease organ dysfunction. Its effects are myriad, but one effect is inhibition of nitric oxide synthase.

Angiotensin II is part of the renin-angiotensin system and is a potent vasoconstrictor. When compared with placebo, patients with vasodilatory shock on high doses of conventional vasopressors were significantly more likely to achieve an MAP of 75 mm Hg with angiotensin II and were more likely to be able to lower catecholamine requirements to meet a target MAP between 65 and 75 mm Hg.

References:

1. Edmund S, Kwok H, Howers D. Use of methylene blue in sepsis: a systematic review. *J Intensive Care Med.* 2006;21:359-363.
2. Roderique JD, VanDyck K, Holman B, et al. The use of high-dose hydroxocobalamin for vasoplegic syndrome. *Ann Thorac Surg.* 2014;97:1785-1786.
3. Zabet MH, Mohammadi M, Ramezani M, et al. Effect of high-dose ascorbic on vasopressor's requirement in septic shock. *J Res Pharm Pract.* 2016;5:94-100.
4. Marik P, Khangoora V, Rivera R, et al. Hydrocortisone, vitamin C, and thiamine for the treatment of severe sepsis and septic shock. *Chest.* 2017;151:1229-1238.
5. Khanna A, English SW, Wang XS, et al. Angiotensin II for the treatment of vasodilatory shock. *N Engl J Med.* 2017;377:419-430.

42. **Correct answer: A**

Postoperative atrial fibrillation is common after pulmonary surgery. It usually occurs on postoperative days 2 to 4. Treatment consists of agents to control heart rate or to convert the rhythm back to sinus.

β-Blockers and calcium channel blockers are commonly used for rate control. β-Blockers such as metoprolol, propranolol, and esmolol reduce ventricular rate within 5 minutes of IV administration and maintain heart rate in 70%-75% of patients. Diltiazem administered as a bolus followed by a continuous infusion can control ventricular response in 70%-90% of patients. Both β-blockers and calcium channel blockers can cause hypotension and bradycardia and should not be used in patients with accessory conduction pathways.

Digoxin can also be used for rate control. Its onset of action is slower (30 min-2 h), and potential for toxicity is increased in patients with hypokalemia, hypomagnesemia, hypercalcemia, and renal dysfunction.

Amiodarone is administered as a bolus followed by continuous infusion. It is effective for both rate and rhythm control. Higher doses of amiodarone have been associated with pulmonary toxicity, namely acute respiratory distress syndrome in pneumonectomy patients. However, studies have also shown that lower doses of IV amiodarone are safe in patients undergoing smaller lung resections.

One trial in postoperative cardiac surgery patients showed no difference in number of hospital days, complication rates, and rate of persistent atrial fibrillation in patients treated with a rate control strategy compared with patients treated with a rhythm control strategy.

Phenylephrine is a selective α1-adrenergic agent that increases blood pressure. It may cause a reflex bradycardia. Use of phenylephrine may be preferred over catecholaminergic agents in hypotensive patients with atrial fibrillation.

References:
1. Frendl G, Sodickson AC, Chung MK, et al. AATS guidelines for the prevention and management of perioperative atrial fibrillation and flutter for thoracic surgical procedures. *J Thorac Cardiovasc Surg*. 2014;148:e153-e193.
2. Gillinov AM, Bagiella E, Moskowitz AJ, et al. Rate control versus rhythm control for atrial fibrillation after cardiac surgery. *N Engl J Med*. 2016;374:1911-1921.

43. Correct answer: D

The MAP is the driving pressure of tissue perfusion. The Surviving Sepsis guidelines recommend an initial target MAP of 65 mm Hg in patients with septic shock requiring vasopressors. In the High versus Low Blood-Pressure Target in Patients with Septic Shock study, patients with septic shock were randomized to either a target MAP of 65-70 mm Hg or a target MAP of 80-85 mm Hg. The patients were also stratified according to whether they had a history of chronic hypertension because the authors postulated that the patients with chronic hypertension would benefit more from a higher target pressure. There was no significant difference between the groups in terms of 28-day mortality, the primary outcome. There were also no significant differences in the secondary outcomes: need for mechanical ventilation, length of ICU and hospital stay, and the Sequential Organ Failure Assessment (SOFA) score at day 7. However, patients with chronic hypertension in the low-target MAP group were significantly more likely to double their plasma creatinine and be on renal replacement therapy compared with the patients in the high-target MAP group. Thus, the Surviving Sepsis guidelines recommend individualizing the target MAP once there is a better understanding of the patient's underlying health conditions.

References:
1. Asfar P, Meziani F, Hamel JF, et al. High versus low blood-pressure target in patients with septic shock. *N Engl J Med*. 2014;370:1583-1593.
2. Rhodes A, Evans LE, Alhazzani W, et al. Surviving Sepsis Campaign: International Guidelines for Management of Sepsis and Septic Shock: 2016. *Crit Care Med*. 2017;45:486-552.

44. Correct answer: B

The Surviving Sepsis guidelines suggest using dobutamine in patients who show evidence of persistent hypoperfusion despite adequate fluid resuscitation and the use of vasopressor agents. However, there are no randomized controlled trials comparing outcomes in patients receiving dobutamine versus placebo. Thus, the recommendation is graded as weak with low quality of evidence.

Milrinone inhibits phosphodiesterase-3 and prevents the degradation of cyclic adenosine monophosphate (cAMP). The downstream effects if increased cAMP result in increased contractility and vasodilatation. The combination of increased contractility and decreased afterload results in increased cardiac output. One meta-analysis and systematic review concluded that the use of milrinone in critically ill adult patients with cardiac dysfunction could be neither recommended or refuted because of risks of both bias and random error in the current evidence.

Levosimendan binds to cardiac troponin C and increases contractility by increasing the sensitivity of myocytes to calcium. Like milrinone, it also has a vasodilatory effect by opening ATP-dependent potassium channels. One trial comparing levosimendan with placebo in patients with sepsis found no difference in organ dysfunction scores and mortality. Patients receiving levosimendan had more supraventricular tachyarrhythmias than patients receiving placebo.

A prospective, randomized trial comparing epinephrine with norepinephrine plus dobutamine titrated to maintain an MAP of 70 mm Hg or more in patients with septic shock found no difference in mortality between the 2 groups.

References:
1. Rhodes A, Evans LE, Alhazzani W, et al. Surviving Sepsis Campaign: International Guidelines for Management of Sepsis and Septic Shock: 2016. *Crit Care Med*. 2017;45:486-552.
2. Annane D, Vignon P, Renault A, et al. Norepinephrine plus dobutamine versus epinephrine alone for management of septic shock: a randomised trial. *Lancet*. 2007;370:676-684.

3. Koster G, Bekema HJ, Wetterslev J, et al. Milrinone for cardiac dysfunction in critically ill adult patients: a systematic review of randomized clinical trials with meta-analysis and trial sequential analysis. *Int Care Med.* 2016;42:1322-1335.
4. Gordon AC, Perkins GD, Singer M, et al. Levosimendan for the prevention of acute organ dysfunction in sepsis. *N Engl J Med.* 2016;375:1638-1648.

45. Correct answer: C

Clevidipine is a dihydropyridine calcium channel blocker and therefore acts on vascular smooth muscle. It is metabolized by blood and tissue esterases and, thus, has a short onset time and duration of action. Clevidipine is poorly soluble in water and thus is dissolved in an emulsion of soybean oil and purified egg yolk phospholipids. Thus, it is contraindicated in patients with allergies to soybeans, soy products, eggs, or egg products as well as patients with defective lipid metabolism.

The ECLIPSE trials were 3 randomized trials comparing clevidipine with nitroprusside, nitroglycerin, and nicardipine for the treatment of perioperative hypertension associated with cardiac surgery. The incidence of death, stroke, myocardial infarction, and renal dysfunction at 30 days was not significantly different in a pooled analysis of clevidipine and the comparator treatment arms. However, when compared with nitroprusside, clevidipine demonstrated a significant mortality advantage. In post hoc analyses, clevidipine was superior for blood pressure control compared with nitroglycerin and nitroprusside but comparable to nicardipine.

Clevidipine has a terminal half-life of 15 minutes, and thus, rebound hypertension may occur if the patient has not been transitioned to other antihypertensive agents.

References:
1. Espinosa A, Ripolles-Melchor J, Casans-Frances R, et al. Perioperative use of clevidipine: a systematic review and meta-analysis. *PLoS One. Public Library of Science.* 2016. Available from: http://journals.plos.org/plosone/article?id=10.1371%2Fjournal.pone.0150625#abstract0.
2. Aronson S, Dyke CM, Stierer KA, et al. The ECLIPSE trials: comparative studies of clevidipine to nitroglycerin, sodium nitroprusside, and nicardipine for acute hypertension treatment in cardiac surgery patients. *Anesth Analg.* 2008;107:1110-1121.

46. Correct answer: C

The CDC places bioterrorism agents into 3 categories, depending on how easily they can be spread and the severity of illness or death they cause.

1. Category A agents are those that pose the highest risk to the public and national security because (1) they can be transmitted easily from person to person, (2) they are associated with high mortality, (3) they may cause public panic and social disruption, or (4) they require special action for public health preparedness. Examples of these agents include *B anthracis* (anthrax), *Clostridium botulinum* toxin (botulism), Variola major (smallpox), and agents that cause viral hemorrhagic fevers (eg, Ebola).
2. Category B agents are those that (1) are moderately easy to spread, (2) result in moderate morbidity and mortality, or (3) require specific enhancements of CDC's laboratory capacity and enhanced disease monitoring. Examples of these agents include *Brucella* species (brucellosis), agents that threaten the safety of food or water (eg, *Vibrio cholerae*, *Escherichia coli* O157:H7, *Shigella*), *Burkholderia mallei* (glanders), and *Chlamydia psittaci* (psittacosis).
3. Category C agents are emerging pathogens that could be engineered for mass spread in the future and have the potential for high morbidity and mortality rates and major health impact. Examples include emerging infectious diseases such as Nipah virus and hantavirus.

Reference:
1. *Emergency Preparedness and Response: Bioterrorism Agents/Diseases.* 2017. Retrieved from: https://emergency.cdc.gov/agent/agentlist-category.asp.

47. Correct answer: B

C botulinum produces potent neurotoxins (types A-G). Exposure to the toxin can occur by ingestion of toxin, inhalation of toxin, or local production of toxin by *C botulinum* in the GI tract or in wounded, devitalized tissue. The toxin blocks acetylcholine release into the synaptic cleft, affecting both nicotinic and muscarinic receptors. The hallmarks of botulism consist of an acute, afebrile, symmetric, descending flaccid paralysis with prominent bulbar palsies (diplopia, dysarthria, dysphonia, and dysphagia) in a patient with a clear sensorium. Postural hypotension, nausea, and vomiting from ileus may also occur due to blockade of muscarinic receptors. Involvement of the respiratory muscles including the diaphragm can result in respiratory failure and the need for intubation and mechanical ventilation. The diagnosis of botulism must be done on a clinical basis, as laboratory testing is specialized and requires several days to complete. Treatment is largely supportive. Antitoxin is available through the CDC and needs to be administered in a timely basis (most effective if given within 24 h). The antitoxin will limit the severity of disease and subsequent nerve damage but will not reverse existent paralysis.

Features suggestive of bioterrorism as cause of an outbreak of botulism include a large number of cases, such as outbreak with an unusual botulinum toxin type, outbreak in a location without a common dietary exposure, and multiple outbreaks at the same time without common source.

References:
1. Arnon SS, Schechter R, Inglesby TV, et al. Botulinum toxin as a biological weapon: medical and public health management. *JAMA*. 2001;285:1059-1070.
2. Karma M, Currie B, Kvetan V. Bioterrorism: Preparing for the impossible or the improbable. *Crit Care Med*. 2005;33:S75-S95.

48. Correct answer: C

Naturally occurring smallpox was declared eradicated by the WHO in 1980. However, there remains concerns for use of smallpox as a bioterrorism agent because it is highly infectious, it has a high mortality rate (30% for variola major), and there is an increasing number of people without immunity to smallpox. Smallpox spreads from person to person through the respiratory tract. The incubation period is 10-14 days. Patients usually experience high fevers, chills, headache, and muscle aches 1-4 days before the appearance of a rash. Lesions typically appear first on the oral mucosa and palate, face, and forearms. Lesions are distributed centrifugally, on the face and distal limbs with relative sparing of the trunk. The lesions evolve from macules to papules to pustules slowly with each stage lasting 1-2 days, and all the lesions are in the same stage of development. Care is supportive, as the skin lesions can result in fluid loss, bacterial infection, and sepsis.

The WHO recommends a surveillance and containment strategy to prevent widespread outbreak of smallpox. Cases of smallpox should be identified based on clinical features and confirmatory laboratory testing. Patients with smallpox should be placed under strict airborne and contact isolation in a negative pressure room. The virus is transmitted at the onset of the rash. Therefore, individuals who had face-to-face contact with the patient at that time (first-ring contacts) should be identified and vaccinated as vaccination within 3-4 days of exposure is effective in preventing smallpox. These individuals should be followed closely and isolated if they develop a fever. Finally, contacts of first-ring contacts (second-ring contacts) should be identified and vaccinated. Identification of smallpox should be reported to local, state, and national health authorities.

References:
1. Moore ZS, Seward JF, Lane JM. Smallpox. *Lancet*. 2006;367(9508):425-435.
2. Henderson DA, Inglesby TV, Bartlett JG. Smallpox as a biological weapon: medical and public health management. *JAMA*. 1999;281(22):2127-2137.

49. Correct answer: A

Properties of hazards of biological weapons determine how they are managed. Toxicity (the toxic effects of the biologic agent) and latency (the time between exposure and appearance of symptoms) determine the management of the victim. The management of an incident is determined by the agent's persistency (the ability of the biologic agent to remain in the environment) and transmissibility (ability to be spread from the environment to humans or from human to human).

Reference:
1. Karwa M, Currie B, Kvetan V. Bioterrorism: preparing for the impossible or the improbable. *Crit Care Med*. 2005;33:S75.

50. Correct answer: B

B anthracis is an encapsulated, gram-positive, spore-forming bacterium that can cause pulmonary, meningeal, cutaneous, and GI disease. Aerosolized anthrax spores may be used as a biological weapon. The spores are inhaled, phagocytized by alveolar macrophages, and carried to mediastinal lymph nodes where they germinate and cause disease through the production of toxins leading to systemic disease and shock.

Early symptoms are nonspecific with fever, cough, myalgia, and malaise and mimic viral illnesses. However, after a short period of apparent recovery, fever, respiratory failure, acidosis, and shock develop.

The earliest clue to diagnosis may be radiographic findings of a widened mediastinum and pleural effusions that rapidly progress to a large size. Anthrax meningitis results from hematogenous seeding and occurs in up to 50% of patients with inhalational anthrax. Patients with anthrax meningitis may need steroids and antiepileptic agents to control edema and seizures. The mortality rate is as high as 67%-88% even with antimicrobial or antiserum treatment. Diagnostic testing should include blood for culture and polymerase chain reaction (PCR) assay, plasma for antitoxin detection, and pleural fluid/CSF for culture and PCR.

If anthrax is suspected, antibiotic treatment should be started immediately while awaiting results of diagnostic testing. In patients with systemic disease, the CDC recommends treatment with 2 or more antimicrobial drugs. One of these drugs should have bactericidal activity, and the other should be a protein synthesis inhibitor to reduce toxin production. First-line drugs with bactericidal activity include fluoroquinolones and carbapenems. Protein synthesis inhibitors include linezolid or clindamycin. Treatment should be continued for 2 or more weeks or until the patient is clinically stable. Because of β-lactam resistance, cephalosporins are contraindicated for the treatment of anthrax.

Because disease is caused by toxins produced by *B anthracis*, early treatment with antibodies directed against anthrax toxins is recommended. Raxibacumab is a monoclonal antibody directed against protective antigen component of the anthrax toxin. Anthrax immune globulin is derived from the plasma of individuals who have been vaccinated against anthrax and is also directed against protective antigen. Anthrax does not spread from person to person; therefore, standard precautions are sufficient for infection control.

References:

1. Swartz MN. Recognition and management of anthrax – an update. *N Engl J Med*. 2001;345:1621-1626.
2. Adalja AA, Toner E, Inglesby TV. Clinical management of potential bioterrorism-related conditions. *N Engl J Med*. 2015;372: 954-962.
3. Beeching NJ, Dance DAB, Miller AR, Spencer RC. Biological warfare and bioterrorism. *BMJ*. 2002;324:336-339.

22

ANESTHESIA FOR AMBULATORY SURGERY

Rebecca I. Kalman

1. **A 69-year-old woman presents to an outpatient surgical center for elbow arthroscopy under regional anesthesia. Her medical history is significant for well-controlled hypertension on 2 antihypertensive agents, type 2 diabetes on metformin with a most recent HbA1c of 6, and obesity with a body mass index of 35. During preoperative assessment, she reports a good functional capacity, able to carry heavy loads of laundry up and down stairs from the basement. When asked, she admits that she has been told she snores loudly, has had witnessed apneic episodes, and is frequently tired during the day. What should the attending anesthesiologist do?**

   A. Cancel the surgery because she is at high risk for having obstructive sleep apnea (OSA) and refer her for a sleep study.
   B. Cancel the surgery because she is at high risk for having OSA and refer her to have to procedure done at an inpatient facility.
   C. Proceed with the surgery despite the fact that she is at high risk for having OSA because her comorbidities are well controlled and she will have a regional anesthetic.
   D. Proceed with the surgery, as she is not at high risk for having OSA.
   E. Cancel the surgery because of her obesity and hypertension.

2. **A 22-year-old woman presents to the same-day surgery clinic for a rhinoplasty revision. Upon meeting her in the preoperative area, you note she is chewing gum. When you ask her about it, she immediately swallows the gum. Upon further questioning she admits that this is the fifth piece of gum she has chewed and swallowed this morning. Which of the following is the most appropriate action?**

   A. Proceed with the surgery as scheduled because chewing gum has little effect on gastric volume or pH.
   B. Delay the surgery for 2 hours because chewing gum is considered similar to liquids according to ASA guidelines.
   C. Delay the surgery for 4 hours because chewing gum is considered similar to breast milk according to ASA guidelines.
   D. Delay the surgery for 6 hours because the gum she swallowed qualifies as a solid/light meal.
   E. Cancel the surgery because she did not follow directions.

3. A nurse calls you from the preoperative area of an outpatient surgical center to tell you about a 35-year-old man with type 1 diabetes scheduled for knee arthroscopy. She notes he has vomited once, is tachycardic, and is constantly asking either to use the bathroom or to be able to drink water. He told her that he has not taken insulin in 2 days, so she took his blood glucose level and it is 467. Which of the following is the best course of action?

A. Proceed with surgery and treat the hyperglycemia intraoperatively with IV regular insulin.
B. Ask the nurse to give the patient his normal dose of NPH and proceed with surgery treating intraoperative hyperglycemia with IV regular insulin.
C. Evaluate the patient yourself and proceed with surgery only if he understands how to treat his hyperglycemia postoperatively.
D. Evaluate the patient yourself. Explain to him that you are concerned that he is showing signs and symptoms of diabetic ketoacidosis, cancel the surgery, draw appropriate laboratory test results, and send him to a tertiary care center for further evaluation and treatment.
E. Counsel the nurse that she should not have checked the blood glucose level without discussing it with you first.

4. A 23-year-old woman presents for same-day surgery for hysteroscopy for a misplaced intrauterine device. She is very anxious about anesthesia. On your preoperative assessment, you note she gets carsick frequently and is a nonsmoker. Which statement is true regarding the most appropriate approach to prevent postoperative nausea and vomiting (PONV) in this patient?

A. Based on her Apfel score, she has 3 risk factors of PONV, giving her a 60% risk of PONV. A multimodal approach using antiemetics of 2 or 3 different classes is appropriate.
B. Her anxiety confers additional risk for PONV.
C. Both avoiding nitrous oxide and minimizing neostigmine dose can help reduce her risk of PONV.
D. Scopolamine patch and ondansetron are most effective when administered before surgery.
E. The use of haloperidol as an antiemetic requires doses the same as or higher than those that are used to treat psychiatric disorders.

5. A 40-year-old woman presents to an ambulatory surgical center for knee arthroscopy. She tells you she needs to get home as soon as possible after the surgery because she has "important things to take care of." What is the best anesthetic plan to ensure the shortest time from arrival to discharge?

A. General anesthesia
B. Regional anesthesia with a "3-in-1" block technique
C. Spinal anesthesia
D. All of the above techniques can be used to affect a short time to discharge
E. Knee arthroscopy is not an appropriate surgery for an ambulatory center

6. A 23-year-old woman is having nausea and vomiting in the postanesthesia care unit (PACU) after hysteroscopy. She was deemed to be at high risk for PONV and received dexamethasone, ondansetron, and haloperidol as PONV prophylaxis intraoperatively. Which of the following is the best next step in management?

A. Repeat the same dose of ondansetron.
B. Repeat the same dose of dexamethasone.
C. Repeat the same dose of haloperidol.
D. Give a higher dose of ondansetron.
E. Administer perphenazine or promethazine.

7. All of the following are common reasons for delay in ambulatory surgical patient discharge EXCEPT which one?

A. Drowsiness
B. Nausea
C. Vomiting
D. Anxiety
E. Pain

8. A 31-year-old man complains of 7/10 pain in the PACU after hemorrhoidectomy under general anesthesia. Which is the most appropriate intervention to treat his pain and facilitate a shorter time to discharge home?

A. Assume his complaint is due to discomfort from something else such as hypoxemia, hypercapnia, or full bladder rather than surgical pain.
B. Administer IV hydromorphone.
C. Administer IV morphine.
D. Administer IV fentanyl.
E. Evaluate for other sources of discomfort such as hypoxemia, hypercapnia, or full bladder. Once these are eliminated, administer IV fentanyl and a nonsteroidal anti-inflammatory drug.

9. A 65-year-old man is recovering from general anesthesia for umbilical hernia repair. You go to evaluate him and note he is sleeping with an oxygen saturation of 94% on room air. When you call his name, he takes a deep breath, coughs, and yells at you for interrupting his nap. You note his blood pressure is 166/70. He kicks his blanket off and throws it at you, yelling "that's what it always is!"

A. His modified Aldrete score is 5 and he is NOT ready for discharge.
B. His modified Aldrete score is 9 and he is ready for discharge.
C. He is hypertensive and therefore is not ready for discharge.
D. He is angry and therefore is not ready for discharge.
E. He was sleeping and therefore is not ready for discharge.

10. A 21-year-old man is in the PACU after receiving general anesthesia for excision and grafting of a small burn he sustained to his right lower extremity several days ago. He is demanding to be discharged home, but the nurse tells him he must urinate and eat crackers first. Which of the following is true regarding the need to void and eat/drink before discharge home?

A. It is absolutely necessary for all patients to urinate and demonstrate that they can eat and drink before discharge home from the PACU.
B. It is never necessary for patients to urinate and demonstrate that they can eat and drink before discharge home from the PACU.
C. All patients who received general anesthesia need to demonstrate that they can eat and drink before discharge home. Only patients who had neuraxial blocks are required to urinate.
D. Requiring all patients to void before discharge home is necessary from a medicolegal standpoint.
E. Requiring patients who are at low risk to void and to eat and drink before discharge home is not necessary.

11. Which of the following is the expected physiologic response to electroconvulsive therapy (ECT), beginning with the electrical stimulus?

A. Initial sympathetic discharge followed by parasympathetic response
B. Initial parasympathetic discharge followed by sympathetic response
C. Initial sympathetic discharge without parasympathetic response
D. Initial prominent sympathetic discharge leading to arrhythmia
E. No physiologic response

12. Which of the following agents CANNOT be used safely and effectively for induction of anesthesia for ECT?

A. Methohexital
B. Propofol
C. Ketamine
D. Etomidate
E. None of the above, all can be used safely and effectively

13. A 52-year-old woman presents for ECT for refractory depression. You note she is on multiple psychiatric medications, including a selective serotonin reuptake inhibitor, a tricyclic antidepressant, and a monoamine oxidase inhibitor (MAOI). Which of the following is false regarding MAOIs and ECT?

   A. Patient's taking MAOIs are at increased risk for hypertensive crisis if direct- or indirect-acting sympathomimetic drugs are given.
   B. If the decision is made to continue MAOI therapy, the patient should be on a stable dose before ECT.
   C. If the decision is made to discontinue the MAOI, it should be held for 3 days before ECT.
   D. If the decision is made to discontinue the MAOI, it should be held for 2 weeks before ECT.
   E. The decision to either stop or continue MAOIs for ECT should be made on an individual patient-by-patient basis.

14. In which of the following patients would you be MOST concerned about ECT?

   A. A 55-year-old man who had a cerebral aneurysm coiled last year, stable on follow-up imaging.
   B. An 87-year-old woman with multivessel coronary artery disease and ejection fraction on 35%
   C. A 41-year-old man with untreated pheochromocytoma
   D. A 71-year-old woman with severe osteoporosis
   E. A 65-year-old man with Parkinson disease

15. A 27-year-old woman with depression who has not responded well to medical management presents for ECT. You are about to go over the consent for anesthesia with her when a nurse tells you "not to bother," consent is implied because she is depressed and therefore cannot consent for herself. Which of the following is the most appropriate response?

   A. Thank her for reminding you and do not consent the patient.
   B. Thank her for reminding you and call the patient's mother to obtain consent.
   C. Cancel the ECT.
   D. Assess the patient to evaluate if she understands the information relevant to consenting for anesthesia for ECT, and if she does, continue with the consent process.

16. All of the following are advantages of an office-based procedure EXCEPT which one?

   A. Cost containment
   B. Patient convenience
   C. Surgeon convenience
   D. Increased patient exposure to nosocomial infections
   E. Improved patient privacy

17. Which of the following equipment is NOT required to be available for the safe delivery of office-based anesthesia?

   A. Pulse oximeter
   B. Capnography
   C. Anesthesia machine
   D. Suction equipment
   E. Dantrolene and malignant hyperthermia supplies

18. According to the ASA Closed Claims Project database, which of the following were the most common adverse events during office-based procedures?

   A. Respiratory events
   B. Cerebrovascular events
   C. Equipment-related injuries
   D. Gastrointestinal-related events
   E. Postanesthetic events

19. **All of the following patients are considered poor candidates for an office-based procedure EXCEPT which one?**

    A. A 30-year-old woman with type 1 diabetes mellitus and HbA1c 9
    B. A 20-year-old man with history of intravenous drug use on Suboxone
    C. A 40-year-old woman with body mass index of 43
    D. A 70-year-old woman with osteoporosis
    E. A 50-year-old man without an escort

20. **The last patient of the day is recovering from her general anesthetic for liposuction at a plastic surgery office. The anesthesiologist and a medical assistant are the only people who remain in the office after a long day. The anesthesiologist tells the administrative assistant she has to leave and asks him if he can give the patient's escort the postoperative care instructions when he gets there. Which of the following statements is correct?**

    A. This is inappropriate because the anesthesiologist must stay until the last patient has left the office.
    B. This is appropriate only if the medical assistant is ACLS/PALS-certified.
    C. This is appropriate because the anesthesiologist has to leave.
    D. This is inappropriate because the anesthesiologist is taking advantage of the medical assistant.
    E. This is inappropriate because the anesthesiologist should remain to answer the escort's questions about postsurgical care.

21. **The 3-step paradigm to nonoperating room anesthesia describes a systematic approach that addresses which of the following?**

    A. The patient, the procedure, and the environment
    B. The patient, the proceduralist, and the anesthesiologist
    C. The proceduralist, the anesthesiologist, and the ASA classification
    D. The anesthesiologist, the environment, and the equipment
    E. The proceduralist, the environment, and the equipment

22. **You are delivering general anesthesia in the interventional radiology suite for fluoroscopy-guided radiofrequency ablation of hepatocellular carcinoma. All of the following steps can be taken to minimize exposure to radiation EXCEPT which one?**

    A. Leaving the procedure room when active radiation is in use
    B. Wearing a lead-lined protective garment
    C. Working behind a lead-lined glass shield
    D. Working on the side of the table on which the X-ray source originates
    E. Limiting the length of time of the procedure

23. **You are performing a general anesthesia for a 4-year-old undergoing an MRI. After induction of anesthesia, you take all of the following steps to ensure safety in the MRI EXCEPT which one?**

    A. Ear protection is placed in the patient's ears.
    B. IV tubing and cables are wound neatly in loops at the patient's skin.
    C. Ensure absence of ferromagnetic equipment such as IV poles, gas cylinders, and pens.
    D. The patient achieves adequate tidal volumes after moving into the scanner.
    E. The patient is adequately anesthetized.

24. **After inducing general anesthesia, you observe your patient as she moves into the MRI scanner. After ensuring MRI safety standards have been met and she is adequately anesthetized and hemodynamically stable, you move to the monitoring room. When you are in the monitoring room, you are in which zone?**

    A. Zone I
    B. Zone II
    C. Zone III
    D. Zone IV
    E. Zone V

25. **ASA standards for nonoperating room anesthetizing locations include all of the following EXCEPT which one?**

   A. Adequate and reliable suction is available.
   B. Easy and expeditious access to the patient is required, but limited access to the anesthesia machine and monitoring equipment is acceptable.
   C. Defibrillator, emergency drugs, and cardiopulmonary resuscitation equipment are all immediately available.
   D. There is adequate illumination of the patient, anesthesia machine, and monitoring equipment with a battery-operated backup light source.
   E. Electrical outlets are sufficient for both the anesthesia machines and monitors.

Chapter 22 ▪ Answers

1. Correct answer: C

Obesity in itself is not associated with an increase in adverse outcomes during general anesthesia; however, patient selection, especially those with known or suspected OSA, must be considered carefully in the outpatient setting. It is, for the most part, acceptable to proceed in the setting of suspected sleep apnea if the procedure is typically performed in the outpatient setting and if local or regional anesthesia is used. Currently, there is insufficient evidence to warrant canceling a planned procedure to obtain a sleep study, and the benefit of implementing preoperative continuous positive airway pressure in this setting is unclear, as there is no agreement of the time period of continuous positive airway pressure use needed to achieve a decrease in perioperative risk; thus A is incorrect. B is incorrect because this is a procedure that is typically performed in the outpatient setting and local or regional anesthesia is planned. D is incorrect because according to the STOP-BANG scoring system as well as the ASA scoring system, she is at high risk for OSA. E is incorrect because it is generally accepted that patients of all ASA status can be considered for ambulatory surgery as long as their systemic disease is medically stable, as is the case here. In addition, the procedure, an inguinal hernia repair, is appropriate for ambulatory surgery, there is a low rate of postoperative complications, and the postoperative care can be easily managed at home.

Reference:

1. Stierer TL, Collop NA. Perioperative assessment and management for sleep apnea in the ambulatory surgical patient. *Chest*. 2015;148(2):559-565.

2. Correct answer: D

Because she has swallowed the gum, it should be considered a solid, and therefore, according to ASA guidelines, a 6-hour fasting time is recommended before anesthesia.

ASA Fasting Guidelines:

> 2 hours—clear liquids (not including alcohol)
> 4 hours—breastmilk
> 6 hours—nonhuman milk, infant formula, light meal
> 8 hours—meat, fried or fatty food

With regard to chewing gum in the preoperative period, studies have found a small, but statistically significant, increase in gastric fluid volume without an associated change in gastric pH. The clinical significance of such a small increase in gastric fluid volume is most likely insignificant. Guidelines in respect to the chewing gum vary and are in flux. For instance, the European Society of Anesthesiologists allows chewing gum up until the time of surgery. The Association of Anesthesiologists in Great Britain and Ireland considers gum as a clear liquid and recommends a 2-hour fasting period.

References:

1. Ouanes JP, Bicket MC, Togioka B, et al. The role of perioperative chewing gum on gastric fluid volume and gastric pH: a meta-analysis. *J Clin Anesth*. 2015;27:146.
2. Smith I, Kranke P, Murat I, et al. Perioperative fasting in adults and children: guidelines from the European Society of Anaesthesiology. *Eur J Anaesthesiol*. 2011;28:556.
3. Practice guidelines for preoperative fasting and the use of pharmacologic agents to reduce the risk of pulmonary aspiration: application to healthy patients undergoing elective procedures: an updated report by the American Society of Anesthesiologists Task Force on preoperative fasting and the use of pharmacologic agents to reduce the risk of pulmonary aspiration. *Anesthesiology*. 2017;126:376.
4. Association of Anaesthetists of Great Britain and Ireland. AAGBI safety guideline. Pre-operative assessment and patient preparation. The role of the anaesthetist. January 2010. London. http://www.aagbi.org/sites/default/files/preop2010.pdf. Accessed on May 10, 2017.

3. Correct answer: D

There have been many studies evaluating perioperative glucose control in hospitalized patients, critically ill patients, and those undergoing major surgical procedures. However, there are little data on how to best address perioperative glucose control in the ambulatory setting. With regard to hyperglycemia, there is no one preoperative glucose level that necessitates postponing elective surgery. However, surgery should be postponed if the patient exhibits signs of symptomatic/complication for hyperglycemia such as dehydration, ketoacidosis, or hyperosmolar state. This young man has nausea, excessive urination, and thirst, concerning for dehydration and ketoacidosis, and thus his procedure should be postponed and he should be referred for appropriate work-up and management.

In general, the primary goals of perioperative glucose management are to avoid hypoglycemia and maintain adequate glucose control. There is no consensus on the best method for achieving these goals. Perioperative glucose goals may depend on multiple factors such as how well the patient's glucose is controlled in general, duration of surgery, and expected time to resume oral intake and antidiabetic management postoperatively. Thus, answer choices A, B, and C may be appropriate in different clinical situations; however, in this case the patient is showing complications of hyperglycemia, and therefore the surgery should be postponed.

Reference:

1. Joshi GP, Chung F, Vann MA, et al. Society for Ambulatory Anesthesia consensus statement on perioperative blood glucose management in diabetic patients undergoing ambulatory surgery. *Anesth Analg.* 2011;111:1378-1387.

---

4. **Correct answer: A**

The Apfel score gives each of the following risk factors 1 point: female sex, nonsmoker, history of PONV or motion sickness, and need of postoperative opioids. The incidence of PONV with 0, 1, 2, 3, and 4 risk factors is 10%, 20%, 40%, 60%, and 80%, respectively. Based on most algorithms, this patient would be considered at high or medium-high risk for PONV, and a multimodal approach to prevention using antiemetics with differing mechanisms of action is recommended.

Anxiety is considered not to be clinically relevant as a predictor of PONV; thus answer choice B is incorrect. Avoiding nitrous oxide can reduce the risk of PONV, but minimizing neostigmine dose has not been found to be helpful, making answer choice C incorrect. Scopolamine patch is most effective when placed the prior evening or 2 hours before surgery, but ondansetron is most effective when given at the end of surgery, making answer choice D incorrect. Answer choice E is incorrect because haloperidol has antiemetic properties when used in much lower doses than those used to treat psychiatric disorders.

References:

1. Gan TJ, Diemunsch P, Habib AS, et al. Consensus guidelines for the management of postoperative nausea and vomiting. *Anesth Analg.* 2014;118(1):85-113.
2. Lichtor JL. Ambulatory anesthesia. In: Barash PG, Cullen BF, Stoelting RK, et al, eds. *Clinical Anesthesia.* Philadelphia: Lippincott; 2013:844-859.

---

5. **Correct answer: D**

All of these techniques can be used to affect a short time to discharge depending on the agents used. The use of short-acting induction and maintenance agents as well as close attention to anesthetic depth can allow for a general anesthesia with a minimal period of impairment. Using a short-acting local anesthesia for a spinal such as chloroprocaine or mepivacaine can allow a faster recovery from neuraxial blockade. Performing blocks takes longer than inducing general anesthesia and the incidence of failure is higher; thus a regional anesthetic does not necessarily lead to a shorter duration of stay. A meta-analysis looking at time to discharge for ambulatory patients found no difference between those who underwent general, neuraxial, or regional anesthesia. Knee arthroscopies are routinely performed as same-day surgeries at ambulatory centers.

References:

1. Lichtor JL. Ambulatory anesthesia. In: Barash PG, Cullen BF, Stoelting RK, et al, eds. *Clinical Anesthesia.* Philadelphia: Lippincott; 2013:844-859.
2. Liu S, Strodtbeck W, Richman J, et al. A comparison of regional versus general anesthesia for ambulatory anesthesia: a meta-analysis of randomized controlled trials. *Anesth Analg.* 2005;101:1634-1642.

---

6. **Correct answer: E**

PONV should be treated with an antiemetic from a different class than the prophylactic antiemetic given. Perphenazine and promethazine are phenothiazines and therefore are more likely to be effective than repeating a type of drug already administered. Thus, answer choice E is correct and answer choices A, B, C, and D are incorrect. In general, smaller doses of 5-HT_3 antagonists such as ondansetron are effective when used for treatment of nausea and vomiting as opposed to those used for prophylaxis; thus answer choice D is incorrect.

Reference:

1. Gan TJ, Diemunsch P, Habib AS, et al. Consensus guidelines for the management of postoperative nausea and vomiting. *Anesth Analg.* 2014;118(1):85-113.

7. Correct answer: D

Drowsiness from residual anesthesia, nausea, vomiting, and pain are the most common reasons for delay in discharge for ambulatory patients. Anxiety has not been shown to be a common reason for delay.

Reference:

1. Lichtor JL. Ambulatory anesthesia. In: Barash PG, Cullen BF, Stoelting RK, et al, eds. *Clinical Anesthesia.* Philadelphia: Lippincott; 2013:844-859.

8. Correct answer: E

It is important to differentiate pain from other sources of discomfort, as treating these symptoms with opiates may actually increase time to discharge by exacerbating the symptom (hypercapnia) or leading to oversedation when the stimulus for discomfort is removed (full bladder). In the ambulatory setting, use of a shorter-acting intravenous opiate along with an adjunct, such as a nonsteroidal anti-inflammatory drug, can lead to a longer duration of pain relief and is associated with less nausea and vomiting than with longer-acting IV agents. Undertreating pain can lead to a prolonged PACU stay and is not the best patient care. Administration of a shorter-acting intravenous opiate, fentanyl, is encouraged over longer-acting IV agents such as morphine or hydromorphone in the ambulatory setting.

Reference:

1. Lichtor JL. Ambulatory anesthesia. In: Barash PG, Cullen BF, Stoelting RK, et al, eds. *Clinical Anesthesia.* Philadelphia: Lippincott; 2013:844-859.

9. Correct answer: B

The modified Aldrete score is one of the commonly used scoring systems for discharge from the PACU. It involves evaluation of 5 factors: respiration, oxygen saturation, level of consciousness, circulation, and activity. Each factor is scored from 0 to 2. In general, a score of 9 or above is acceptable for discharge, which this patient has. See table below. In general, a blood pressure within 20 mm Hg of preoperative/baseline measurement is acceptable.

Although scoring systems can be used to simplify and standardize discharge criteria, there is no one set of fixed discharge criteria that ensures safe PACU discharge home for every patient. Each patient should be evaluated individually, taking into consideration the severity of underlying disease, anesthetic and recovery course, and resources at home. A plan for postdischarge symptoms and follow-up should be in place.

Modified Aldrete Scoring System

	RESPIRATION	O_2 SATURATION	CONSCIOUSNESS	CIRCULATION	ACTIVITY
0	Apnea	<90% with supplemental O_2	Not responding	BP ± 50 mm Hg of preoperative	Unable to move extremities
1	Dyspnea/shallow breathing	Requires O_2 to maintain SpO_2 > 90%	Arousable on calling	BP ± 20-50 mm Hg of preoperative	Able to move 2 extremities
2	Able to take deep breath and cough	Maintains SpO_2 > 92% on RA	Fully awake	BP ± 20 mm Hg of preoperative	Able to move 4 extremities

Reference:

1. Lichtor JL. Ambulatory anesthesia. In: Barash PG, Cullen BF, Stoelting RK, et al, eds. *Clinical Anesthesia.* Philadelphia: Lippincott; 2013:844-859.

10. **Correct answer: E**

There is no one set of fixed discharge criteria that ensures safe PACU discharge home for every patient. Each patient should be evaluated individually, taking into consideration the severity of underlying disease, anesthetic, and recovery course. Postoperative nausea may be greater for some patients if they are required to eat before discharge. Although it is warranted to require patients, who underwent urologic procedures and/or had spinal or epidural anesthesia to void before discharge, requiring patients who are at low risk for urinary retention to urinate before discharge is not necessary and can lead to prolonged PACU stay.

Reference:

1. Lichtor JL. Ambulatory anesthesia. In: Barash PG, Cullen BF, Stoelting RK, et al, eds. *Clinical Anesthesia*. Philadelphia: Lippincott; 2013:844-859.

11. **Correct answer: B**

The electrical stimulus causes an initial parasympathetic discharge usually lasting 10-15 seconds. This is usually followed by a more prominent sympathetic response. In some cases, this is followed by another parasympathetic response. Parasympathetic discharges can lead to bradycardia, hypotension, and less commonly, asystole. Sympathetic responses can lead to cardiac arrhythmia and an increase in heart rate, blood pressure, and myocardial oxygen demand.

Reference:

1. Uppal V, Dourish J, Macfarlane A. Anaesthesia for electroconvulsive therapy. *Contin Educ Anaesth Crit Care Pain*. 2010;10(6):192-196.

12. **Correct answer: E**

All of these induction agents can be and are used to induce anesthesia for ECT.

Methohexital is an ultrashort-acting barbiturate that is often described as the "gold standard" for ECT because of its long history of use, rapid onset and recovery, and very modest anticonvulsant properties.

Propofol is also short acting; however, it has more anticonvulsant properties and may raise the seizure threshold or shorten the seizure.

Ketamine is a noncompetitive NMDA antagonist. It may take longer for patients to achieve the appropriate depth of anesthesia for ECT after a bolus dose than with propofol or methohexital. Ketamine also has sympathomimetic properties, which may not be ideal for some patients. At high doses, there is evidence that ketamine can increase seizure duration and quality.

Etomidate is short acting, may reduce the seizure threshold, and has been shown to increase seizure duration; thus it is sometimes used in patients with resistant seizures. Etomidate does suppress corticosteroid synthesis, which theoretically may be of consequence for patients receiving multiple treatments. It is also associated with increased nausea.

References:

1. Bryson E, Aloysi A, Farber K, Kellner C. Individualized anesthetic management for patients undergoing electroconvulsive therapy: a review of current practice. *Anesth Analg*. 2017;124(6):1943-1956.
2. Uppal V, Dourish J, Macfarlane A. Anaesthesia for electroconvulsive therapy. *Contin Educ Anaesth Crit Care Pain*. 2010;10(6):192-196.

13. **Correct answer: C**

The decision to either stop or continue MAOIs for ECT should be made on an individual patient-by-patient basis. If MAOIs are to be stopped, patients should stop taking them for 2 weeks before ECT. If they are continued, patients should be on a stable dose. Sympathomimetic agents and meperidine should be avoided.

Reference:

1. Bryson E, Aloysi A, Farber K, Kellner C. Individualized anesthetic management for patients undergoing electroconvulsive therapy: a review of current practice. *Anesth Analg*. 2017;124(6):1943-1956.

14. **Correct answer: C**

ECT is frequently used as a treatment in elderly people with significant comorbidities. Although all of these patients have comorbidities that need to be considered carefully during evaluation for ECT, the only absolute contraindication is the presence of an untreated pheochromocytoma. Other populations have done well when medically maximized. Despite the cardiovascular effects, ECT is often tolerated well in patients with significant cardiac disease. During ECT, cerebral oxygen consumption, blood flow, and intracranial pressure all increase. For these reasons, patients with intracranial pathology should be seen by a neurologist before undergoing ECT. However, there are multiple reports of successful ECT in patients with intracranial aneurysms. Although patients with severe osteoporosis are at increased risk for fracture with ECT, adequate muscle relaxation can often prevent this. It is not uncommon for patients with Parkinson disease to present for ECT, and many have been treated successfully.

References:

1. Bryson E, Aloysi A, Farber K, Kellner C. Individualized anesthetic management for patients undergoing electroconvulsive therapy: a review of current practice. *Anesth Analg.* 2017;124(6):1943-1956.
2. Uppal V, Dourish J, Macfarlane A. Anaesthesia for electroconvulsive therapy. *Contin Educ Anaesth Crit Care Pain.* 2010;10(6):192-196.

15. **Correct answer: D**

Although illnesses that require ECT can feature significant impairment of mental capacity, carrying a diagnosis of a mental illness in itself does not mean that a patient lacks capacity to make medical decisions and provide consent for procedures. Most patients presenting for ECT do in fact have capacity. You must assess whether she can understand the nature, purpose, and likely risks and benefits pertaining to the treatment. If she can, then she has capacity to consent for ECT.

Reference:

1. Uppal V, Dourish J, Macfarlane A. Anaesthesia for electroconvulsive therapy. *Contin Educ Anaesth Crit Care Pain.* 2010;10(6):192-196.

16. **Correct answer: D**

The major advantages of office-based procedures are cost containment, patient and surgeon convenience, improved patient privacy, and DECREASED patient exposure to nosocomial infections.

Reference:

1. Hausman LM, Rosenblatt MA. Office based anesthesia. In: Barash PG, Cullen BF, Stoelting RK, et al, eds. *Clinical Anesthesia.* 7th ed. Philadelphia: Lippincott; 2013:860-876.

17. **Correct answer: C**

Offices are required to have a means to deliver positive pressure ventilation. A bag valve mask and adequate oxygen supply are sufficient. The availability of a ventilator or anesthesia machine is not necessary. Pulse oximetry, capnography, suction equipment, and dantrolene/malignant hyperthermia supplies are all required.

Reference:

1. Hausman LM, Rosenblatt MA. Office based anesthesia. In: Barash PG, Cullen BF, Stoelting RK, et al, eds. *Clinical Anesthesia.* 7th ed. Philadelphia: Lippincott; 2013:860-876.

18. **Correct answer: A**

According to the ASA Closed Claims project, approximately one-half of the adverse events during office-based anesthesia were respiratory in nature (airway obstruction, bronchospasm, inadequate oxygenation/ventilation, unrecognized esophageal intubation). Oversedation during minimum alveolar concentration anesthesia leading to respiratory depression was an important mechanism of patient injury. The second most common cause were medication-related events. Cardiovascular and equipment-related injuries accounted for a smaller percentage. The majority of events occurred intraoperatively.

References:

1. Hausman LM, Rosenblatt MA. Office based anesthesia. In: Barash PG, Cullen BF, Stoelting RK, et al, eds. *Clinical Anesthesia.* 7th ed. Philadelphia: Lippincott; 2013:860-876.
2. Desai M. Office-based anesthesia: new frontiers, better outcomes, and emphasis on safety. *Curr Opin Anaesthesiol.* 2008;21(6):699-703.

19. **Correct answer: D**

Patient selection criteria for office-based anesthesia are multifactorial. The ideal patient is an ASA 1 or 2; however, it may be appropriate for an ASA 3 patient to have an office-based anesthetic after thorough anesthesia evaluation and consultation. In general, patients with poorly controlled diabetes (A), history of substance use (B), morbid obesity (C), and those without an escort (E) are poor candidates for office-based procedures. Patients should not be excluded from office-based procedures based solely on age.

Reference:
1. Hausman LM, Rosenblatt MA. Office based anesthesia. In: Barash PG, Cullen BF, Stoelting RK, et al, eds. *Clinical Anesthesia*. 7th ed. Philadelphia: Lippincott; 2013:860-876.

20. **Correct answer: B**

It is recommended that there be at least 1 ACLS/PALS-certified member of the health care team present until the last patient has left the office.

Reference:
1. Hausman LM, Rosenblatt MA. Office based anesthesia. In: Barash PG, Cullen BF, Stoelting RK, et al, eds. *Clinical Anesthesia*. 7th ed. Philadelphia: Lippincott; 2013:860-876.

21. **Correct answer: A**

Anesthesiologists delivering care outside of the operating room may find themselves in an unfamiliar environment, lacking familiar equipment, and interacting with staff with varying amounts of familiarity with anesthesia care. The simple 3-step paradigm consisting of PATIENT, PROCEDURE, and ENVIRONMENT is recommended to address these issues.

Reference:
1. Souter KJ, Pittaway AJ. Nonoperating room anesthesia (NORA). In: Barash PG, Cullen BF, Stoelting RK, et al, eds. *Clinical Anesthesia*. Philadelphia: Lippincott; 2013:876-890.

22. **Correct answer: D**

The power of reflected radiation is inversely related to the angle between the radiation beam and the target. At the same distance from the field, the exposure on the side of the X-ray source far exceeds that on the side of the image intensifier, which allows an image to be displayed on a monitor. For this reason, an anesthesiologist standing on the side of the table next to the source of the X-ray beam receives more radiation than if he/she were standing on the side of the image display. Methods for decreasing radiation exposure include increasing the distance from the source of radiation, using protective shielding, and limiting the time of exposure to radiation.

References:
1. Souter KJ, Pittaway AJ. Nonoperating room anesthesia (NORA). In: Barash PG, Cullen BF, Stoelting RK, et al, eds. *Clinical Anesthesia*. Philadelphia: Lippincott; 2013:876-890.
2. Wang R, Kumar A, Tanaka P. Occupational radiation exposure of anesthesia providers: a summary of key learning points and resident-led radiation safety projects. *Semin Cardiothorac Vasc Anesth*. 2017;21(2):165-171.

23. **Correct answer: B**

Cables and wires should not be wound in loops, as this can cause an induction heating effect and thermal injury. Considerable noise is generated by the MRI, which can exceed occupational exposure limits; thus ear protection should be placed in the patient's ears. Ferromagnetic equipment such as IV poles, gas cylinders, and pens can become lethal projectiles when too close to the magnetic field. You should ensure the patient is adequately anesthetized and their airway is secure. Endotracheal tubes or laryngeal mask airways may kink or dislodge if there is a close fit into the MRI scanner.

References:
1. Souter KJ, Pittaway AJ. Nonoperating room anesthesia (NORA). In: Barash PG, Cullen BF, Stoelting RK, et al, eds. *Clinical Anesthesia*. Philadelphia: Lippincott; 2013:876-890.
2. Apfelbaum J, Singleton MA, Ehrenwerth J, et al. Practice advisory on anesthetic care for magnetic resonance imaging: an updated report by the American Society of Anesthesiologists Task Force on Anesthetic Care for MRI. *Anesthesiology*. 2015;122:495-520.

24. **Correct answer: C**

Zone I includes all areas that are freely accessible to the general public and is typically outside of the MR environment.

Zone II is the area that serves as the interface between the publically accessible uncontrolled zone I and the more strictly controlled zone III. This is typically where patients are greeted by MR personnel and where screening questions take place.

Zone III is the region in which free access by unscreened non-MR personnel or ferromagnetic objects can result in injury or death. There may be exposure to the MRI scanner's static and varying magnetic fields. Access to zone III is strictly restricted.

Zone IV is the MRI scanner magnet room, the MR magnet, and its associated magnetic field.

There is no zone V.

Reference:

1. Apfelbaum J, Singleton MA, Ehrenwerth J, et al. Practice advisory on anesthetic care for magnetic resonance imaging: an updated report by the American Society of Anesthesiologists Task Force on Anesthetic Care for MRI. *Anesthesiology*. 2015;122:495-520.

25. **Correct answer: B**

Easy and expeditious access to the patient, anesthesia machine, and monitoring equipment are all required.

Reference:

1. Souter KJ, Pittaway AJ. Nonoperating room anesthesia (NORA). In: Barash PG, Cullen BF, Stoelting RK, et al, eds. *Clinical Anesthesia*. Philadelphia: Lippincott; 2013:876-890.

23

GERIATRICS

Alexandra Plichta, Christoph Nabzdyk, Nathan Lee, Alexander Nagrebetsky,
Alexandra Raisa Adler, and Jerome Crowley

1. **, , Of the following choices, which opioid has consistently been associated with delirium when used for postoperative pain management in the elderly?**

   A. Fentanyl
   B. Morphine
   C. Hydromorphone
   D. Meperidine

2. **Which of the following changes that occur with increasing age can account for the possible increase of morphine's duration of action in the elderly?**

   A. Increased adipose tissue
   B. Increased lean body mass
   C. Increased total body water
   D. Decreased gastric pH

3. **Which of the following opioids would be most appropriate to treat pain in an elderly patient on fluoxetine?**

   A. Tramadol
   B. Meperidine
   C. Fentanyl
   D. Oxycodone

4. **When comparing an 80-year-old patient with a 20-year-old patient with the same lean body mass, which of the following statements about remifentanil is false?**

   A. A reduction of the bolus dose will be required in the 80-year-old to have the same therapeutic effect as in the 20-year-old.
   B. A reduction of the maintenance infusion rate will be required in the 80-year-old to have the same therapeutic effect as in the 20-year-old.
   C. The 80-year-old patient may have a delayed emergence after receiving a remifentanil infusion.
   D. The 20-year-old patient may have a delayed emergence after receiving a remifentanil infusion.

5. **An 80-year-old man is scheduled for radical prostatectomy. He denies any significant medical history other than hypertension, for which he takes hydrochlorothiazide. He reports a good exercise tolerance and is able to climb 4 flights of stairs without difficulty. What would be the expected minimum alveolar concentration (MAC) of sevoflurane to prevent movement to surgical stimulation assuming the patient has a response to anesthesia in line with the median population?**

A. 1.8%

B. 1.6%

C. 1.4%

D. 1.2%

6. **A 90-year-old man with no significant cardiopulmonary history, other than hypertension, is undergoing an elective right hemicolectomy. After induction of general anesthesia, the patient is noted to be requiring escalating doses of phenylephrine to maintain a mean arterial pressure (MAP) >65 mm Hg. ECG shows normal sinus rhythm, and airway pressures are within normal limits. End tidal carbon dioxide is stable. He is being maintained on desflurane with an expired concentration of 6%. Which of the following is the most appropriate next step?**

A. Decrease the desflurane with a goal expired concentration of 5.5%.

B. Decrease the desflurane with a goal expired concentration of 4.6%.

C. Tolerate a MAP of 55 mm Hg.

D. Administer midazolam with the goal of creating a balanced anesthetic.

7. **Which of the following statements regarding cardiovascular physiology in the elderly is true?**

A. Vascular stiffening leads to a decrease in pulse pressure.

B. Diastolic dysfunction is present in half of those diagnosed with congestive heart failure.

C. Nitric oxide production is increased to balance increases in systemic vascular resistance.

D. Cardiac output is maintained by increased stroke volume and ventricular contractility.

8. **Which of the following cardiovascular changes associated with aging is false?**

A. Reduced ventricular compliance

B. Decreased blood vessel contractility

C. Desensitization of carotid and aortic baroreceptors

D. Preserved sympathetic and vagal resting tone

9. **Which of the following statements regarding cardiovascular pathology in elderly patients is false?**

A. Out of every 3 patients older than 70 years, 1 patient will develop significant coronary artery disease.

B. Hypertension can develop in the setting of normal systemic vascular resistance.

C. In the developing world, rheumatic heart disease affecting the aortic valve is the most common cause of valvular heart disease.

D. In the absence of disease, resting systolic cardiac function can be preserved even in octogenarians.

10. **Which of the following statements regarding autonomic physiology in the elderly is true?**

A. α-Adrenergic sensitivity and response to α-agonists are increased.

B. β-Adrenergic sensitivity and response to β-agonists are increased.

C. Adrenal tissues atrophy, resulting in a decrease in circulating norepinephrine and epinephrine levels.

D. Maintenance of MAP is dependent on increases in vascular resistance.

11. A 84-year-old man is admitted to the hospital after a fall from standing, striking his left chest on a night stand. The patient's medical history includes hypertension, coronary artery disease with multiple drug eluting stent placements in the left and right coronary arteries, non-ST elevation myocardial infarction (5 years ago), and heart failure with a left ventricular (LV) ejection fraction of 35%. He is taking aspirin, clopidogrel, and apixaban (factor Xa [FXa] inhibitor), as well as ibuprofen as needed for intermittent back pain. The patient's laboratory test results reveal the following: Na 134, K 3.2, Cl 100, HCO$_3$ 21, BUN 6, and Cr 0.81. Laboratory results from the following day reveal Na 132, K 3.0, Cl 97, HCO$_3$ 16, BUN 12, and Cr 1.98. The patient's hourly urine output is 25 cc. Which of the following statements about the patient's kidney function is most accurate?

A. Andexanet alfa administration is associated with acute kidney injury (AKI).
B. Ibuprofen (NSAID) caused acute interstitial nephritis by inhibition of local prostaglandin production.
C. The patient's urine output was inadequate.
D. The degree of the patient's increase in creatinine is associated with an increased risk of hospital death.

12. A 82-year-old woman with a medical history of hypertension, hyperlipidemia, and chronic kidney disease (CKD) (baseline Cr 1.4) is brought to the emergency department by ambulance from her retirement home with altered mental status. The patient's vital signs are as follows: T 39.3°C, HR 121, BP 72/45, RR 38, Sao$_2$ 88%, and Fio$_2$ 1.0 via nonrebreather mask. The patient is admitted to the intensive care unit with subsequent intubation and initiation of norepinephrine (4 µg/min) infusion. The patient's P/F ratio is 102 and serum lactate is 3. Which of the following statements is false?

A. The patient meets criteria for septic shock according to Sepsis-3 consensus.
B. Nondialysis requiring CKD in septic and septic shock patients is associated with increased mortality.
C. Titration of vasopressors to a mean arterial perfusion pressure of 75-85 mm Hg increases mortality.
D. The patient's expected in-hospital mortality is approximately 40%.

13. A 85-year-old woman with a history of hypertension, atrial fibrillation, type II diabetes mellitus (DM), hypercholesterolemia, CKD stage IV (glomerular filtration rate 15-29 mL/min; baseline creatinine 2.3), a recent ST-elevation myocardial infarction, and osteoporosis on hormone replacement therapy returns to the hospital with chest pain and dyspnea. Her home medications include aspirin, clopidogrel, apixaban, and lisinopril. She states she was recently started on exenatide (glucagonlike peptide-1 [GLP-1] receptor agonist). The patient shows clinical signs of congestive heart failure. A diagnosis of pericarditis was made. The patient receives diclofenac for pain control and furosemide for a diagnosis of pulmonary edema. Which of the following statements with regard to this patient is true?

A. CKD in women is characterized by low estradiol levels, but estrogen replacement might be associated with progressive renal loss.
B. Exenatide is a preferred oral antiglycemic in patients with severe CKD.
C. Androgens may protect renal function through prevention of parenchymal, fibrotic remodeling.
D. Apixaban is relatively contraindicated in patients with atrial fibrillation and end-stage CKD.

14. An 83-year-old man with obesity, poorly controlled hypertension, hyperlipidemia, type II DM, and nonalcoholic fatty liver disease (NAFLD) presents to the emergency department with abdominal pain, nausea, and vomiting. Vitals are as follows: T 38.3°C, HR 113, BP 81/51, RR 32, Sao$_2$ 94%, and Fio$_2$ 0.4. The patient's WBC count is 17, Hgb 12, Plt 102, Na 145, K 3.4, Cl 104, CO$_2$ 15, BUN 34, Cr 1.6, INR 1.6, PTT 41, and albumin 2.3. Which of the following statements is true?

A. Hypoalbuminemia is associated with increased perioperative morbidity but not mortality.
B. Preoperative albumin administration in patients with hypoalbuminemia may increase the incidence of AKI.
C. NAFLD lowers the risk of CKD by decreasing renal artery vascular resistance.
D. The patient is at increased risk of thromboembolic complications due to increased circulating levels of vitamin K–dependent and vitamin K–independent clotting factors.

15. An 87-year-old man with a history of perforated diverticulitis is now transferred to the intensive care unit after a >12 hour operation secondary to prolonged sedation and inability to extubate. The patient's intraoperative anesthetic consisted of propofol and sufentanil infusions. The patient was hypotensive for the majority of the case in the absence of large blood loss, requiring varying degrees of vasopressor infusion support. Which aging related changes to liver/renal physiology/anatomy help explain the patient's clinical presentation?

   A. Although absolute liver weight decreases in patients older than 50 years, liver blood flow stays largely constant.
   B. Drugs with a high hepatic extraction ratio are less affected by the age-related hepatic enzyme changes compared with drugs with a low hepatic extraction ratio.
   C. The geriatric population is relatively protected from drug-induced liver injury because of decreased mitochondrial radical oxygen species production.
   D. Changes in the medullary vasculature, increased renin-angiotensin-aldosterone system activity, and increased tubular ammonium ion excretion are key features of renal aging.

16. A 72-year-old man is scheduled for an elective ankle fracture repair. He has a history of anxiety and panic attacks. He prefers not to have a nerve block but is concerned that general anesthesia will considerably increase his risk of developing dementia. You decide to do which of the following?

   A. Convince the patient that regional anesthesia is a safer option in this case.
   B. Suggest a third option—fracture repair under monitored anesthesia care.
   C. Agree that general anesthesia increases risk of dementia and address specific concerns about the nerve block.
   D. Explain that there is no convincing evidence that general anesthesia increases the risk of dementia.

17. A 78-year-old woman is participating in a study that is assessing pain perception. A cryoprobe on her forearm is gradually cooled to produce a painful stimulus. She has undergone a similar experiment at the age of 27 years. Compared with the results of the experiment obtained in younger age, the findings are likely to elicit which of the following?

   A. Increased pain threshold but decreased pain tolerance
   B. Unchanged pain threshold and pain tolerance
   C. Decreased pain threshold and tolerance
   D. Prominent local vasodilatation due to cold-reacting agglutinins

18. A 71-year-old man is scheduled for elective surgical removal of a posterior neck cyst. He is overall healthy but reports occasional dizziness when sitting up in bed after he wakes up in the morning. Of the following choices, which is the most likely the cause of his dizziness in light of his age?

   A. Decreased baroreceptor reflex
   B. Decreased sympathetic system activity
   C. Decreased venous capacitance
   D. Decreased brain volume

19. A 73-year-old woman is scheduled for hip arthroplasty. She has a history of hypertension, hyperlipidemia, depression, and type 2 DM. She mentions that after a cholecystectomy 3 years ago, as she was recovering in PACU, she saw another elderly patient who was "acting crazy." She asks you if she will "act crazy" after her surgery. Of the following choices, which statement is the most appropriate reply in response to her concerns?

   A. This is unlikely to happen, as she has an excellent mental status before surgery.
   B. It is uncommon for patients who are fit enough to undergo a hip arthroplasty to have postoperative delirium.
   C. If she develops postoperative delirium, you expect it to resolve quickly.
   D. She may have postoperative delirium, which can affect her recovery from surgery.

20. **Which of the following lung volumes, or combination of lung volumes, changes most significantly over the lifetime of an adult?**

    A. Total lung capacity (TLC)
    B. Closing capacity (CC)
    C. Functional residual capacity (FRC)
    D. Tidal volume

21. **Which of the following statements regarding oxygenation and ventilation in the elderly is false?**

    A. The resting Pao_2 in a 20-year-old is similar to that in an 80-year-old.
    B. They have a decreased ventilatory response to hypercapnia.
    C. They have a decreased ventilatory response to hypoxia.
    D. The muscles of the upper airway atrophy.

22. **All of the following statements regarding oxygenation and ventilation in the elderly (as compared with the average adult) are correct EXCEPT which one?**

    A. FEV1 (forced expiratory volume in 1 s) is decreased.
    B. Diffusing capacity is decreased.
    C. The amount of physiologic dead space is increased.
    D. Their ventilation/perfusion matching is relatively preserved.

23. **All of the following changes in respiratory mechanics are seen in the geriatric population EXCEPT which one?**

    A. Decreased compliance of the chest wall
    B. Increased compliance of the lung parenchyma
    C. Increased curvature of the diaphragm
    D. Decreased mass of accessory muscles

24. **The pattern that most accurately describes the change in CC over time starting from age 30 years and progressing to age 80 years is which of the following?**

    A. An asymptotic increase, followed by a plateau
    B. An exponential increase
    C. An approximately linear increase
    D. An approximately linear, steep increase until middle age (50 y old), followed by a more gradual decrease

25. **The increase in CC seen with aging can BEST be attributed to which of the following?**

    A. A relatively more positive intrapleural pressure compressing alveoli
    B. A functional extrathoracic large airway obstruction
    C. The loss of cartilage from large airways
    D. The loss of elastin from surrounding tissues, which once tethered open small airways

Chapter 23 ▪ Answers

1. Correct answer: D

Postoperative delirium is a complication that especially affects the elderly following surgery and can be a major contributor to morbidity and mortality. Unfortunately, both undertreated pain and its treatment can play a role in the development of this condition. While there have not been any differences in cognitive outcomes seen when using fentanyl, morphine, or hydromorphone in the postoperative setting, meperidine does appear to have an association with the development of postoperative delirium. A systematic review of the literature examining the use of different opioid regimens on postoperative delirium found that meperidine was consistently associated with an increased risk of delirium. Of course, these data are difficult to interpret given the myriad of contributors to postoperative delirium (for example, it is difficult to prove that pain control was equal with all the opioids studied).

Meperidine is no longer frequently used for pain control. Its metabolite, normeperidine, which is cleared renally, stimulates the central nervous system and can lead to seizures or delirium. However, meperidine is still used at a subanalgesic dose for treatment of postoperative shivering. It is not known if there is a dose effect in the association between meperidine and the development of postoperative delirium.

References:
1. Fong HK, Sands LP, Leung JM. The role of postoperative analgesia in delirium and cognitive decline in elderly patients: a systematic review. *Anesth Analg.* 2006;102:1255-1266.
2. Siber F, Pauldine R. Geriatric anesthesia. In: Miller RD, Eriksson L, Fleisher L, et al. *Miller's Anesthesia.* 8th ed. Philadelphia: Elsevier; 2015:2407-2422.

2. Correct answer: A

Many pharmacokinetic and pharmacodynamic changes occur with aging. However, the clinical relevance of these effects varies greatly between individuals and may not always be clinically significant.

In the elderly, there is an increase in adipose tissue, a decrease in lean body mass, a decrease in total body water, and an increase in the volume of distribution of lipid soluble drugs. In the elderly, because there is a decrease in total body water, there is a decrease in the volume of distribution of water-soluble drugs, which leads to higher serum levels. However, the volume of distribution of lipophilic drugs actually increases (along with increased adipose tissue), which can prolong their half-life. Other factors that contribute to altered drug metabolism and effects include reduced hepatic blood flow, impaired phase I metabolism reactions, and reduced renal blood flow. Increased, not decreased, gastric pH can be found in the elderly because of the common use of antacids, proton pump inhibitors, and H_2-receptor blockers. However, this would affect absorption of the drug, not necessarily its duration of action.

References:
1. Mangoni AA, Jackson SHD. Age-related changes in pharmacokinetics and pharmacodynamics: basic principles and practical applications. *Br J Clin Pharmacol.* 2003;57(1):6-14.
2. Chau DL, Walker V, Pai L, Cho LM. Opiates and elderly: use and side effects. *Clin Interv Aging.* 2008;3(2):273-278.

3. Correct answer: D

It is not unusual for elderly patients to be on a myriad of medications. Thus, it is essential for the anesthesiologist to understand important interactions. Fluoxetine, a selective serotonin reuptake inhibitor, can, in combination with some drugs, lead to an increased risk of serotonin syndrome. Many anesthetic drugs, including opioids, increase serotonin levels. These include tramadol, meperidine, and fentanyl. Oxycodone has not been associated with an increased risk of serotonin syndrome. Serotonin syndrome can be fatal and is characterized by a triad of features: neuromuscular hyperactivity (such as tremor, clonus, and hyperreflexia), autonomic hyperactivity (such as fever, tachycardia, and diaphoresis), and change in mental status (agitation followed by confusion and eventually coma).

References:
1. Chau DL, Walker V, Pai L, Cho LM. Opiates and elderly: use and side effects. *Clin Interv Aging.* 2008;3(2):273-278.
2. Naples JG, Gellad WF, Hanlon JT. Managing pain in older adults: the role of opioid analgesics. *Clin Geriatr Med.* 2016;23(4):725-735.
3. Gillman PK. Monoamine oxidase inhibitors, opioid analgesics and serotonin toxicity. *Br J Anaesth.* 2005;95(4):434-441.

4. **Correct answer: D**

Age affects many aspects of metabolism. Remifentanil is a synthetic opioid that is metabolized by non-specific tissue esterases and is thereby not affected by hepatic or renal failure. It also has a very short context-sensitive half-time. Despite the fact that remifentanil does not rely on hepatic or renal metabolism, its dosing to achieve a therapeutic effect does differ in the elderly. Pharmacokinetic and pharmacodynamic modeling studies have shown that a reduced bolus dose of remifentanil (reduced by up to 50%) was required to reach a similar target concentration in the plasma of elderly patients as compared with younger patients. This effect was also seen using EEG monitoring. The same is true for maintenance infusions, which may require a 30%-50% reduction in infusion rate. Finally, despite the ultrashort context-sensitive half-time of remifentanil, there is variation in the rate of decrease of remifentanil in the elderly such that they may have delayed emergence.

References:

1. Spanjer MRK, Bakker NA, Absalom AR. Pharmacology in the elderly and newer anaesthesia drugs. *Best Pract Res Clin Anaesthesiol.* 2011;25:355-365.
2. Glass PSA, Tong GJ, Howell S. A review of the pharmacokinetics and pharmacodynamics of remifentanil. *Anesth Analg.* 1999;89(4S):7.

5. **Correct answer: C**

The MAC to prevent surgical stimulation decreases by ~6% with each decade after 40 years of age. For this 80-year-old patient, this translates into a predicted MAC at the 50th percentile to be ~1.4%. This is important, as overly deep anesthetics in elderly patients may have significant cardiovascular and neurocognitive effects. The reason for this phenomenon is likely due to age-related changes leading to altered activity of ion channels, synaptic activity, or receptor sensitivity.

References:

1. Bentov I, Rooke GA. Anesthesia for the older patient. In: Barash PG, Cullen BF, Stoelting RK, et al, eds. *Clinical Anesthesia.* 8th ed. Philadelphia: Lippincott; 2017:897-913.
2. Siber F, Pauldine R. Geriatric anesthesia. In: Miller RD, Eriksson L, Fleisher L, et al. *Miller's Anesthesia.* 8th ed. Philadelphia: Elsevier; 2015:2407-2422.
3. Nickalls RW, Mapleson WW. Age-related iso-MAC charts for isoflurane, sevoflurane and desflurane in man. *Br J Anaesth.* 2003;91(2).

6. **Correct answer: B**

This patient is likely overly deep under anesthesia leading to excessive vasodilation and hence increased vasoconstrictor requirements. The estimated MAC of desflurane to prevent movement to surgical stimulation is 4.6%. The MAC to prevent surgical stimulation decreases by ~6% with each decade after 40 years of age. The MAC of desflurane at age 40 years is 6.6%; for a 90-year-old patient, the reduction translates to 4.6%. Tolerating a lower MAP is not preferable in an elderly patient with chronic hypertension. Adding midazolam is not ideal in an elderly patient, as benzodiazepines are associated with an increased risk of postoperative cognitive dysfunction.

References:

1. Bentov I, Rooke GA. Anesthesia for the older patient. In: Barash PG, Cullen BF, Stoelting RK, et al, eds. *Clinical Anesthesia.* 8th ed. Philadelphia: Lippincott; 2017:897-913.
2. Siber F, Pauldine R. Geriatric anesthesia. In: Miller RD, Eriksson L, Fleisher L, et al. *Miller's Anesthesia.* 8th ed. Philadelphia: Elsevier; 2015:2407-2422.
3. Nickalls RW, Mapleson WW. Age-related iso-MAC charts for isoflurane, sevoflurane and desflurane in man. *Br J Anaesth.* 2003;91(2).

7. **Correct answer: B**

Diastolic dysfunction is present in approximately half of patients older than 65 years with a known diagnosis of congestive heart failure. It manifests as pulmonary congestion following ventricular overload, as well as exercise intolerance.

Vascular stiffening in older age leads to a gradual increase in systolic pressure, a decrease in diastolic pressure, and, overall, increased pulse pressure. The increase in impedance to LV outflow increases LV work and ultimately results in LV hypertrophy. The myocardium becomes stiffer, and diastolic filling is impaired. Furthermore, the diminished diastolic pressure leads to a decrease in coronary blood flow and higher risk of cardiac ischemia. Owing to decreased response to β-adrenergic stimulation, cardiac output is maintained by an enhanced stroke volume resulting from an increase in end-diastolic volume rather than increased contractility. Decreased production of nitric oxide occurs with aging, resulting in impairment of flow in the microvasculature and increasing risk for organ dysfunction.

References:

1. Rooke GA. Cardiovascular aging and anesthetic implications. *J Cardiothorac Vasc Anesth*. 2003;17(4):512-523.
2. Phillip B, Pastor D, Bellows W, Leung JM. The prevalence of preoperative diastolic filling abnormalities in geriatric surgical patients. *Anesth Analg*. 2003;97(5):1214-1221.
3. Ungvari Z, Kaley G, de Cabo R, Sonntag WE, Csiszar A. Mechanisms of vascular aging: new perspectives. *J Gerontol A Biol Sci Med Sci*. 2010;65A(10):1028-1041.

8. Correct answer: D

There is an age-related increase in resting sympathetic nerve activity, with elevated plasma norepinephrine levels and an increase in burst discharge rate on muscle sympathetic fibers as measured by microneurography. However, decreasing β-adrenergic receptor reactivity limits the heart's ability to increase cardiac output by increasing its rate, so the patient is more reliant on vascular tone and preload. Orthostatic and postprandial hypotension occur more frequently with age and may be associated with baroreflex impairment. Studies have demonstrated decreases in vagal component of heart rate variability, decreased response to anticholinergics, and slower conduction speed of the vagus nerve.

With aging, the heart muscle itself gradually becomes replaced with collagen and fat, becoming stiffer and less compliant. Amyloid deposits and calcification may be present, disrupting the conduction system of the heart and increasing risk of arrhythmias. Smooth muscle loss in blood vessels and gradual replacement of elastin by collagen decreases their contractility, raising systemic vascular resistance. Untreated hypertension leads to LV strain, hypertrophy, and, ultimately, systolic and diastolic dysfunction. Stiffening of the large arteries desensitizes carotid and aortic baroreceptors, disrupting the compensatory chronotropic and ionotropic cardiac response to hypotension.

References:

1. Rooke GA. Cardiovascular aging and anesthetic implications. *J Cardiothorac Vasc Anesth*. 2003;17(4):512-523.
2. Hotta H, Uchida S. Aging of the autonomic nervous system and possible improvements in autonomic activity using somatic afferent stimulation. *Geriatr Gerontol Int*. 2010;10(S1):S127-S136.
3. Ungvari Z, Kaley G, de Cabo R, Sonntag WE, Csiszar A. Mechanisms of vascular aging: new perspectives. *J Gerontol A Biol Sci Med Sci*. 2010;65A(10):1028-1041.

9. Correct answer: C

In the developing world, rheumatic heart disease is the most common cause of valvular heart disease with approximately 60% of cases involving the mitral valve. The cardiac inflammation and scarring by group A streptococci can cause valvular fibrosis, resulting in stenosis and/or insufficiency. The valves most affected are, in order, mitral, aortic, tricuspid, and pulmonary. In the Western world, calcification of the aortic valve leading to aortic sclerosis is more prevalent, seen in up to 40% of patients aged ≥75 years. Although it does not cause ventricular obstruction or other symptoms, aortic sclerosis has been associated with increased incidence, chances of developing myocardial infarction, and even death.

The rest of the answers are accurate. Coronary artery disease is the most common cause of heart disease in the elderly, especially smokers and diabetics. All elderly patients undergoing anesthesia should be considered as having increased risk for cardiovascular ischemia. Cardiac afterload due to vascular impedance can increase even in the setting of normal systemic vascular resistance, resulting in hypertension. Healthy patients can have preserved resting LV systolic function even into the 10th decade of life.

References:

1. Jackson CF, Wenger NK. Cardiovascular disease in the elderly. *Rev Esp Cardiol*. 2011;64(8):697-712.
2. Nichols WW, O'Rourke MF, Avolio AP, Yaginuma T, Pepine CJ, Conti CR. Ventricular/vascular interaction in patients with mild systemic hypertension and normal peripheral resistance. *Circulation*. 1986;74(3):455-462.
3. Aronow WS, Stein PD, Sabbah HN, Koenigsberg M. Resting left ventricular ejection fraction in elderly patients without evidence of heart disease. *Am J Cardiol*. 1989;63(5):368-369.

10. Correct answer: D

Unlike young adults, who rely on increases in heart rate and contractility to maintain cardiac output, elderly patients rely much more on increases in vascular resistance to maintain MAP. Impairment of baroreflex stimulation and vagal tone results in decreased heart rate variability and ability to control a constant cardiac output in the setting of hypovolemia, hypotension, or hypoxia.

As the human body ages, there is a state of β-adrenergic insensitivity with a concomitant decrease in response to β-agonists. This is likely secondary to a decrease in intracellular coupling with adenylate cyclase, rather than a decline in the number of β-receptors. The diminished chronotropic and inotropic response of the heart to β-receptor stimulation alters the heart's ability to respond to both intrinsic and exogenous catecholamine stimulation. α-Adrenergic sensitivity is maintained or decreased, and response to α-agonists is impaired likely secondary to stiffened vascular system. Adrenal tissues will atrophy, but circulating norepinephrine and epinephrine levels increase 2-fold to 4-fold to compensate for β-insensitivity. There is both an increase in norepinephrine release from nerve terminals and a decrease in metabolism and reuptake.

References:
1. Ziegler MG, Lake CR, Kopin IJ. Plasma noradrenaline increases with age. *Nature*. 1976;261(5558):333-335.
2. Shannon RP, Maher KA, Santinga JT, Royal HD, Wei JY. Comparison of differences in the hemodynamic response to passive postural stress in healthy subjects >70 years and <30 years of age. *Am J Cardiol*. 1991;67(13):1110-1116.
3. Rooke GA. Cardiovascular aging and anesthetic implications. *J Cardiothorac Vasc Anesth*. 2003;17(4):512-523.

11. Correct answer: D

Andexanet alfa is a novel antidote to reverse the anticoagulation effects of FXa inhibitors. It has not shown to cause AKI in a randomized controlled study.

NSAIDs are known to inhibit prostaglandin synthesis leading to impaired renal parenchymal perfusion and also are known to induce acute interstitial nephritis. NSAID-mediated inhibition of prostaglandin production may contribute to a prerenal AKI, as prostaglandins regulate renal blood blow. However, the mechanism NSAID-induced acute interstitial nephritis is believed to occur independently of prostaglandin production inhibition.

The patient's creatinine more than doubled since admission (~24 h) consistent with AKI. Given the patient's cachectic state (low muscle mass), serum creatinine in the absence of CKD is expected to be low normal at baseline.

Given the patient's weight (~40 kg), a urine output of 0.5 cc/kg/h is acceptable.

Increases of serum creatinine of ≥0.5 mg/dL have been associated with an increased risk of death, increased length of stay, and increased hospital costs.

References:
1. Siegal DM, Curnutte JT, Connolly SJ, et al. Andexanet alfa for the reversal of Factor Xa inhibitor activity. *N Engl J Med*. 2015;373(25):2413-2424.
2. Whelton A. Nephrotoxicity of nonsteroidal anti-inflammatory drugs: physiologic foundations and clinical implications. *Am J Med*. 1999;106(5B):13S-24S.
3. Clarkson MR, Giblin L, O'Connell FP, et al. Acute interstitial nephritis: clinical features and response to corticosteroid therapy. *Nephrol Dial Transplant*. 2004;19(11):2778-2783.
4. Mangoni AA, Jackson SH. Age-related changes in pharmacokinetics and pharmacodynamics: basic principles and practical applications. *Br J Clin Pharmacol*. 2004;57(1):6-14.

12. Correct answer: C

CKD in septic or septic shock patients is associated with increased mortality.

In most patients with septic shock, an MAP target of 65 mm Hg is sufficient, though an MAP of 75-85 mm Hg appears to decrease the incidence of AKI in patients with chronic arterial hypertension. Raising the target MAP to 75-85 mm Hg does not increase mortality but increases the incidence of atrial fibrillation, possibly a result of increased catecholamine administration.

In the elderly (≥60 y of age), recent "Eighth Joint National Committee (JNC 8)" hypertension guidelines recommend the following blood pressure goals: <150/90 in the absence of DM or CKD and <140/90 mm Hg with the presence of either DM and/or CKD. Aggressive blood pressure control (mean systolic blood pressure 132 vs 140 mm Hg) in outpatients with hypertension and CKD is associated with decreased mortality.

The patient meets Sepsis-3 consensus definitions of septic shock. According to the consensus statement, the new definition of septic shock confers an in-hospital mortality of ~40%, whereas the diagnosis of "sepsis" confers an in-hospital mortality of approximately 10%.

Following are "The Third International Consensus Definitions for Sepsis and Septic Shock (Sepsis-3)":

Sepsis should be defined as life-threatening organ dysfunction caused by a dysregulated host response to infection. For clinical operationalization, organ dysfunction can be represented by an increase in the Sequential [Sepsis-related] Organ Failure Assessment (SOFA) score of 2 points or more, which is associated with an in-hospital mortality greater than 10%. Septic shock should be defined as a subset of sepsis in which particularly profound circulatory, cellular, and metabolic abnormalities are associated with a greater risk of mortality than with sepsis alone. Patients with septic shock can be clinically identified by a vasopressor requirement to maintain a mean arterial pressure of 65 mm Hg or greater and serum lactate level greater than 2 mmol/L (>18 mg/dL) in the absence of hypovolemia. This combination is associated with hospital mortality rates greater than 40%. In out-of-hospital, emergency department, or general hospital ward settings, adult patients with suspected infection can be rapidly identified as being more likely to have poor outcomes typical of sepsis if they have at least 2 of the following clinical criteria that together constitute a new bedside clinical score termed quick-SOFA (qSOFA): respiratory rate of 22/min or greater, altered mentation, or systolic blood pressure of 100 mm Hg or less.

References:

1. Mansur A, Mulwande E, Steinau M, et al. Chronic kidney disease is associated with a higher 90-day mortality than other chronic medical conditions in patients with sepsis. *Sci Rep.* 2015;5:10539.
2. Maizel J, Deransy R, Dehedin B, et al. Impact of non-dialysis chronic kidney disease on survival in patients with septic shock. *BMC Nephrol.* 2013;14:77.
3. Leone M, Asfar P, Radermacher P, et al. Optimizing mean arterial pressure in septic shock: a critical reappraisal of the literature. *Crit Care.* 2015;19:101.
4. James PA, Oparil S, Carter BL, et al. 2014 evidence-based guideline for the management of high blood pressure in adults: report from the panel members appointed to the Eighth Joint National Committee (JNC 8). *JAMA.* 2014;311(5):507-520.

13. Correct answer: A

Data suggest that estrogens may elicit protective effects with regard to renal aging in women, whereas in men androgens may cause renal dysfunction possibly due to increased fibrosis and mesangial matrix production.

Endogenous estrogen positively modulates renin-angiotensin-aldosterone system. Estrogen has been shown to increase angiotensinogen and possibly angiotensin I and II levels, whereas renin, angiotensin-converting enzyme, and angiotensin receptor 1 are either not affected or downregulated. Estrogen also favorably modulates transforming growth factor-β affecting parenchymal remodeling.

In animal experiments, estrogen therapy and androgen deprivation protected them from CKD progression. However, hormone replacement therapy with estrogen in postmenopausal women is controversial with opposing results published. According to one large retrospective study, exogenous estradiol is associated with progressive renal loss. Two systematic reviews and meta-analyses evaluating the role of hormone replacement therapy in women with CKD are ongoing.

GLP-1 receptor agonists such as exenatide or liraglutide have been associated with AKI, and administration in patients with severe CKD and/or at risk for AKI should be carefully considered. Dehydration may have contributed in these cases. Elderly are at high risk for dehydration given a decreased thirst perception. Thus, elderly patients with CKD receiving GLP-1 agonists warrant close monitoring for proper hydration and acute changes in renal function.

Interestingly, in otherwise stable outpatients with CKD, liraglutide showed renoprotective effects. One systematic review and meta-analysis of GLP-1 agonists in type II DM patients with moderate to severe CKD showed safety and efficacy, though wide confidence intervals precluded definitive conclusions regarding progression of renal disease or mortality.

Perioperative management of GLP-1 agonists in comparison with insulin is currently being investigated (PILGRIM trial) though patients with renal dysfunction (Cr > 1.5 mg/dL) have been excluded.

Apixaban is a novel oral anticoagulant and direct FXa inhibitor approved for patients with atrial fibrillation and concomitant CKD. Apixaban is also approved for patients with end-stage renal disease and on dialysis.

References:

1. Baylis C. Sexual dimorphism: the aging kidney, involvement of nitric oxide deficiency, and angiotensin II overactivity. *J Gerontol A Biol Sci Med Sci.* 2012;67(12):1365-1372.
2. Weinstein JR, Anderson S. The aging kidney: physiological changes. *Adv Chronic Kidney Dis.* 2010;17(4):302-307.
3. O'Donnell E, Floras JS, Harvey PJ. Estrogen status and the renin angiotensin aldosterone system. *Am J Physiol Regul Integr Comp Physiol.* 2014;307(5):R498-R500.
4. Ahmed SB, Ramesh S. Sex hormones in women with kidney disease. *Nephrol Dial Transplant.* 2016;31(11):1787-1795.

14. **Correct answer: D**

Hypoalbuminemia as a result of malnutrition is common in the elderly and is associated with adverse surgical/in-hospital outcomes.

Serum albumin is associated with perioperative morbidity and mortality. In a prospective, single-center, randomized, parallel-arm double-blinded trial preoperative albumin administration prevented AKI in patients with an albumin of <4 mg/dL undergoing heart surgery.

NAFLD is a common disease in the geriatric population, and it is defined as fat accumulation exceeding 5%-10% by the weight of the liver. In this patient population, it confers an increased risk of nonalcoholic steatohepatitis (NASH), cirrhosis, and hepatocellular carcinoma compared with younger patients. Obesity, DM, and hyperlipidemia are associated with NAFLD. NAFLD can result in a variety of extrahepatic manifestations. FEV1 and forced vital capacity appear to inversely correlate with degree of NAFLD. NAFLD is associated with an increased development of CKD. NAFLD and NASH are also believed to be risk factors for atherosclerosis. Patients with NAFLD showed increased activities of FIX, FXI and FXII independent of age, gender, and BMI. Separately, NAFLD patients were shown to have increased levels of factor VIII and decreased levels of protein C. Patients with NASH were found to have decreased levels of protein S compared with patients with NAFLD.

References:

1. Shirasu T, Hoshina K, Nishiyama A, et al. Favorable outcomes of very elderly patients with critical limb ischemia who undergo distal bypass surgery. *J Vasc Surg.* 2016;63(2):377-384.
2. Rich MW, Keller AJ, Schechtman KB, et al. Increased complications and prolonged hospital stay in elderly cardiac surgical patients with low serum albumin. *Am J Cardiol.* 1989;63(11):714-718.
3. Ganai S, Lee KF, Merrill A, et al. Adverse outcomes of geriatric patients undergoing abdominal surgery who are at high risk for delirium. *Arch Surg.* 2007;142(11):1072-1078.
4. Lee EH, Kim WJ, Kim JY, et al. Effect of exogenous albumin on the incidence of postoperative acute kidney injury in patients undergoing off-pump coronary artery bypass surgery with a preoperative albumin level of less than 4.0 g/dl. *Anesthesiology.* 2016;124(5):1001-1011.
5. Peng TC, Kao TW, Wu LW, et al. Association between pulmonary function and nonalcoholic fatty liver disease in the NHANES III study. *Medicine (Baltimore).* 2015;94(21):e907.

15. **Correct answer: B**

Although liver weight remains largely unchanged throughout most of adulthood, in patients older than 50 years, liver weight progressively decreases from approximately 2.5% to 1.6% of body weight by age 90 years. Between ages 25 and 65 years, there is a progressive 40% decrease in hepatic blood flow.

Hepatic drug extraction ratio is considered high (>0.7), intermediate (0.3-0.7), or low (<0.3) according to the fraction of drug removed after 1 pass through the liver. The clearance of high-extraction drugs depends on blood flow and is considered flow limited. Thus, high-extraction-ratio drug clearance decreases 30%-40% in older patients according to the decrease in hepatic blood flow. Low-extraction drugs are cleared based on the liver's intrinsic enzymatic capacity (function of liver size and enzyme availability), which also may decrease with age, although human data vary greatly depending on CYP enzyme isoform and gender examined. In fact, some data suggest that overall hepatic enzymatic activity is preserved well into the advanced age. Phase I metabolism may show a selective age-associated impairment, whereas phase II metabolism does not show a significant reduction in healthy elderly. Frailty has been associated with decreased phase II metabolism.

Drugs with a high hepatic extraction ratio include nitroglycerin, isoproterenol, propranolol, labetalol, verapamil, morphine, fentanyl, propofol, lidocaine, meperidine, sufentanil, and ketamine.

Drugs with a low hepatic extraction ratio include warfarin, phenytoin, diazepam, digitoxin, erythromycin, phenobarbital, theophylline, acetaminophen, naproxen, and metronidazole. Renal mass decreases with age, which is reflected by a decrease in the number of nephrons. Intrarenal vascular changes affect mostly the afferent arterioles in the cortex. However, medullary vasculature is generally not affected. Renal plasma flow and glomerular filtration rate decline with age. The aging kidney excretes decreased amounts of ammonium and thus is less capable of managing a sudden acid load. Renin and aldosterone levels are decreased in the elderly. However, the deficit in urine-concentrating ability in the elderly reflects intrinsic renal causes and not a lack of circulating vasopressin.

References:

1. Lortat-Jacob B, Servin F. Pharmacology of intravenous drugs in the elderly. In: Sieber FE, ed. *Geriatric Anesthesia.* New York: McGraw-Hill; 2006:91-103.
2. Rivera R, Antognini JF. Perioperative drug therapy in elderly patients. *Anesthesiology.* 2009;110(5):1176-1181.

3. Salem F, Abduljalil K, Kamiyama Y, et al. Considering age variation when coining drugs as high versus low hepatic extraction ratio. *Drug Metab Dispos.* 2016;44(7):1099-1102.
4. Wynne HA, Cope LH, Herd B, et al. The association of age and frailty with paracetamol conjugation in man. *Age Ageing.* 1990;19(6):419-424.
5. Rogge MC, Solomon WR, Sedman AJ, et al. The theophylline-enoxacin interaction: II. Changes in the disposition of theophylline and its metabolites during intermittent administration of enoxacin. *Clin Pharmacol Ther.* 1989;46(4):420-428.

16. Correct answer: D

A recent warning issued by the FDA suggested that repeated or lengthy general anesthesia and sedative medications in children may affect brain development. This warning was widely covered in mass media and has provoked increasing concern among the general public regarding possible cognitive decline after general anesthesia. Anesthesiologists should be prepared to address such concerns based on existing scientific data.

At present, there is no convincing evidence that general anesthesia leads to cognitive decline. Most of the studies that have explored the subject are retrospective and did not support the association between general anesthesia and dementia. Although some studies suggest the possibility of long-term cognitive decline, such effects are yet to be confirmed.

References:

1. Rasmussen LS, Johnson T, Kuipers HM, et al. Does anaesthesia cause postoperative cognitive dysfunction? A randomised study of regional versus general anaesthesia in 438 elderly patients. *Acta Anaesthesiol Scand.* 2003;47(3):260-266.
2. Seitz DP, Shah PS, Herrmann N, et al. Exposure to general anesthesia and risk of Alzheimer's disease: a systematic review and meta-analysis. *BMC Geriatr.* 2011;11:83.

17. Correct answer: A

Pain control is an important marker of the quality of anesthesia care. Elderly patients may have decreased behavioral and verbal expression of pain, but perioperative pain should be anticipated and addressed to the same standards as in other age groups.

Aging is typically associated with structural changes in the myelin sheath of peripheral nerves. Changes in myelination may lead to decreasing conductivity and increasing thresholds of perception of a number of stimuli, including pain. Thus, the threshold at which the experimental stimulus becomes painful is likely to increase with age; therefore, answer choices B and C are incorrect. However, experimental data suggest that the maximum duration or intensity of the painful stimulus that the person can tolerate is likely to decrease or remain unchanged with aging.

Cold agglutinins (answer choice D) are antibodies that cause agglutination of red blood cells but do not result in vasodilation.

References:

1. Cole LJ, Farrell MJ, Gibson SJ, et al. Age-related differences in pain sensitivity and regional brain activity evoked by noxious pressure. *Neurobiol Aging.* 2010;31(3):494-503.
2. Lautenbacher S. Experimental approaches in the study of pain in the elderly. *Pain Med.* 2012;13(suppl 2):S44-S50.
3. Paladini A, Fusco M, Coaccioli S, et al. Chronic pain in the elderly: the case for new therapeutic strategies. *Pain Physician.* 2015;18(5):E863-E876.

18. Correct answer: A

Aging is associated with a decrease in baroreceptor sensitivity and effectiveness of the baroreceptor reflex. These changes are most likely due to age-related functional and biochemical changes in the central nervous system, such as alterations in secondary messenger systems. Furthermore, increased arterial stiffness in the elderly people limits the effectiveness of vasoconstriction. Impaired regulation of systemic blood pressure and heart rate is an important consideration because most analgesic, sedative, and hypnotic agents result in vasodilatation.

Age-related changes in the neuronal conduction systems result in limited adaptability of the cardiovascular system and in limited ability to tolerate hemodynamic stress. Answer choice B is incorrect: There is an increase in baseline sympathetic activity with aging. Decreased venous capacitance would be likely to improve venous return and thus counteract orthostatic hypotension (C). Brain volume (D) does decrease with age, but this is unlikely to result in orthostatic hypotension.

References:

1. Turnheim K. When drug therapy gets old: pharmacokinetics and pharmacodynamics in the elderly. *Exp Gerontol.* 2003;38(8):843-853.
2. Nordquist D, Halaszynski TM. Perioperative multimodal anesthesia using regional techniques in the aging surgical patient. *Pain Res Treat.* 2014;2014:902174.

19. **Correct answer: D**

A combination of this patient's age, history of depression, and major orthopedic surgery put her at high risk for postoperative delirium. In one case series of patients older than 70 years, the incidence of delirium after femoral fracture repair was more than 60%. In these patients, delirium increased the duration of hospital stay and affected rehabilitation; therefore, answer choice C is incorrect.

Answer choices A and B are incorrect. Postoperative delirium is a common complication after major surgery even in elderly patients with excellent baseline cognitive function and physical health.

References:
1. Nordquist D, Halaszynski TM. Perioperative multimodal anesthesia using regional techniques in the aging surgical patient. *Pain Res Treat.* 2014;2014:902174.
2. Olofsson B, Lundström M, Borssén B, et al. Delirium is associated with poor rehabilitation outcome in elderly patients treated for femoral neck fractures. *Scand J Caring Sci.* 2005;19(2):119-127.

20. **Correct answer: B**

There is a slight decrease in total lung capacity and slight increase in FRC. There is a slight increase in tidal volume, but the biggest change with aging is the increase in CC. In fact, CC typically surpasses FRC in the mid-60s.

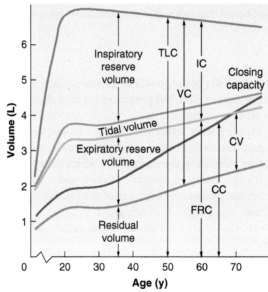

Effect of aging on lung volumes. (From Smith TC. Respiratory system: aging, adversity, and anesthesia. In: McLeskey CH, ed. *Geriatric Anesthesiology.* 1st ed. Baltimore: Williams & Wilkins; 1997:85, with permission.)

Reference:
1. Bentov I, Rooke GA. Anesthesia for the older patient. In: Barash PG, Cullen BF, Stoelting RK, et al, eds. *Clinical Anesthesia.* 8th ed. Philadelphia: Lippincott; 2017:897-913.

21. **Correct answer: A**

With increased age, there is a slight decrease in the resting Pao_2. This is due to a slight decrease in the surface area of alveoli as well as increased ventilation-perfusion ($\dot{V}/\dot{Q}$) mismatching (due to loss of elastin from lung tissue). As one ages, there is generalized wasting of muscles of the upper airway, including the hypopharyngeal and genioglossal muscles, thereby putting this population at increased risk for upper airway obstruction. There is about a 50% decrease in the hypercapneic ventilatory response and an even greater decrease in the hypoxic ventilatory response.

Reference:
1. Bentov I, Rooke GA. Anesthesia for the older patient. In: Barash PG, Cullen BF, Stoelting RK, et al, eds. *Clinical Anesthesia.* 8th ed. Philadelphia: Lippincott; 2017:897-913.

22. Correct answer: D

Owing to the loss of elastin and the resultant loss of lung tissue stiffness, V/Q mismatching increases in the elderly. In the geriatric population, it is also true that FEV1 decreases as airways that were once stented open begin to collapse with the loss of outward pulling forces; DLCO decreases as the alveolar surface available for gas exchange is destroyed, and dead space increases.

Reference:

1. Bentov I, Rooke GA. Anesthesia for the older patient. In: Barash PG, Cullen BF, Stoelting RK, et al, eds. *Clinical Anesthesia*. 8th ed. Philadelphia: Lippincott; 2017:897-913.

23. Correct answer: C

The diaphragm actually flattens with aging, which makes it more difficult to generate a negative intrapleural pressure (which in turn provides the gradient that drives air movement from the atmosphere into the lungs). The chest wall becomes increasingly stiff, which results in an increased work of breathing as well as a more barrel-shaped thoracic cavity. This barrel shape promotes a *flattening*, not curving, of the diaphragm. With increased age, there is progressively more elastin lost from lung parenchyma, resulting in a lung with relatively *more* compliance than that of a young adult with a higher elastin content.

Reference:

1. Bentov I, Rooke GA. Anesthesia for the older patient. In: Barash PG, Cullen BF, Stoelting RK, et al, eds. *Clinical Anesthesia*. 8th ed. Philadelphia: Lippincott; 2017:897-913.

24. Correct answer: C

CC gradually increases in a linear manner from approximately 2 L in a 30-year-old to more than 4 L in an 80-year-old as depicted by the graph in the answer to question 20 earlier.

Reference:

1. Bentov I, Rooke GA. Anesthesia for the older patient. In: Barash PG, Cullen BF, Stoelting RK, et al, eds. *Clinical Anesthesia*. 8th ed. Philadelphia: Lippincott; 2017:897-913.

25. Correct answer: D

The patency of small airways in young adults is maintained by surrounding tissue. With age, there is loss of elastin from the surrounding tissues, compromising the structural integrity of the support system that ordinarily serves to pull the small airways outward. They are therefore more prone to collapse at a given volume than those of a younger adult. Alternatively, a larger volume of air is needed (as a counterforce) to maintain this patency of the airway (definition of CC). This phenomenon can also be reflected in a decreased FEV1 observed on spirometry.

Reference:

1. Bentov I, Rooke GA. Anesthesia for the older patient. In: Barash PG, Cullen BF, Stoelting RK, et al, eds. *Clinical Anesthesia*. 8th ed. Philadelphia: Lippincott; 2017:897-913.

24

CRITICAL CARE

Lydia Miller

1. All of the following patients with respiratory failure may be candidates for noninvasive positive pressure ventilation (NIPPV) EXCEPT which one?

   A. Decompensated heart failure and SpO_2 85% on room air
   B. HIV-positive patient with bilateral opacities on chest X-Ray and PaO_2/FiO_2 150
   C. Urosepsis requiring norepinephrine with tachypnea and SpO_2 90% on 6 L nasal cannula
   D. Acute chronic obstructive pulmonary disease (COPD) exacerbation and $PaCO_2$ 70 mm Hg
   E. Immediately following extubation in a patient at high risk for reintubation

2. You are called to intubate a patient with a COPD exacerbation. Following intubation, you confirm bilateral breath sounds and presence of carbon dioxide by capnogram. You manually ventilate with an Ambu bag while waiting for the ventilator circuit. The automated blood pressure cuff is unable to read a blood pressure, and the pulse oximeter tracing is lost while the blood pressure cuff repeatedly cycles on the ipsilateral arm. ECG shows sinus bradycardia in the 60s. You are unable to palpate a carotid pulse. Your team initiates chest compressions and administers epinephrine. Which of the following is the next maneuver?

   A. Increase minute ventilation.
   B. Remove endotracheal tube and reintubate.
   C. Needle decompression in second intercostal space.
   D. Disconnect patient from Ambu bag.
   E. Place an arterial line.

3. A patient with acute respiratory distress syndrome (ARDS) is being mechanically ventilated with the following settings on volume control ventilation: tidal volume 480 cc, respiratory rate 20 breaths per minute, PEEP (positive end-expiratory pressure) 12 cm H_2O, FiO_2 50%, plateau pressure 33 cm H_2O, and peak inspiratory pressure 35 cm H_2O. His ideal body weight is 70 kg. The most recent arterial blood gas test shows PaO_2 80 mm Hg, $PaCO_2$ 48 mm Hg, and pH 7.33. What change should you make to the ventilator settings?

   A. No change.
   B. Decrease PEEP.
   C. Decrease tidal volume.
   D. Increase FiO_2.
   E. Switch to pressure support ventilation.

4. **When preparing to extubate an ICU patient, all of the following criteria should be met EXCEPT which one?**

   A. Rapid shallow breathing index (RSBI) of less than 100
   B. Minimal secretions
   C. Presence of cuff leak
   D. Successful spontaneous breathing trial (SBT) lasting 30 minutes using continuous positive airway pressure of 5 cm H_2O
   E. Ability to follow commands

5. **Which of the following hypotensive patients could potentially show improvement in their hemodynamics with the administration of positive pressure ventilation?**

   A. Large myocardial infarction in left anterior descending territory
   B. Acute liver failure (ALF)
   C. Acute pulmonary embolism
   D. Induction of anesthesia
   E. Sepsis

6. **What is the static thoracic compliance on the following volume control ventilation settings?**

   Tidal volume 450 mL
   Peak inspiratory pressure 25 cm H_2O
   Plateau pressure 20 cm H_2O
   PEEP 5 cm H_2O

   A. 18 mL/cm H_2O
   B. 22 mL/cm H_2O
   C. 30 mL/cm H_2O
   D. 33 mL/cm H_2O
   E. 50 mL/cm H_2O

   The next 2 questions are based on the following scenario:
   An elderly man who was found down is brought to the ICU intubated for respiratory failure of unknown etiology. His ideal body weight is 80 kg. Initial settings on volume control ventilation are as follows:

   Tidal volume 480 mL
   Peak inspiratory pressure 25 cm H_2O
   Plateau pressure 15 cm H_2O
   Respiratory rate 16 breaths per minute
   PEEP 5 cm H_2O
   I:E 1:2

   His ventilator flow tracing is shown below.

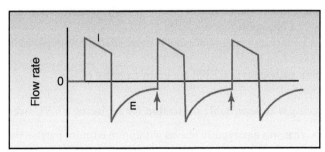

(From Marino PL. *Marino's The ICU Book*. 4th ed. Philadelphia: Wolters Kluwer Health/Lippincott Williams & Wilkins; 2014, with permission.)

7. **Based on this information, which of the following is the most likely cause of his respiratory failure?**

   A. Obstructive lung disease
   B. Restrictive lung disease
   C. Acute respiratory distress syndrome
   D. Opioid overdose
   E. Unable to determine

8. **Which of the following changes should be made to his ventilator settings?**

   A. Increase respiratory rate.
   B. Change I:E to 1:1.
   C. Increase inspiratory flows.
   D. Decrease tidal volume.
   E. Increase PEEP.

9. **Which of the following differentiates pressure support from assist-control pressure control ventilation?**

   A. Delivered tidal volume increases with increased patient effort.
   B. Cycling depends on change in inspiratory flow.
   C. Ability of a patient to trigger breaths.
   D. Lung injury is unlikely on pressure support ventilation.
   E. Delivered tidal volume depends on thoracic compliance.

10. **Which of the following parameters determines the tidal volume delivered in volume control ventilation?**

    A. Peak inspiratory pressure
    B. Lung compliance
    C. Airway resistance
    D. Inspiratory flow
    E. Patient effort

11. **All of the following interventions are recommended to reduce the risk of ventilator-associated pneumonia (VAP) EXCEPT which one?**

    A. Elevation of head of bed at least 30°
    B. Early tracheostomy
    C. Daily SBTs
    D. Noninvasive positive pressure ventilation
    E. Minimizing sedation

12. **Which of the following statements regarding catheter-related bloodstream infections (CRBSIs) is true?**

    A. Central venous catheters (CVCs) should be replaced weekly.
    B. CRBSI is diagnosed when blood cultures drawn from the catheter are positive.
    C. Arterial lines carry a negligible risk of CRBSI.
    D. Skin preparation with chlorhexidine/alcohol is more effective than povidone iodine in preventing CRBSI.
    E. The most common pathogens in CRBSI are gram-negative rods.

13. **Which of the following is an acceptable indication for replacing a CVC over a guidewire?**

    A. Replacing a CVC that was emergently placed without maximum barrier precautions
    B. Loss of blood return
    C. After 14 days of catheter use
    D. Fever
    E. CVC should never be replaced over a guidewire

14. **Which of the following statements regarding catheter-associated urinary tract infection (CAUTI) is true?**

    A. External urinary catheters have similar rates of complications compared with indwelling catheters.
    B. Asymptomatic catheter-associated bacteriuria should be treated to reduce the risk of developing systemic infection.
    C. Intermittent catheterization does not reduce the risk of CAUTI.
    D. Indwelling catheters should be replaced at regular intervals to reduce the risk of CAUTI.
    E. Screening for bacteriuria is not effective in reducing CAUTI.

15. **Alcohol-based hand rubs are effective in removing all of the following pathogens EXCEPT which one?**

    A. Methicillin-resistant *Staphylococcus aureus* (MRSA)
    B. Vancomycin-resistant enterococci
    C. *Clostridium difficile*
    D. *Mycobacterium tuberculosis* (MTB)
    E. They are effective for all pathogens

16. **All of the following statements regarding *Clostridium difficile* prevention are true EXCEPT which one?**

    A. Tighter regulations on antibiotic use have decreased the incidence of *C. difficile*.
    B. Only chlorine-containing cleaning products should be used for environmental decontamination.
    C. Monotherapy with metronidazole is appropriate for mild cases of *C. difficile*.
    D. Contact precautions can be lifted when diarrhea resolves.
    E. Limiting acid suppression therapy can reduce the risk of *C. difficile*.

17. **Which of the following personal protective equipment items (PPEs) is sufficient for a provider to wear before performing endotracheal intubation?**

    A. Goggles
    B. Mask
    C. Face shield
    D. Gown
    E. No PPE required if low suspicion for respiratory infection

18. **An HIV-positive patient is admitted to the ICU with respiratory failure requiring intubation. Mycobacterium tuberculosis (MTB) disease is suspected. All of the following statements regarding MTB precautions are true EXCEPT which one?**

    A. The patient should be placed in a negative-pressure isolation room.
    B. Empiric therapy for MTB disease with a 4-drug regimen should be initiated immediately.
    C. Contact precautions are not necessary.
    D. Airborne precautions can be discontinued if a tuberculin skin test is negative.
    E. A bacterial filter should be placed on the ventilator circuit.

19. **While caring for a patient with acute hepatitis B virus (HBV), an anesthesia resident sustains a needle stick injury. The resident received the HBV vaccine series as an adolescent. Which of the following is true regarding his need for postexposure prophylaxis for HBV?**

    A. He does not require any HBV prophylaxis or further testing because he has been vaccinated.
    B. Anti-HBs titers should be checked.
    C. His risk of acquiring HBV is 30%.
    D. He should receive 1 dose of hepatitis B immune globulin and be revaccinated.
    E. He should undergo baseline testing for anti-HBc now and repeat testing at 6 months.

20. A 75-year-old man presents with fever, cough, and infiltrate on chest X-ray. His oxygen saturation is 90% on room air and he is subsequently admitted to the floor for treatment of a presumed pneumonia. He was previously healthy except for hypertension and has not had recent hospital admissions or antibiotic therapy. He has no smoking history. Which of the following empiric antibiotic regimens is appropriate while awaiting the results of sputum culture?

    A. Vancomycin and cefepime
    B. Piperacillin/tazobactam monotherapy
    C. Ceftriaxone and azithromycin
    D. Meropenem and levofloxacin
    E. Vancomycin, piperacillin/tazobactam, and fluconazole

21. You are called to evaluate a 65-year-old woman with known lung cancer who was admitted to the hospital for a COPD exacerbation. She appears somnolent and tachypneic with the following vital signs: BP 65/40, HR 120, SpO_2 85% on room air. There are diffuse ST depressions on 12-lead ECG. Focused bedside cardiac ultrasonography demonstrates the following:

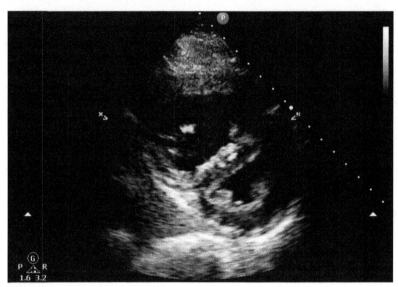

(Reproduced with permission from Miller L, Shelton K. Critical care ultrasound. In: Parsons PE, Wiener-Kronish JP, Stapleton RD, Berra R, eds. *Critical Care Secrets*. 6th ed. Philadelphia: Elsevier; 2019:107-113.)

What is the most likely etiology of this patient's shock?

    A. Distributive
    B. Hypovolemic
    C. Cardiogenic
    D. Obstructive
    E. Unable to determine at this time

22. Additional echocardiography views reveal McConnell sign. Which of the following is the next step in the management of this patient?

    A. Cardiac catheterization
    B. Systemic fibrinolytic therapy
    C. Rapid infusion of 2 L crystalloid
    D. Initiation of heparin infusion
    E. CT scan

23. **You are taking care of a patient in the cardiac ICU who underwent an uncomplicated coronary artery bypass grafting several hours ago. His norepinephrine requirement is steadily increasing. Bedside cardiac ultrasonography reveals the following:**

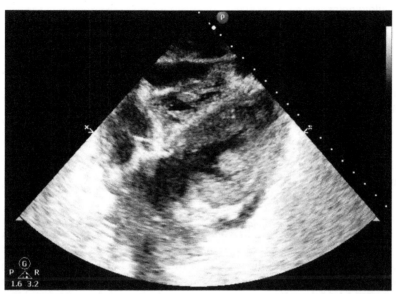

(Reproduced with permission from Miller L, Shelton K. Critical care ultrasound. In: Parsons PE, Wiener-Kronish JP, Stapleton RD, Berra R, eds. *Critical Care Secrets*. 6th ed. Philadelphia: Elsevier; 2019:107-113.)

What Would the PA Catheter Show?

	HR	CVP	PA	CO (L/min)	SVR (dyn × s × cm⁻⁵)
A.	120	1	12/8	3	1800
B.	80	7	20/10	5	1300
C.	50	25	45/25	2	1800
D.	120	25	45/25	3	2000
E.	150	2	12/8	7	500

24. **Which of the following is the next step with regard to the appropriate management of this patient's immediate problem?**

   A. Pericardiocentesis
   B. Immediately returning to OR for redo sternotomy
   C. Rapid fluid bolus
   D. Ordering a transesophageal echocardiography for further evaluation
   E. Cardiac catheterization

25. A 70-year-old man presents to the hospital with chest pain and dyspnea. ECG shows 2-mm ST elevations in V2-V4. His vital signs are as follows: HR 85, BP 100/55, Spo$_2$ 95% on room air. Laboratory test results are remarkable for troponin 3.5 ng/mL and lactate 6 mmol/L. Emergent cardiac catheterization is planned. What other treatment should be initiated at this time?

   A. Dopamine
   B. 1 L crystalloid bolus
   C. Dobutamine
   D. Norepinephrine
   E. No other intervention necessary besides immediate cardiac catheterization

26. Data from a pulmonary artery catheter (PAC) can be used to derive all of the following hemodynamic and oxygen transport parameters EXCEPT which one?

   A. Stroke volume
   B. Mixed venous oxygen saturation
   C. Systemic vascular resistance
   D. Oxygen consumption
   E. Left ventricle (LV) ejection fraction

27. You are called to evaluate a 60-year-old woman with a history of nephrolithiasis and urinary tract infections who is in the PACU recovering from ureteroscopy and ureteral stone extraction 1 hour ago. Her vital signs are as follows: temperature 37.8°C, HR 110, BP 95/50, and respiratory rate 25 breaths per minute. She appears to be shivering and drowsy but does answer questions appropriately. Which of the following is the next step in your management of this patient?

   A. This is likely due to residual effects of anesthetics and pain; continue observation in PACU for now.
   B. Discharge to phase II PACU with a prescription for ciprofloxacin.
   C. Transfer to ICU.
   D. Start vancomycin and cefepime and continue observation in PACU.
   E. Suggest her urologist repeat ureteroscopy for possible retained stone.

28. The patient continues to have mean arterial pressures (MAPs) in the low 60s despite 3 L of lactated ringers and initiation of broad spectrum antibiotics. Laboratory test results are notable for the following:

   WBC 18 000
   Lactate 3.5 mmol/L

Which of the following is the most appropriate next step in management of this patient?

   A. Administer a 500 cc bolus of 5% albumin.
   B. Place a central line and initiate norepinephrine.
   C. Initiate peripheral phenylephrine.
   D. Consider adding antifungal coverage to your antibiotic regimen.
   E. MAP is adequate; continue to observe.

29. A 25-year-old man is admitted to the ICU after a surfing accident. Primary survey is notable
     for GCS 15, absence of sensation below clavicles, and inability to move legs and arms except
     for weak arm flexion bilaterally. He has weak cough and intermittent desaturations that
     resolve with deep nasal suctioning. Chest and abdominal CTs are remarkable for a 5 mm
     pneumothorax and grade 2 splenic laceration. His BP is 70/30 and HR 50s. Cervical spine MRI
     reveals the following:

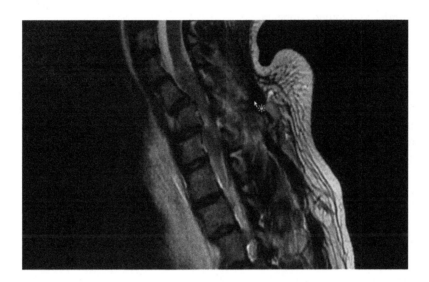

Which of the following is the primary etiology of his hemodynamic instability?

   A. Spinal shock
   B. Neurogenic shock
   C. Obstructive shock
   D. Septic shock
   E. Hypovolemic shock

30. Which of the following is the most appropriate regarding the next step in management of this
     patient?

   A. Fiberoptic intubation and mechanical ventilation
   B. Blood transfusion
   C. High-dose steroids
   D. OR for spinal decompression and fusion
   E. Initiation of bilevel positive airway pressure (BiPAP)

31. All of the following practices may reduce the risk of ICU-acquired weakness (ICUAW) EXCEPT
     which one?

   A. Treatment of hyperglycemia
   B. Minimizing use of steroids
   C. Minimizing use of neuromuscular blockers
   D. Passive exercises in sedated patients
   E. Early diagnosis with electrophysiology studies

32. **Which of the following statements regarding venous thromboembolism (VTE) prevention and treatment is true?**

    A. Upperextremity deep venous thromboses (DVTs) associated with CVCs do not require systemic anticoagulation.
    B. VTE is very unlikely in patients receiving appropriate pharmacologic prophylaxis.
    C. Low-molecular-weight heparin (LMWH) is preferred to subcutaneous heparin for patients at high risk of DVT.
    D. Prophylactic LMWH is preferred to subcutaneous heparin because it does not carry the risk of heparin-induced thrombocytopenia.
    E. An IVC filter should be considered for all trauma patients.

33. **Which of the following statements regarding nutrition in the ICU is true?**

    A. Gastric residual volumes should be frequently measured to monitor for feeding intolerance.
    B. Initiation of enteral nutrition should be delayed until signs of return of bowel function.
    C. Early enteral nutrition decreases mortality.
    D. Protein has the lowest respiratory quotient.
    E. A postpyloric tube should be placed for enteral feeding.

34. **Diagnosis of brain death requires all of the following criteria EXCEPT which one?**

    A. Absence of spontaneous respirations at $Paco_2$ of 60 or greater
    B. Complete absence of motor function
    C. Absent brainstem reflexes
    D. Normotension
    E. Establishing etiology of coma

35. **Which of the following statements regarding the performance of ancillary testing in patients with suspected brain death is true?**

    A. Isoelectric EEG using frontal leads identifies brain death.
    B. Absence of cerebral vessel filling on cerebral angiography is the gold standard ancillary test.
    C. At least 1 ancillary test is required in addition to clinical testing for determination of brain death.
    D. Noncontrast CT showing extensive edema and herniation can serve as an ancillary test.
    E. Evoked potentials are not used as ancillary tests.

36. **A 21-year-old man is admitted to the ICU with a massive subarachnoid hemorrhage and is displaying signs of herniation. He arrives intubated from the emergency department (ED) and is not receiving any sedative agents. His initial physical examination demonstrates GCS 3, absence of brainstem reflexes and no spontaneous respirations with a $Paco_2$ 65. There are 4 strong twitches on train-of-four monitoring on the ulnar nerve. His temperature is 37.5°C. His laboratory test results are unremarkable. He is requiring norepinephrine to maintain SBP >100. He is evaluated by neurosurgery and determined not to be a candidate for surgical intervention. Which of the following is the next appropriate step in management?**

    A. Declare brain death and withdraw ventilator support.
    B. Declare brain death and contact organ bank.
    C. Increase norepinephrine to goal SBP >120.
    D. Perform cerebral angiography.
    E. Repeat brain death examination in 6 hours.

37. **A 30-year-old man with no known medical history is admitted to the ICU after being found on the side of the road following a motor vehicle collision. His GCS is 6 upon arrival and he is promptly intubated. Mannitol was administered just before leaving the ED en route to the ICU. Laboratory test results on admission to the ICU are notable for hyponatremia to 121 mEq/L and serum osmolarity 320 mOsm/kg. Which of the following is the next step in management of his hyponatremia?**

   A. Send urine electrolytes and urine osmolarity.
   B. Administer hypertonic saline bolus
   C. Observe.
   D. Administer furosemide.
   E. Begin fluid restriction

38. **A 70-year-old man is admitted to the ICU following a thoracotomy and lobectomy for lung cancer. Over the next few days, he develops progressively worsening hyponatremia. He is alert and tolerating oral intake. Maintenance IV fluids have been stopped.**

Laboratory test results are notable for the following:

   Na 127 mEq/L
   Serum osmolarity 270 mOsm/kg
   Urine sodium 50 mEq/L
   Urine osmolarity 800 mOsm/kg
   Glucose 130 mg/dL
   Serum potassium 3.8 mEq/L
   Serum BUN 12 mg/dL
   Serum creatinine 1.2 mg/dL

Which of the following is the most likely etiology of his hyponatremia?

   A. Syndrome of inappropriate antidiuretic hormone secretion (SIADH)
   B. Hypovolemia
   C. Pseudohyponatremia
   D. Cerebral salt wasting
   E. Mineralocorticoid deficiency

39. **Which of the following is the most appropriate regarding the next step in management of this patient?**

   A. 3% saline
   B. 500 cc normal saline bolus
   C. Fluid restriction
   D. Vasopressin receptor antagonist
   E. Salt tablets

40. A young trauma patient is admitted to the ICU with multiple orthopedic injuries. Admission laboratory test results several hours ago show creatine kinase 20 000 IU/L, potassium 5.2 mEq/L, ionized calcium 1.1 mmol/L, magnesium 1.5 mEq/L, bicarbonate 16 mEq/L, and creatinine 1.5 mg/dL. Over the next few hours, he develops worsening oliguria. A repeat electrolyte panel is pending. ECG shows the following:

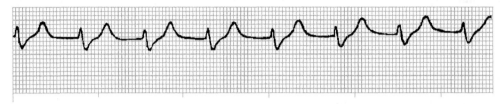

(From Badescu GC, Sherman B, Zaidan JR, et al. Appendix 1 Atlas of electrocardiography. In: Barash PG, Cullen BF, Stoelting RK, et al, eds. *Clinical Anesthesia*. 7th ed. Philadelphia: Wolters Kluwer; 2013.)

Which of the following is the most appropriate next step in management?

A. Administer Furosemide
B. Dialysis
C. Administer Magnesium
D. Administer Bicarbonate
E. Administer Calcium chloride

41. Which of the following clinical scenarios is *least* likely to be associated with the following ECG?

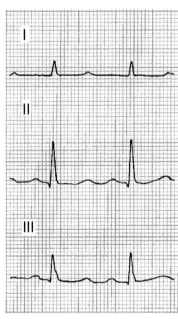

(From Badescu GC, Sherman B, Zaidan JR, et al. Appendix 1 Atlas of electrocardiography. In: Barash PG, Cullen BF, Stoelting RK, et al, eds. *Clinical Anesthesia*. 7th ed. Philadelphia: Wolters Kluwer; 2013.)

A. Use of erythromycin
B. Primary hyperparathyroidism
C. Massive transfusion during the anhepatic phase of liver transplantation
D. Vitamin D deficiency
E. Tumor lysis syndrome

42. A 55-year-old man with a history of alcohol dependence is admitted to the ICU for management of acute pancreatitis. Enteral feeding is initiated on hospital day 2. Laboratory test results the following day are notable for phosphate 0.8 mg/dL, total calcium 6.5 mg/dL, magnesium 1 mEq/L, potassium 2.8 mEq/L, and albumin 1.5 g/dL. Which of the following is the most appropriate regarding the next step in management of this patient?

   A. Increase enteral feeds.
   B. Temporarily stop enteral feeding.
   C. Switch to total parenteral nutrition.
   D. Initiate work-up for hyperparathyroidism.
   E. Increase phosphate, magnesium, and potassium content in enteral feeds.

43. A 6-year-old child is rescued from a pool and is found to be unresponsive and pulseless. His skin is cool and cyanotic. There is one Basic Life Support-certified rescuer present. All of the following resuscitation maneuvers should be performed EXCEPT:

   A. Chest compressions
   B. Rescue breaths
   C. Heimlich maneuver
   D. Vigorous warming
   E. Attach Automated external defibrillator (AED) pads

44. Which of the following is true regarding the management of a comatose drowning victim after return of spontaneous circulation (ROSC)?

   A. Therapeutic hypothermia is contraindicated.
   B. PEEP should be minimized to reduce alveolar injury.
   C. Prophylactic antibiotics are indicated if the patient was rescued from a natural body of water.
   D. Hypothermic drowning victims may have a better prognosis.
   E. Fluid restriction and diuretics are indicated.

45. A 21-year-old woman with a history of major depression disorder is brought to the ED by her roommate. Her roommate states she found an empty bottle of acetaminophen next to the patient in her bedroom. She is lethargic and vomiting. Which of the following is the first step in management?

   A. Measure serum APAP levels.
   B. Administer IV N-acetylcysteine (NAC).
   C. Administer activated charcoal.
   D. Observe clinically for now while trending liver function tests.
   E. Transfer to a liver transplant institution.

46. All of the following are risk factors for APAP hepatoxicity EXCEPT which one?

   A. Chronic alcohol use
   B. Elderly
   C. Malnutrition
   D. Pregnancy
   E. Concurrent use of certain herbal medications

47. Which of the following drug-antidote combinations is incorrect?

   A. Metoprolol-glucagon
   B. Nortriptyline-sodium bicarbonate
   C. Ethanol-fomepizole
   D. Diltiazem-insulin
   E. Sarin gas-glycopyrrolate

48. A middle-aged woman is brought to the ED after being rescued from a house fire. She is tachypneic and agitated. She has first- and second-degree burns affecting her right leg (total body surface area 9%). Examination of her airway and nasal passages does not demonstrate any signs of smoke inhalation. Pulse oximetry is 95% on room air. Laboratory test results are notable for pH 7.19, lactate 10 mmol/L, and P_{CO_2} 24 mm Hg. Which of the following is/are the most appropriate initial therapy(ies)?

    A. Hydroxocobalamin
    B. Oxygen at 10 L/min via nonrebreather facemask
    C. Intubation
    D. Aggressive resuscitation with crystalloid
    E. A and B

    Questions 49 and 50 are based on the following scenario.
    You are called urgently for an intubation in the ED for a young woman who was found stumbling out of a subway terminal confused and with labored breathing. She has copious secretions and she has clearly recently vomited. As you prepare to intubate, the patient has a seizure. You hear of other patients arriving from the same subway station with a similar presentation and suspect a terrorist attack with a biologic or chemical weapon.

49. **Which of the following is most likely the agent?**

    A. Sarin
    B. Chlorine
    C. Phosgene
    D. Cyanide
    E. Anthrax

50. **All of the following symptoms are expected to improve with atropine EXCEPT which one?**

    A. Wheezing
    B. Vomiting
    C. Weakness
    D. Salivation
    E. Blurred vision

Chapter 24 ■ Answers

1. **Correct answer: C**

NIPPV can avoid intubation in carefully selected patients with hypoxemic and/or hypercapnic respiratory failure. NIPPV has significant benefits compared with intubation, including lower risk of nosocomial pneumonia and avoidance of sedation. Well-accepted indications for NIPPV include acute cardiogenic pulmonary edema, acute COPD exacerbation, respiratory failure in immunosuppressed patients, and postextubation in patients at risk of failing extubation ("prophylactic" NIPPV).

Meticulous patient selection for NIPPV is essential, as there are several important contraindications to NIPPV. Patients must able to protect their airway and tolerate a tight-fitting facemask; patients with copious secretions, recent vomiting, or who are uncooperative are poor candidates. Hemodynamic instability is a contraindication to NIPPV. NIPPV may cause gastric distention, especially if pressures exceed lower esophageal sphincter opening pressure (20 mm Hg). Patients with recent esophageal or gastric surgery or requiring high inspiratory pressures should not receive NIPPV. Patients should be frequently reassessed for contraindications while receiving NIPPV (eg, change in mental status, vomiting, hemodynamic instability).

Checklist for Noninvasive Ventilation

	YES	NO
A. Does the patient have:		
1. Signs of respiratory distress?	☑	☐
2. Pao$_2$/Fio$_2$ < 200 and/or Paco$_2$ > 45 mm Hg?	☑	☐
B. If the answer is YES to both, answer the following questions.		
C. Does the patient have:		
1. Respiratory failure that is an immediate threat to life?	☐	☑
2. A life-threatening circulatory disorder (eg, shock)?	☐	☑
3. Coma, severe agitation, or uncontrolled seizures?	☐	☑
4. Inability to protect the airways?	☐	☑
5. Hematemesis or recurrent vomiting?	☐	☑
6. Laryngeal edema, facial trauma, or recent head and neck surgery?	☐	☑
D. If the answer is NO to all of the above questions, the patient is a candidate for noninvasive ventilation.		

From Marino PL. Marino's The ICU Book. 4th ed. Philadelphia: Wolters Kluwer Health/Lippincott Williams & Wilkins; 2014, with permission.

References:
1. Hibbert KA, Hess DR. Mechanical ventilation. In: Wiener-Kronish JP, Bagchi A, Charnin JE, et al, eds. *Critical Care Handbook of the Massachusetts General Hospital*. 6th ed. Philadelphia: Wolters Kluwer; 2016:66-87.
2. Marino PL. Alternate modes of ventilation. In: *Marino's The ICU Book*. 4th ed. Philadelphia: Wolters Kluwer; 2014:521-534.

2. **Correct answer: D**

Intrinsic PEEP, also known as auto-PEEP or air trapping, is a serious complication of mechanical ventilation and can lead to significant hemodynamic instability. Patients with obstructive airway disease with reduced expiratory flow (eg, asthma, COPD) are at especially high risk for auto-PEEP with mechanical ventilation. Auto-PEEP reduces cardiac preload and can culminate in obstructive shock and cardiac arrest similar to a tension pneumothorax. Cardiac arrest following intubation and mechanical ventilation, particularly in patients with obstructive lung disease, should raise suspicion for auto-PEEP. Disconnecting from the Ambu bag or ventilator should be the first intervention in cases of suspected auto-PEEP.

Increasing respiratory rate or tidal volume would worsen auto-PEEP and should be avoided. The endotracheal tube was likely placed correctly based on the presence of breath sounds and carbon dioxide on the capnogram, and reintubation should not be attempted. Patients with COPD are at increased risk for pneumothorax with positive pressure ventilation because of bleb rupture, and empiric needle decompression could be considered if there are other signs of tension pneumothorax (unilateral absence of breath sounds, absence of lung sliding on bedside ultrasound). Given the absence of other signs of pneumothorax in this patient and the risks of unnecessary needle decompression (ie, causing a pneumothorax!), empiric treatment for auto-PEEP should be the first step. Placing an arterial line may be helpful for assessing the quality of chest compressions and monitoring for ROSC but is not a priority (and is very difficult!) in a cardiac arrest.

Reference:

1. Hallman MR, Treggiari MM, Deem S. Critical care medicine. In: Barash PG, Cullen BF, Stoelting RK, et al, eds. *Clinical Anesthesia*. 7th ed. Philadelphia: Wolters Kluwer; 2013:1580-1610.

3. Correct answer: C

Low-tidal volume ventilation is the standard of care in critically ill patients with ARDS. In a landmark ARDS Network randomized controlled trial, low-tidal volume ventilation starting at 6 mL/kg ideal body weight and titrated to a plateau pressure less than 30 cm H_2O (range 4-8 mL/kg tidal volumes) was associated with significantly reduced mortality compared with starting with 12 mL/kg tidal volumes and titrating to a goal plateau pressure less than 50 cm H_2O. Patients with ARDS are at especially high risk for ventilation-induced lung injury because their remaining healthy lung receives proportionally more ventilation compared with diseased, atelectatic lung. Low-tidal volume ventilation is now advocated for almost all critically ill patients.

Another important principle in ARDS ventilation is optimizing PEEP to enhance lung recruitment and reduce atelectrauma. In the ARDSNet trial, PEEP and Fio_2 were titrated to maintain a goal Spo_2 88%-95% (Pao_2 55-80 mm Hg).

In this case, the patient's plateau pressure exceeds 30 cm H_2O and needs to be reduced. The tidal volume of 450 cc amounts to about 7 mL/kg; this can be reduced potentially as low as 4 mL/kg as per the ARDSNet trial. Oxygenation is within goal; therefore PEEP and Fio_2 are sufficient. Pressure support ventilation would not be appropriate until ARDS resolves because of the inability to control tidal volumes.

References:

1. Brower RG, Matthay MA, Morris A, et al; The acute respiratory distress syndrome network. Ventilation with lower tidal volumes as compared with traditional tidal volumes for acute lung injury and the acute respiratory distress syndrome. *N Engl J Med*. 2000;342(18):1301-1308.
2. Hallman MR, Treggiari MM, Deem S. Critical care medicine. In: Barash PG, Cullen BF, Stoelting RK, et al, eds. *Clinical Anesthesia*. 7th ed. Philadelphia: Wolters Kluwer; 2013:1580-1610.

4. Correct answer: E

Key criteria for extubation in the ICU include resolution of the indication for intubation, adequate gas exchange, ability to protect the airway (including strong cough and minimal secretions), stable hemodynamics, and absence of airway obstruction. The ability to follow commands is not a requirement for extubation. Delirium, dementia, or other neurologic disorders may impair a patient's ability to follow commands but are not indications for intubation so long as the patient is able to protect the airway.

The amount of pressure support, if any, to provide during a spontaneous breathing trial (SBT) and the duration of the trial is controversial. Disconnecting from the ventilator and breathing with a T-piece requires the most patient effort. However, studies comparing SBT with a T-piece versus low pressure support ventilation showed no difference in the rate of reintubation. Recent CHEST/ATS guidelines for ventilator weaning now recommend inspiratory pressure support (5-8 cm H_2O) over T-piece or continuous positive airway pressure during SBT. A study comparing SBT lasting 30 minutes versus 2 hours showed no difference in rate of reintubation. However, these findings may not apply to patients at high risk of reintubation, and it has been suggested that high-risk patients should meet more stringent criteria for extubation (eg, prolonged T-piece trial).

The RSBI, calculated by respiratory rate divided by tidal volume, is helpful in identifying patients likely to fail extubation. RSBI greater than 100 is associated with extubation failure. The absence of a cuff leak implies airway obstruction, and extubation should not be attempted in the absence of leak. However, the presence of a cuff leak does not eliminate the possibility of significant airway obstruction after extubation.

References:

1. Esteban A, Alía I, Gordo F, et al. Extubation outcome after spontaneous breathing trials with T-tube or pressure support ventilation. The Spanish Lung Failure Collaborative Group. *Am J Respir Crit Care Med*. 1997;156(2 Pt 1):459-465.
2. Perren A, Domenighetti G, Mauri S, et al. Protocol-directed weaning from mechanical ventilation: clinical outcome in patients randomized for a 30-min or 120-min trial with pressure support ventilation. *Intensive Care Med*. 2002;28(8):1058-1063.

3. Thille AW, Richard JC, Brochard L. The decision to extubate in the intensive care unit. *Am J Respir Crit Care Med.* 2013;187(12):1294-1302.

4. Ouellette DR, Patel S, Girard TD, et al. Liberation from mechanical ventilation in critically ill adults: an official American College of Chest Physicians/American Thoracic Society clinical practice guideline. *Chest.* 2017;151(1):166-180.

5. Correct answer: A

Positive pressure ventilation can have significant hemodynamic effects through changes in cardiac function and pulmonary vascular pressure. The overall effect on hemodynamic function depends on underlying pathology. An increase in intrathoracic pressure reduces the gradient for venous return to the right heart and therefore decreases right-sided preload. In patients with reduced preload due to hypovolemia or decreased SVR (hemorrhage, sepsis, liver failure, anesthetic agents), the addition of positive pressure ventilation will further decrease preload and worsen hypotension. Increased alveolar pressure increases pulmonary vascular resistance and therefore increases right heart afterload. In general, right-sided cardiac output declines under positive pressure ventilation. Patients with pulmonary hypertension and right ventricle (RV) failure (eg, acute PE) will therefore develop worsening hemodynamics with positive pressure ventilation.

In contrast to the right heart, left heart function can improve with positive pressure ventilation. Positive intrathoracic pressure decreases left ventricle (LV) transmural pressure and wall tension according to the Law of Laplace. This in turn reduces LV afterload. Assuming the LV preload is adequate, cardiac output may improve due to reduced afterload. This becomes especially apparent in patients with cardiogenic shock. LV failure should always be considered in the differential of ventilator weaning failure.

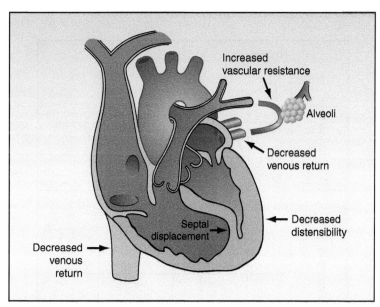

Hemodynamic effects of positive pressure ventilation. (From Marino PL. *Marino's The ICU Book.* 4th ed. Philadelphia: Wolters Kluwer Health/Lippincott Williams & Wilkins; 2014, with permission.)

Reference:
1. Marino PL. Positive pressure ventilation. In: *Marino's The ICU Book.* 4th ed. Philadelphia: Wolters Kluwer; 2014:487-504.

6. Correct answer: C

Static thoracic compliance is a measure of the combined lung and chest wall compliance in the absence of airflow. It is calculated by tidal volume/(plateau pressure − PEEP). Normal static compliance is about 50-80 mL/cm H_2O. Compliance measurements are best made on volume control ventilation and are important in determining optimal PEEP for a given patient. (The PEEP at which compliance is highest is the "best PEEP.") Reduced static compliance can be seen in the setting of pulmonary edema, ARDS, or restrictive lung disease.

$$\text{Static lung compliance} = \text{tidal volume} / [\text{plateau pressure} - \text{PEEP}]$$
$$30 = 450 / [20 - 5]$$

Reference:
1. Marino PL. Positive pressure ventilation. In: *Marino's The ICU Book*. 4th ed. Philadelphia: Wolters Kluwer; 2014:487-504.

7. **Correct answer: A**

Same explanation and references as question 8.

8. **Correct answer: C**

In this ventilator flow tracing, flow at end expiration does not return to baseline before the next breath is delivered, concerning for air trapping (also known as dynamic hyperinflation) and auto-PEEP. Air trapping should raise suspicion for obstructive airway disease, such as COPD or asthma. Restrictive lung disease or ARDS would show decreased compliance and that is not seen here (the static compliance is 48 mL/cm H_2O, which is nearly normal). Opioid overdose would show hypoventilation, which we cannot detect on volume control ventilation. Another clue to obstructive airway disease is the large difference between peak inspiratory and plateau pressures.

In obstructive lung disease, the goal is to increase expiratory time to prevent air trapping and auto-PEEP. This can be accomplished through several ways: (1) reducing respiratory rate, (2) prolonging expiratory time by changing the I:E ratio, (3) prolonging expiratory time by increasing inspiratory flows, (4) minimizing tidal volume. In this case, tidal volume is 6 cc/kg, and other maneuvers should be attempted before it is lowered further. Extrinsic PEEP may need to be eliminated in patients with obstructive lung disease who show signs of air trapping.

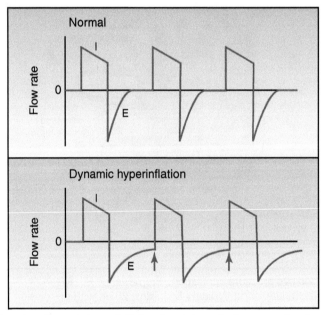

Ventilator flow tracing showing dynamic hyperinflation (or air trapping), concerning for obstructive lung disease. (From Marino PL. *Marino's The ICU Book*. 4th ed. Philadelphia: Wolters Kluwer Health/Lippincott Williams & Wilkins; 2014, with permission.)

References:
1. Marino PL. Asthma and COPD in the ICU. In: *Marino's The ICU Book*. 4th ed. Philadelphia: Wolters Kluwer; 2014:465-486.
2. Hibbert KA, Hess DR. Mechanical ventilation. In: Wiener-Kronish JP, Bagchi A, Charnin JE, et al, eds. *Critical Care Handbook of the Massachusetts General Hospital*. 6th ed. Philadelphia: Wolters Kluwer; 2016:66-87.

9. **Correct answer: B**

In both pressure support and pressure control ventilation, the ventilator delivers a set inspiratory pressure, and tidal volume is determined by the amount of pressure delivered, thoracic compliance, airway resistance, and patient inspiratory effort. The key difference between the 2 settings is what terminates a breath (ie, cycling). In assist-control ventilation modes (both volume and pressure control), the duration of inspiration is set by the I:E time (time-cycled ventilation). In pressure support ventilation, inspiratory time is variable and depends on the patient's efforts. Inspiration is triggered when the ventilator senses the patient's inspiratory effort and is terminated when the ventilator senses a decrease in inspiratory flow.

In both pressure support and assist-control pressure control ventilation, the patient can **trigger** breaths that will be delivered by the ventilator. In pressure control, these triggered breaths are identical to mandatory breaths with a fixed I:E ratio and set pressure achieved. In both modes, lung injury can occur due to inability to control tidal volumes. For this reason, volume control ventilation is usually preferred in patients with ARDS.

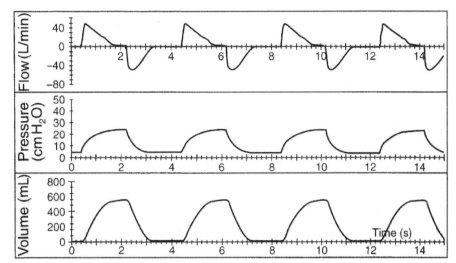

Pressure control ventilation. (From Hibbert KA, Hess DR. Mechanical ventilation. In: Wiener-Kronish JP, Bagchi A, Charnin JE, et al, eds. *Critical Care Handbook of the Massachusetts General Hospital.* 6th ed. Philadelphia: Wolters Kluwer; 2016:66-87, with permission.)

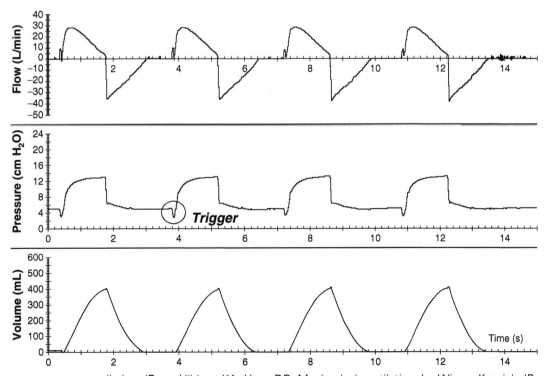

Pressure support ventilation. (From Hibbert KA, Hess DR. Mechanical ventilation. In: Wiener-Kronish JP, Bagchi A, Charnin JE, et al, eds. *Critical Care Handbook of the Massachusetts General Hospital.* 6th ed. Philadelphia: Wolters Kluwer; 2016:66-87, with permission.)

Reference:
1. Hibbert KA, Hess DR. Mechanical ventilation. In: Wiener-Kronish JP, Bagchi A, Charnin JE, et al, eds. *Critical Care Handbook of the Massachusetts General Hospital*. 6th ed. Philadelphia: Wolters Kluwer; 2016:66-87.

10. **Correct answer: D**

In volume control ventilation, tidal volume is determined by a set inspiratory flow. As a result of a set inspiratory flow, tidal volumes do not change with patient effort, lung compliance, or airway resistance. Any decrease in thoracic compliance or increase in airway resistance will lead to increased airway pressures. By contrast, flow (and therefore tidal volume) is variable in pressure control and pressure support ventilation and determined by lung compliance, airway resistance, and patient effort. The fixed inspiratory flow in volume control ventilation could potentially contribute to patient-ventilator dyssynchrony; switching to pressure modes is often the first move in attempts to increase synchrony.

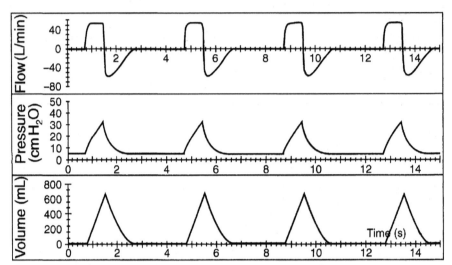

Volume control ventilation. (From Hibbert KA, Hess DR. Mechanical ventilation. In: Wiener-Kronish JP, Bagchi A, Charnin JE, et al, eds. *Critical Care Handbook of the Massachusetts General Hospital*. 6th ed. Philadelphia: Wolters Kluwer; 2016:66-87, with permission.)

Reference:
1. Hibbert KA, Hess DR. Mechanical ventilation. In: Wiener-Kronish JP, Bagchi A, Charnin JE, et al, eds. *Critical Care Handbook of the Massachusetts General Hospital*. 6th ed. Philadelphia: Wolters Kluwer; 2016:66-87.

11. **Correct answer: B**

Ventilator-associated pneumonia (VAP) is diagnosed in 5%-15% of patients on mechanical ventilation and carries significant morbidity and mortality. VAP increases the duration of mechanical ventilation and ICU length of stay and has a mortality of about 10%.

The most effective way to prevent VAP is to minimize duration of mechanical ventilation. Recent evidence-based recommendations for VAP prevention include the following:

- Use NIPPV if possible.
- Decrease duration of mechanical ventilation by minimizing sedation and daily SBTs.
- Elevate head of bed 30°-45°.
- Administer oral hygiene with chlorhexidine.
- Use endotracheal tubes with subglottic secretion drainage ports if patients are likely to be intubated for more than 2-3 days.

Interventions that are *not* recommended for VAP prevention include early tracheostomy, stress ulcer prophylaxis, and monitoring gastric residual volumes. Monitoring for regurgitation or vomiting is sufficient for detection for feeding intolerance and risk of aspiration.

Reference:
1. Klompas M, Branson R, Eichenwald EC, et al. Strategies to prevent ventilator-associated pneumonia in acute care hospitals: 2014 update. *Infect Control Hosp Epidemiol*. 2014;35(8):915-936.

12. **Correct answer: D**

CRBSIs carry significant morbidity and cost. Diagnosis requires a positive blood culture from the catheter *and* a matching positive blood culture obtained from another site. The catheter must have been in place for at least 48 hours before positive blood cultures, and other sources of bacteremia should be ruled out. A positive blood culture from the catheter with negative blood culture from another site is suggestive of line colonization or contaminant. The most common pathogens are coagulase-negative staphylococci, *Staphylococcus aureus*, enterococci, and *Candida*; gram-negative rods are responsible for only about 20% of infections. A recent meta-analysis showed that arterial lines do in fact carry a risk of CRBSI with an incidence of 3.4/1000 arterial catheters.

Key recommendations in recent CDC guidelines for CRBSI prevention include the following:

- Do not replace CVCs unless clinically indicated; routine replacement of CVCs does not reduce the risk of CRBSI.
- Maximal sterile barrier precautions are required for CVC insertion and guidewire exchange and include sterile gown and gloves, mask, cap, and full body drape.
- Avoid femoral line placement in adult patients.
- Avoid subclavian placement in patients with end-stage renal disease owing to risk of causing subclavian vein stenosis.
- Chlorhexidine with alcohol for skin disinfection is more effective compared with povidone iodine or alcohol.
- Replace dressings on CVC at minimum of every 7 days unless loose or soiled.
- Placement of peripheral arterial lines requires a cap, mask, sterile gloves, small sterile drape, and chlorhexidine for skin preparation. Femoral and axillary arterial lines require maximal sterile barrier precautions described above for CVCs.

References:

1. Hallman MR, Treggiari MM, Deem S. Critical care medicine. In: Barash PG, Cullen BF, Stoelting RK, et al, eds. *Clinical Anesthesia*. 7th ed. Philadelphia: Wolters Kluwer; 2013:1580-1610.
2. O'Horo JC, Maki DG, Krupp AE, et al. Arterial catheters as a source of bloodstream infection: a systematic review and meta-analysis. *Crit Care Med*. 2014;42(6):1334-1339.
3. O'Grady NP, Alexander M, Burns LA, et al. *Guidelines for the Prevention of Intravascular Catheter-Related Infections*. 2011. https://www.cdc.gov/infectioncontrol/guidelines/bsi/background/prevention-strategies.html.

13. **Correct answer: B**

CVCs should not be replaced unless clinically indicated—that is, if there is concern for catheter infection or the catheter is malfunctioning. Catheter replacement using a guidewire is more comfortable for patients and carries lower risk of complications compared with a fresh percutaneous insertion. However, if there is any possibility of catheter infection (eg, positive blood cultures or nonsterile placement), the catheter should *not* be replaced over a guidewire because the skin tract to vein is potentially colonized. Catheter replacement using a guidewire is only appropriate for malfunctioning catheters, eg, obstruction as evidenced by loss of blood return.

Fever alone is not an indication to replace a CVC, particularly if another source of infection is found, blood cultures are negative, or a noninfectious cause of fever is considered more likely.

Reference:

1. O'Grady NP, Alexander M, Burns LA, et al. *Guidelines for the Prevention of Intravascular Catheter-Related Infections*. 2011. https://www.cdc.gov/infectioncontrol/guidelines/bsi/background/prevention-strategies.html.

14. **Correct answer: E**

Catheter-associated urinary tract infection (CAUTI) is the most preventable health care–acquired infection. The most effective method to prevent CAUTI is to remove indwelling catheters as soon as they are no longer indicated. Each day a urinary catheter in place carries up to 10% risk of developing bacteriuria. There are several alternatives to an indwelling urinary catheter. Intermittent straight catheterization carries lower risk of CAUTI compared with indwelling catheters and is recommended in patients with urinary retention. External catheters ("condom catheters") have a reduced rate of complications compared with indwelling catheters and are recommended in male patients with incontinence. Routine catheter exchange in the absence of infection does not reduce the risk of CAUTI and is not recommended.

Symptomatic CAUTI should be treated with antibiotics. Asymptomatic catheter-associated bacteriuria should *not* be treated with antibiotics. Monitoring for asymptomatic bacteriuria is not recommended.

Acceptable indications for indwelling urinary catheters according to CDC guidelines:

- Acute urinary retention
- Close monitoring of urine output in critically ill patients
- Incontinence in setting of open sacral or perineal wounds (incontinence is otherwise not an indication for indwelling catheters)
- Comfort care at end of life

References:

1. Tenke P, Köves B, Johansen TE. An update on prevention and treatment of catheter-associated urinary tract infections. *Curr Opin Infect Dis*. 2014;27(1):102-107.
2. Centers for Disease Control and Prevention. *Guideline for Prevention of Catheter-Associated Urinary Tract Infections*. 2009. https://www.cdc.gov/infectioncontrol/guidelines/cauti/evidence-review.html.

15. Correct answer: C

Alcohol-based hand rubs (ABHRs) have broad germicidal activity against most bacteria and viruses including MRSA, vancomycin-resistant enterococci, MTB, HIV, influenza, hepatitis, HSV, and fungi. ABHR should contain 60%-95% ethanol or isopropanol and work by denaturing proteins. ABHR increases adherence to hand hygiene and reduces the spread of serious hospital-acquired infections. Recent CDC guidelines in fact recommend using ABHR over handwashing with antimicrobial soaps for routine hand hygiene. (Handwashing is still indicated if hands are visibly contaminated.)

An important exception to this rule is *Clostridium difficile*. *C. difficile* is transmitted by spores, which are highly resistant to alcohol and many standard hospital cleaning products. Gloves and gown should be worn during any patient contact, and hands should be washed with soap and water to mechanically remove spores. Isolation and contact precautions should be initiated while test results are pending. Chloride-containing products (eg, bleach) are required for cleaning medical equipment and rooms.

References:

1. Boyce JM, Pittet D. Centers for Disease Control and Prevention. Guideline for Hand Hygiene in Health-Care Settings: Recommendations of the Healthcare Infection Control Practices Advisory Committee and the HICPAC/SHEA/APIC/IDSA Hand Hygiene Task Force. *MMWR*. 2002;51(No. RR-16).
2. Cooper CC, Jump RL, Chopra T. Prevention of infection due to *Clostridium difficile*. *Infect Dis Clin N Am*. 2016;30(4):999-1012.

16. Correct answer: D

Clostridium difficile is the leading cause of gastroenteritis-related mortality in the United States. *C. difficile* is acquired through ingestion of spores, which are resistant to alcohol-based handrubs and many hospital cleaning products. Only chloride-containing cleaning products (ie, bleach) should be used for environmental decontamination when there is suspicion for *C. difficile*.

Monotherapy with metronidazole is acceptable for mild to moderate cases of *C. difficile*; oral vancomycin should be added for severe cases. Antibiotic therapy should be continued for 10-14 days and not stopped with resolution of diarrhea. (Spread of spores can continue despite clinical improvement.) Unfortunately, up to 50% of these patients will continue to be asymptomatic carriers despite treatment.

The leading risk factor for *C. difficile* infection is antibiotic use. Antibiotics disrupt normal gut flora and allow spore proliferation and toxin production. Tighter regulation of antibiotic use has successfully decreased *C. difficile* infection rates. Acid suppression therapy, particularly proton pump inhibitors, has been associated with increased risk of *C. difficile*, and careful prescribing of acid suppression therapy has been recommended as a means to reduce *C. difficile* infection.

References:

1. Cooper CC, Jump RL, Chopra T. Prevention of infection due to *Clostridium difficile*. *Infect Dis Clin N Am*. 2016;30(4):999-1012.
2. Ofosu A. *Clostridium difficile* infection: a review of current and emerging therapies. *Ann Gastroenterol*. 2016;29(2):147-154.

17. Correct answer: C

Endotracheal intubation and bronchoscopy can expose health care providers to infected respiratory secretions. Mucous membranes must be shielded during these procedures. CDC guidelines recommend the following options for PPE during procedures with exposure to respiratory secretions: (1) face shield, (2) mask with attached eye shield, and (3) mask with goggles. Gown and gloves should be worn as well.

Reference:

1. Siegel JD, Rhinehart E, Jackson M, et al. *Guideline for Isolation Precautions: Preventing Transmission of Infectious Agents in Healthcare Settings*. 2007. https://www.cdc.gov/infectioncontrol/guidelines/isolation/recommendations.html.

18. Correct answer: D

MTB outbreaks in health care facilities have been attributed to delayed diagnosis and inadequate precautions. MTB is transmitted through respiratory droplets. The risk of transmission is especially high for health care workers in close contact with respiratory secretions, including intubation, suctioning, and bronchoscopy. When MTB disease is suspected, airborne precautions should be instituted immediately, including admitting the patient to a negative pressure room and requiring health care workers to wear fitted N95 respirators. Before each use of an N95 respirator, the user should confirm a tight mask seal by positive and negative pressure leak tests. In the positive pressure leak test, the wearer exhales with hands around the corners of the mask; if airflow is detected, there is a leak around the mask. In the negative pressure leak test, the wearer inhales deeply; the mask should move closer to the face, indicating a tight seal. A bacterial filter should be applied to the ventilator circuit.

Airborne precautions should only be discontinued when (1) the patient is found to have another condition that explains the symptoms or (2) there are 3 negative sputum AFB smears obtained 8-24 hours apart. A tuberculin skin test is unreliable in patients with active MTB disease and/or HIV due to anergy and cannot be used to rule out MTB in these patients.

MTB is not acquired through surfaces; contact precautions are therefore not necessary. If the suspicion for MTB disease is high and the patient is critically ill, empiric therapy for MTB disease should begin with a 4-drug regimen to prevent development of resistance.

Reference:

1. Centers for Disease Control and Prevention. Guidelines for preventing the transmission of *Mycobacterium tuberculosis* in health-care settings, 2005. *MMWR.* 2005;54(No. RR-17).

19. Correct answer: B

HBV is highly infectious and can be acquired through percutaneous, mucosal, or nonintact skin exposure with blood or body fluids. The risk of seroconversion following a percutaneous exposure to HBV ranges from 30% to 60% (compared with about 2% for HCV and 0.3% for HIV). CDC recommends all health care workers be vaccinated for HBV. (Other recommended vaccines are mumps, measles, rubella, varicella, pertussis, and influenza.)

The HBV vaccine is recombinant HBV surface antigen and requires 3 doses over a 6-month period. Seroprotection should be confirmed by measuring anti-HBs titers 2 months after the last vaccine; levels >10 mIU/mL are considered adequate for lifelong immunity. Health care workers should have anti-HBs titers checked upon starting their jobs to confirm immunity and receive additional doses of the vaccine if titers <10 mIU/mL.

The resident should undergo testing of anti-HBs titers immediately postexposure because his response to prior vaccination is unknown. If he were found to have inadequate anti-HBs titers (ie, <10 mIU/mL), he should receive hepatitis B immune globulin and HBV vaccine. If he were found to have adequate titers of anti-HBs, then no prophylaxis is necessary. If the resident had been tested for HBV immunity in the past (as he should have been!), no HBV testing or prophylaxis is necessary after exposure to HBV.

Reference:

1. Weber DJ, Rutala WA. Occupational health update: focus on preventing the acquisition of infections with pre-exposure prophylaxis and postexposure prophylaxis. *Infect Dis Clin North Am.* 2016;30(3):729-757.

20. Correct answer: C

Although it may be tempting to start with broad-spectrum antibiotics in a patient requiring hospital admission for community-acquired pneumonia (CAP), inappropriate empiric use of broad-spectrum antibiotics is harmful, including drug toxicity, superinfection with *C difficile* and *Candida*, increased cost, and development of antibiotic resistance. Empiric CAP coverage should include antibiotics with activity against pneumococcus (the most common cause of CAP) and atypical organisms. Ceftriaxone is an excellent choice for pneumococcal coverage. A macrolide or fluoroquinolone should be added for atypical coverage.

This patient has no recent hospitalizations and is not likely to be immunocompromised. Empiric coverage for hospital-acquired pneumonia (HAP) should include coverage of gram-negative rods and MRSA. Vancomycin (which adds MRSA coverage) and cefepime (which adds pseudomonal coverage) would be reasonable empiric coverage for HAP or immunosuppressed patients. Piperacillin/tazobactam monotherapy (which also covers pseudomonas) would not be appropriate because it does not cover atypicals, is unnecessarily broad spectrum, and is associated with risk of renal injury (and therefore should only be used if necessary). Meropenem is also unnecessarily broad spectrum and should be reserved for cases of suspected extended-spectrum β-lactamase-producing organisms. Fungal coverage with fluconazole is not necessary in CAP.

Reference:
1. Levine AR, Kadri SS. Infectious disease- empiric and emergency treatment. In: Wiener-Kronish JP, Bagchi A, Charnin JE, et al, eds. *Critical Care Handbook of the Massachusetts General Hospital*. 6th ed. Philadelphia: Wolters Kluwer; 2016:397-428.

21. **Correct answer: D**

Focused bedside cardiac ultrasonography can be extremely valuable in the rapid evaluation of patients presenting with shock. This is a parasternal short-axis view, which can be obtained by placing the ultrasound probe in the left third to fifth intercostal spaces with the marker facing the left shoulder. Normally, the RV should be smaller than the LV, and the interventricular septum should bow into the RV because of the higher filling pressures of the LV. This image is notable for a dilated RV and flattened interventricular septum resulting in a D-shaped LV, findings highly concerning for pulmonary embolism in the setting of acute hemodynamic instability. Live images may show McConnell sign: akinesis of RV freewall with preserved apical function. Pulmonary embolism is one etiology of obstructive shock. Other etiologies of obstructive shock include tension pneumothorax and cardiac tamponade.

Distributive shock (eg, due to sepsis or anaphylaxis) would show underfilled and hyperdynamic ventricles, not signs of RV overload seen here. Cardiogenic shock is a possibility, given evidence of cardiac ischemia on ECG; however, the absence of a dilated LV makes this less likely. The ST depressions in this case are more likely demand ischemia in the setting of hypoperfusion.

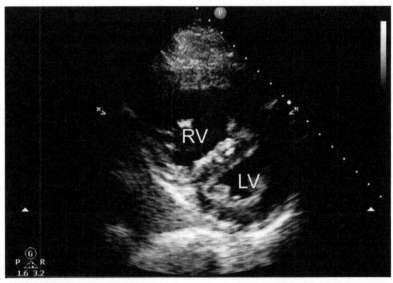

(Reproduced with permission from Miller L, Shelton K. Critical care ultrasound. In: Parsons PE, Wiener-Kronish JP, Stapleton RD, Berra R, eds. *Critical Care Secrets*. 6th ed. Philadelphia: Elsevier; 2019:107-113.)

Reference:
1. Shelton K, Riddell K. Use of ultrasound in critical illness. In: Wiener-Kronish JP, Bagchi A, Charnin JE, et al, eds. *Critical Care Handbook of the Massachusetts General Hospital*. 6th ed. Philadelphia: Wolters Kluwer; 2016:33-44.

22. **Correct answer: B**

McConnell sign on echocardiography (akinesis of RV free wall with preserved apical function) is highly concerning for acute PE. This patient is currently too unstable to have a CT scan of her chest to help guide and/or confirm diagnosis, and therefore, empiric systemic fibrinolytic therapy with tissue plasminogen activator should be considered. Systemic thrombolysis is indicated for massive PE (defined by hypotension with SBP less than 90). Important contraindications to systemic fibrinolysis include active bleeding, intracranial lesions, history of intracranial hemorrhage, ischemic CVA <3 months ago, recent head trauma or brain or spinal surgery. Patients with a massive PE and absolute contraindications to systemic fibrinolysis may be candidates for surgical embolectomy.

Rapid infusion of 2 L crystalloid would be appropriate in the setting of distributive shock (sepsis or anaphylaxis) but could worsen acute RV strain caused by PE. Cardiac catheterization may be appropriate for cardiogenic shock.

Reference:

1. Witkin AS, Channick RN. Deep venous thrombosis and pulmonary embolism in the intensive care unit. In: Wiener-Kronish JP, Bagchi A, Charnin JE, et al, eds. *Critical Care Handbook of the Massachusetts General Hospital*. 6th ed. Philadelphia: Wolters Kluwer; 2016:276-284.

23. Correct answer: D

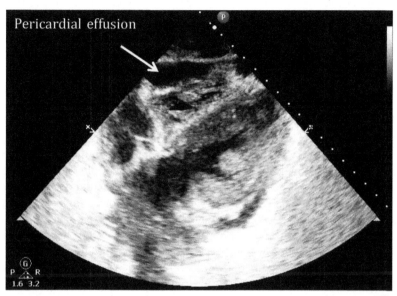

(Reproduced with permission from Miller L, Shelton K. Critical care ultrasound. In: Parsons PE, Wiener-Kronish JP, Stapleton RD, Berra R, eds. *Critical Care Secrets*. 6th ed. Philadelphia: Elsevier; 2019:107-113.)

This subcostal view shows a pericardial effusion with RV collapse, which is highly concerning for tamponade in the presence of hemodynamic instability. A PA line would show elevated and theoretically "equal" CVP and PA diastolic pressures because of impaired ventricle filling and elevated systemic vascular resistance (a compensatory response to obstructive shock). HR would be elevated as a compensatory response to maintain cardiac output in the setting of reduced stroke volume. Physical examination findings might include muffled heart sounds, distended neck veins, and pulsus paradoxus (Beck triad).

Answer choice A is consistent with hypovolemic shock with low CVP, PA pressures, and compensatory elevated HR and SVR. Although the ventricles appear underfilled on echocardiography, this is more likely due to restricted filling. It can also be difficult to assess ventricular filling on long-axis views; the parasternal short-axis midpapillary view is most reliable for volume assessment. Answer choice B consists of normal values. Answer choice C is consistent with cardiogenic shock with an inappropriately low HR (perhaps in the setting of conduction block or β-blocker use). Answer choice E is consistent with distributive shock with low CVP, PA pressures, and SVR and compensatory elevated HR and cardiac output.

Hemodynamic Patterns in Different Types of Shock

PARAMETER	HYPOVOLEMIC SHOCK	CARDIOGENIC SHOCK	VASOGENIC SHOCK
CVP or PAWP	Low	High	Low
Cardiac output	Low	Low	High
SVR	High	High	Low

PAWP, pulmonary artery wedge pressure. From Marino PL. Marino's The ICU Book. 4th ed. Philadelphia: Wolters Kluwer Health/Lippincott Williams & Wilkins; 2014, with permission.

References:

1. Shelton K, Riddell K. Use of ultrasound in critical illness. In: Wiener-Kronish JP, Bagchi A, Charnin JE, et al, eds. *MGH Critical Care Handbook*. 6th ed. Philadelphia: Wolters Kluwer; 2016:33-44.
2. Marino PL. The pulmonary artery catheter. In: *Marino's The ICU Book*. 4th ed. Philadelphia: Wolters Kluwer; 2014:135-150.

24. **Correct answer: B**

Postcardiac surgery tamponade must be treated immediately with removal of pericardial blood and repair of the source of bleeding. This is most effectively accomplished with redo sternotomy; pericardiocentesis would not allow for repair of the source of bleeding. A rapid fluid bolus would likely not significantly increase cardiac output in cardiac tamponade because of severely restricted filling. Ordering a transesophageal echocardiography for further evaluation would not change management and just delay treatment; the patient needs to go to the OR immediately. Cardiac catheterization to evaluate graft patency would not be indicated, as the much more likely etiology of shock is tamponade.

Reference:

1. Hallman MR, Treggiari MM, Deem S. Critical care medicine. In: Barash PG, Cullen BF, Stoelting RK, et al, eds. *Clinical Anesthesia*. 7th ed. Philadelphia: Wolters Kluwer; 2013:1580-1610.

25. **Correct answer: C**

This patient likely has cardiogenic shock due to an acute myocardial infarction. He has evidence of organ hypoperfusion, given his elevated lactate, and would benefit from an inotropic agent while undergoing revascularization. Dobutamine is a β1- and β2-agonist with inotropic and chronotropic effects and is the preferred agent in cardiogenic shock. Dobutamine can cause a mild decrease in SVR because of its β2-agonism, and patients should be monitored closely for development of hypotension. Norepinephrine has β1 effects as well but increases afterload and therefore can adversely affect cardiac output secondary to its α1-agonism. Norepinephrine is therefore not the preferred inotrope in cardiogenic shock but could be used in addition to dobutamine to counteract persistent hypotension.

A fluid bolus is not likely to be beneficial in cardiogenic shock, as cardiac filling pressures are typically elevated. A fluid bolus may even be harmful by worsening any pulmonary edema that could be present. Dopamine is associated with significantly increased risks of dysrhythmias and should be avoided in cardiogenic shock. A recent randomized controlled trial found increased mortality in patients with cardiogenic shock who were treated with dopamine when compared with those treated with norepinephrine.

References:

1. De Backer D, Biston P, Devriendt J, et al. Comparison of dopamine and norepinephrine in the treatment of shock. *N Engl J Med*. 2010;362(9):779-789.
2. Hallman MR, Treggiari MM, Deem S. Critical care medicine. In: Barash PG, Cullen BF, Stoelting RK, et al, eds. *Clinical Anesthesia*. 7th ed. Philadelphia: Wolters Kluwer; 2013:1580-1610.

26. **Correct answer: E**

Data from a PAC can be used to derive more than 10 hemodynamic and oxygen transport parameters. These parameters can be very useful in identifying the etiology of shock. Cardiac output is measured by thermodilution. The pulmonary artery occlusion pressure (or wedge pressure) approximates left atrial and LV end-diastolic pressure (assuming there is no mitral valve pathology). The mixed venous oxygen saturation is measured on a blood sample drawn from the PA port (central venous saturation is obtained from the CVP port). Several important oxygen transport parameters can be calculated when the cardiac output and mixed venous saturations are known (listed below). SVR can be calculated knowing the MAP, CVP, and cardiac output. Stroke volume can be calculated knowing the cardiac output and HR. Calculating the LV ejection fraction requires the LV end-diastolic volume and is measured by echocardiography, not a PAC.

Oxygen transport parameters derived from a PAC and knowing oxygen content of blood:

Oxygen content arterial blood (Cao_2) = $1.3 \times Hgb \times Sao_2$

Oxygen content mixed venous blood (Cvo_2) = $1.3 \times Hgb \times Mvo_2$

Oxygen delivery (Do_2) = $CO \times Cao_2$

Oxygen consumption (Vo_2) = $CO \times (Cao_2 - Cvo_2)$

Oxygen extraction = Vo_2/Do_2

$SVR = (MAP - CVP)/CO$

$SV = CO/HR$

$EF = SV/LVEDV$

References:
1. Connor CW, et al. Commonly used monitoring techniques. In: Barash PG, Cullen BF, Stoelting RK, et al, eds. *Clinical Anesthesia.* 7th ed. Philadelphia: Wolters Kluwer; 2013:699-722.
2. Marino PL. The pulmonary artery catheter. In: *Marino's The ICU Book.* 4th ed. Philadelphia: Wolters Kluwer; 2014:135-150.

27. **Correct answer: D**

This patient's presentation is concerning for postoperative urosepsis, and therefore empiric broad spectrum antibiotic therapy should be initiated immediately. She may continue to be observed in the PACU while awaiting results of further work-up, with the plan for ICU transfer should she become hemodynamically unstable and/or begin to warrant a higher level of care. Patients undergoing surgical procedures to remove kidney stones are at risk for urosepsis secondary to manipulation of the urinary tract. Signs of sepsis frequently surface within 6 hours of the surgical procedure.

The latest Sepsis-3 guidelines offer the Quick SOFA (qSOFA) criteria as a simple bedside screening tool for evaluating patients with possible sepsis. The qSOFA criteria are based on physical examination and vital signs: respiratory rate ≥22 breaths per minute, altered mental status, SBP ≤100 mm Hg. A qSOFA score ≥2 in a patient with suspected infection (as this patient has) should prompt further work-up for sepsis and organ dysfunction, including cultures, complete blood count, metabolic panel, and lactate. The cornerstone of sepsis treatment is timely initiation of broad-spectrum antibiotics (ideally within 1 h). Vancomycin and cefepime would be reasonable in this patient, given her history of urinary tract infections and likely recent exposure to antibiotics (which increases the risk of colonization with resistant organisms). It is important to obtain blood cultures and cultures from sites of possible infection (in this case, urine) before initiating antibiotics.

Sepsis is considered a medical emergency, and treatment should not be delayed while making triage decisions. It would be inappropriate to discharge a patient home when sepsis is suspected. She should not be discharged to the floor until empiric antibiotics have been administered and she has remained hemodynamically stable after an extended period of observation. She may require ICU admission if her hemodynamics do not improve or laboratory work shows evidence of significant organ dysfunction. Although pain and residual anesthetics could explain her signs and symptoms (shivering, tachypnea, tachycardia), this patient is at risk for infection and should be treated for presumed sepsis until proven otherwise. Postoperative urosepsis following stone removal surgery can occur simply from manipulation of the urinary tract and does not necessarily indicate a retained stone. Returning to the OR for repeat ureteroscopy is not currently indicated for this patient at this time.

References:
1. Singer M, Deutschman CS, Seymour CW, et al. The third international consensus definitions for sepsis and septic shock (Sepsis-3). *JAMA.* 2016;315(8):801-810.
2. Mariappan P, Tolley DA. Endoscopic stone surgery: minimizing the risk of post-operative sepsis. *Curr Opin Urol.* 2005;15(2): 101-105.

28. **Correct answer: B**

This patient now meets criteria for septic shock based on lactate >2 mmol/L and hypotension despite fluid resuscitation.

Along with early antibiotic therapy, aggressive fluid resuscitation is a cornerstone of early sepsis treatment. Guidelines recommended at least 30 cc/kg of crystalloid for initial resuscitation, followed by additional fluid based on evaluation of fluid responsiveness using dynamic over static (eg, CVP) variables. Systolic or pulse pressure variation with respiration is the most well-accepted marker of fluid responsiveness, but keep in mind that this has only been validated in patients receiving positive pressure ventilation. In a spontaneously breathing patient, performing a straight leg raise or bedside ultrasound evaluation of heart filling and IVC size can be used to assess fluid responsiveness.

While attempts are underway to assess fluid responsiveness in this patient, it would be reasonable to initiate vasopressors. Norepinephrine is the first-line vasopressor in septic shock and should be titrated to a goal MAP 65. The addition of vasopressin should be considered given the relative "vasopressin deficiency" that is seen in patients with septic shock. Norepinephrine is preferred to dopamine (which carries risk of tachyarrhythmias) and phenylephrine (lack of data in sepsis). Crystalloid is preferred over colloid for initial fluid resuscitation. It would be premature to broaden antibiotics after 1 dose; vasopressor support should be added first.

References:
1. Singer M, Deutschman CS, Seymour CW, et al. The third international consensus definitions for sepsis and septic shock (Sepsis-3). *JAMA*. 2016;315(8):801-810.
2. Rhodes A, Evans LE, Alhazzani W, et al. Surviving Sepsis Campaign: International Guidelines for Management of Sepsis and Septic Shock: 2016. *Crit Care Med*. 2017;45(3):486-552.

29. Correct answer: B

This patient's MRI shows a C6 subluxation injury with resulting spinal cord compression and edema at C4-C7. Given these imaging and clinical findings and absence of significant bleeding, his hemodynamic instability is most likely due to neurogenic shock. Cervical spinal cord injury interrupts input to the sympathetic neurons in the spinal cord (located T1-L2) so that there is loss of cardioaccelerator fibers, inotropy, and peripheral vasoconstriction. Bradycardia and hypotension resolve over time as the spinal cord sympathetic neurons develop automaticity.

Neurogenic shock, which refers to the hemodynamic changes seen with a sympathectomy, is often confused with spinal shock. Spinal shock describes transient flaccid muscle weakness following spinal cord injury. Obstructive shock could be seen in tension pneumothorax, but a small pneumothorax is unlikely to cause the degree of hemodynamic instability seen here. Hypovolemic shock is also unlikely to explain his degree of hemodynamic instability. In pure hypovolemic shock, 30%-40% of blood volume must be lost before hypotension results (class III shock), and a grade 2 splenic laceration would be unlikely to cause this degree of bleeding. Hypovolemic and obstructive shock would also be accompanied by compensatory tachycardia, not seen here. Although trauma patients are certainly at risk for infection, septic shock would be unlikely to have developed this early.

Reference:
1. Mccunn M, Grissom TE, Dutton RP. Anesthesia for trauma. In: Miller RD, Cohen NH, Eriksson LI, et al, eds. *Miller's Anesthesia*. 8th ed. Philadelphia; 2015:2423-2459.

30. Correct answer: A

This patient is showing signs of impending respiratory failure, given his weak cough and intermittent desaturations, which are likely due to mucous plugging and atelectasis. Patients with cervical spinal cord injury below C4 have preserved diaphragm function and are able to take adequate resting tidal volumes but lose their accessory muscles (intercostals, scalenes, and abdominal muscles), which are crucial for producing an adequate cough and deep breathing. His airway should be secured before he decompensates and requires urgent intubation. Intubation in patients with cervical spinal cord injury carries a risk of worsening their current spinal cord injury with neck manipulation. For this reason, it is best to perform intubation in controlled nonurgent circumstances whenever possible. In a patient who is calm and cooperative, awake fiberoptic intubation while keeping the cervical collar in place is the safest option. If a patient is unable to tolerate awake intubation, manual in-line stabilization during asleep intubation is crucial.

Signs of significant bleeding have not been identified at this time, and an empiric blood transfusion is not currently indicated. Recent studies have shown that high-dose steroids do not have a significant benefit in long-term motor recovery in spinal cord injury and are therefore no longer recommended. Although BiPAP would increase his minute ventilation, his inability to manage secretions currently contraindicates its use. Although he will need to go to the OR for spinal cord decompression and fusion as soon as possible, he should be intubated first in a safe and controlled manner while his respiratory status is relatively stable.

References:
1. Mccunn M, Grissom TE, Dutton RP. Anesthesia for trauma. In: Miller RD, Cohen NH, Eriksson LI, et al, eds. *Miller's Anesthesia*. 8th ed. Philadelphia; 2015:2423-2459.
2. Velmahos GC, Toutouzas K, Chan L, et al. Intubation after cervical spinal cord injury: to be done selectively or routinely? *Am Surg*. 2003;69(10):891-894.
3. Evaniew N, Belley-Côté EP, Fallah N, et al. Methylprednisolone for the treatment of patients with acute spinal cord injuries: a systematic review and meta-analysis. *J Neurotrauma*. 2016;33(5):468-481.

31. Correct answer: E

ICU-acquired weakness (ICUAW) encompasses polyneuropathy, myopathy, and/or muscle atrophy. ICUAW is definitively diagnosed by muscle biopsy and electrophysiology testing, including sensory and motor nerve conduction studies and electromyography. These studies are rarely done, however, because the tests are uncomfortable and—because there is no specific treatment for ICUAW—usually do not change management. ICUAW may affect up to 80% of ICU patients and has been associated with decreased functional status after recovery from critical illness.

There is currently no specific treatment for ICUAW other than aggressive physical therapy, and therefore attempting to prevent this debilitating condition is crucial. Severity of critical illness is the most well-established risk factor for ICUAW. There is good evidence that hyperglycemia and immobilization are risk factors. Possible risk factors include corticosteroids and neuromuscular blockers (data are conflicting). Early mobilization and physical therapy (including passive exercises in patients unable to participate in physical therapy) is currently our best prevention and treatment of ICUAW. Minimizing the use of high-dose steroids and neuromuscular blocking drugs and treating hyperglycemia may be beneficial.

Reference:

1. Jolley SE, Bunnell AE, Hough CL. ICU-acquired weakness. *Chest*. 2016;150(5):1129-1140.

32. Correct answer: C

ICU patients are at increased risk of VTE because of immobilization, recent trauma or surgery, and presence of indwelling CVCs. VTE prophylaxis is therefore extremely important in the ICU. LMWH is more potent and has more predictable activity compared with subcutaneous heparin and should be used in patients at high risk for VTE without renal failure. Pharmacologic prophylaxis does not eliminate the possibility of VTE; VTE can occur in 5%-30% of patients receiving pharmacologic prophylaxis! Evaluation for VTE or empiric anticoagulation should proceed expeditiously in patients with signs of VTE receiving pharmacologic prophylaxis.

Upper-extremity DVTs associated with CVCs can lead to pulmonary embolism and require therapeutic anticoagulation. The use of IVC filters is controversial and should only be considered in high-risk patients with contraindications to anticoagulation. LMWH does carry a risk of HIT, although significantly lower than heparin.

Risk Factors for Venous Thromboembolism

Strong Risk Factors (Odds Ratio > 10)

- Fracture (hip or leg)
- Hip or knee replacement
- Major trauma
- Spinal cord injury

Moderate Risk Factors (Odds Ratio 2-9)

- Arthroscopic knee surgery
- Central venous lines
- Chemotherapy
- Congestive heart or respiratory failure
- Hormone replacement therapy
- Malignancy
- Oral contraceptive therapy
- Paralytic stroke
- Pregnancy/postpartum
- Previous venous thromboembolism
- Thrombophilia

Weak Risk Factors (Odds Ratio < 2)

- Bed rest >3 d
- Immobility due to sitting (eg, prolonged car or air travel)
- Increasing age
- Laparoscopic surgery (eg, cholecystectomy)
- Obesity
- Pregnancy/antepartum
- Varicose veins

From Anderson Jr FA, Spencer FA. Risk factors for venous thromboembolism. Circulation. 2003;107:I9-16, with permission.

Reference:

1. Witkin AS, Channick RN. Deep venous thrombosis and pulmonary embolism in the intensive care unit. In: Wiener-Kronish JP, Bagchi A, Charnin JE, et al, eds. *Critical Care Handbook of the Massachusetts General Hospital.* 6th ed. Philadelphia: Wolters Kluwer; 2016:276-284.
2. Marino PL. Venous thromboembolism. In: *Marino's The ICU Book.* 4th ed. Philadelphia: Wolters Kluwer; 2014:97-122.
3. Hallman MR, Treggiari MM, Deem S. Critical care medicine. In: Barash PG, Cullen BF, Stoelting RK, et al, eds. *Clinical Anesthesia.* 7th ed. Philadelphia: Wolters Kluwer; 2013:1580-1610.

33. Correct answer: C

Early enteral nutrition in the ICU has been shown to reduce the risk of infection and mortality. Enteral nutrition promotes gut integrity, which provides a barrier to infection. Enteral nutrition is strongly preferred to parenteral nutrition, which carries risk of infection, hypertriglyceridemia, and liver dysfunction. Parenteral nutrition may be unavoidable in cases of severe malabsorption (eg, short gut syndrome).

The most recent ASPEN guidelines advocate strongly for early enteral feeding in the ICU within 24-48 hours of admission and address concerns related to enteral feeding. Initiation of enteral nutrition should not be delayed until there are clear "signs of contractility," namely bowel sounds, flatus, or stool. A postpyloric tube is not required for all patients receiving enteral nutrition but should be considered in patients at high risk for aspiration or with signs of gastric feeding intolerance. Guidelines recommend against routinely checking gastric residual volumes as a way to assess feeding tolerance. The head of the bed should be elevated to 30°-45° to reduce aspiration risk, and prokinetic agents, such as erythromycin and metoclopramide, could be considered in patients with feeding intolerance.

Reference:

1. McClave SA, Taylor BE, Martindale RG, et al. Guidelines for the Provision and Assessment of Nutrition Support Therapy in the Adult Critically Ill Patient: Society of Critical Care Medicine (SCCM) and American Society for Parenteral and Enteral Nutrition (A.S.P.E.N.). *J Parenter Enteral Nutr.* 2016;40(2):159-211.
2. Hallman MR, Treggiari MM, Deem S. Critical care medicine. In: Barash PG, Cullen BF, Stoelting RK, et al, eds. *Clinical Anesthesia.* 7th ed. Philadelphia: Wolters Kluwer; 2013:1580-1610.

34. Correct answer: B

Brain death is defined as the irreversible loss of brain function. The protocol for determining brain death is not universal across countries or even hospitals within the United States. However, some basic steps in diagnosing brain death include (1) identifying the etiology of coma, (2) ruling out potential confounders, and (3) clinical examination demonstrating absent consciousness (GCS 3) and brainstem reflexes, including apnea testing. Absence of brainstem reflexes is the key distinguishing factor between persistent vegetative state (absence of cerebral cortical functioning) and brain death.

Ruling out potential reversible causes of coma is essential in diagnosing brain death. Potential confounders include CNS depressant drugs and neuromuscular blocking agents, hypothermia (temperature must be greater than 36°C to declare brain death), and severe electrolyte, acid/base, or endocrine disorders. Cerebral hypoperfusion in the setting of hypotension can also confound a brain death examination; all brain death testing must therefore be conducted in the presence of normotension (SBP >100) using vasopressors if needed.

Motor function can be seen in brain dead patients and is attributed to spinal reflexes; spinal cord function is often preserved in brain death. For this reason, neuromuscular blockers are often required during organ procurement surgery.

Reference:

1. Shingu K, Nakao S. Brain death. In: Miller RD, Cohen NH, Eriksson LI, et al, eds. *Miller's Anesthesia.* 8th ed. Philadelphia; 2015:2307-2327.

35. **Correct answer: B**

In the United States, brain death can be determined based on clinical criteria alone; ancillary testing is not mandatory but recommended if the clinical examination is equivocal or cannot be completed (eg, hemodynamic instability develops during apnea testing). Brain death is confirmed when ancillary tests demonstrate absence of cerebral blood flow or neural activity. When intracranial pressure exceeds MAP, blood flow to the brain ceases. Absence of flow on 4-vessel cerebral angiography is considered the gold standard ancillary test because results are not susceptible to potential confounders such as medications and hypothermia. Other imaging options include CT angiography, single-photon emission computed tomography, transcranial Doppler ultrasound, and positron emission tomography.

Isoelectric EEG strongly supports a clinical diagnosis of brain death but—as any anesthesiologist knows—is subject to confounders such as CNS depressants and hypothermia. There are strict guidelines for EEG testing in brain death, including number and location of channels (using frontal leads alone would be inadequate). Evoked testing including brainstem auditory evoked potentials and somatosensory evoked potentials can be used as ancillary tests.

Imaging tests showing devastating neurologic injury with herniation are helpful in identifying the cause of coma but are not considered ancillary tests to determine brain death; ancillary tests must demonstrate lack of either cerebral blood flow or neuronal activity.

Reference:

1. Shingu K, Nakao S. Brain death. In: Miller RD, Cohen NH, Eriksson LI, et al, eds. *Miller's Anesthesia.* 8th ed. Philadelphia; 2015:2307-2327.

36. **Correct answer: E**

Brain death is defined as the *irreversible* loss of brain function. A determination of brain death therefore requires at least 2 clinical examinations at least 6 hours apart and performed by 2 separate physicians. Invasive ancillary testing such as cerebral angiography should not be performed unless a second brain death clinical examination has been attempted and the second examination is equivocal or cannot be completed. If the patient is declared brain dead and he is not going to be an organ donor, it is appropriate to withdraw ventilator support.

Reference:

1. Shingu K, Nakao S. Brain death. In: Miller RD, Cohen NH, Eriksson LI, et al, eds. *Miller's Anesthesia.* 8th ed. Philadelphia; 2015:2307-2327.

37. **Correct answer: C**

Sodium is the major plasma solute (recall serum osmolarity = Na × 2 + glucose/18 + BUN/2.3). Alcohols, sugars (including mannitol), and dyes will cause an increased osmolarity gap (measured – calculated osmolarity).

The first step in the work-up of hyponatremia is to check serum osmolarity. If serum osmolarity is normal or elevated, it is likely pseudohyponatremia because of the presence of solutes (eg, glucose, mannitol, alcohols) that draw water into the extracellular fluid, thereby causing dilutional hyponatremia. Serum sodium will normalize over several hours with clearance of the solute (in this case, excretion of mannitol). Treatment of pseudohyponatremia with hypertonic saline, diuretics, or fluid restriction is not indicated. If plasma sodium remains low several hours after mannitol, then further work-up of hyponatremia is indicated (repeat serum osmolarity, urine osmolarity, and urine sodium).

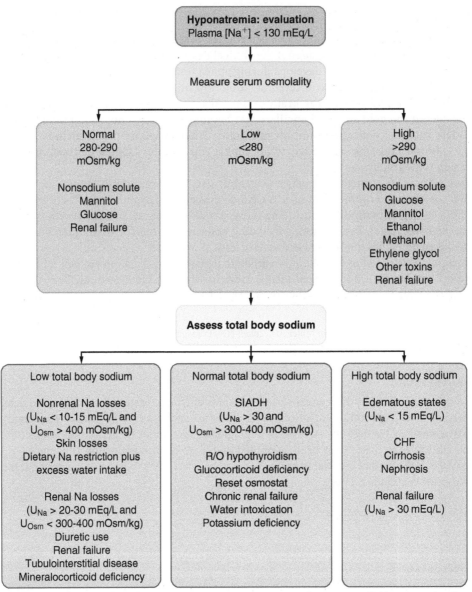

SIADH, syndrome of inappropriate antidiuretic hormone secretion; R/O, rule out; CHF, congestive heart failure. (From Prough DS, Funston JS, Svensén, Wolf SW. Fluids, electrolytes, and acid-base physiology. In: Barash PG, Cullen BF, Stoelting RK, et al, eds. *Clinical Anesthesia*. 7th ed. Philadelphia: Wolters Kluwer Health/Lippincott Williams & Wilkins; 2013:342, with permission.)

Reference:
1. Prough DS, Funston JS, Svensen CH, et al. Fluids, electrolytes and acid-base physiology. In: Barash PG, Cullen BF, Stoelting RK, et al, eds. *Clinical Anesthesia*. 7th ed. Philadelphia: Wolters Kluwer; 2013:327-361.

38. Correct answer: A

The most common electrolyte abnormality in hospitalized patients is hyponatremia (Na <130 mEq/L). The most feared complication of hyponatremia is cerebral edema, leading to coma and seizures. Cerebral edema is more likely in the setting of acute hyponatremia with rapid water shifts into cells and severe hyponatremia (Na <120 mEq/L).

Hyponatremia in the presence of serum hypo-osmolarity—"true hyponatremia"—has a wide differential, but in the postoperative setting it is most frequently due to SIADH or hypovolemia. SIADH can be caused by postoperative pain, anxiety and nausea, pulmonary and cerebral pathologies, and malignancy. Postoperative SIADH is usually not severe and not associated with neurologic symptoms.

It is important to distinguish SIADH (which is associated with euvolemia) from hypovolemic hyponatremia because the treatment is opposite (fluid restriction vs fluids). This requires urine studies (urine osmolarity and sodium) and careful clinical assessment of volume status. In both cases, urine osmolarity will be elevated (>400 mOsm/kg) because of free water uptake stimulated by ADH. In hypovolemic hyponatremia, urine sodium will be low (<10-15 mEq/L) because of the renin-angiotensin-aldosterone system stimulating urine sodium uptake. (The exception here is hypovolemic hyponatremia due to renal sodium losses, in which case urine Na is >20 mEq/L.) In SIADH, urine sodium is not low (>20 mEq/L).

This patient's urine studies are most consistent with SIADH with elevated urine osmolarity and sodium. His BUN/Cr ratio of 10 is also not consistent with hypovolemia. This patient has no neurologic injury that could be causing cerebral salt wasting (which is also associated with hypovolemia). Pseudohyponatremia is excluded by his low serum osmolarity. Mineralocorticoid deficiency is unlikely based on the absence of hyperkalemia.

Diagnostic Criteria for Syndrome of Inappropriate Antidiuretic Hormone Secretion

Hyponatremia with appropriately low plasma osmolality

Urinary osmolality greater than plasma osmolality

Renal sodium excretion >2 mmol/L

Absence of hypotension, hypovolemia, and edematous states

Normal renal and adrenal functions

Absence of drugs that directly influence renal water and sodium handling

Modified from Ball SG. Vasopressin and disorders of water balance: the physiology and pathophysiology of vasopressin. Ann Clin Biochem. *2007;44:417-431, with permission.*

References:
1. Prough DS, Funston JS, Svensen CH, et al. Fluids, electrolytes and acid-base physiology. In: Barash PG, Cullen BF, Stoelting RK, et al, eds. *Clinical Anesthesia.* 7th ed. Philadelphia: Wolters Kluwer; 2013:327-361.
2. Lai Y, Bagchi A. Fluids, electrolytes and acid-base management. In: Wiener-Kronish JP, Bagchi A, Charnin JE, et al, eds. *Critical Care Handbook of the Massachusetts General Hospital.* 6th ed. Philadelphia: Wolters Kluwer; 2016:113-134.

39. Correct answer: C

The first step in SIADH treatment is to remove sources of excess free water and treat any reversible causes (such as postoperative pain, anxiety, and nausea). A fluid bolus with normal saline is not indicated because this patient does not have evidence of hypovolemic hyponatremia as explained above. Giving normal saline (which has an osmolarity of 308 mOsm/L) would in fact worsen his hyponatremia because his urine osmolarity exceeds the osmolarity of normal saline, which means he would retain free water from the normal saline bolus. Salt tablets could be the next step in SIADH treatment if free water restriction fails.

Hypertonic saline (3% NaCl) is not indicated because his hyponatremia is mild and asymptomatic, but could be considered for correction of severe or symptomatic hyponatremia. If hypertonic saline is required, great care must be taken to not correct sodium too quickly, which can lead to the osmotic demyelination syndrome, particularly in patients with long-standing hyponatremia. Rate of sodium correction should not exceed 1-2 mEq/L per hour until sodium reaches 120 mEq/L; rate of correction should then be slowed to 0.5-1 mEq/L per hour. Vasopressin receptor antagonist (vaptans) would not be first line for mild asymptomatic hyponatremia in the postoperative setting (but could be considered for treatment of chronic hyponatremia).

References:
1. Prough DS, Funston JS, Svensen CH, et al. Fluids, electrolytes and acid-base physiology. In: Barash PG, Cullen BF, Stoelting RK, et al, eds. *Clinical Anesthesia.* 7th ed. Philadelphia: Wolters Kluwer; 2013:327-361.
2. Lai Y, Bagchi A. Fluids, electrolytes and acid-base management. In: Wiener-Kronish JP, Bagchi A, Charnin JE, et al, eds. *Critical Care Handbook of the Massachusetts General Hospital.* 6th ed. Philadelphia: Wolters Kluwer; 2016:113-134.

40. **Correct answer: E**

This patient is developing renal failure because of rhabdomyolysis. The ECG is highly concerning for hyperkalemia based on peaked T waves, loss of P wave, and prolonged QRS. An ECG concerning for hyperkalemia in the appropriate clinical setting (worsening oliguria and rhabdomyolysis in this case) is an emergency and warrants empiric treatment for hyperkalemia. The first step is to administer calcium chloride or gluconate to stabilize the myocardium. The second step is to give temporizing treatments that shift potassium into cells. This is usually accomplished with IV insulin and dextrose. β-Agonists and sodium bicarbonate could also be considered. These temporizing measures must be followed by treatment to lower total body potassium; furosemide is usually first line. If patients are hypovolemic, fluid can be given with furosemide. Dialysis should be initiated if medical management of hyperkalemia fails. Urgent magnesium administration would be indicated if the ECG showed torsades de pointes, which is not the case.

Increasing hyperkalemia is associated with progressive ECG changes:
Mild hyperkalemia (5.5-6.5 mEq/L): peaked T waves, prolonged PR
Moderate (6.5-8.0 mEq/L): disappearance of P wave, prolonged QRS, ST elevation, ectopy
Severe (>8.0 mEq/L): Sine wave, ventricular fibrillation, asystole

Severe Hyperkalemia[a] Treatment
Reverse Membrane Effects
Calcium (10 mL of 10% calcium chloride IV over 10 min)
Transfer extracellular [K^+] into cells
Glucose and insulin ($D_{10}W$ + 5-10 U regular insulin per 25-50 g glucose)
Sodium bicarbonate (50-100 mEq over 5-10 min)
β_2-Agonists
Remove potassium from body
Diuretics, proximal or loop
Potassium-exchange resins (sodium polystyrene sulfonate)
Hemodialysis
Monitor ECG and serum [K^+] level

[a]Potassium concentration ([K^+]) >7 mEq/L or electrocardiographic changes.
$D_{10}W$, 10% dextrose in water; ECG, electrocardiogram; IV, intravenous.
From Prough DS, Funston JS, Svensén, Wolf SW. Fluids, electrolytes, and acid-base physiology. In: Barash PG, Cullen BF, Stoelting RK, et al, eds. Clinical Anesthesia. 7th ed. Philadelphia: Wolters Kluwer Health/Lippincott Williams & Wilkins; 2013:342, with permission.

References:
1. Prough DS, Funston JS, Svensen CH, et al. Fluids, electrolytes and acid-base physiology. In: Barash PG, Cullen BF, Stoelting RK, et al, eds. *Clinical Anesthesia*. 7th ed. Philadelphia: Wolters Kluwer; 2013:327-361.
2. Lai Y, Bagchi A. Fluids, electrolytes and acid-base management. In: Wiener-Kronish JP, Bagchi A, Charnin JE, et al, eds. *Critical Care Handbook of the Massachusetts General Hospital*. 6th ed. Philadelphia: Wolters Kluwer; 2016:113-134.

41. **Correct answer: B**

This ECG is notable for a prolonged QT interval. The medication list should be examined for QT-prolonging medications (such as erythromycin), and hypocalcemia should be ruled out. Hypocalcemia can be caused by chelation, such as citrate toxicity during massive transfusion in the setting of liver failure and hyperphosphatemia in tumor lysis syndrome. Vitamin D deficiency leads to decreased calcium absorption from the gut and bone. Primary hyperparathyroidism would cause hypercalcemia, which would shorten the QT interval.

Symptoms of hypocalcemia include paresthesias of fingers, toes, and perioral area. Symptoms can progress to hypotension, muscle spasm (including laryngeal spasm), and mental status changes.

References:

1. Prough DS, Funston JS, Svensen CH, et al. Fluids, electrolytes and acid-base physiology. In: Barash PG, Cullen BF, Stoelting RK, et al, eds. *Clinical Anesthesia*. 7th ed. Philadelphia: Wolters Kluwer; 2013:327-361.
2. Lai Y, Bagchi A. Fluids, electrolytes and acid-base management. In: Wiener-Kronish JP, Bagchi A, Charnin JE, et al, eds. *Critical Care Handbook of the Massachusetts General Hospital*. 6th ed. Philadelphia: Wolters Kluwer; 2016:113-134.

42. Correct answer: B

This patient has severe hypophosphatemia and other electrolyte disturbances coinciding with initiation of nutrition, which is concerning for refeeding syndrome. His history of alcoholism and low serum albumin suggest he is chronically malnourished and puts him at high risk for refeeding syndrome. When refeeding syndrome is suspected, the first step is to temporarily stop feeding while aggressively repleting electrolytes.

Although exact criteria for refeeding syndrome have not been established, it can be broadly defined as severe electrolyte and fluid shifts following initiation of nutrition (most commonly hypophosphatemia, hypomagnesemia, and hypokalemia). Electrolyte depletion occurs due to sudden increased utilization. Clinical symptoms of refeeding syndrome include encephalopathy, heart failure, edema, respiratory failure, and arrhythmias. Refeeding syndrome typically begins within the first 72 hours after initiating nutrition. Malnourished patients are at high risk for refeeding syndrome; risk factors include alcoholism, anorexia nervosa, low BMI, and low prealbumin.

Enteral feeds should not be increased if refeeding syndrome is suspected. Electrolyte content can be adjusted when feeding is restarted, but electrolyte repletion should be given intravenously initially. Feeds should be restarted at a lower rate or calorie content. Hypophosphatemia can be seen in hyperparathyroidism, but refeeding syndrome is more likely in this scenario. This patient's calcium level is also not consistent with hyperparathyroidism. (Note: His corrected calcium level for low albumin is 8.5, which is normal.)

References:

1. Friedli N, Stanga Z, Sobotka L, et al. Revisiting the refeeding syndrome: results of a systematic review. *Nutrition*. 2017;35:151-160.
2. Kalman RI, Yeh DD. Nutrition in critical illness. In: Wiener-Kronish JP, Bagchi A, Charnin JE, et al, eds. *Critical Care Handbook of the Massachusetts General Hospital*. 6th ed. Philadelphia: Wolters Kluwer; 2016:154-163.

43. Correct answer: C

The cause of cardiac arrest in drowning is hypoxia until proven otherwise. Although chest compressions are usually the priority in CPR (C-A-B sequence), the A-B-C sequence should be used for drowning victims because cardiac arrest is most likely due to hypoxia. After 2 rescue breaths, perform a pulse check; if a pulse cannot be detected, chest compressions should be started, alternating with breaths.

An AED can be attached during CPR, but shockable rhythms are rare in drowning victims and this should not be the first move in resuscitation. Abnormal cardiac rhythm in drowning victims is almost always due to hypoxia and typically progresses from bradycardia to pulseless electrical activity (PEA) to asystole.

Drowning victims may also suffer from hypothermia. Wet clothes should be removed and external warming should be initiated. Although warming is important in resuscitation efforts, CPR is the first step. In cases of severe hypothermia (T <30°C) and cardiac arrest, the patient should be aggressively rewarmed, possibly with cardiopulmonary bypass. Resuscitation efforts should continue until the patient is warmed. Oral suctioning is appropriate; more aggressive efforts to expel swallowed water (eg, Heimlich) are not recommended because this can cause vomiting and aspiration.

References:

1. Vanden Hoek TL, Morrison LJ, Shuster M, et al. 2010 American Heart Association guidelines for cardiopulmonary resuscitation and emergency cardiovascular care. Part 12: cardiac arrest in special situations. *Circulation*. 2010;122(18 Suppl 3):S829-S861.
2. Szpilman D, Bierens JJ, Handley AJ, et al. Drowning. *N Engl J Med*. 2012;366(22):2102-2110.

44. Correct answer: D

Hypothermic drowning patients may have lower risk of neurologic injury, likely due to the effects of hypothermia in reducing cerebral oxygen consumption. Although warming is important in resuscitation efforts (resuscitation efforts should not be stopped until the patient is normothermic), therapeutic hypothermia should be considered in drowning victims with poor neurologic function post-ROSC.

Drowning victims may suffer from severe lung injury. Aspiration of water leads to loss of surfactant and alteration of the osmotic gradient across the alveolar-capillary membrane causing pulmonary edema, V/Q mismatch, atelectasis, and bronchospasm. Respiratory failure in drowning victims should be managed similar to ARDS with lung-protective ventilation. PEEP is encouraged for management of hypoxemia.

Pneumonia is actually uncommon in drowning victims; prophylactic antibiotics are therefore not recommended. Fluid restriction and diuretics have not been shown to be beneficial for treatment of pulmonary edema associated with drowning.

Reference:

1. Szpilman D, Bierens JJ, Handley AJ, et al. Drowning. *N Engl J Med*. 2012;366(22):2102-2110.

45. Correct answer: B

Acetaminophen (APAP) overdose accounts for nearly half of all cases of acute liver failure (ALF). Early symptoms of APAP overdose are nonspecific, including nausea, vomiting, and lethargy. Transaminases usually begin to rise after 24 hours. Signs of fulminant liver failure typically appear after 72-96 hours with massive transaminitis (possibly >10 000 IU/L), jaundice, encephalopathy, coagulopathy, lactic acidosis, and renal failure.

Early diagnosis of APAP overdose is essential, as early treatment with NAC can reduce the risk of ALF and death. APAP hepatotoxicity is caused by its metabolite N-acetyl-para-benzo-quinone imine (NAPQI). NAC contains a sulfhydryl group, which reduces NAPQI.

Immediate administration of NAC should be the first step in the management of any patient presenting with suspected APAP overdose of unknown quantity or timing. If the time of ingestion is known, APAP levels should be measured starting 4 hours postingestion and plotted on the Rumack-Matthew nomogram, which depicts time since ingestion versus APAP levels and indicates toxic levels and need for NAC administration. If the time of ingestion or quantity is unknown (as in this case), NAC should be given empirically. NAC should also be administered for late presentations when signs of ALF have appeared.

Gastrointestinal decontamination via activated charcoal is an option for early presentations of APAP overdose (usually within the first 4 h). Activated charcoal should not be the first step in this patient's management, as she is at increased risk of aspiration because of her altered mental status, and immediate NAC administration is potentially lifesaving. If this patient develops signs of ALF, she should be transferred to a liver transplant facility.

References:

1. Yoon E, Babar A, Choudhary M, et al. Acetaminophen-induced hepatotoxicity: a comprehensive update. *J Clin Transl Hepatol*. 2016;4(2):131-142.
2. Blackney K, Lee J. Drug overdose, poisoning, and adverse drug reactions. In: Wiener-Kronish JP, Bagchi A, Charnin JE, et al, eds. *Critical Care Handbook of the Massachusetts General Hospital*. 6th ed. Philadelphia: Wolters Kluwer; 2016:470-483.

46. Correct answer: D

The lethal APAP dose is estimated to be greater than 150 mg/kg (about 10 g in a 70-kg patient), although hepatotoxicity has been reported with lower doses. Although the dose of APAP and "time to NAC" are the most important determinants of APAP hepatotoxicity, several other risk factors for hepatotoxicity have been identified, including chronic alcohol use, chronic liver disease, advanced age, malnutrition, and certain medications, including herbals. The increased risk of hepatotoxicity in these cases is likely due to alterations in APAP metabolism.

APAP hepatotoxicity is due to production of a toxic metabolite, and alteration of APAP metabolism can increase the risk of hepatotoxicity. APAP metabolism is depicted in the figure below. The majority of APAP is metabolized by glucuronidation and sulfation to nontoxic metabolites. A small fraction is metabolized by CYP2E1 to the hepatotoxic metabolite NAPQI. NAPQI is reduced by glutathione to nontoxic metabolites. Upregulation of CYP2E1 or depletion of glutathione stores increases levels of NAPQI and the risk of hepatotoxicity.

Pregnancy is not known to increase the risk of APAP hepatotoxicity. Of note, APAP crosses the placenta, and therefore the fetus is at risk for hepatotoxicity in cases of maternal overdose.

The FDA recommends a maximum daily APAP dose of 4 g; however, this has been questioned recently, and some pharmaceutical companies now recommend a maximum daily dose of 3-3.25 g per day. Patients with chronic liver disease should limit APAP use to 2 g per day.

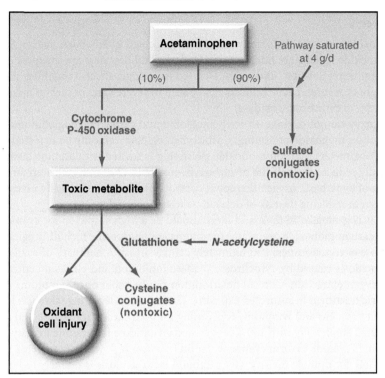

(From Marino PL. *Marino's The ICU Book*. 4th ed. Philadelphia: Wolters Kluwer Health/Lippincott Williams & Wilkins; 2014, with permission.)

Reference:
1. Yoon E, Babar A, Choudhary M, et al. Acetaminophen-induced hepatotoxicity: a comprehensive update. *J Clin Transl Hepatol.* 2016;4(2):131-142.

47. **Correct answer: C**

Fomepizole is indicated for the treatment of methanol and ethylene glycol poisoning. Methanol and ethylene glycol toxicity is due to their metabolism to toxic metabolites, beginning with alcohol dehydrogenase. These toxic metabolites inhibit cellular respiration, leading to severe metabolic acidosis, renal failure (ethylene glycol), and blindness (methanol). Fomepizole inhibits alcohol dehydrogenase, therefore reducing production of toxic metabolites. Dialysis is the definitive therapy to remove methanol and ethylene glycol. In contrast to methanol and ethylene glycol ingestions, treatment of ethanol intoxication is supportive, and fomepizole is not indicated.

Beta-blocker (BB) and calcium channel blocker (CCB) overdose causes bradycardia and cardiogenic shock (more so with nondihydropyridine CCBs verapamil and diltiazem compared with dihydropyridines). High-dose insulin infusions are effective in treating cardiogenic shock from both BB and CCB overdose through several proposed mechanisms, including increased myocardial glucose. IV dextrose should be started with insulin infusion. Glucagon is effective in BB overdose by bypassing β-receptors to increase cAMP production. Atropine can be given for bradycardia in BB and CBB overdose but unfortunately may not be very effective.

Tricyclic antidepressant overdose is treated with sodium bicarbonate. Sarin gas is an organophosphate that works by inhibiting acetylcholinesterase. The mainstay of organophosphate toxicity treatment is administration of anticholinergics, including atropine or glycopyrrolate.

References:
1. Graudins A, Lee HM, Druda D. Calcium channel antagonist and beta-blocker overdose: antidotes and adjunct therapies. *Br J Clin Pharmacol.* 2015;81(3):453-461.
2. King AM, Aaron CK. Organophosphate and carbamate poisoning. *Emerg Med Clin North Am.* 2015;33(1):133-151.
3. Blackney K, Lee J. Drug overdose, poisoning, and adverse drug reactions. In: Wiener-Kronish JP, Bagchi A, Charnin JE, et al, eds. *Critical Care Handbook of the Massachusetts General Hospital.* 6th ed. Philadelphia: Wolters Kluwer; 2016:470-483.

48. Correct answer: E

Carbon monoxide and cyanide toxicity should be suspected in any burn victim. Signs and symptoms of carbon monoxide toxicity are nonspecific. Headache and dizziness are the most common symptoms, followed by confusion, seizures, and coma. Delayed neurologic effects (cognitive, parkinsonism) can be seen after severe exposures. Lactic acidosis can be seen in severe cases of carbon monoxide toxicity and is due to inhibition of cytochrome oxidase.

Pulse oximetry cannot distinguish oxyhemoglobin and carboxyhemoglobin and is unreliable in assessing for carbon monoxide poisoning. Carboxyhemoglobin can only be detected by an 8-wavelength oximeter (CO-oximeter). Carbon monoxide poisoning is treated with administration of 100% oxygen, which markedly reduces the half-life of carboxyhemoglobin (320 min on room air vs 74 min on 100% Fio_2). The use of hyperbaric oxygen therapy is controversial; there is currently no evidence it is superior to 100% oxygen in reducing the risk of delayed neurologic sequelae.

Cyanide gas is generated in fires, and there should be a high suspicion for cyanide exposure in burn victims. Like carbon monoxide, signs and symptoms are nonspecific including agitation and tachypnea, followed by loss of consciousness and ultimately cardiac arrest. A hallmark of cyanide poisoning is profound lactic acidosis caused by cytochrome oxidase inhibition and elevated central venous saturation due to low oxygen extraction. Clinical deterioration can be rapid once symptoms appear necessitating prompt empiric treatment in suspected exposure. (Serum cyanide testing takes too long.)

This patient has signs and symptoms concerning for both carbon monoxide and cyanide toxicity. She should be treated empirically with 100% oxygen and an antidote for cyanide toxicity. Hydroxocobalamin (CyanoKit) binds cyanide to form cyanocobalamin (vitamin B_{12}), which is excreted in the urine. It is the first-line antidote for cyanide toxicity. Her profound lactic acidosis is unlikely to be explained by hypovolemia alone, and fluid boluses are unlikely to fully correct it. Intubation may be required, particularly if there are signs of smoke inhalation, but she appears to be ventilating well ($Paco_2$ 24), so immediate empiric treatment of cyanide and carbon monoxide toxicity is the priority.

References:

1. Blackney K, Lee J. Drug overdose, poisoning, and adverse drug reactions. In: Wiener-Kronish JP, Bagchi A, Charnin JE, et al, eds. *Critical Care Handbook of the Massachusetts General Hospital.* 6th ed. Philadelphia: Wolters Kluwer; 2016:470-483.
2. Marino PL. Nonpharmaceutical toxidromes. In: *Marino's The ICU Book.* 4th ed. Philadelphia: Wolters Kluwer; 2014:981-994.

49. Correct answer: A

This patient's presentation is concerning for organophosphate exposure. Organophosphates are found in pesticides, although the use has decreased in the United States per the Environmental Protection Agency. Organophosphates used as chemical weapons are called nerve agents and include tabun, sarin, and soman. Nerve agent exposure can occur via inhalation, skin exposure, or ingestion. Organophosphates inhibit acetylcholinesterase. Excessive stimulation of muscarinic receptors produces signs of parasympathetic stimulation: defecation, urination, miosis, bradycardia, bronchorrhea, bronchospasm, emesis, lacrimation, and salivation (mnemonic DUMBBBELS). It is important to remember that anticholinergic crisis can include signs of sympathetic stimulation due to activation of nicotinic receptors in the sympathetic ganglia. Stimulation of nicotinic receptors at the neuromuscular junction produces fasciculations and weakness progressing to paralysis (similar to succinylcholine). The signs of nicotinic stimulation can be remembered by the mnemonic "Monday-Tuesday-Wednesday-Thursday-Friday" (mydriasis-tachycardia-weakness-hypertension-fasciculations). CNS symptoms of organophosphate toxicity include headache, agitation, confusion, seizures, and coma. Death is usually caused by respiratory insufficiency (aspiration, bronchospasm, CNS depression, or weakness) or seizures.

Chlorine and phosgene gases cause respiratory failure resembling ARDS and are managed supportively. Cyanide can be aerosolized as used as a chemical weapon; its hallmark is severe lactic acidosis caused by inhibition of cytochrome oxidase. *Bacillus anthracis* is a gram-positive spore-producing bacillus (anthrax) that can be used as biologic weapon. Inhalation of anthrax spores is highly lethal and produces a flulike syndrome progressing to dyspnea, hemoptysis, and chest pain with widened mediastinum on chest X-ray.

References:

1. Murray MJ, et al. Emergency preparedness for and disaster management of casualties from natural disasters and chemical, biologic, radiologic, nuclear and high-yield explosive (CBRNE) events. In: *Clinical Anesthesia.* 7th ed. Philadelphia: Wolters Kluwer; 2013: 1535-1554.
2. King AM, Aaron CK. Organophosphate and carbamate poisoning. *Emerg Med Clin North Am.* 2015;33(1):133-151.

50. **Correct answer: C**

Severe organophosphate poisoning is a clinical diagnosis and should be treated empirically emergently (laboratory testing takes too long!). Decontamination is the first step, followed by antidotes. Atropine treats both CNS and peripheral muscarinic toxicity but is ineffective in treating symptoms resulting from nicotinic receptor stimulation (eg, weakness). Glycopyrrolate will only treat peripheral muscarinic effects and not treat CNS muscarinic symptoms but could be used if there is atropine shortage. Pralidoxime (2-PAM) reactivates anticholinesterase and therefore unlike antimuscarinics, it will also treat nicotinic effects including weakness. Benzodiazepines are the first-line antiepileptics for seizures occurring in setting of organophosphate poisoning.

Reference:

1. King AM, Aaron CK. Organophosphate and carbamate poisoning. *Emerg Med Clin North Am.* 2015;33(1):133-151.

25

ETHICS, PROFESSIONALISM AND PATIENT SAFETY

Aditi Balakrishnan

1. **Which of the following statements is false of anesthesiologists with chemical dependence?**

   A. 50% are younger than 35 years old.
   B. The most frequently abused drugs are nonopiate anesthetics.
   C. One-third of these individuals have a family history of addiction.
   D. Rates of chemical abuse among residents are higher than among attending anesthesiologists.
   E. One-third to one-half of individuals abuse multiple classes of drugs.

2. **Which of the following behaviors is *inconsistent* with an anesthesiologist with chemical dependence?**

   A. Withdrawal from friends and family
   B. Mood swings, with increased anger and hostility
   C. Calling in sick and avoiding call
   D. Requesting frequent bathroom breaks
   E. Signing out more narcotics than appropriate for given case

3. **After admission to a treatment center or facility to address chemical dependence, which of the following factors does NOT predispose a clinician to relapse?**

   A. Family history of substance abuse
   B. Main drug of abuse being a major opiate
   C. Having a coexisting psychiatric disorder
   D. Returning to practice in anesthesia
   E. No previous history of relapse

4. **Which of the following legal statutes provides protection for anesthesiologists as they age?**

   A. Age Discrimination Act
   B. Americans with Disabilities Act
   C. Equal Pay Act
   D. Medical and Family Leave Act
   E. Fair Labor Standards Act

5. **Which of the following statements is false about the Americans with Disabilities Act of 1990?**

    A. Reasonable accommodations for employees with disabilities are required.
    B. If a condition is episodic, it cannot be considered a disability under this act.
    C. Blindness, deafness, and mobility impairments are included.
    D. Conditions that often result in illegal activity (eg, kleptomania, pedophilia) are not covered.
    E. Mental health conditions (eg, posttraumatic stress disorder, obsessive-compulsive disorder, schizophrenia) may be considered under this act.

6. **The American Society of Anesthesiology Statement on Professionalism states that professionalism involves "the application of ethical principles...". Which of the following is not delineated in their guidelines for the Ethical Practice of Anesthesiology?**

    A. Anesthesiologists have ethical responsibilities to their patients.
    B. Anesthesiologists have ethical responsibilities to medical colleagues.
    C. Anesthesiologists have ethical responsibilities to the health care facilities in which they practice.
    D. Anesthesiologists have ethical responsibilities to their families.
    E. Anesthesiologists have ethical responsibilities to their community and to society.

7. **Which of the following test(s) need to be passed before an anesthesia provider can be considered licensed?**

    A. USMLE Steps 1, 2, and 3
    B. ABA BASIC
    C. ABA ADVANCED
    D. ABA APPLIED
    E. B, C, and D

8. **Which information is not collected in the National Practitioner Data Bank?**

    A. Malpractice payments
    B. License actions by medical boards
    C. Clinical privilege actions taken by hospitals or other health care bodies
    D. Participation in substance abuse rehabilitation
    E. Actions taken by the Drug Enforcement Agency

9. **You are a primary care physician caring for a 72-year-old woman with multiple comorbid illnesses. She asks you about creating a living will. Which of the following subjects would not usually be covered in this document?**

    A. Wishes regarding CPR
    B. Naming a health care proxy
    C. Nutritional support (tube feeding)
    D. Blood transfusions
    E. Respiratory support

10. **You are taking care of a 62-year-old man with early-onset dementia who has a subdural hematoma after a fall at home. After looking through his records, you discover he has a court-appointed guardian who is a different individual than his health care proxy. His brother, sister, wife, and children are in the waiting area. Which of the following people possesses the authority to provide consent for nonemergency procedures?**

    A. Court-appointed guardian
    B. Health care proxy/durable power of attorney for health care decisions
    C. Spouse
    D. Children
    E. Siblings

11. **Which of the following statements is false regarding the treatment of a Jehovah's Witness?**

   A. Some means of blood sequestration or preservation are allowed by some members of the faith.
   B. A physician may decline to care for such a patient.
   C. Individuals of this faith may differ in which blood products they refuse to receive.
   D. Parents of this faith may elect to prevent the use of blood products for their child.
   E. Discussions regarding blood product administration should be documented in detail in the chart.

12. **A 75-year-old man with stage IV lung cancer comes in for a rigid bronchoscopy with stenting. He has an existing DNR/DNI order in place. Which of the following is/are automatically allowed when he consents for general anesthesia?**

   A. Intubation
   B. Defibrillation
   C. Chest compressions
   D. All of the above
   E. None of the above

13. **Which of the following is an accepted reason by professional societies for an anesthesiologist to participate in executions?**

   A. Participation is a separate activity from routine clinical practice so should not be considered as part of one's normal clinical work.
   B. Being involved is "beneficent," in that one's involvement may facilitate a more humane death.
   C. Executions are legal, so participation by clinicians should not be limited.
   D. Anesthesiologists are most facile with some of the medications used, so they are obligated to ensure they are used appropriately.
   E. None of the above.

14. **You are an anesthesia resident on an acute pain rotation who stops by the coffee cart in the hospital lobby between consults. Your patient list falls out of your scrub pocket to the floor as you leave. The list is found shortly thereafter by an unrelated health care provider. You go back to look for it when you realize your mistake, but it is gone. Does this constitute a HIPAA (Health Insurance Portability and Accountability Act of 1996) violation, and what is the minimum fine given this situation?**

   A. $0 because it is not a violation
   B. $0 because it was an "unknowing" violation
   C. $100 because it was an "unknowing" violation
   D. $10 000 because it constitutes willful neglect
   E. $50 000 because the information was "knowingly" disclosed

15. **You are participating in data collection and analysis for a study to examine the efficacy of a new noninvasive cardiac output monitor. Which of the following is not a HIPAA compliant means of storing study data?**

   A. Hospital-encrypted flash drive
   B. Unencrypted flash drive in hospital-designated locked drawer
   C. Hospital-encrypted laptop
   D. Password-protected shareable Google spreadsheet
   E. Unencrypted laptop with deidentified data

16. **A 45-year-old woman is diagnosed with metastatic lung cancer. She declines chemotherapy and other interventions and opts instead for hospice care. Allowing the patient to decline all medical conditions upholds which of the following ethical principles?**

   A. Autonomy
   B. Justice
   C. Nonmaleficence
   D. Beneficence
   E. Integrity

17. An 86-year-old man with hypertension, chronic obstructive pulmonary disorder, and benign prostatic hyperplasia presents to the emergency department after slipping on a sidewalk during his morning walk. He is found to have a hip fracture and needs surgery. Which of the following diagnoses would rule out his capacity to give informed consent?

   A. Schizoaffective disorder
   B. Substance use disorder
   C. Alzheimer disease
   D. Depression
   E. None of the above

18. A 42-year-old man presents for liver transplantation. During the procedure, laboratory test results are checked, and ionized calcium is noted to be low. The anesthesia provider begins to administer calcium chloride but after giving 0.5 mL from the syringe realizes that he picked up epinephrine instead. The patient's blood pressure increases but is quickly controlled, and no harm comes to the patient. How is this event qualified?

   A. Preventable adverse event
   B. Ameliorable adverse event
   C. Adverse event due to negligence
   D. Near miss
   E. Error

19. According to closed claims analysis, which of the following is the most common site of peripheral nerve injury after anesthetic care?

   A. Brachial plexus
   B. Ulnar nerve
   C. Lumbosacral nerve root
   D. Common peroneal nerve
   E. Cervical nerve root

20. Which of the following is a commonly used means of identifying medication errors and resultant adverse events?

   A. Chart review
   B. Computerized monitoring
   C. Claims data
   D. Reporting systems
   E. All of the above

21. Which of the following does NOT qualify as a "sentinel event" that requires reporting to The Joint Commission?

   A. Wrong site surgery
   B. Suicide within 7 days of discharge from the hospital
   C. Hemolytic transfusion reaction due to administration of incorrect blood group
   D. Retained sponge after surgery
   E. Infant abduction

22. You are an anesthesia provider involved in commission of a medical error that results in harm to a patient. Which of the following is your next step?

   A. Ameliorate harm and say nothing to patient and family.
   B. Immediate full disclosure and apology to patient and family.
   C. Consult hospital liability group and risk manager, and/or administrator before moving forward with an apology.
   D. Retain a personal lawyer and say nothing to patient and family.
   E. Adjust medical record such that personal culpability is minimized.

23. **A resident places a radial arterial line before thoracotomy. Which of the following ACGME (Accreditation Council for Graduate Medical Education) competencies does this illustrate?**

   A. Patient care
   B. Medical knowledge
   C. Professionalism
   D. Interpersonal and communication skills
   E. Systems-based practice

24. **Within the ACGME "Milestones" framework of resident assessment, which "Level" is seen as the graduation target?**

   A. Level 1
   B. Level 2
   C. Level 3
   D. Level 4
   E. Level 5

25. **An anesthesia provider has achieved certification by the American Board of Anesthesiology (ABA). Which "Level" (Milestones framework) has the individual achieved and in which "core competency?"**

   A. Patient care, Level 3
   B. Medical knowledge, Level 5
   C. Practice-based learning, Level 4
   D. Interpersonal and communication skills, Level 5
   E. Systems-based practice, Level 3

Chapter 25 ▪ Answers

1. Correct answer: B

The most frequently abused agent for anesthesiologists entering a substance abuse treatment program was an opiate (76%-90%), with fentanyl and sufentanil as the most commonly abused medication. Other drugs, such as ketamine, propofol, nitrous oxide, lidocaine, sodium thiopental, and potent volatile agents, are also abused, albeit less frequently. The rate of alcohol abuse among anesthesiologists is similar to the general population.

The rest of the answer choices are true. It has been reported in numerous studies that addiction is common among anesthesia providers. The degree of this—and whether the incidence is truly higher within this specialty—varies between studies.

References:

1. Bryson EO, Silverstein JH. Addiction and substance abuse in anesthesiology. *Anesthesiology.* 2008;109(5):905-917.
2. Task Force on Chemical Dependence of the Committee on Occupational Health of Operating Room Personnel. *Chemical Dependence in Anesthesiologists: What You Need to Know When You Need to Know It.* Park Ridge, IL: American Society of Anesthesiologists; 1998.
3. Katz JD, Holzman RS. Occupational health. In: Barash PG, Cullen BF, Stoelting RK, et al., eds. *Clinical Anesthesia.* 7th ed. Philadelphia, PA: Wolters Kluwer Health; 2013:61-89.

2. Correct answer: C

Addicts often try to be close to their drug source. For those with dependency to narcotics available in the hospital, this means spending long hours in the hospital, even volunteering for additional call or spending time there when not working. In contrast, those with alcohol dependency may need to spend more time outside the hospital, in proximity to bars or their home.

Signs of Substance Abuse and Dependence

WHAT TO LOOK FOR OUTSIDE THE HOSPITAL

1. Addiction is a disease of loneliness and isolation. Addicts quickly withdraw from family, friends, and leisure activities.
2. Addicts have unusual changes in behavior, including wide mood swings and periods of depression, anger, and irritability alternating with periods of euphoria.
3. Unexplained overspending, legal problems, gambling, extramarital affairs, and increased problems at work are commonly seen in addicts.
4. An obvious physical sign of alcoholism is the frequent smell of alcohol on the breath.
5. Domestic strife, fights, and arguments may increase in number and intensity.
6. Sexual drive may significantly decrease.
7. Children may develop behavioral problems.
8. Some addicts frequently change jobs over a period of several years in an attempt to find a "geographic cure" for their disease or to hide it from coworkers.
9. Addicts need to be near their drug source. For a health care professional, this means long hours at the hospital, even when off duty. For alcoholics, it means calling in sick to work. Alcoholics may disappear without any explanation to bars or hiding places to drink secretly.
10. Addicts may suddenly develop the habit of locking themselves in the bathroom or other rooms while they are using drugs.
11. Addicts frequently hide pills, syringes, or alcohol bottles around the house.
12. Persons who inject drugs may leave bloody swabs and syringes containing blood-tinged liquid in conspicuous places.
13. Addicts may display evidence of withdrawal, especially diaphoresis (sweating) and tremors.
14. Narcotic addicts often have pinpoint pupils.
15. Weight loss and pale skin are also common signs of addiction.
16. Addicts may be seen injecting drugs.
17. Tragically, some addicts are found comatose or dead before any of these signs have been recognized by others.

WHAT TO LOOK FOR INSIDE THE HOSPITAL

1. Addicts sign out ever-increasing quantities of narcotics.
2. Addicts frequently have unusual changes in behavior, such as wide mood swings and periods of depression, anger, and irritability alternating with periods of euphoria.
3. Charting becomes increasingly sloppy and unreadable.
4. Addicts often sign out narcotics in inappropriately high doses for the operation being performed.
5. They refuse lunch and coffee relief.
6. Addicts like to work alone to use anesthetic techniques without narcotics, falsify records, and divert drugs for personal use.
7. They volunteer for extra cases, often where large amounts of narcotics are available (eg, cardiac cases).
8. They frequently relieve others.
9. They are often at the hospital when off duty, staying close to their drug supply to prevent withdrawal.
10. They volunteer frequently for extra call.
11. They are often difficult to find between cases, taking short naps after using.
12. Addicted anesthesia personnel may insist on personally administering narcotics in the recovery room.
13. Addicts make frequent requests for bathroom relief. This is usually where they use drugs.
14. Addicts may wear long-sleeved gowns to hide needle tracks and also to combat the subjective feeling of cold they experience when using narcotics.
15. Narcotic addicts often have pinpoint pupils.
16. An addict's patients may come into the recovery room complaining of pain out of proportion to the amount of narcotic charted on the anesthesia records.
17. Weight loss and pale skin are also common signs of addiction.
18. Addicts may be seen injecting drugs.
19. Untreated addicts are found comatose.
20. Undetected addicts are found dead.

Adapted from Farley WJ, Arnold WP. Videotape: Unmasking Addiction: Chemical Dependency in Anesthesiology. Produced by Davids Productions, Parsippany, NJ, funded by Janssen Pharmaceutica, Piscataway, NJ; 1991. Reprinted with permission from American Society of Anesthesiologists: Task Force on Chemical Dependence of the Committee on Occupational Health of Operating Room Personnel. Chemical Dependence in Anesthesiologists: What You Need to Know When You Need to Know It. Park Ridge, IL: American Society of Anesthesiologists; 1998.

References:
1. Bryson EO, Silverstein JH. Addiction and Substance abuse in Anesthesiology. *Anesthesiology.* 2008;109(5):905-917.
2. Katz JD, Holzman RS. Occupational health. In: Barash PG, Cullen BF, Stoelting RK, et al., eds. *Clinical Anesthesia.* 7th ed. Philadelphia, PA: Wolters Kluwer Health; 2013:61-89.

3. Correct answer: E

One small retrospective study of health care professionals identified an overall relapse rate of 25% among those undergoing treatment. The hazard ratio with family history of substance abuse was 2.3, and use of a "major opiate" (ie, injecting fentanyl versus using oral oxycodone) in the setting of a coexisting psychiatric disorder corresponded to a hazard ratio of 5.8. When all 3 were present, the hazard ratio was 13.3 , indicating that patients with all three risk factors have a risk of relapsing 13.3 times higher than if they did not have these risk factors. Hazard ratio for anesthesiologists who returned to practice was 8.5 when compared with those who did not return to practice. Previous relapse was also shown to increase the incidence of future relapse.

In general, physicians with chemical dependency should be referred to a state-affiliated physician's health program where they can begin inpatient treatment, which later transitions to outpatient therapy. Overall relapse rates in the general population approach 60%; there is some evidence that because physicians are highly motivated, these rates may be better, with some studies suggesting rates around 40% for anesthesiologists (roughly equivalent to other physicians) and sustained recovery >2 years around 80%. However, there was another study that demonstrated a relapse rate of 66% among anesthesia residents, with a 17% over dose or death rate. Another study (by Collins et al) demonstrated that 46% of anesthesia residents completed their training after treatment (9 of these 100 died), 34% entered a program in another specialty, and 16% left medicine. There is a paucity of clear "guidelines" with regard to the safest reentry path, but it may be that returning to another specialty may be safer for those physicians.

References:
1. Domino KB, Hornebin TF, Polissar NL, et al. Risk factors for relapse in health care professionals with substance use disorders. *JAMA.* 2005;293(12):1453-1460. doi:10.1001/jama.293.12.1453.
2. Katz JD, Holzman RS. Occupational health. In: Barash PG, Cullen BF, Stoelting RK, et al., eds. *Clinical Anesthesia.* 7th ed. Philadelphia, PA: Wolters Kluwer Health; 2013:61-89.

4. **Correct answer: A**

The Age Discrimination in Employment Act of 1967 forbids employment discrimination against anyone over the age of 40 years; this also applies to the standards of pensions and benefits provided by employers. At present, no specific regulations exist with regard to the age of an anesthesiologist and his/her licensure. Retiring occurs largely at the discretion of the anesthesiologist and his/her self-evaluation.

The Americans with Disabilities Act of 1990 prohibits discrimination based on disability. Mental and physical medical conditions are covered by this act; these conditions do not need to be severe or permanent to qualify. Although several age-related comorbidities may qualify, age itself is not covered by this act.

The Equal Pay Act of 1963 prohibits employers from discriminating based on gender in determining pay for jobs that require equal skill, effort, and responsibility unless based on seniority, merit, quality metrics, or other non–gender-based differentials.

The Medical and Family Leave Act of 1993 requires employers to provide employees with job-protected and unpaid leave for qualifying medical and family reasons, including personal/family illness, family military leave, pregnancy, adoption, or foster care placement of a child.

The Fair Labor Standards Act of 1938 created the 40-hour work week (along with the concept of overtime pay in certain jobs), established a national minimum wage, and prohibited most child labor; in its initial form, it applied to employees engaged in interstate commerce primarily.

References:

1. *Age Discrimination in Employment Act of 1967, 29 U.S.C. § 621 to 29 U.S.C. § 634.*
2. *Americans with Disabilities Act of 1990, Pub. L. 101-336. 104 Stat. 327, codified as amended at 42 U.S.C. § 12101.*
3. *Equal Pay Act of 1963, Pub. L. 88-38. 77 Stat. 56, codified as amended at 29 U.S.C. § 206.*
4. *Medical and Family Leave Act of 1993, Pub. L 103-3. 107 Stat. 6.*
5. *Fair Labor Standards Act of 1938, Pub. L 75-718. 29 U.S.C. Ch. 8.*
6. Katz JD, Holzman RS. Occupational health. In: Barash PG, Cullen BF, Stoelting RK, et al., eds. *Clinical Anesthesia.* 7th ed. Philadelphia, PA: Wolters Kluwer Health; 2013:61-89.

5. **Correct answer: B**

The Americans with Disabilities Act of 1990 prohibits discrimination based on disability. "Episodic" conditions can be considered disabilities based on what the person's symptoms would be in the absence of "mitigating measures." An example of an episodic condition that could qualify for protection under this act is substance dependence. The rest of the answer choices are true. This act provides protection for a wide array of physical or mental medical conditions. Those conditions that often result in illegal activity are not covered so as to avoid abuse of the law.

References:

1. *Americans with Disabilities Act of 1990, Pub. L. 101-336. 104 Stat. 327, codified as amended at 42 U.S.C. § 12101.*
2. Katz JD, Holzman RS. Occupational health. In: Barash PG, Cullen BF, Stoelting RK, et al., eds. *Clinical Anesthesia.* 7th ed. Philadelphia, PA: Wolters Kluwer Health; 2013:61-89.

6. **Correct answer: D**

The ASA's Guidelines for the Ethical Practice of Anesthesiology spells out guidelines for professional behavior under each of those categories except for D; the one additional category that is described is an ethical responsibility to oneself. The guidelines also include the American Medical Association's 2001 Principles of Medial Ethics, which include such similar standard, including providing care with "compassion and respect for human dignity and rights," maintaining "a commitment to medical education," and supporting "access to medical care for all people."

References:

1. *Guidelines for the Ethical Practice of Anesthesiology.* 2013. Retrieved from: https://www.asahq.org/~/media/sites/asahq/files/public/resources/standards-guidelines/guidelines-for-the-ethical-practice-of-anesthesiology.pdf?la=en.
2. *Statement on professionalism.* 2014. Retrieved from: https://www.asahq.org/resources/~/media/Sites/ASAHQ/Files/Public/Resources/standards-guidelines/statement-on-professionalism.pdf.

7. **Correct answer: A**

The designation of "licensing" in the United States requires passing the USMLE (United States Medical Licensing Examination) or COMLEX (Comprehensive Osteopathic Medical Licensing Examination). States also may have licensing requirements, which generally involve proof of passing these tests and other proof of credentials. The American Board of Anesthesia examinations are necessary to become certified as an anesthesiologist. Maintenance of Certification requires taking the MOCA (Maintenance of Certification in Anesthesia) examinations at prespecified intervals. Individual hospitals and other care institutions also have standards for granting clinical privileges to care providers that may be individually determined. These credentialing processes are geared toward upholding a certain standard of clinical acumen among providers and ensuring that incompetent individuals or criminal/deviant providers cannot practice.

References:

1. Eichhorn JH, Grider JS. Scope of practice. In: Barash PG, Cullen BF, Stoelting RK, et al., eds. *Clinical Anesthesia.* 7th ed. Philadelphia: Wolters Kluwer Health; 2013:28-60.
2. n.d. Retrieved from: http://www.theaba.org/.

8. Correct answer: D

The National Practitioner Data Bank is a nationwide system that helps licensing organizations and health care entities keep track of information that might reflect negative performance on the part of a physician. The National Practitioner Data Bank was created by Congress to help promote quality of physicians and protect the public from providers who would relocate from state to state to avoid issues with local licensing due to poor outcomes.

Health care organizations are obligated to make reports to and inquiries of the Data Bank when dealing with current or prospective employees. Answer choices A-C, E, and Medicare/Medicaid exclusions are all required inputs to the Data Bank. Unless a physician's substance abuse resulted in one of those issues, it would not in and of itself be flagged in the Data Bank. If a report is submitted, the physician is alerted to be able to verify or dispute the veracity of the claim.

The general public cannot access the Data Bank but can be provided to hospitals, health care organizations, licensing and certification boards, and organizations that administer federal or state health care programs. Individual practitioners also have the ability to access their own records.

References:

1. Posner KL, Adeogba S, Domino KB. Anesthetic risk, quality improvement and liability. In: Barash PG, Cullen BF, Stoelting RK, et al., eds. *Clinical Anesthesia.* 7th ed. Philadelphia, PA: Wolters Kluwer Health; 2013:90-103.
2. n.d. Retrieved from: https://www.npdb.hrsa.gov/index.jsp.

9. Correct answer: B

Living wills are legal documents created by patients before becoming incapacitated to express what their goals and preferences for care would be—including the refusal of life-sustaining treatment—in the event that they are not able to communicate these wishes themselves. These documents do not automatically determine a health care proxy or power of attorney; however, in some states, the paperwork is combined. The term "advance directive" encompasses both living wills and documents that describe naming a health care proxy or durable power of attorney.

References:

1. Living Wills, Health Care Proxies, Advance Health Care Directives. n.d. Retrieved from: http://www.americanbar.org/groups/ real_property_trust_estate/resources/estate_planning/living_wills_health_care_proxies_advance_health_care_directives.html.
2. Posner KL, Adeogba S, Domino KB. Anesthetic risk, quality improvement and liability. In: Barash PG, Cullen BF, Stoelting RK, et al., eds. *Clinical Anesthesia.* 7th ed. Philadelphia, PA: Wolters Kluwer Health; 2013:90-103.

10. Correct answer: A

When a court-appointed guardian exists, his/her authority supersedes all others in terms of making a decision for a patient. Next, a health care proxy—a person named by the patient to make medical decisions in their stead—carries the most weight. After this, most states have a predetermined hierarchy of family members who should serve as decision makers for a patient. The spouse is generally first in order; however, if the spouse is deceased or incapacitated, a patient's children are usually next. If they are not in agreement, or if they do not exist, the parents and then the siblings of a patient are next in line. Some states also specifically prioritize grandchildren, other living relatives, close friends, and some will give decision-making authority to the treating physicians. If none of these individuals exists or no consensus can be reached, the courts will usually appoint someone.

These decision makers are charged with acting in "substituted judgment" for the patient, meaning that they are supposed to determine what the patient would have wanted and act on that preference. This is meant to help preserve patient's autonomy. Of note, this standard is considered somewhat controversial, and some have argued that an alternative standard such as acting in the patient's "best interests" may be more consistent with the goal of autonomy.

References:

1. Default Surrogate Consent Statutes. 2016. Retrieved from: http://www.americanbar.org/content/dam/aba/administrative/law_aging/2014_default_surrogate_consent_statutes.authcheckdam.pdf.
2. Torke AM, Alexander GC, Lantos J. Substituted judgment: the limitations of autonomy in surrogate decision making. *J Gen Intern Med*. 2008;23(9):1514-1517. doi:10.1007/s11606-008-0688-8.

11. Correct answer: D

Jehovah's Witnesses have a religious doctrine with stated implications regarding that transfusion of blood or blood products into their body will preclude them from a blessed afterlife. However, as with any faith-based tenet, there are multiple interpretations of an edict, so individuals may differ in whether they are willing to accept certain types of products (eg, albumin) or blood that has exited their body but has remained in continuity with it through tubing (eg, cell saver). Having explicit and thoroughly documented conversations with patients about their specific allowances before surgery is very important to preserve patient autonomy and ensure medicolegal protection. Should a provider feel that they are hindered in their ability to provide safe and effective care in an elective situation, they are not obligated to do so. Although there is ample support in case law to allow adult patients the freedom to refuse blood products, parents cannot make this decision for minors. A court order is often needed to facilitate transfusion in these circumstances.

Reference:

1. Posner KL, Adeogba S, Domino KB. Anesthetic risk, quality improvement and liability. In: Barash PG, Cullen BF, Stoelting RK, et al., eds. *Clinical Anesthesia*. 7th ed. Philadelphia, PA: Wolters Kluwer Health; 2013:90-103.

12. Correct answer: E

Although many practitioners believe that consent for anesthesia automatically suspends DNR orders, this is not the case. Practice guidelines by multiple bodies (including the ASA) recommend strongly that careful reconsideration and discussion of those orders in the perioperative period is undertaken.

ASA guidelines describe reviewing the patient's directive in advance and modifying the plan based on the patient's preferences. They describe 3 levels of resuscitative efforts that may be appropriate based on the patient's wishes. Full Attempt at Resuscitation would fully suspend the DNR order and allow all involved procedures. Limited Attempt at Resuscitation Defined with Regard to Specific Procedures would more granularly define which procedures would and would not be acceptable (eg, compressions vs defibrillation vs intubation) based on which procedures may or may not be essential to the success of anesthesia. Limited Attempt at Resuscitation Defined with Regard to the Patient's Goals and Values would allow the anesthesia and surgical team to use clinical judgment in determining which efforts would be in line with furthering the patient's values.

Duration of suspension should also be clarified in advance, be it for the immediate perioperative period (eg, discharge from recovery) or the entire perioperative period (when the patient has "fully recovered" from a procedure at a later date).

References:

1. Posner KL, Adeogba S, Domino KB. Anesthetic risk, quality improvement and liability. In: Barash PG, Cullen BF, Stoelting RK, et al., eds. *Clinical Anesthesia*. 7th ed. Philadelphia, PA: Wolters Kluwer Health; 2013:90-103.
2. *Ethical Guidelines for the Anesthesia Care of Patients with Do-Not-Resuscitate Orders or Other Directives that Limit Treatment*. 2013. Retrieved from: http://www.asahq.org/~/media/Sites/ASAHQ/Files/Public/Resources/standards-guidelines/ethical-guidelines-for-the-anesthesia-care-of-patients.pdf.

13. Correct answer: E

The ASA's Statement on Physician Nonparticipation in Legally Authorized Executions states that "Although lethal injection mimics certain technical aspects of the practice of anesthesia, *capital punishment in any form is not the practice of medicine*" and "strongly discourages participation by anesthesiologists in executions." Meanwhile, the ABA has stated that "an anesthesiologist should not participate in an execution by lethal injection and that violation of this policy is inconsistent with the Professional Standing criteria required for ABA Certification and Maintenance of Certification in Anesthesiology or any of its subspecialties. As a consequence, ABA certificates may be revoked if the ABA determines that a diplomate participates in an execution by lethal injection. What constitutes participation is clearly defined by the AMA's policy."

References:
1. American Board of Anesthesiology Professional Standing Policy. *Anesthesiologists and Capital Punishment.*
2. *American Medical Association Code of Medical Ethics, Opinion E-2.06-Capital Punishment.* 2000. Retrieved from: https://www.ama-assn.org/delivering-care/ama-code-medical-ethics.
3. *Statement on Physician Nonparticipation in Legally Authorized Executions.* 2016. From: https://www.asahq.org/resources/~/media/Sites/ASAHQ/Files/Public/Resources/standards-guidelines/statement-on-physician-nonparticipation-in-legally-authorized-executions.pdf.

14. Correct answer: C

The Health Insurance Portability and Accountability Act was created in 1996 to both protect health insurance coverage when individuals lose or change jobs and create standards for privacy and electronic health care transactions. Providers more commonly focus on this second issue, with upholding privacy standards being the most relevant to day-to-day life.

This example does violate HIPAA, given that multiple of the 18 HIPAA identifiers that comprise personally identifiable information (and are thus part of protected health information, or PHI) are likely present on this patient list. These identifiers include pieces of information such as name, address, all elements of dates related to individual (birth date, admission/discharge date, death date), telephone numbers, email address, SSN, medical record number, and photographic image.

Should HIPAA noncompliance be deemed to be present and not satisfactorily resolved, the Office for Civil Rights within the Department of Justice can choose to impose civil money penalties. Criminal violations (which generally comprise those instances in which information was knowingly or maliciously obtained or disclosed) are handled by the DOJ.

With regard to civil penalties, an "unknowing" violation is subject to a minimum fine of $100 per violation, with an annual maximum of $25 000 for repeat violations. "Reasonable Cause" violations are subject to a minimum fine of $1000 per violation, with an annual maximum of $100 000 for repeat offenses. Willful neglect that is corrected within 30 days is subject to a minimum fine of $10 000, with an annual maximum of $250 000 for repeat offenses. Willful neglect that is not corrected is subject to a minimum fine of $50 000, with an annual maximum of $1.5 million for repeat offenses. All of these types of violations can be subject to a maximum fine of $50 000 per violation, with an annual maximum of $1.5 million if so decided by the state's attorney general.

Criminal penalties tend to be higher and include prison time. Those who "knowingly" obtain/disclose PHI can face a $50 000 fine and 1 year imprisonment; "false pretenses" bump this to $100 000, with 5 years in prison; and the intent to sell, transfer, or use PHI for commercial advantage, personal gain, or malicious harm increases these penalties to $250 000 and 10 years in prison.

References:
1. Health Information Privacy. 2015. Retrieved from: https://www.hhs.gov/hipaa/.
2. *HIPAA Violations & Enforcement.* n.d. Retrieved from: https://www.ama-assn.org/practice-management/hipaa-violations-enforcement.

15. Correct answer: D

Password protection in itself is not sufficient enough to uphold the standards of data protection, especially when the server on which information is being stored may not be compliant with the security rule of the Health Insurance Portability and Accessibility Act.

Data security standards apply to a collection of information that contains any of the 18 patient identifiers that comprise PHI as set out by HIPAA: name, address, all elements of dates related to an individual (birth date, admission/discharge date, death date, exact age if above 89 y), telephone number, fax number, email address, social security number, medical record number, health plan beneficiary number, account number, certificate or license number, any vehicle or device serial number, web URL, IP address, finger/voice print, photographic image, and any other characteristics that could uniquely identify the individual.

The security rule comprises 3 parts: technical safeguards, physical safeguards, and administrative safeguards, all of which have implementation specifications. Much of this applies more to organizing the larger health system, but the principles have relevance to what individual practitioners do as well.

With regard to technical safeguards, required standards are related to access control (eg, unique user identification), audit control (monitoring access), data integrity (monitoring manipulation of PHI), user authentication, and transmission security. With regard to physical safeguards, standards are related to facility access, workstation use, workstation security, and device/media controls (disposal of devices, data storage on devices, reuse of devices). With regard to administrative safeguards, standards include rigorous security management processes, assigning security responsibility, creating workforce security systems, maintaining information access management systems, creating security awareness and training, creating security incident procedures, having contingency plans for violations, evaluation of institutional standards, and maintaining appropriate contracts with business associates who may have access to PHI.

Reference:

1. Secretary HO, (OCR) OF. 2013. *Summary of the HIPAA Security Rule*. Retrieved from: https://www.hhs.gov/hipaa/for-professionals/security/laws-regulations/.

16. Correct answer: A

Philosophers Tom Beauchamp and James Childress outlined what is now the most common framework for medical ethics utilized in our health system—the "four principles"—in their textbook *Principles of Biomedical Ethics*. First among these values is respect for a patient's autonomy; this means that a patient has the right to agree to or refuse any given treatment. In the case of the example above, this is the value being upheld by respecting her decision. Justice is the requirement of fairness and equality in determining who gets what in a world of scarce resources. Beneficence requires that a provider act in the best interest of a patient. Nonmaleficence essentially means "do no harm." Integrity is not one of the 4 principles that commonly guide medical ethics in this framework.

These principles play a major role in the process of informed consent, which requires balancing a patient's autonomy with the provider's goal of beneficence and nonmaleficence.

Reference:

1. Beauchamp TL, Childress JF. *Principles of Biomedical Ethics*. New York: Oxford University; 1983.

17. Correct answer: E

A psychiatric or neurologic diagnosis cannot determine whether or not an individual has capacity to make an informed decision. Capacity requires 4 decision-making abilities be present; if present, even when a comorbid diagnosis exists, the individual has capacity. These 4 abilities are understanding the substance of information (often options for treatment) that is presented to them, appreciating how the information applies to them, reasoning through the presented options, and expressing a clear and consistent choice.

Reference:

1. Grisso T, Appelbaum PS, Mulvey EP, Fletcher K. The MacArthur Treatment Competence Study. II: Measures of abilities related to competence to consent to treatment. *Law Hum Behav*. 1995;19(2):127-148.

18. Correct answer: D

A near miss is defined as exposure to a dangerous situation that does not result in harm to the patient as a result of early detection or circumstance, here given that the patient did not have a negative outcome as a result of the mistake. An error is another term to describe a situation that does not result in harm; an error is a broader term that refers to either a commission (doing an incorrect thing) or omission (failure to do a correct thing) that exposes a patient to potential harm. An adverse event is a situation in the course of care that does result in harm. Preventable adverse events are defined as those that happened because accepted strategies for prevention were not used. Ameliorable adverse events are those that were not preventable but could have been less harmful with different care. Adverse events due to negligence are those that happened in the setting of lower than standard-of-care practice.

Reference:

1. *Adverse Events, Near Misses, and Errors*. n.d. Retrieved from: https://psnet.ahrq.gov/primers/primer/34/adverse-events-near-misses-and-errors.

19. **Correct answer: B**

Nerve injury is a common cause of malpractice claims in anesthesia. Ulnar neuropathy is the most frequently cited injury. The incidence of ulnar neuropathy has been estimated at 3.7-50 per 10 000 patients; in contrast, lower-extremity neuropathy after lithotomy positioning has been noted in 2.7 of 10 000 patients. Males, obese patients, preexisting ulnar nerve dysfunction, and long hospitalization have been found to be risk factors for development of this as well.

References:
1. Cheney FW, Domino KB, Caplan RA, Posner KL. Nerve injury associated with anesthesia. *Anesthesiology.* 1999;90(4): 1062-1069.
2. Posner KL, Adeogba S, Domino KB. Anesthetic risk, quality improvement and liability. In: Barash PG, Cullen BF, Stoelting RK, et al., eds. *Clinical Anesthesia.* 7th ed. Philadelphia, PA: Wolters Kluwer Health; 2013:90-103.
3. Warner MA, Warner DO, Matsumoto JY, Harper MC, Schroeder DR, Maxson PM. Ulnar neuropathy in surgical patients. *Anesthesiology.* 1999;90(1):54-59.

20. **Correct answer: E**

The National Coordinating Council for Medication Error Reporting and Prevention defines medication error as "any preventable event that may cause or lead to inappropriate medication use or patient harm while the medication is in the control of the health care professional, patient, or consumer. Such events may be related to professional practice, health care products, procedures, and systems, including prescribing, order communication, product labeling, packaging, and nomenclature, compounding, dispensing, distribution, administration, education, monitoring, and use."

In the current clinical system, detecting medication errors and resultant adverse events tends to occur in the following ways: retrospective chart review, computerized monitoring (generally by pharmacists), analysis of administrative databases, looking at claims data, direct observation of medication administration, reporting systems (voluntary and mandatory), and patient surveys/monitoring.

Each of these means of detecting errors comes with its own limitations with regard to timeliness of error detection and required resource commitment. Designing a system to encourage a safety culture likely requires using multiple of these methods simultaneously to identify errors and then be able to address them.

When errors are identified, one way to improve the systems that allowed the error is a process called a clinical audit. This is a quality improvement activity that uses the "Plan-Do-Study-Act" (PDSA) system devised by Edwards Deming. An audit should aim to identify the underlying problem, define "best practice" protocols, determine means of assessing performance when compared with those standards, and plan ways to bridge those gaps. These are generally interdisciplinary processes that may require multiple cycles to achieve desired effect.

References:
1. Montesi G, Lechi A. Prevention of medication errors: detection and audit. *Br J Clin Pharmacol.* 2009;67(6):651-655.
2. *About Medication Errors.* 2015. Retrieved from: http://www.nccmerp.org/about-medication-errors.

21. **Correct answer: B**

A sentinel event is defined as any unexpected outcome involving death or serious physical or psychologic injury or risk thereof. In order for patient suicide to qualify as a sentinel event, it must occur within 72 hours of discharge from the hospital.

When these events occur, The Joint Commission requires a "root cause analysis" to be undertaken. This type of analysis requires that the events surrounding the error be deconstructed to identify any and all systematic problems that lead to the error. The Joint Commission publishes a sentinel event alert to promote learning from these experiences and avoid similar errors.

Reference:
1. Posner KL, Adeogba S, Domino KB. Anesthetic risk, quality improvement and liability. In: Barash PG, Cullen BF, Stoelting RK, et al., eds. *Clinical Anesthesia.* 7th ed. Philadelphia, PA: Wolters Kluwer Health; 2013:90-103.

22. **Correct answer: C**

When a serious adverse event occurs, it can be difficult for both the affected patient/family and the anesthesia provider involved. Disclosure of error and apology for said error is becoming increasingly supported, with some states adopting "I'm sorry!" legislation to limit explanation or the apology from being used as part of a malpractice suit to encourage disclosure after such an event. However, there remain medicolegal and administrative ramifications of immediate full disclosure, particularly when information about what occurred may be limited. As a result, it is important for individual practitioners to ensure that they have the appropriate support to undertake such an explanation and apology.

The anesthesia patient safety foundation has created an adverse event protocol to help guide practitioners. Their "Basic Plan" prescribes (1) getting help during the acute event, (2) continuing patient care, (3) designating an "Incident Supervisor" to oversee the event, appropriately manage resources, and ensure that the equipment involved is not altered so that relevant inspection can be undertaken if necessary to determine the cause of the event, (4) contacting administrators, risk managers, insurance company, attorneys if needed, (5) arranging for support for patient/family and sharing as much information as possible and deemed appropriate based on conversations with groups mentioned in 4, (6) designating a follow-up supervisor to ensure appropriate reporting and investigation is completed, (7) documentation of the event in as much detail as possible, (8) reviewing formal reports created by the institution, and (9) continuing involvement as needed.

References:
1. Posner KL, Adeogba S, Domino KB. Anesthetic risk, quality improvement and liability. In: Barash PG, Cullen BF, Stoelting RK, et al., eds. *Clinical Anesthesia*. 7th ed. Philadelphia, PA: Wolters Kluwer Health; 2013:90-103.
2. Eichhorn JH. *Adverse Event Protocol*. 2015. Retrieved from: http://apsf.org/resources_safety_protocol.php.

23. **Correct answer: A**

This is an example of a competency in patient care. The ACGME started an initiative in the 1998 to focus residency training on a competency-based model called the Outcome Project.

Six core competencies were identified: patient care (providing compassionate, appropriate, effective treatment), medical knowledge (knowledge about established and evolving biomedical, clinical, and epidemiologic/social-behavioral sciences, and application of this knowledge), practice-based learning and improvement (investigating/evaluating their practices and improving such practices based on scientific evidence), interpersonal and communication skills (having the ability to effectively exchange information with patients, families, and team members), professionalism (commitment to professional responsibilities, ethical principles, and treatment of a diverse patient population), and systems-based practice (being aware of and able to respond to the larger context of the health care system and providing high-value care).

Reference:
1. Swing SR. The ACGME outcome project: retrospective and prospective. *Med Teach*. 2007;29(7):648-654.

24. **Correct answer: D**

The ACGME developed specialty-specific outcomes-based milestones as a means of assessing performance within the 6 core competencies previously described. Programs can use the milestones in a semiannual review of resident performance to report to the ACGME about resident progress. Per the ACGME's anesthesia-specific milestone document, the levels are defined as follows:

Level 1: The resident demonstrates milestones expected of a resident who has completed one postgraduate year of education in either an integrated anesthesiology program or another preliminary education year prior to entering the CA1 year in anesthesiology.
Level 2: The resident demonstrates milestones expected of a resident in anesthesiology residency prior to significant experience in the subspecialties of anesthesiology.
Level 3: The resident demonstrates milestones expected of a resident after having experience in the subspecialties of anesthesiology.
Level 4: The resident substantially fulfills the milestones expected of an anesthesiology residency, and is ready to transition to independent practice. This level is designed as the graduation target.
Level 5: The resident has advanced beyond performance targets defined for residency, and is demonstrating "aspirational" goals which might describe the performance of someone who has been in practice for several years. It is expected that only a few exceptional residents will reach this level for selected milestones.

Reference:
1. *The Anesthesiology Milestone Project.* 2015. Retrieved from: https://www.acgme.org/Portals/0/PDFs/Milestones/AnesthesiologyMilestones.pdf.

25. **Correct answer: B**

ABA certification is a reflection of medical knowledge and would allow the individual to practice independently, placing them in Level 5.

Please see explanations given for questions 23 and 24 for more details.

References:
1. Swing SR. The ACGME outcome project: retrospective and prospective. *Med Teach.* 2007;29(7):648-654.
2. *The Anesthesiology Milestone Project.* 2015. Retrieved from: https://www.acgme.org/Portals/0/PDFs/Milestones/AnesthesiologyMilestones.pdf.

INDEX

Note: Page numbers followed by "f" indicate figures.